Cellular Regulation
of Secretion and Release

This is a volume in
CELL BIOLOGY
A series of monographs

Editors: D. E. Buetow, I. L. Cameron, G. M. Padilla, and A. M. Zimmerman

A complete list of the books in this series appears at the end of the volume.

Cellular Regulation of Secretion and Release

Edited by

P. MICHAEL CONN

Department of Pharmacology
Duke University Medical Center
Durham, North Carolina

1982

ACADEMIC PRESS

A Subsidiary of Harcourt Brace Jovanovich, Publishers

New York London
Paris San Diego San Francisco São Paulo Sydney Tokyo Toronto

ACADEMIC PRESS, INC.
111 Fifth Avenue, New York, New York 10003

United Kingdom Edition published by
ACADEMIC PRESS, INC. (LONDON) LTD.
24/28 Oval Road, London NW1 7DX

Library of Congress Cataloging in Publication Data
Main entry under title:

Cellular regulation of secretion and release.

  (Cell biology)
  Includes index.
  1. Cellular control mechanisms. 2. Secretion.
I. Conn, Michael P. II. Series. [DNLM: 1. Cells--
Physiology. 2. Hormones--Physiology. QH 604
C3936]
QH604.C45   574.87'6   82-6652
ISBN 0-12-185058-7   AACR2

PRINTED IN THE UNITED STATES OF AMERICA

82 83 84 85   9 8 7 6 5 4 3 2 1

Another error is an impatience of doubting and a blind hurry of asserting without a mature suspension of judgement . . . if we begin with certainties, we shall end in doubts; but if we begin with doubts, and are patient in them, we shall end in certainties.

Bacon, ADVANCEMENT OF LEARNING

Contents

Part I   Stimulus: Receptor Occupancy and Regulation

1   Receptor Regulation by Hormones: Relevance to Secretion and Other Biological Functions
ELI HAZUM

Part III   Subcellular Architecture: Its Role in Secretion

Part V Mechanisms and Modulation of Secretion and Release

Contributors

Numbers in parentheses indicate the pages on which the authors' contributions begin.

ELI Y. ADASHI[1] (495), Department of Reproductive Medicine, University of California, San Diego, La Jolla, California 92093

MARIO ASCOLI (409), Division of Endocrinology, Vanderbilt University Medical School, Nashville, Tennessee 37232

A. E. BOYD III (223), Departments of Medicine and Cell Biology, Baylor College of Medicine, Texas Medical Center, Houston, Texas 77030

WILLIAM A. BRADLEY (301), Department of Medicine, Baylor College of Medicine, Texas Medical Center, and The Methodist Hospital, Houston, Texas 77030

MARGARET M. BRIGGS (23), Departments of Medicine and Biochemistry, Duke University Medical Center, Durham, North Carolina 27710

JAMES G. CHAFOULEAS (445), Department of Cell Biology, Baylor College of Medicine, Texas Medical Center, Houston, Texas 77030

LAWRENCE CHAN (301), Departments of Cell Biology and Medicine, Baylor College of Medicine, Texas Medical Center, Houston, Texas 77030

DAVID J. CHASE (355), Departments of Obstetrics and Gynecology and Biological Chemistry, Reproductive Endocrinology Program, The University of Michigan, Ann Arbor, Michigan 48109

P. MICHAEL CONN (459), Department of Pharmacology, Duke University Medical Center, Durham, North Carolina 27710

---

[1]Present address: Department of Obstetrics and Gynecology, University of Maryland, Baltimore, Maryland 21201.

PRICILLA S. DANNIES (529), Department of Pharmacology, Yale
    University School of Medicine, New Haven, Connecticut 06510
EMANUEL J. DILIBERTO, Jr. (147), Department of Medicinal Bio-
    chemistry, Wellcome Research Laboratories, Research Triangle
    Park, North Carolina 27709
BERNARD DUFY (107), INSERM-U176, 33077 Bordeaux, France
RAYMOND S. GREENBERG (323), School of Public Health, Univer-
    sity of North Carolina, Chapel Hill, North Carolina 27514
VINCE GUERRIERO, Jr. (445), Department of Cell Biology, Baylor
    College of Medicine, Texas Medical Center, Houston, Texas 77030
PETER F. HALL (195), Worcester Foundation for Experimental Biolo-
    gy, Shrewsbury, Massachusetts 01545
ELI HAZUM (3), Department of Hormone Research, The Weizmann
    Institute of Science, Rehovot, Israel
AARON J. W. HSUEH (495), Department of Reproductive Medicine,
    University of California, San Diego, La Jolla, California 92037
SUZANNE G. LAYCHOCK (53), Department of Pharmacology, Medi-
    cal College of Virginia, Richmond, Virginia 23293
ROBERT J. LEFKOWITZ (23), Department of Medicine, Duke Univer-
    sity Medical Center, Durham, North Carolina 27710
RICHARD A. MAURER (267), Department of Physiology and Bio-
    physics, Iowa College of Medicine, University of Iowa, Iowa City,
    Iowa 52242
ANTHONY R. MEANS (445), Department of Cell Biology, Baylor Col-
    lege of Medicine, Texas Medical Center, Houston, Texas 77030
PETER J. O'SHAUGHNESSY (355), Department of Obstetrics and
    Gynecology, Reproductive Endocrinology Program, The Univer-
    sity of Michigan, Ann Arbor, Michigan 48109
ANITA H. PAYNE (355), Departments of Obstetrics and Gynecology
    and Biological Chemistry, Reproductive Endocrinology Program,
    The University of Michigan, Ann Arbor, Michigan 48109
MERRILY POTH (323), Department of Pediatrics, Pediatric Endo-
    crinology Division, Uniformed Services University of the Health
    Sciences, Bethesda, Maryland 20814
JAMES W. PUTNEY, Jr. (53), Department of Pharmacology, Medical
    College of Virginia, Richmond, Virginia 23298
S. WILLIAM TAM (529), Stine Laboratory, E. I. du Pont de Nemours,
    and Company, Newark, Delaware 19711
JEAN-DIDIER VINCENT (107), INSERM-U176, 33077 Bordeaux,
    France

Preface

Recent technical and conceptual breakthroughs have allowed us to examine secretory and release processes with increased resolution and in a new perspective. Video image intensification, for example, has allowed us to measure internalization of ligands previously thought to interact only with the outer face of the plasma membrane. Speculation about the role of the plasma membrane in secretion now includes the concept of receptors as proteins afloat in the lipid bilayer; we now also recognize the importance of the plasma membrane as a regulator of cellular electrical potentials. The discovery and characterization of calmodulin has elevated calcium to the status of a "second messenger" in many secretory systems. Cyclic nucleotides have retained this status in some systems and major advances have been made in understanding the molecular basis of regulation of these compounds. Our view of the intracellular space has been modified to include the microskeleton among other levels of increased organization. Considerable information is now available to describe the synthesis and intracellular targeting of secretory products. The ability to measure the expression of single genes has offered us a chance to learn about regulation of the accumulation of mRNA's for secretory proteins.

It is clear that the methodologies for studying secretion and release transcend the disciplines of genetic control, protein processing and targeting, receptor regulation, intracellular messengers, cellular organization, membrane cycling, and neuroendocrine control. Accordingly, the authors of the following chapters are well known for research contributions in biochemistry, electrophysiology, endocrinology, genetics, immunology, pharmacology, medicine, and ultrastructure. The need to bring together these different research areas in a single volume dealing with secretion and release was a prime reason for this book. To emphasize the similarity in cell function, the volume has been organized according to function rather than by individual model systems. In order to suggest the similarities between different systems, the volume is heavily cross-indexed.

We have intentionally encouraged an in-depth discussion of particular individual model systems because they provide demonstrations of more general concepts. Thus, we hope to have produced a volume which is current enough to be useful for the "specialist" in secretion, yet one which offers a sufficient overview for all scientists and students whose work touches upon this area. It is hoped that the cross-disciplinary nature of the volume will suggest new research approaches to some readers.

The cooperation of the authors and publisher has permitted rapid publication so that the material is current. The authors have been kept aware of each others' progress from the outset, which has allowed us to prevent overlap and encourage appropriate citation within the volume.

I wish to acknowledge NIH grants HD13220, AG1204, and RCDA HD00337, and the Mellon Foundation (Rockefeller–Ford–Mellon Program for Targeted Research in Reproduction) which supported the editor and his laboratory during the preparation of this volume.

P. Michael Conn

Introduction

Cellular communication is necessary for the organization of multi-cellular systems. Because communication allows integration of function, it is central to the stability and maintenance of the multicellular state; it forms the basis of homeostasis. Organized cells produce chemicals that have informational value for other cells. The processes subject to regulation are "secretion" (an energy-requiring process usually involving a granule) and "release" (a passive process). Another process, "excretion" (removal of toxic waste products), is regulated by substantially different processes and is outside the scope of this volume. It should be noted, however, that even the quantity and type of excreted products can convey some information about cellular status.

Secretion and release processes are found in virtually all multicellular life forms and, yet, retain surprising similarities at the molecular level. As an integrator of cell function, secretion and release must occur in response to a signal from either inside the cell or the immediate environment. This process is generally mediated by a specific receptor molecule embedded in the plasma membrane or, in the case of permeant or intracellular signals, within the cell. Transduction of the signal into a response is a particularly interesting area because in many systems the precise mechanism remains a "black box."

This volume is organized into five sections dealing with events in cellular perception of stimuli and response to them. The first section, "Stimulus: Receptor Occupancy and Regulation," begins with a chapter that describes the technique of video image intensification. Dr. Hazum describes how this technique has allowed us to use an electronically processed image of a fluorescing ligand in order to develop models for receptor regulation following exposure to a stimulus. He compares information gained in several systems and its meaning in terms of cellular regulation. Drs. Briggs and Lefkowitz describe the β-adrenergic receptor system and new insights into the manner in which receptor occupancy and other regulators control adenylate cyclase activity.

The second section presents several "Early Responses of Secretory Cells." These events include changes in phospholipid metabolism (Drs. Laychock and Putney), in electrophysiological events (Drs. Vincent and Dufy), and in macromolecular carboxymethylation (Dr. Diliberto). Rapid changes in these parameters can be measured following exposure of cells to stimuli. Accordingly, study of these phenomena may offer insight into the manner in which cells couple receptor occupancy to the mechanism of response.

The third section, "Subcellular Architecture: Its Role in Secretion," describes the stage in which secretion and release occur. Dr. Hall and Dr. Boyd describe important structural components of the skeleton of the cell. They include discussions describing how extant knowledge about the function of these components can be used to devise testable hypotheses concerning secretion mechanisms.

The fourth section describes the means by which the cells are able to produce and accumulate secretory products. Dr. Maurer describes a model for regulation of specific gene expression and mechanisms in which cells respond to some stimuli by altered transcription. Drs. Chan and Bradley provide a summary of mechanisms by which specific proteins can be destined for storage and secretion by the cell. Dr. Poth describes how secretory disease states arise when regulatory mechanisms fail; she summarizes the physiological consequence of these events.

The final section offers detailed descriptions of several individual secretory and release systems for which some aspects have become especially clear in recent years. For steroidogenesis, the stimulus primarily regulates biosynthesis, and the product appears to diffuse from the cell. Drs. Payne, Chase, and O'Shaughnessy describe this cyclic nucleotide-dependent process in the Leydig cells of the testes; Dr. Ascoli's chapter concentrates on how tumor cells have provided especially useful models for examining specific events in the steroidogenic process. Drs. Chafouleas, Guerriero, and Means' chapter describes the role of a newly appreciated intracellular calcium-binding protein, calmodulin, and indicates that this molecule appears to hold a pivotal position for regulation of both cyclic nucleotide and calcium metabolism. They indicate potential roles for this protein and an enzyme it regulates, myosin light chain kinase, in secretion. Our own chapter describes a system in which calcium plays a role as a second messenger and discusses how information about receptor function can be used to develop a model for secretory function in one system. Drs. Hsueh and Adashi discuss modulators of secretion in this same model. Dr. Dannies brings to bear information about regulation of release in a system that secretes spontaneously under normal conditions; the best-characterized regulators act to prevent this spontaneous secretion.

The authors join me in hoping that the reader finds the following chapters interesting and useful in catalyzing further experimentation in other systems.

P. Michael Conn

PART I
STIMULUS: RECEPTOR OCCUPANCY AND REGULATION

1

Receptor Regulation by Hormones: Relevance to Secretion and Other Biological Functions

ELI HAZUM

3

I. INTRODUCTION

One of the major goals in modern biology is understanding the mechanism by which hormones control secretion and other biological functions via receptor-mediated events. Recent advances in the field of cell biology have made it possible to study receptor redistribution induced by hormones in living cells. These studies have indicated that, in general, the occupied receptors for polypeptide hormones appear to be initially distributed uniformly over the cell surface and then rapidly form clusters that are subsequently internalized.

This chapter summarizes recent studies related to receptor redistribution induced by hormones and speculates on its possible relevance to secretion and other biological functions. Two models are presented. In the first, receptor microaggregation or cross-linking is important for hormonal action and is independent of internalization; in the second, internalization of receptor-bound proteins may serve as a selective transport system that directs specific ligands to specific subcellular organelles, or internalization and degradation of hormone–receptor complexes may produce a "second messenger."

II. PITUITARY GONADOTROPIN-RELEASING HORMONE RECEPTORS

A. Introductory Remarks

Gonadotropin-releasing hormone (GnRH) is a hypothalamic decapeptide (pGlu-His-Trp-Ser-Tyr-Gly-Leu-Arg-Pro-Gly-NH$_2$), which stimulates gonadotropin release from the anterior pituitary. The first step in GnRH action (Conn *et al.*, 1981b; Chapter 14 in this volume) is its recognition by specific binding sites (receptors) at the surface of gonadotrope cells of the anterior pituitary. The interaction of GnRH with pituitary membrane preparations or cultured pituitary cells has been studied in detail by using radioiodinated, metabolically stable GnRH analogs (Clayton *et al.*, 1978; Conne *et al.*, 1979; Clayton and Catt, 1980; Marian and Conn, 1980; Naor *et al.*, 1980; Hazum, 1981; Marian *et al.*, 1981; Meidan and Koch, 1981). These studies have indicated the presence of a single class of high-affinity binding sites for both agonists and antagonists of GnRH.

B. Internalization of GnRH by Pituitary Gonadotropes

Internalization of GnRH by dissociated pituitary cells was first reported after electron microscopic studies (Hopkins and Gregory, 1977)

C. GnRH Receptor Clustering and Internalization Are Not a Requirement for Gonadotropin Release

It has been shown that an immobilized GnRH analog ([D-Lys^6]GnRH coupled by its epislon amino group, through a 10-Å spacer, to agarose matrix) can stimulate luteinizing hormone (LH) release from pituitary cells (Conn *et al.*, 1981a). This immobilized analog is stable under various conditions, including exposure to cell cultures, thus excluding the possibility of leakage from the matrix. As shown in Table I, the apparent potency of the immobilized analog (which cannot be internalized) is one-quarter that of the free hormone. Nevertheless, it is still capable of evoking a full LH secretory response (Conn *et al.*, 1981a). These studies indicate that internalization of GnRH is not required for stimulation of gonadotropin release from pituitary cells.

Three different approaches have also been described that indicate that GnRH–receptor internalization as well as cluster formation are not required for GnRH-stimulated LH release from pituitary cells (Conn and Hazum, 1981). The first approach utilized the immobilization technique (Table I). A more potent GnRH agonist, [D-Lys^6-des-Gly^{10}-ethylamide]GnRH, immobilized at a higher hormone/bead ratio (providing additional evidence for the stability of the immobilized ago-

TABLE I

Stimulation of LH Release from Pituitary Cells Cultured under Various Conditions of Hormone–Receptor Distribution[a]

Condition	ED$_{50}$ for LH release (M)	Hormone–receptor complex pattern
[D-Lys^6]GnRH	2×10^{-9}	—
Immobilized [D-Lys^6]GnRH	8×10^{-9}[b]	No internalization
[D-Lys^6-des-Gly^{10}-ethylamide]GnRH	8×10^{-10}	—
Immobilized [D-Lys^6-des-Gly^{10}-ethylamide]GnRH	2×10^{-7}[b]	No internalization
Rhod–GnRH	—	Internalization
Rhod–GnRH + 0.1 mM vinblastine	—	Uniform distribution
GnRH	3×10^{-9}	—
GnRH + 0.1 mM vinblastine	3×10^{-9}	—
[D-Lys^6-des-Gly^{10}-ethylamide]GnRH	8×10^{-10}	—
[D-Lys^6-des-Gly^{10}-ethylamide] GnRH + 0.1 mM vinblastine	8×10^{-10}	—

[a] Data from Hazum *et al.* (1980b), Conn *et al.* (1981a), and Conn and Hazum (1981).
[b] The quantity of LH release is restricted by the number of beads added and the ratio of ligand/bead largely determines the lower bound of ED$_{50}$ (see also text).

nist) also induced LH release with full efficacy. In these highly derivatized beads, the quantity of LH release is restricted by the number of
beads added as a result of the fact that the hormone is exposed to only a
small number of cells. In the second approach, it has been shown that
the removal of external GnRH from the cells at different times
throughout the GnRH stimulation results in a prompt return of LH
release to basal levels. Thus, under conditions in which internalization
takes place, continuous release of LH can only occur when external
GnRH is present. These results again indicate that LH release with
full efficacy does not require internalization of the hormone–receptor
complex.

Finally, comparative studies on receptor distribution and LH release
have been undertaken. As indicated in Table I, cluster formation and
internalization of Rhod–GnRH are not observed in the presence of 0.1
mM vinblastine, and the fluorescence is evenly distributed over the
cell surface of gonadotropes. Under these conditions, gonadotropin secretion by GnRH or its agonist is not affected (Table I). This result
suggests that cluster formation, as well as large-scale clusters of
GnRH receptors, are not important in eliciting the biological effects of
GnRH. These studies do not exclude the possibility that microaggregation of receptors (Section V) is required for LH release. However, the
conversion of a GnRH antagonist to an agonist and the potency enhancement of a GnRH agonist by bridging two molecules within a
critical distance d ($15 \text{ Å} < d < 150 \text{ Å}$) suggest that receptor cross-
linking as such is sufficient to activate the effector system in pituitary
cells to evoke release (Conn *et al.*, 1982a,b). The internalization of
GnRH (and presumably its receptor) may have some other intracellular action or it may be simply degraded or recycled. Nevertheless, this
could explain the decrease in gonadotrope responsiveness to the hormone after chronic treatment with GnRH (Conn *et al.*, 1982).

III. OPIATE (ENKEPHALIN) RECEPTORS IN NEUROBLASTOMA CELLS

A. Characterization of Enkephalin Receptors in Neuroblastoma Cells

The enkephalins and endorphins are naturally occurring peptides
with morphine-like activity. The discovery of these opioid peptides has
led to the classification of multiple types of opiate receptors (Chang
and Cuatrecasas, 1979; Chang *et al.*, 1979, 1980). Two subtypes of
opiate receptors have been described biochemically in brain membrane

preparations. One site has higher affinity for morphine and is referred to as morphine (mu) receptor, and the other has higher affinity for enkephalins and is referred to as enkephalin (delta) receptor. In contrast to brain membranes, which contain two classes of opiate receptors, cultured neuroblastoma cells bind enkephalins with high affinity and opiates with low affinity and thus contain only enkephalin receptors. The interaction of enkephalins with receptors in neuroblastoma cells has been studied in detail by using a ^{125}I-labeled derivative of the metabolically stable enkephalin analog [D-Ala^2,D-Leu^5]enkephalin (Chang *et al.*, 1978; Miller *et al.*, 1978). Neuroblastoma–glioma hybrid cells (NG108-15) and N4TG1 neuroblastoma cells bind enkephalins specifically and with high affinity (1 nM) and have approximately 100,000 and 20,000 enkephalin-binding sites per cell, respectively.

B.   Clustering of Enkephalin Receptors

As shown in Fig. 2b, incubation of N4TG1 neuroblastoma cells (or NG108-15 neuroblastoma glioma hybrid cells) with 10^{-8} M bioactive rhodamine-enkephalin derivative, [D-Ala^2,D-Leu^5]enkephalin-Lys-N^ε-rhodamine (Hazum *et al.*, 1979a), for 30 minutes at 25°C results in many patch-type areas of fluorescence (Hazum *et al.*, 1979b,c, 1980a). These patches are localized both on the cell body and on processes and are highly concentrated in the area where the connections of the neurons are assembled. These fluorescent clusters are not seen in the presence of 10^{-6} M [D-Ala^2, Leu^5]enkephalin or with other cell lines that lack opiate receptors. At 4°C, no discrete clusters can be seen, even after incubation for as long as 2 hours (Fig. 2a). In the presence of 0.1 M NaCl, only a few clusters are detected. These results are consistent with the known characteristics of opiate receptors (for review, see Snyder and Childers, 1979) and with studies describing the interaction of ^{125}I-labeled [D-Ala^2,D-Leu^5]enkephalin with receptors in neuroblastoma cells (Chang *et al.*, 1978; Miller *et al.*, 1978). Thus, the fluorescent clusters most likely represent specific binding sites (receptors) for enkephalin.

It is of interest that the enkephalin-labeled receptor patches, in contrast to other systems (Section IV), appear only slowly and do not become internalized (Hazum *et al.*, 1979b). The visible patches begin to appear after 20 minutes and reach their maximum number after 40 minutes at 25°C; no further changes are detected after longer incubation (2 hours) at 37°C. Furthermore, most of the patches disappear if the cells are washed and incubated at 37°C to allow the cell-bound enkephalin to dissociate. Similarly, binding studies have indicated (Miller *et al.*, 1978) that more than 95% of the cell-bound ^{125}I-labeled

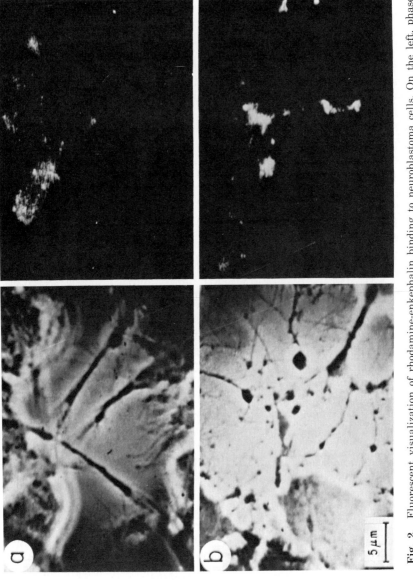

Fig. 2. Fluorescent visualization of rhodamine-enkephalin binding to neuroblastoma cells. On the left, phase micrographs; on the right, fluorescence micrographs of the same field. (a) Uniform distribution of receptors; (b) cluster of receptors. Modified from Hazum *et al.* (1980a).

a

b

5 μm

[D-Ala^2,D-Leu^5]enkephalin can dissociate from the cells even if the binding has taken place at 37°C for 2 hours. Thus, it is likely that enkephalin receptors in neuroblastoma cells form surface clusters that do not internalize. Nevertheless, the possibility of very slow internalization or extremely rapid recycling of occupied receptors cannot be completely ruled out.

C. Mechanism of Cluster Formation: Differences between Clusters Induced by Agonists and Antagonists

Sulfhydryl groups are involved in the binding of opiates to brain membranes and may affect differentially the binding of agonists and antagonists (Pasternak *et al.*, 1975; Simon and Groth, 1975). Preincubation of neuroblastoma cells with specific sulfhydryl reagents under conditions identical to those used for binding assays (Table II) results in the uniform distribution of the fluorescently labeled receptors and no formation of clusters (similar to Fig. 2a). The diffuse patterns observed are probably due to the modification of free sulfhydryl

TABLE II

Effect of Sulfhydyl, Disulfide, and Miscellaneous Reagents on ^{125}I-Labeled [D-Ala^2,D-Leu^5]Enkephalin Binding and Clustering in N4TG1 Cells[a]

Reagent	Reagent conc. (mM)	Specific binding (% control)	Hormone–receptor complex pattern
Iodoacetate	1	89	Uniform distribution
Iodoacetamide	0.1	89	Uniform distribution
N-Ethylmaleimide	0.01	95	Uniform distribution
Dithiothreitol	0.01	94	Uniform distribution
Hydrogen peroxide	0.1	100	Clusters
Dithiothreitol	0.01[b]	95	Clusters
+ hydrogen peroxide	0.1	95	Clusters
Sodium azide	1	82	Clusters
Sodium azide	10	67	Clusters
Dinitrophenol	0.5	100	Clusters
Dinitrophenol	1	98	Clusters
Methylamine·HCl	1	81	Clusters
Methylamine·HCl	10	76	Small reduction in the number of clusters

[a] Data from Hazum *et al.* (1979c). Adapted by permission from *Nature (London)* **282**, 626–628. Copyright 1981, Macmillan Journals Limited.
[b] Reagent applied for 40 minutes before application of hydrogen peroxide.

groups and are probably not due to a reduction in the number of binding sites, because under these conditions the cells retain their ability to bind ^{125}I-labeled [D-Ala^2,D-Leu^5]enkephalin (Table II).

When the rhodamine-enkephalin derivative is added to the cells in the presence of 10^{-5} M dithiothreitol, no bright patches are seen and the fluorescence is distributed evenly over the cell surface (similar to Fig. 2a). This diffuse pattern (10^{-5} M dithiothreitol, 40 minutes at 25°C) is quickly (10 minutes) modified to one containing clusters by oxidation with 10^{-4} M hydrogen peroxide (as in Fig. 2b). These results suggest that in neuroblastoma cells there are reactive sulfhydryl and disulfide groups that are essential for cluster formation, but not for binding, and the possibility exists that a sulfhydryl–disulfide exchange reaction may be involved in this process (Hazum et al., 1979c).

The formation of clusters is independent of the generation of metabolic energy because sodium azide and dinitrophenol do not affect cluster formation (Table II). In addition, various amines (e.g., methylamine; Table II) do not prevent clustering, suggesting that the enzyme transglutaminase is not involved in the formation of clusters. This calcium-requiring enzyme has been postulated to be involved in the clustering of α_2-macroglobulin and epidermal growth factor (Section IV,A,2).

Indirect studies in this system have indicated (Hazum et al., 1980a) that both agonists and antagonists can induce cluster formation. However, these clusters seem to differ in that those induced by agonists (morphine and enkephalins) can be dispersed by dithiothreitol in the absence of agonists, whereas clusters induced by antagonists (naloxone and nalorphine) cannot. These data suggest that in the case of clusters induced by agonists, the disulfide bonds, which are stabilized by or directly involved in receptor clustering, are exposed to reduction when the hormone is absent. However, substantial protection (60–80%) is achieved upon reduction in the presence of agonist, suggesting that the disulfide bonds are protected when the agonist is bound to the receptor. In the antagonist-induced clusters, the disulfide bonds are probably buried, or the clusters are formed by different mechanisms.

D. Receptor Pattern and Relationships to Inhibition of Adenylate Cyclase

Opiates and opioid peptides inhibit both basal and prostaglandin E$_1$-stimulated adenylate cyclase activity in homogenates of NG108-15 cells and decrease cAMP concentrations in intact NG108-15 cells, whereas naloxone has no effect (Sharma et al., 1975; Traber et al., 1975; Lampert et al., 1976). Enkephalins are more potent than morphine in inhibiting adenylate cyclase activity, in harmony with the binding data to enkephalin receptors.

To further investigate the mechanisms of opiate action, the possible relationship of receptor clustering to modulation of adenylate cyclase activity has been studied (Hazum *et al.*, 1980a, 1981). As shown in Table III, there is no alteration in the inhibitory effect of enkephalins on both basal and PGE_1-stimulated adenylate cyclase activity when cluster formation is prevented by sulfhydryl-blocking reagents. Under these conditions, PGE_1 is still able to stimulate adenylate cyclase, indicating that sulfhydryl blockade does not affect the enzyme. This suggests that the inhibitory effect of enkephalins and opiates can occur when the receptors are in a diffused state. Whether microaggregation or cross-linking of receptors (Section V) is required for these inhibitory effects of opiates remains to be shown. Nevertheless, studies (Hazum *et al.*, 1982) utilizing synthetic dimers of both opiates and enkephalins have indicated that dimerization of ligands can increase their biological activity and suggest that receptor cross-linking may be important for the biological functions of opiates and opioid peptides.

IV. RECEPTOR INTERNALIZATION AS A POSSIBLE MECHANISM FOR BIOLOGICAL RESPONSES

A. Epidermal Growth Factor

1. *Internalization of Epidermal Growth Factor*

A highly fluorescent rhodamine derivative of epidermal growth factor (EGF), ^{125}I-labeled EGF, and ferritin-labeled EGF have been used to study the pattern and the mobility of receptors on fibroblastic cells (Gorden *et al.*, 1978; Schlessinger *et al.*, 1978; McKanna *et al.*, 1979; Schlessinger, 1980). It has been found that EGF receptors are initially distributed uniformly (4°C) and quickly (few minutes at 23° or 37°C) form patches that are subsequently internalized (30 minutes at 37°C). The latter step is found to be temperature dependent and presumably takes place only within specialized coated regions (coated pits and vesicles) of the plasma membranes (Gorden *et al.*, 1978; Maxfield *et al.*, 1978; Goldstein *et al.*, 1979; McKanna *et al.*, 1979). The coated vesicles that are formed ultimately fuse with lysosomes, where the hormone and its receptor are degraded. Coated pits and vesicles are involved in the processes of endocytosis and membrane transport within the cell (see also Section IV,B). These structures consist of a lipid vesicle surrounded by a basket of protein that is organized in a network of hexagons and pentagons. The coat of the coated vesicles is composed pre-

TABLE III

Effects of Sulfhydryl-Blocking Reagents on the Inhibition of Adenylate Cyclase Activity by Enkephalin[a]

| | Adenylate cyclase activity (%) | | |
| | | Pretreatment | |
Addition	No treatment	N-Ethylmaleimide $(10^{-5}\ M)$	Iodoacetamide $(10^{-4}\ M)$ or iodoacetate $(10^{-3}\ M)$
Control	100	101	95
[D-Ala^2,D-Leu^5] En-kephalin $(10^{-7}\ M)$	80	77	64
PGE$_1$ $(10^{-6}\ M)$	210	231	208
PGE$_1$ $(10^{-6}\ M)$ + [D-Ala^2, D-Leu^5]en-kephalin $(10^{-7}\ M)$	182	203	166

[a] Data from Hazum *et al.* (1980a).

dominantly of a single protein named clathrin (molecular weight 180,000).

2. Mechanism and Role of Cluster Formation and Internalization

It has been shown that the clustering and subsequent internalization of occupied EGF receptors require calcium and can be inhibited by various amines (Maxfield *et al.*, 1979; Davies *et al.*, 1980). These observations suggest several potential mechanisms of inhibition, including the possibility that the enzyme transglutaminase is involved in these processes. This enzyme requires calcium for activity and catalyzes the cross-linking of adjacent glutamyl and lysyl residues.

Biochemical studies (King *et al.*, 1980, 1981) as well as studies with ferritin–EGF conjugates and ^{125}I-labeled EGF (Gorden *et al.*, 1978; McKanna *et al.*, 1979) have indicated that the internalization of EGF is not blocked by alkylamines. Rather, these amines, which inactivate lysosomal hydrolases, inhibit the intracellular processing of hormone–receptor complexes and this results in their accumulation within the cells in dense membrane vesicles. Furthermore, it has been suggested (Schlessinger *et al.*, 1981; Yarden *et al.*, 1981) that amines only slow down the formation of visible patches of EGF receptors but do not affect the rate and the extent of internalization.

Studies concerning the biological activity have indicated that stimulation of DNA synthesis by EGF is inhibited by alkylamines only when present for the duration of the stimulatory preincubation (20–24 hours). This suggests that continuous internalization and degradation of hormone–receptor complexes may be involved in inducing mitogenesis (King *et al.*, 1981). These results support the endocytic activation hypothesis, which suggests that processing of the hormone–receptor complexes of EGF may produce a "second messenger" in the action of the hormone (Fox and Das, 1979). Although internalization may be regarded as an integral part of the transduction mechanism, the possibility that signaling by the EGF–receptor complex begins with microaggregation on the cell surface should be considered (Section V,A).

B.   Studies with Low-Density Lipoprotein

One of the best-studied systems in which internalization of receptors is important for biological activity is that for low-density lipoprotein (LDL). The receptor-mediated endocytosis of LDL coordinates the transport of cholesterol from plasma into the cells (for reviews, see Brown and Goldstein, 1979; Goldstein *et al.*, 1979; Brown *et al.*, 1981). The biochemical steps in the LDL receptor pathway are initiated by the binding of the LDL to specific surface receptors located in coated pits. These pits invaginate into the cell and pinch off to form endocytic vesicles that carry the LDL to lysosomes. The protein of LDL is hydrolyzed to amino acids and the cholesterol esters are converted, by a specific enzyme, to cholesterol, which crosses the lysosomal membrane and enters the cytoplasmic component. LDL receptors that enter cells in coated vesicles can be recycled and they are not destroyed when the vesicles fuse with lysosomes. Interestingly, morphological and kinetic evidence indicate that the whole pathway of insertion of receptors, clustering in coated pits, internalization, and recycling occurs continuously whether or not LDL is present (Brown and Goldstein, 1979; Goldstein *et al.*, 1979; Brown *et al.*, 1981).

V.   RECEPTOR CROSS-LINKING AS A POSSIBLE MECHANISM FOR BIOLOGICAL RESPONSES

Several studies suggest that receptor microaggregation or cross-linking, perhaps independent of internalization, may be important for certain biological responses in some systems such as those involving insulin, epidermal growth factor, and immunoglobulin E (IgE).

A. Insulin and EGF

Studies with insulin have shown that bivalent antibodies to the insulin receptor block insulin binding, bind to insulin receptors, and trigger many of the same biological responses caused by insulin (Jacobs et al., 1978; Kahn et al., 1978). Monovalent Fab' fragments compete for insulin binding to the receptor but are unable to initiate a biological response. However, addition of anti-Fab' antibodies to cross-link the Fab'–receptor complexes restores the insulin-like activity (Kahn et al., 1978). Furthermore, under certain conditions, bivalent, but not univalent, antibodies directed to insulin and EGF can dramatically enhance the activity of very low concentrations of these hormones in fibroblasts (Shechter et al., 1979a,b). In addition, other multivalent compounds such as lectins (Cuatrecasas, 1973; Cuatrecasas and Tell, 1973) have been shown to mimic insulin actions.

A biologically inactive analog of EGF (cyanogen bromide-cleaved EGF) has been described (Shechter et al., 1979b). This analog retains 10% of the binding capacity of EGF and only 0.3% of its ability to stimulate DNA synthesis. In contrast to rhodamine–EGF, which readily aggregates on the cell surface (Section IV,A,1), the rhodamine derivative of this analog appears to be diffusely distributed on the cell surface. However, addition of bivalent anti-EGF antibodies restores both the bioactivity and the morphological cross-linking (patch formation) of this derivative toward that observed with the native hormone. Addition of monovalent anti-EGF Fab' fragment does not restore the ability of the analog to induce patching or DNA synthesis. Thus, receptor occupation alone is not sufficient for signal generation. More recently, the generation of monoclonal antibodies directed against the EGF receptor of human epidermoid carcinoma cell line has been described (Schreiber et al., 1981). These antibodies inhibit the binding of radiolabeled EGF. Moreover, the antibodies, like EGF, enhance the phosphorylation of endogenous membrane proteins and stimulate DNA synthesis.

These data suggest that microaggregation or cross-linking of receptors may be necessary for early and delayed biological responses of EGF and insulin. The possibility exists that a primary function of a hormone may be to induce and maintain a state of receptor self-aggregation that is by itself sufficient to trigger the subsequent biochemical events of hormone action.

B. Receptor Cross-Linking and Histamine Release

Considerable evidence for the importance of receptor microaggregation is available from basophil and mast cell systems, which require
cross-linking of their Fc receptors for induction of histamine release
(Siraganian et al., 1975; Segal et al., 1977; Izerski et al., 1978). It has
been shown that a series of divalent antigens capable of bridging two
receptor-bound IgE molecules can activate basophils, whereas the
monovalent compounds cannot. Anti-receptor antibodies cause histamine release; Fab' fragments bind to the IgE receptor but are inactive, whereas cross-linking the Fab'–receptor complexes restores activity. In addition, dimerization of receptors rather than the formation
of large aggregates is needed to initiate biological responses. Mathematical analyses (DeLisi and Siraganian, 1979) relating the number of
antigen-induced IgE clusters to the amount of histamine release have
indicated that the number of IgE clusters required to initiate local
release of histamine is small and is independent of the size of a cluster.
These studies suggest that microaggregation or cross-linking of a
small number of receptors may be essential for the immediate biological responses of at least certain systems.

C. The Bivalent Ligand Model

Based on the experimental data with insulin and EGF, a model for
hormone action has been proposed (Minton, 1981). It is suggested that
the hormone can interact with two distinct regions: a specific and high-
affinity site (receptor) and a response site having lower affinity and
specificity (effector). According to the model, the formation of hormone–receptor complex increases the apparent affinity of the effector
site to hormone, and the steady-state response is proportional to the
amount of hormone bound to effector (substantially less than receptor
sites). The hormone may simultaneously bind to, and thereby cross-
link, receptor and effector, in both the absence and presence of cross-
linking agents such as lectins and anti-receptor antibodies. Thus, activation is achieved upon the interaction between the response deter-
minant of the hormone and the complementary binding site on the
effector. According to the bivalent ligand model, the cross-linking of a
hormone by anti-hormone antibodies only increases the apparent affinity of the hormone for cell surface by a process of localization,
whereas only the hormone itself cross-links receptor and effector. The
hormone-like effects of anti-receptor antibodies are interpreted by the
presence of anti-effector antibodies.

MODEL A

Binding → Cross-linking of receptors → biological response → Internalization of H–R complexes → Degradation of H–R complexes

MODEL B

Binding → Internalization of H–R complexes → Degradation of H–R complexes → biological response

Fig. 3. Two models for the mode of action of hormones. In model A, cross-linking of receptors is important for biological response, whereas in Model B, internalization and degradation of hormone–receptor (H–R) complexes is involved in the biological response.

VI. CONCLUSIONS: MODELS FOR HORMONE ACTION

Receptors for polypeptide hormones appear to have a common topological redistribution. The occupied receptors are initially evenly distributed over the cell surface and quickly form clusters that are subsequently internalized. However, there are two possibilities in the subsequent events that could mediate hormone action as shown in the models in Fig. 3. In model A, the binding of ligand to receptors leads to cross-linking of receptors (or receptor–effector) at the cell surface, which is by itself sufficient to trigger the subsequent biochemical events of hormone action. Although ligand internalization and degradation may occur, it is not a prerequisite for ligand function. In model B, however, internalization and degradation of hormone–receptor complexes are important for biological activity. Thus, internalization may serve as a selective transport mechanism, or processing of the hormone–receptor complexes may produce a "second messenger" in the action of the hormone.

ACKNOWLEDGMENT

I wish to thank Mrs. M. Kopelowitz for excellent secretarial assistance.

REFERENCES

Brown, M. S., and Goldstein, J. L. (1979). Receptor-mediated endocytosis: Insights from the lipoprotein receptor system. *Proc. Natl. Acad. Sci. U.S.A.* **76**, 3330–3337.
Brown, M. S., Kovanen, P. T., and Goldstein, J. L. (1981). Regulation of plasma cholesterol by lipoprotein receptors. *Science* **212**, 628–635.

Chang, K. J., and Cuatrecasas, P. (1979). Multiple opiate receptors: Enkephalins and morphine bind to receptors of different specificity. *J. Biol. Chem.* **254,** 2610–2618.

Chang, K. J., Miller, R. J., and Cuatrecasas, P. (1978). Interaction of enkephalin with opiate receptors in intact cultured cells. *Mol. Pharmacol.* **14,** 961–970.

Chang, K. J., Cooper, B. R., Hazum, E., and Cuatrecasas, P. (1979). Multiple opiate receptors: Different regional distribution in the brain and differential binding of opiates and opioid peptides. *Mol. Pharmacol.* **16,** 91–104.

Chang, K. J., Hazum, E., and Cuatrecasas, P. (1980). Multiple opiate receptors. *Trends NeuroSci.* **3,** 160–162.

Clayton, R. N., and Catt, K. J. (1980). Receptor-binding affinity of gonadotropin-releasing hormone analogs: Analysis by radioligand receptor assay. *Endocrinology (Baltimore)* **106,** 1154–1159.

Clayton, R. N., Shakespear, R. A., and Marshall, J. C. (1978). LHRH binding to purified plasma membranes: Absence of adenylate cyclase activation. *Mol. Cell. Endocrinol.* **11,** 63–78.

Conn, P. M., and Hazum, E. (1981). LH release and GnRH-receptor internalization: Independent actions of GnRH. *Endocrinology (Baltimore),* **109,** 2040–2045.

Conn, P. M., Smith, R., and Rogers, D. C. (1981a). Stimulation of pituitary gonadotropin release does not require internalization of gonadotropin-releasing hormone. *J. Biol. Chem.* **256,** 1098–1100.

Conn, P. M., Marian, J., McMillian, M., Stern, J., Rogers, D., Hamby, M., Penna, A., and Grant, E. (1981b). Gonadotropin–releasing hormone action in the pituitary: A three step mechanism. *Endocrine Rev.* **2,** 174–185.

Conn, P. M., Rogers, D. C., Stewart, J. M., Niedel, J., and Sheffield, T. (1982a). Conversion of a gonadotropin-releasing hormone antagonist to an agonist. *Nature (London)* **296,** 653–655.

Conn, P. M., Rogers, D. C., and McNeil, R. (1982b). Potency enhancement of a GnRH agonist: GnRH–receptor microaggregation stimulates gonadotropin release. *Endocrinology* (in press).

Conne, B. S., Aubert, M. L., and Sizoneko, P. C. (1979). Quantification of pituitary receptor sites for LHRH: Use of superactive analog as a tracer. *Biochem. Biophys. Res. Commun.* **90,** 1249–1256.

Cuatrecasas, P. (1973). Interaction of concanavalin A and wheat germ agglutinin with the insulin receptor of fat cells and liver. *J. Biol. Chem.* **248,** 3528–3534.

Cuatrecasas, P., and Tell, G. P. E. (1973). Insulin-like activity of concanavalin A and wheat germ agglutinin: Direct interaction with insulin receptors. *Proc. Natl. Acad. Sci. U.S.A.* **70,** 485–489.

Dacheux, F. (1981). Ultrastructural localization of gonadotropin-releasing hormone in porcine gonadotrophic cells. *Cell Tissue Res.* **216,** 143–150.

Davies, P. J. A., Davies, D. R., Levitzki, A., Maxfield, F. R., Milhaud, P., Willingham, M. C., and Pastan, I. (1980). Transglutaminase is essential in receptor mediated endocytosis of α_2-macroglobulin and polypeptide hormones. *Nature (London)* **283,** 162–167.

DeLisi, C., and Siraganian, R. P. (1979). Receptor cross-linking and histamine release. I. The quantitative dependence of basophil degranulation on the number of receptor doublets. *J. Immunol.* **122,** 2286–2292.

Duello, T. M., and Nett, T. M. (1980). Uptake, localization, and retention of gonadotropin–releasing hormone and gonadotropin–releasing hormone analogs in rat gonadotrophs. *Mol. Cell. Endocrinol.* **19,** 101–112.

Fox, C. F., and Das, M. (1979). Internalization and processing of the EGF receptor in the induction of DNA synthesis in cultured fibroblasts: The endocytic activation hypothesis. *J. Supramol. Struc.* **10,** 199–214.

Goldstein, J. L., Anderson, R. G. W., and Brown, M. S. (1979). Coated pits, coated vesicles, and receptor-mediated endocytosis. *Nature (London)* **279,** 679–685.

Gorden, P., Carpentier, J. L., Cohen, S., and Orci, L. (1978). Epidermal growth factor: Morphological demonstration of binding, internalization, and lysosomal association in human fibroblasts. *Proc. Natl. Acad. Sci. U.S.A.* **75,** 5025–5029.

Hazum, E. (1981). Some characteristics of GnRH-receptors in rat pituitary membranes: Differences between an agonist and an antagonist. *Mol. Cell. Endocrinol.,* **23,** 275–281.

Hazum, E., Chang, K. J., Shechter, Y., Wilkinson, S., and Cuatrecasas, P. (1979a). Fluorescent and photo-affinity enkephalin derivatives: Preparation and interaction with opiate receptors. *Biochem. Biophys. Res. Commun.* **88,** 841–846.

Hazum, E., Chang, K. J., and Cuatrecasas, P. (1979b). Opiate (enkephalin) receptors of neuroblastoma cells: Occurrence in clusters on the cell surface. *Science* **206,** 1077–1079.

Hazum, E., Chang, K. J., and Cuatrecasas, P. (1979c). Role of disulphide and sulphydryl groups in clustering of enkephalin receptors in neuroblastoma cells. *Nature (London)* **282,** 626–628.

Hazum, E., Chang, K. J., and Cuatrecasas, P. (1980a). Cluster formation of opiate (enkephalin) receptors in neuroblastoma cells: Differences between agonists and antagonists and possible relationships to biological functions. *Proc. Natl. Acad. Sci. U.S.A.* **77,** 3038–3041.

Hazum, E., Cuatrecasas, P., Marian, J., and Conn, P. M. (1980b). Receptor-mediated internalization of gonadotropin–releasing hormone by pituitary gonadotropes. *Proc. Natl. Acad. Sci. U.S.A.* **77,** 6692–6695.

Hazum, E., Chang, K. J., and Cuatrecasas, P. (1981). Receptor redistribution induced by hormones and neurotransmitters: Possible relationships to biological functions. *Neuropeptides* **1,** 217–230.

Hazum, E., Chang, K. J., Leighton, H. J., Lever, O. W., and Cuatrecasas, P. (1982). Increased biological activity of dimers of oxymorphone and enkephalin: Possible role of receptor cross-linking. *Biochem. Biophys. Res. Commun.* **104,** 347–353.

Hopkins, C. R., and Gregory, H. (1977). Topographical localization of the receptors for luteinizing hormone-releasing hormone on the surface of dissociated pituitary cells. *J. Cell Biol.* **75,** 528–540.

Izerski, C., Taurog, J. D., Poy, G., and Metzger, H. (1978). Triggering of cultured neoplastic mast cells by antibodies to the receptor for IgE. *J. Immunol.* **121,** 549–558.

Jacobs, S., Chang, K. J., and Cuatrecasas, P. (1978). Antibodies to purified insulin receptor have insulin-like activity. *Science* **200,** 1283–1284.

Kahn, C. R., Baird, K. L., Jarrett, D. B., and Flier, J. S. (1978). Direct demonstration that receptor cross-linking or aggregation is important in insulin action. *Proc. Natl. Acad. Sci. U.S.A.* **75,** 4209–4213.

King, A. C., Hernaez-Davis, L., and Cuatrecasas, P. (1980). Lysomotropic amines cause intracellular accumulation of receptors for epidermal growth factor. *Proc. Natl. Acad. Sci. U.S.A.* **77,** 3283–3287.

King, A. C., Hernaez-Davis, L., and Cuatrecasas, P. (1981). Lysosomotropic amines inhibit mitogenesis induced by growth factors. *Proc. Natl. Acad. Sci. U.S.A.* **78,** 717–721.

Lampert, A., Nirenberg, M., and Klee, W. A. (1976). Tolerance and dependence evoked by an endogenous opiate peptide. *Proc. Natl. Acad. Sci. U.S.A.* **73**, 3165–3167.

McKanna, J. A., Haigler, H. T., and Cohen, S. (1979). Hormone receptor topology and dynamics: Morphological analysis using ferritin-labeled epidermal growth factor. *Proc. Natl. Acad. Sci. U.S.A.* **76**, 5689–5693.

Marian, J., and Conn, P. M. (1980). The calcium requirement in GnRH-stimulated LH release is not mediated through a specific action on receptor binding. *Life Sci.* **27**, 87–92.

Marian, J., Cooper, R. L., and Conn, P. M. (1981). Regulation of the rat pituitary gonadotropin-releasing hormone receptor. *Mol. Pharmacol.* **19**, 399–405.

Maxfield, F. R., Schlessinger, J., Shechter, Y., Pastan, I., and Willingham, M. C. (1978). Collection of insulin, EGF, and α_2-macroglobulin in the same patches on the surface of cultured fibroblasts and common internalization. *Cell* **14**, 805–810.

Maxfield, F. R., Willingham, M. C., Davies, P. J. A., and Pastan, I. (1979). Amines inhibit the clustering of α_2-macroglobulin and EGF on the fibroblast cell surface. *Nature (London)* **277**, 661–663.

Meidan, R., and Koch, Y. (1981). Binding of luteinizing-hormone releasing hormone analogues to dispersed pituitary cells. *Life Sci.* **28**, 1961–1968.

Miller, R. J., Chang, K. J., Leighton, J., and Cuatrecasas, P. (1978). Interaction of iodinated enkephalin analogues with opiate receptors. *Life Sci.* **22**, 379–388.

Minton, A. P. (1981). The bivalent ligand hypothesis: A quantitative model for hormone action. *Mol. Pharmacol.* **19**, 1–14.

Naor, Z., Clayton, R. N., and Catt, K. J. (1980). Characterization of GnRH receptors in cultured rat pituitary cells. *Endocrinology (Baltimore)* **107**, 1144–1152.

Naor, Z., Atlas, A., Clayton, R. N., Forman, D. S., Amsterdam, A., and Catt, K. J. (1981). Interaction of fluorescent gonadotropin-releasing hormone with receptors in cultured pituitary cells. *J. Biol. Chem.* **256**, 3049–3052.

Pasternak, G. W., Wilson, H. A., and Snyder, S. H. (1975). Differential effects of protein modifying reagents on receptor binding of opiate agonists and antagonists. *Mol. Pharmacol.* **11**, 340–351.

Schlessinger, J. (1980). The mechanism and role of hormone-induced clustering of membrane receptors. *Trends Biochem. Sci. (Pers. Ed.)* **5**, 210–214.

Schlessinger, J., and Elson, E. L. (1980). Quantitative methods for studying the mobility and distribution of receptors on viable cells. *In Recept. Recognition, Ser. B* **11**, 159–170.

Schlessinger, J., Shechter, Y., Willingham, M. C., and Pastan, I. (1978). Direct visualization of binding, aggregation, and internalization of insulin and epidermal growth factor on living fibroblastic cells. *Proc. Natl. Acad. Sci. U.S.A.* **75**, 2659–2663.

Schlessinger, J., Yarden, Y., Barak, L., Lax, I., Gabbay, M., and Geiger, B. (1981). Epidermal growth factor: New facts concerning its mode of action. *Horm. Cell Regul.* **5**, 197–208.

Schreiber, A. B., Lax, I., Yarden, Y., Eshhar, Z., and Schlessinger, J. (1981). Monoclonal antibodies against the receptor for epidermal growth factor induce early and delayed effects of epidermal growth factor. *Proc. Natl. Acad. Sci. U.S.A.,* **78**, 7535–7539.

Segal, D. M., Taurog, J. D., and Metzger, H. (1977). Dimeric immunoglobulin E serves as a unit for mast cell degranulation. *Proc. Natl. Acad. Sci. U.S.A.* **74**, 2993–2997.

Sharma, S. K., Klee, W. A., and Nirenberg, M. (1975). Dual regulation of adenylate cyclase accounts for narcotic dependence and tolerance. *Proc. Natl. Acad. Sci. U.S.A.* **72,** 3092–3096.

Shechter, Y., Chang, K. J., Jacobs, S., and Cuatrecasas, P. (1979a). Modulation of binding and bioactivity of insulin by anti-insulin antibody: Relation to possible role of receptor self-aggregation in hormone action. *Proc. Natl. Acad. Sci. U.S.A.* **76,** 2720–2724.

Shechter, Y., Hernaez, L., Schlessinger, J., and Cuatrecasas, P. (1979b). Local aggregation of hormone–receptor complexes is required for activation by epidermal growth factor. *Nature (London)* **278,** 835–838.

Simon, E. J., and Groth, J. (1975). Kinetics of opiate receptor inactivation by sulfhydryl reagents: Evidence for conformational change in presence of sodium ion. *Proc. Natl. Acad. Sci. U.S.A.* **72,** 2404–2407.

Siraganian, R. P., Hook, W. A., and LeVine, B. B. (1975). Specific *in vitro* histamine release from basophils by bivalent haptens: Evidence for activation by simple bridging of membrane bound antibody. *Immunochemistry* **12,** 149–157.

Snyder, S. H., and Childers, S. R. (1979). Opiate receptors and opioid peptides. *Ann. Rev. Neurosci.* **2,** 35–64.

Sternberger, L. A., and Petrali, J. P. (1975). Quantitative immunocytochemistry of pituitary receptors for luteinizing hormone-releasing hormone. *Cell Tissue Res.* **162,** 141–176.

Traber, J., Fischer, K., Latzin, S., and Lamprecht, B. (1975). Morphine antagonizes action of prostaglandin in neuroblastoma and neuroblastoma X glioma hybrid cells. *Nature (London)* **253,** 120–122.

Yarden, Y., Gabbay, M., and Schlessinger, J. (1981). Primary amines do not prevent the endocytosis of epidermal growth factor into 3T3 fibroblasts. *Biochim. Biophys. Acta* **674,** 188–203.

2

The β-Adrenergic Receptor System: A Model for the Transmembrane Regulation of Adenylate Cyclase

MARGARET M. BRIGGS AND ROBERT J. LEFKOWITZ

I. INTRODUCTION

For a number of years there has been keen interest in discovering the mechanisms by which cells can sense and respond to changing extracellular conditions. Hormones provide one of the major influences in regulating intracellular processes. A number of hormones, including the catecholamines, act by binding to specific cell surface receptors and need not enter the cell to alter intracellular metabolic events.

23

CELLULAR REGULATION OF SECRETION AND RELEASE

Instead, a signal generated by hormone binding is transferred across the plasma membrane, resulting in activation of membrane-bound adenylate cyclase. This enzyme, present at the cytoplasmic side of the plasma membrane, catalyzes the conversion of ATP into cAMP, which is often termed the *second messenger* because it ultimately mediates the action of the hormone (*first messenger*) (Sutherland *et al.*, 1962; Sutherland and Robison, 1966).

Catecholamines influence events in many types of cells and produce the familiar "fight or flight" response. The diverse effects of β-adrenergic agents, such as epinephrine and the synthetic analog isoproterenol, include stimulation of glycogenolysis in liver and lipolysis in fat cells, as well as increase of the rate and force of contraction of the heart. In addition, epinephrine stimulates secretion of a number of proteins and other hormones, such as renin, insulin, glucagon, parathyroid hormone, thyroxine, and calcitonin. All of these effects appear to be mediated by activation of adenylate cyclase and subsequent accumulation of cAMP within the cells.

In recent years much has been learned both about the individual components involved in activation of adenylate cyclase and about their interactions; in fact, in the β-adrenergic-responsive adenylate cyclase system, two of the components (the receptor and guanine nucleotide regulatory protein) have been purified (Northup *et al.*, 1980; Shorr *et al.*, 1981). These advances make it an excellent model system for investigating the molecular details of transmembrane communication and regulation of cellular processes.

A schematic illustration of the components believed to constitute the catecholamine-sensitive adenylate cyclase system is shown in Fig. 1. Three separate proteins have been identified: the receptor (R), the catalytic unit of the enzyme adenylate cyclase (C), and the guanine nucleotide regulatory protein (N). Hormones bind to the specific cell surface receptor proteins, thus setting in motion a series of events resulting in activation of the catalytic unit exposed at the inner face of the membrane. Rodbell and colleagues (1971a,b) first demonstrated that guanine nucleotides are also involved in regulation of both adenylate cyclase activation and hormone binding to receptors in liver plasma membranes. Since then, significant evidence has accumulated showing that these effects of guanine nucleotides may reflect general characteristics of hormone-responsive adenylate cyclase systems. Several lines of evidence have suggested that the guanine nucleotide binding protein is distinct from both receptor and catalytic unit and forms the functional link between hormone occupancy of the receptor and

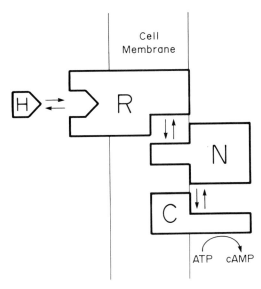

Fig. 1. Schematic model of the components of hormone-sensitive adenylate cyclase. H, Hormone; R, receptor; N, guanine nucleotide regulatory component; C, catalytic unit.

activation of the enzyme (Cassel and Selinger, 1978; Stadel *et al.,* 1981b).

The three components described here are integral membrane proteins that require the fundamental integrity of the membrane bilayer for productive interaction. Modifying the composition or fluidity of the membrane phospholipids can significantly alter or abolish hormone–effector coupling (Puchwein *et al.,* 1974; Orly and Schramm, 1975; Limbird and Lefkowitz, 1976; Bakardjieva *et al.,* 1979). Adenylate cyclase activity is retained in preparations of broken cells and in more purified plasma membranes. However, further disruption of the membrane milieu by detergents (Neer, 1974; Haga *et al.,* 1977; Limbrid and Lefkowitz, 1977), phospholipases (Pohl *et al.,* 1971; Rethy *et al.,* 1972; Limbird and Lefkowitz, 1976), or anesthetics (Voeikov and Lefkowitz, 1979) generally leads to an uncoupling of hormone responsiveness of adenylate cyclase. The individual components can retain their activity after solubilization with certain detergents, allowing resolution from the other components, biochemical characterization, and even purification of the receptor and guanine nucleotide regulatory protein. However, studying the interactions of resolved or purified components will require reconstitution of a suitable membrane environment and progress in this direction will be described in the following sections.

II. IDENTIFICATION AND CHARACTERIZATION OF THE RECEPTOR

A. Receptor Binding Studies

The development of radioligand binding techniques in the early 1970s has greatly facilitated studies of the β-adrenergic receptor, as well as a number of other hormone receptors. Radioactively labeled adrenergic agonists and antagonists, which stimulate or block stimulation of adenylate cyclase, respectively, have been used to bind to membrane-associated sites that show the characteristics expected of the physiologically relevant receptors. An important criterion is that the binding sites should exhibit the specificity and stereospecificity characteristic of the β-adrenergic response. The order of potency of agonists or antagonists in binding to receptor sites should correlate well with the order of potency in either stimulating or blocking stimulation of adenylate cyclase activity. The biologically active (−) stereoisomer should be more potent in binding to the receptor than the corresponding (+) isomer. In addition, the number of binding sites should be finite, i.e., the ligand binding phenomenon should be saturable. For β-adrenergic receptors in purified plasma membrane preparations, there are commonly 0.1–1 pmol/mg protein of receptor binding sites.

The ligands that have been widely used in adrenergic receptor binding studies are (−)-[^{3}H]dihydroalprenolol ([^{3}H]DHA) (Lefkowitz *et al.,* 1974) and ^{125}I-labeled (±)-hydroxybenzylpindolol ([^{125}I]HYP) (Aurbach *et al.,* 1974). These ligands label β-adrenergic receptors in a variety of tissues, including erythrocytes, leukocytes, and heart (Lefkowitz *et al.,* 1974; Aurbach *et al.,* 1974; Williams *et al.,* 1975; Alexander *et al.,* 1975), as well as several cultured cell lines, such as S49 lymphoma and C_6 glioma (Maguire *et al.,* 1976; Ross *et al.,* 1977). Although [^{125}I]HYP has the advantages of higher specific radioactivity and somewhat higher binding affinity, the pure (−) stereoisomer of [^{3}H]DHA enables more straightforward analysis of both kinetic and equilibrium binding data (Bürgisser *et al.,* 1981).

Methods for analyzing radioligand binding to hormone receptors have been developed and refined from the general theories of receptor–ligand interaction based on the law of mass action (that is, $R + L \rightleftharpoons RL$ in which R is receptor, L is the ligand; the equilibrium dissociation constant $K_D = [R][L]/[RL]$). Traditionally, Scatchard's transformation of this equation has been used to determine K_D values and receptor site number from saturation binding data (Scatchard, 1949). However, more versatile methods of analyzing binding data have been developed; these methods involve iterative computer curve fitting to equations based on the law of mass action (Feldman, 1972; Hancock *et al.*, 1979). Requiring fewer assumptions and less data transformation than previous approaches, this type of analysis permits successful dissection of complex binding curves such as those obtained with heart tissue, which contains a mixture of two pharmacologically distinct subtypes of the β-adrenergic receptor, termed β_1 and β_2 (Lands *et al.*, 1967). The two subtypes were differentiated, and values for the individual K_D and amount of each subtype were determined (Hancock *et al.*, 1979). The validity of this method has been tested by mixing known amounts of two types of membranes, each composed of a single receptor subtype, and analyzing the resulting binding data. The values determined by computer curve fitting proved to be essentially identical to predictions based on the known proportions of the individual components (De Lean *et al.*, 1982). These quantitative methods have also been used to analyze complex agonist binding curves, as described later.

An important goal of receptor binding studies is the characterization of agonist binding to the β-adrenergic receptor and the correlation of binding with the subsequent activation of adenylate cyclase. Two approaches have proved successful: direct binding of the radiolabeled agonist $(\pm)$-[³H]hydroxybenzylisoproterenol (HBI) to the receptor (Lefkowitz and Williams, 1977) and competition of unlabeled agonists with antagonists [³H]DHA or [¹²⁵I]HYP for binding to the receptor as described earlier. Both approaches indicate that binding of an agonist to the β-adrenergic receptor is significantly more complex than binding of antagonists (Kent *et al.*, 1980; De Lean *et al.*, 1980). Interaction of the agonist [³H]HBI with the β-adrenergic receptor in the absence of guanine nucleotides appears to induce or stabilize a high-affinity binding state that requires Mg^{2+} and that is very slowly reversible when a competing ligand is added. The ability of a given agonist to form this high-affinity binding state can be correlated with the intrinsic activity or efficacy of that drug. Guanine nucleotides, which are required for agonist activation of adenylate cyclase, cause a transition of this high-affinity state of the receptor to a lower affinity state, causing a rapid dissociation of [³H]HBI bound to receptor (Kent *et al.*, 1980). This effect of guanine nucleotides on agonist binding is also apparent in agonist competition curves as a rightward shift to higher agonist concentration (to lower affinity of the competing ligand) and a steepening of the curve. In contrast to agonist competition curves, antagonist competition curves are steeper and not shifted by guanine nucleotides, which is consistent with direct binding studies indicating that antagonists bind to receptors with a single affinity state and do not induce the alterations in affinity noted earlier for agonists.

These guanine nucleotide-mediated effects on agonist competition binding curves have been quantitatively analyzed by Kent *et al.* (1980) (see Fig. 2). The shallow agonist curve observed without guanine nucleotides can be resolved into two interconvertible affinity states: the agonist-specific, high-affinity state (K_H) also observed with direct agonist binding (R_H), and the lower affinity state (K_L) equivalent to that observed in the presence of guanine nucleotides (R_L). In highly purified plasma membranes from frog erythrocytes, 90% of the β-adrenergic receptors assume the higher affinity state, whereas in less pu-

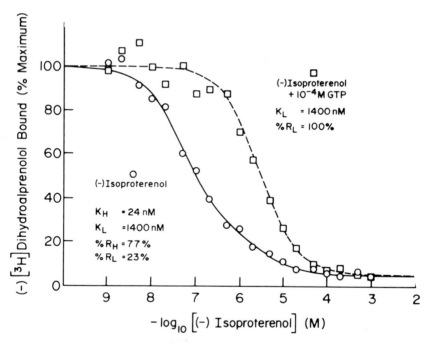

Fig. 2. Competition by (−)-isoproterenol for [³H]DHA binding to the β-adrenergic receptor of frog erythrocytes. The symbols represent data points obtained in the absence (○) or presence (□) of 10^{-4} *M* GTP. The solid and dashed lines correspond to curves generated from the most appropriate model as determined by computer curve fitting procedures described in the text and in Kent *et al.* (1980). Taken from Kent *et al.* (1980).

rified preparations containing more endogenous guanine nucleotides only 60–65% of the receptors accumulate in the high-affinity form. In both cases, exogenous guanine nucleotides shift the competition curve to the right and all the receptors are then found in the lower affinity state. These observations led to the development of a ternary complex model that describes agonist binding to the receptors and that so far is the simplest model that can explain all the data (De Lean *et al.*, 1980). This model will be discussed further in Section VI.

A number of other hormone-coupled adenylate cyclase systems also demonstrate agonist-specific binding characteristics, including modulation by guanine nucleotides. Other β-adrenergic systems that display this phenomenology include the turkey erythrocyte (Stadel *et al.*, 1980), the S49 lymphoma cell (Ross *et al.*, 1977), and the human astrocytoma (Su *et al.*, 1980). Similar observations have also been made for inhibitory α_2 receptors in the platelet (Hoffman *et al.*, 1980) and glucagon receptors in liver (Rodbell *et al.*, 1971b). However, quantitative analysis of these systems is complicated by a number of factors, including a lack of suitable antagonists. The widespread occurrence of agonist-specific binding events and the dual effects of guanine nucleotides on agonist binding and adenylate cyclase activation suggest that these effects are intimately related to coupling of the receptors to adenylate cyclase.

B.   Agonist-Promoted Events

The nature of these agonist-promoted events has been explored on a molecular level by solubilization and characterization of the agonist-occupied receptor protein. Limbird and Lefkowitz (1978) treated frog erythrocyte plasma membranes with the agonist [3H]HBI and solubilized the membrane with digitonin. The resulting agonist–receptor complex was larger in apparent size (assessed by gel exclusion chromatography) than receptors prelabeled with antagonist, and the difference in size was prevented by labeling with [3H]HBI in the presence of guanine nucleotides. This regulation of receptor size and affinity for agonist by guanine nucleotides suggested that the guanine nucleotide regulatory protein might become associated with the receptor.

This possibility was further explored by treating rat reticulocyte membranes with [32P]NAD+ and cholera toxin, which specifically labels one of the subunits (42,000 daltons) of the guanine nucleotide regulatory protein with [32P]ADP-ribose. The membranes were then treated with the agonist [3H]HBI to label the β-adrenergic receptor (Limbird *et al.*, 1980). After solubilization and gel exclusion chromatography as described earlier, the ^{32}P-labeled unit of the guanine nucleotide regulatory protein was found to coelute with the receptor. The guanine nucleotide regulatory protein did not coelute with the receptor when the receptor was occupied with antagonist or unoccupied, indicating that an important result of agonist interaction with receptor is the formation of a ternary complex composed of agonist, receptor, and at least part of the guanine nucleotide regulatory protein.

The existence of such a stable association was corroborated by Stadel *et al.* (1981b), who demonstrated that the agonist–receptor complex (containing the guanine nucleotide regulatory protein) could bind through the receptor to wheat germ agglutinin linked to Sepharose beads. As predicted from the effects of guanine nucleotides on agonist binding to receptor, incubation of the Sepharose beads with the non-hydrolyzable nucleotide analog, guanosine-5′-O-(3-thiotriphosphate) (GDP-γS) reversed the high-affinity complex and released the activated guanine nucleotide regulatory protein from the beads. The amount released was then assayed by reconstitution with adenylate cyclase catalytic units solubilized from turkey erythrocytes. In control experiments, the guanine nucleotide regulatory protein was not retained by nor released from the wheat germ–Sepharose when unoccupied or antagonist-occupied receptors were bound. Thus, agonist binding to receptor stabilizes a high-affinity complex of agonist, receptor, and guanine nucleotide regulatory protein, which can be destabilized by guanine nucleotides.

Although we have so far focused on alterations of agonist binding to receptor by guanine nucleotides, Cassel and Selinger (1977a, 1978) have documented a reciprocal effect, i.e., a change in nucleotide binding to the guanine nucleotide regulatory protein caused by β-adrenergic agonists. They were able to show that guanine nucleotides become associated with membranes from turkey erythrocytes in the presence of agonists and that this binding is sufficiently stable to withstand repeated washing of the membranes and subsequent incubation at 37°C in buffer without agonist. They also demonstrated that subsequent incubation of the membranes with agonist caused specific release of bound nucleotide in the form of GDP, in amounts roughly equivalent to the amount of receptor in these membranes (Cassel and Selinger, 1978). Agonist-induced GDP release has also been observed in frog and turkey erythrocyte membranes (Pike and Lefkowitz, 1981). These experiments emphasize the importance of communication between hormone receptors and the guanine nucleotide regulatory protein and led Cassel and Selinger (1978) to suggest that the function of hormones in activating adenylate cyclase is to promote the release of tightly bound GDP from the guanine nucleotide regulatory protein, thus allowing binding of the activating guanosine triphosphate (GTP) or one of its nonhydrolyzable analogs.

C.   Characterization and Purification

The β-adrenergic receptor is an integral membrane protein that re-quires treatment with detergent to extract it from the membrane. The plant glycoside digitonin has been used successfully in several tissues to solubilize the receptor with retention of the specificity and order of potency of binding ligands observed for the membrane-bound receptor (Caron and Lefkowitz, 1976; Haga et al., 1977). To date, use of other detergents has required prior stabilization of the membrane-bound receptor by ligand occupancy.

Identifying the polypeptide(s) that makes up a hormone receptor is a major step toward a biochemical understanding of receptor function. In several β-adrenergic systems (Atlas and Levitzki, 1978; Rashidbaigi and Ruoho, 1981; Lavin et al., 1981), this goal has been approached by covalently tagging the receptor with a radioactive ligand analog modi-fied with either a chemically reactive or photoactivable group. The covalently labeled polypeptides are then visualized on SDS gels. Atlas and Levitzki (1978) reported labeling two polypeptides (M_r 41,000 and 37,000) in turkey erythrocytes and L6P cells with a tritiated β-adre-nergic   antagonist, N-[2-hydroxy-3-(1-naphthyloxy)propyl]-N'-bro-moacetylethylenediamine. Rashidbaigi and Ruoho (1981) observed la-beling of two polypeptides (M_r 45,000 and 48,500) in duck erythrocytes with the photoactivated pindolol derivative ^{125}I-labeled p-azidobenzyl-pindol. Two irreversible ligands have been used to label β-receptors in the frog erythrocyte, a ^{3}H-labeled bromoacetylated derivative of al-prenolol (Pitha et al., 1980), and ^{125}I-labeled p-azidobenzylcarazolol (Lavin et al., 1981). Both agents are specifically incorporated into a 58,000-M_r polypeptide, which coincides on SDS gels with the β-recep-tor subunit purified from the frog erythrocytes (Shorr et al., 1981), as described later. The reasons for the disparities in reported molecular weights remain unclear, but it may be that they represent differences between species or β-receptor subtypes (β_1 for turkey and duck eryth-rocytes versus β_2 for frog erythrocytes).

Although covalent labeling allows a first glance at the protein(s) that functions as the β-adrenergic receptor, purification of the receptor is the next step toward understanding its function. The receptor bind-ing site of the frog erythrocyte was purified 55,000-fold from frog erythrocyte membranes and retained the affinity, specificity, and stereoselectivity characteristic of the membrane-bound receptor (Shorr *et al.*, 1981). Upon sucrose density gradient centrifugation, the purified receptor (located by binding activity or radioiodination) migrates at the same apparent sedimentation coefficient (9 S) as the binding activity of crude solubilized receptor preparations. Both isoelectric focusing and SDS gel electrophoresis techniques indicate that the purified, iodinated receptor is homogeneous, with a single peak at an isoelectric point of 5.8 and one band on SDS gels at an apparent molecular weight of 58,000. The 9 S sedimentation coefficient is somewhat larger than expected for the lipid–detergent complex associated with a protein of M_r 58,000, suggesting that the receptor may exist as either a monomer or a dimer in the cell membrane.

Progress has been made in the partial purification of the β-receptor from several other sources, including turkey (Vauquelin *et al.*, 1977) and duck (Shing *et al.*, 1980) erythrocytes and mammalian lung (Soiefer and Venter, 1980). Comparison of the characteristics of purified receptors from several sources should provide insight into the structural properties required for binding ligands and conveying that information through the guanine nucleotide regulatory protein to the catalytic unit at the inside of the cell membrane.

III. ADENYLATE CYCLASE

A. Catalytic Unit

In contrast to the receptor, the catalytic unit of adenylate cyclase has so far resisted numerous attempts to characterize and purify it. The task is particularly difficult because the enzyme is extremely labile and, with the exception of modest activity in the presence of low concentrations of manganese ion (Ross *et al.*, 1978), requires interaction with the guanine nucleotide regulatory protein to be activated by any of the normal effectors such as NaF, agonist, or Gpp(NH)p (Pfeuffer, 1977; Ross *et al.*, 1978; Nielson *et al.*, 1980; Downs *et al.*, 1980). Maintenance of activity after solubilization generally required prior irreversible activation by either NaF or agonist plus Gpp(NH)p. Estimations of the molecular weight of the enzymes from a variety of sources were based on sucrose gradient centrifugation or gel permeation chromatography and varied from 50,000 to 1,000,000 (Neer, 1974; Lefkowitz and Caron, 1975; Neer, 1976; Haga *et al.*, 1977; Welton *et al.*, 1978), but these values are difficult to interpret because they include some contribution from the guanine nucleotide regulatory protein, as well as undefined amounts of phospholipid and detergent.

Characterization of the catalytic unit now has become more feasible as a result of the development of reconstitution assays in which solubilized catalytic unit and guanine nucleotide regulatory protein can be combined to interact and reinstate adenylate cyclase activity. Strittmatter and Neer (1980) and Ross (1981) used this approach to monitor the resolution by gel permeation chromatography of the catalytic unit from the guanine nucleotide regulatory protein in brain cortex and rabbit liver membranes, respectively. In both cases, catalytic unit was found to be substantially larger than the guanine nucleotide regulatory protein and exhibited no activation by Gpp(NH)p or NaF unless recombined with guanine nucleotide regulatory protein-containing fractions or partially purified guanine nucleotide regulatory protein. There have also been several other reports of partial separation of the catalytic unit from the guanine nucleotide regulatory protein (Renart et al., 1979; Drummond et al., 1980). These advances should allow more definitive characterization and eventual purification of the catalytic unit of adenylate cyclase.

B. Interactions of the Guanine Nucleotide Regulatory Protein with the Catalytic Unit

Although little information is available on the structure of the catalytic unit, considerable progress has been made in understanding its interactions with the guanine nucleotide regulatory protein. Although the importance of guanine nucleotides in regulating adenylate cyclase activity was recognized a number of years ago (Rodbell et al., 1971a), the discrete protein character of the nucleotide binding component was not established until recently. Pfeuffer (1977) showed that a guanine nucleotide binding factor of pigeon erythrocytes was retained by the affinity matrix GTP-Sepharose and could then be eluted with non-hydrolyzable GTP analogs. The eluted material was shown to restore stimulation of adenylate cyclase activity when added to the inactive pass-through fraction from the affinity column. In addition, Pfeuffer (1977) developed a photoreactive derivative of GTP, [³H](azido-anilido)GTP, which retained biological activity and covalently labeled several proteins in pigeon erythrocyte membranes. Only one, with an M_r of 42,000, remained associated with adenylate cyclase activity upon sucrose density gradient centrifugation. Similar results in turkey erythrocyte membranes were reported by Spiegel et al. (1979). These results suggested that the factor could be separated from and reassociated with the catalytic unit to produce guanine nucleotide activation of adenylate cyclase.

In another approach to identifying the nucleotide binding component, cholera toxin treatment of pigeon erythrocyte membranes with [^{32}P]NAD$^+$ was found to catalyze [^{32}P]ADP ribosylation of a 42,000-M_r protein as assessed by sodium dodecyl sulfate gel electrophoresis (Gill and Meren, 1978; Cassel and Pfeuffer, 1978). This labeled protein has been identified in a variety of other cell types (Kaslow *et al.*, 1979; Limbird *et al.*, 1980; Cooper *et al.*, 1981), and an additional specific band at 52,000 M_r was found in S49 lymphoma and HTC-4 hepatoma cells (Johnson *et al.*, 1978b). The effects of cholera toxin on adenylate cyclase activity include enhanced stimulation by GTP (to the level produced by the slowly hydrolyzed analog Gpp(NH)p) and decreased activation by NaF. The extent of reaction measured by incorporation of [^{32}P]ADP-ribose into the 42,000-M_r protein was proportional to the increase in adenylate cyclase activation by GTP, providing further evidence of association of the labeled protein with the guanine nucleotide regulatory protein and its involvement in activation of adenylate cyclase.

Specific labeling of the regulatory protein provided a marker to demonstrate its actual physical association with the catalytic unit of adenylate cyclase by sucrose density gradient centrifugation (Pfeuffer, 1979). After pigeon erythrocyte membranes were [^{32}P]ADP ribosylated and solubilized, a GTP-binding fraction was isolated by the GTP affinity column procedure described earlier and recombined with the resolved catalytic unit. Reconstituted adenylate cyclase activity had an apparent sedimentation coefficient of 7.6 S, the same value obtained with adenylate cyclase activated with either Gpp(NH)p or NaF prior to solubilization with the same detergent. The sedimentation coefficient of the 42,000-M_r ^{32}P-labeled protein varied according to the guanine nucleotide bound to it, being 3.4 S with GTP-γS bound or 5.5 S with GDP bound. Guillon *et al.* (1979) reported quite similar results for the sedimentation coefficients of both catalytic unit (6.0 S) and Gpp(NH)p-stimulated adenylate cyclase (7.6 S) solubilized from pig kidney medulla, but a lower value for NaF activity (6.0 S). Summarized in Fig. 3, these results indicate that an association between the catalytic unit and the guanine nucleotide regulatory protein is stabilized by persistent activation with nonhydrolyzable guanine nucleotides or NaF and that either the size or the conformation of the guanine nucleotide regulatory protein seems to be determined by the type of guanine nucleotide bound to it.

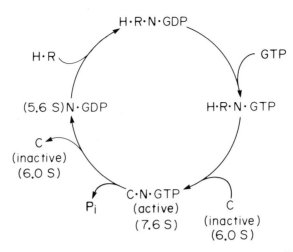

Fig. 3. Interactions of the components of the adenylate cyclase system. H, Hormone; R, receptor; N, guanine nucleotide regulatory protein; C, catalytic unit of adenylate cyclase. Taken from Stadel *et al.* (1982).

The observation of persistent activation of adenylate cyclase by slowly hydrolyzable analogs of GTP suggested that the hydrolysis of GTP might be part of the mechanism that regulates adenylate cyclase activity. Indeed, Cassel and Selinger (1976) reported a catecholamine-stimulated GTPase activity in turkey erythrocyte membranes, which could be inhibited by Gpp(NH)p or cholera toxin. Hormone-stimulated GTPase activity has subsequently been observed with catecholamines in frog erythrocytes (Pike and Lefkowitz, 1980b), glucagon in rat liver (Kimura and Shimada, 1980), and secretin in rat pancreas (Lambert *et al.*, 1979). Cassel and Selinger (1978) also found that the nucleotide released from membranes by hormone treatment was GDP, leading them to propose that hormone treatment caused release of tightly bound GDP and allowed GTP (or nonhydrolyzable analogs) to bind and activate adenylate cyclase. The GTP would then be hydrolyzed to the nonactivating GDP, resulting in the "turn-off" of adenylate cyclase.

An elegant approach to further characterization of the guanine nucleotide regulatory protein is to reconstitute solubilized fractions with membranes from mutant cells that lack all or part of the guanine nucleotide regulatory protein activity. In the *cyc⁻* line of S49 lymphoma cells, the β-adrenergic and prostaglandin receptors are intact, but they lack the nucleotide-sensitive, high-affinity state of agonist binding (Ross *et al.*, 1977). The catalytic unit of adenylate cyclase is also

present, but there is no discernable activation of adenylate cyclase by
either hormone or by effectors such as GTP or NaF, which bypass the
hormone receptors. Addition of guanine nucleotide regulatory protein
solubilized from a variety of sources reconstitutes the adenylate
cyclase response to those activators, as well as guanine nucleotide
regulation of receptor affinity for agonists (Ross and Gilman, 1977;
Ross et al., 1978; Johnson et al., 1978b; Sternweis and Gilman, 1979).
In addition, the 45,000- (also reported as 42,000 with different SDS gel
conditions) and 52,000-M_r substrates for ADP ribosylation by cholera
toxin, which are missing in the cyc^- mutant, are replaced by these
reconstitution procedures (Kaslow et al., 1979). These observations
strongly suggest that basal, hormone, guanine nucleotide and NaF
activation of adenylate cyclase, high-affinity agonist binding, and
cholera toxin effects are all mediated by the same protein.

Definitive support for this assertion requires that a single, purified
protein be used in the reconstitution. This goal has recently been accomplished (Northup et al., 1980). The guanine nucleotide regulatory
protein was purified from plasma membranes from rabbit liver or turkey erythrocytes by a series of ion exchange, gel exclusion, and hydrophobic chromatography steps. The purified protein possesses all functions attributed to the guanine nucleotide regulatory protein earlier
and consists of three bands detected by protein staining of SDS polyacrylamide gels, at M_r 52,000, 45,000, and 35,000 for rabbit liver
(Northup et al., 1980) and at M_r 45,000 and 35,000 for turkey
erythrocyte (Sternweis et al., 1981). The two larger subunits correspond to the substrates for ADP ribosylation described earlier and
apparently form the binding sites for guanine nucleotides. Because the
guanine nucleotide regulatory protein from turkey and human erythrocytes lacks the 52,000-M_r subunit but still reconstitutes adenylate
cyclase activity in cyc^- membranes, it seems likely that the largest
subunit is not essential for most guanine nucleotide regulatory protein
functions. In fact, comparison of the peptide maps derived from proteolysis of the [^{32}P]ADP ribosylated 45,000- and 52,000-M_r subunits
indicates nearly identical patterns, with one additional peptide in the
52,000-M_r (Hudson and Johnson, 1980) unit. This observation raises
the possibility that the subunits are basically identical proteins, but
one has undergone a different covalent modification, or that the
52,000-M_r unit is a precursor of the 45,000-M_r subunit. The functions
of the 52,000-M_r and 35,000-M_r subunits remain to be clarified, as does
the stoichiometry of subunits in the intact guanine nucleotide regulatory protein. The molecular weight of the guanine nucleotide regulatory protein determined by hydrodynamic and gel exclusion techniques

is in the neighborhood of 130,000 daltons, with an apparent decrease of 40,000 daltons observed upon activation of the guanine nucleotide regulatory protein by Gpp(NH)p or NaF prior to solubilization (Howlett and Gilman, 1980). This observation suggests that either a substantial alteration in conformation or an association–dissociation of subunits may be involved in the function of the guanine nucleotide regulatory protein in activating adenylate cyclase. Availability of the purified guanine nucleotide regulatory protein should allow more definitive investigation of these possibilities.

IV.   DESENSITIZATION

The phenomenon of desensitization or refractoriness appears to play an important role in regulating the responsiveness of cells to hormonal stimuli. Prolonged incubation of tissues or cells with a hormone or drug causes a dramatic decrease in the response to that hormone (Lefkowitz et al., 1980). For the hormone-responsive adenylate cyclase systems, desensitization results in attenuation of cAMP production, mainly by decreased activation of adenylate cyclase. These effects have been observed in a wide variety of cells, involving receptors for prostaglandins (Su et al., 1976; Johnson et al., 1978c; Clark and Butcher, 1979), human chorionic gonadotropin and luteinizing hormone (Conti et al., 1977), and thyroid stimulating hormone (Plas and Nunez, 1975), as well as β-adrenergic receptors.

There seem to be several different types of desensitization. In the case of homologous desensitization, only the response to the specific desensitizing hormone is altered, whereas stimulation of adenylate cyclase by other hormones or by NaF is unchanged. Loss or down-regulation of the receptors is often observed in such cases, possibly resulting from internalization of the receptors (Chuang and Costa, 1979; Harden et al., 1980). The other form of desensitization is termed heterologous and is characterized by a general loss of responsiveness of adenylate cyclase to all activators and no down-regulation of receptors. Investigations in a wide variety of cell types have provided some insight into the mechanisms by which desensitization occurs. It seems likely that the recently developed techniques for studying the individual components of the adenylate cyclase system should extend our understanding of adenylate cyclase regulation to a molecular level.

Homologous desensitization by β-adrenergic agonists has been reported in a variety of cell types, among them the S49 lymphoma (Shear et al., 1976), frog erythrocyte (Mukherjee et al., 1975), and human astrocytoma (Johnson *et al.*, 1978c; Su *et al.*, 1980), and in rat kidney (Anderson and Jaworski, 1979). The decrease in receptor-mediated stimulation of adenylate cyclase can be correlated with a reduction in affinity of agonist binding to the β-adrenergic receptor. For the frog erythrocyte, Kent *et al.* (1980) showed that formation of the high-affinity binding state for agonists was impaired after desensitization. In several other systems, such uncoupling of the β-adrenergic receptor from adenylate cyclase can be separated temporally from down-regulation of the receptors (Su *et al.*, 1980). Impairment of high-affinity agonist binding is observed within minutes, followed by a loss of β-adrenergic receptors only after longer incubation. These results suggest that several steps are involved in the process of desensitization: First, the receptor is uncoupled from adenylate cyclase, probably by some modification of one of the components; and second, functional receptors are lost from the membrane in a process likely triggered by the initial modifications.

In order to more clearly define the locus of these alterations, Pike and Lefkowitz (1980a) used cell fusion techniques to add fresh components of adenylate cyclase to frog erythrocytes previously desensitized with isoproterenol. They found that replacing the desensitized β-adrenergic receptor restored the responsiveness of adenylate cyclase to control levels, whereas adding both the guanine nucleotide regulatory protein and catalytic units did not overcome desensitization. When frog erythrocytes were desensitized with both isoproterenol and prostaglandin E_1, reconstitution with cells containing fresh β-adrenergic receptors restored to control levels only the isoproterenol response, indicating that the "resensitization" was not due to nonspecific reversal of desensitization during cell fusion and membrane preparation. These results suggest that the receptor may be the locus of desensitization of the homologous type.

Iyengar *et al.* (1981) have tested the activity of the guanine nucleotide regulatory protein from S49 cells desensitized for 20 minutes, during which time uncoupling, but no receptor loss, occurred. The guanine nucleotide regulatory protein was solubilized with detergent from the plasma membranes of the desensitized donor cells and incubated with the acceptor, the S49 lymphoma mutant *cyc⁻*, which has β-adrenergic receptors and catalytic units but lacks functional guanine nucleotide regulatory protein. The added guanine nucleotide regulatory protein became associated with the acceptor *cyc⁻* membranes to reconstitute hormone-stimulated adenylate cyclase activity. By this technique, it was shown that the guanine nucleotide regulatory protein from desensitized cells retained full reconstitutive activity.

Reports of desensitization in the S49 *cyc*⁻ cell (Green and Clark, 1981) (which can be assayed by reconstitution) and the HC-1 hepatoma cell (Su *et al.*, 1980) (which lacks a functional catalytic unit) indicate that the initial phase of desensitization can take place in the absence of receptor coupling with adenylate cyclase or cAMP synthesis. Interestingly, although desensitized S49 *cyc*⁻ cells exhibit decreased hormone stimulation of adenylate cyclase if the missing guanine nucleotide regulatory protein is replaced by reconstitution, the expected receptor loss does not occur upon longer incubation with hormone (Green and Clark, 1981). This result suggests that the catalytic unit or production of cAMP is required for receptor loss. These lines of experimentation seem to implicate the receptor as a major locus of alteration in homologous desensitization. Further characterization and purification of receptors after desensitization should provide more details.

Heterologous desensitization with a β-adrenergic agonist has been observed in turkey (Hoffman *et al.*, 1979; Stadel *et al.*, 1981a) and pigeon erythrocytes (Simpson and Pfeuffer, 1980), WI38 fibroblasts (Clark and Butcher, 1979), and certain astrocytoma lines (Su *et al.*, 1976; Johnson *et al.*, 1978c). This type of desensitization differs from that discussed earlier in that all activators become less effective in stimulating adenylate cyclase, suggesting that the components altered by desensitization may be distal to the receptor. A reconstitution approach similar to that described earlier has been used to test the effects of desensitization on turkey erythrocytes (M. M. Briggs, J. M. Stadel, R. Iyengar, and R. J. Lefkowitz, in preparation). In this case, the hormone-stimulated adenylate cyclase activity reconstituted with the guanine nucleotide regulatory protein solubilized from desensitized cells was lower than control levels, suggesting that the guanine nucleotide regulatory protein may be modified in cells that undergo heterologous desensitization. Further investigation should help determine whether other modifications occur as a result of desensitization.

V. RECONSTITUTION

Developing a detailed picture of the mechanism of stimulation of adenylate cyclase by hormones will require purification of each component and then reconstitution of functional interactions among them. Although this goal remains to be attained, significant progress has been made, and more importantly, these efforts have provided valuable insight into individual steps in the hormone-induced interactions of receptor, guanine nucleotide regulatory protein, and catalytic unit.

Several approaches to reconstitution have been described in Sections III and IV and will only be briefly mentioned here. Reconstitutions of solubilized components from turkey erythrocytes provided strong evidence for the independent existence of the guanine nucleotide regulatory protein (Spiegel *et al.*, 1979) and for its ability to act as a shuttle between the receptor and cyclase (Stadel *et al.*, 1981b). Another approach, pioneered by Gilman and colleagues, was to reconstitute solubilized guanine nucleotide regulatory protein into membranes of the S49 lymphoma cell *cyc⁻*, which is a mutant possessing normal receptors and catalytic unit but lacking functional guanine nucleotide regulatory protein. These experiments have been extremely useful in identifying, characterizing, and purifying the guanine nucleotide regulatory protein (Ross and Gilman, 1977; Johnson *et al.*, 1978a; Ross *et al.*, 1978; Sternweis and Gilman, 1979) and were described in Section III.

Cell fusion provides a way of engineering the protein composition of a cell membrane with relatively little perturbation. Orly and Schramm (1976) inactivated the catalytic unit of turkey erythrocytes with *N*-ethyl maleimide and fused the treated cells with Friend erythroleukemia cells, which are reported to lack β-adrenergic receptors. Only the hybrid cells, but neither individual cell type, exhibited isoproterenol stimulation of adenylate cyclase, demonstrating that the receptor and adenylate cyclase from two different cells could undergo lateral diffusion in the plasma membrane to interact effectively. Those studies were extended to show that receptors for hormones such as glucagon, prostaglandin, and vasoactive intestinal peptide could all interact with adenylate cyclase from various sources, suggesting that the structural features of the receptors allowing interaction with the other components of adenylate cyclase are remarkably well conserved (Schramm *et al.*, 1977; Schramm, 1979; Laburthe *et al.*, 1979). Cell fusion of frog erythrocytes (Pike *et al.*, 1979) demonstrated that the pharmacological specificity of β_1 and β_2 subtypes is determined by the receptor, but the intrinsic activity or maximal stimulation of adenylate cyclase by agonists depends on the character of the more distal components as well.

The information obtainable from fusion of whole cells is limited as a result of the heterogeneity of the systems. Attempts are currently being made to reconstitute resolved or partially purified components in a better-defined milieu, such as phospholipid vesicles. Some progress has been made in reconstituting adenylate cyclase into phospholipids (Hebdon *et al.*, 1979), as well as partially purified receptors (Fleming and Ross, 1981). Dopamine-sensitive adenylate cyclase solubilized from caudate nucleus has been reconstituted by addition of phospholipids and removal of the detergent (Hoffman, 1979). Citri and Schramm (1980) described reconstitution of receptor and guanine nucleotide regulatory protein from turkey erythrocytes and subsequent activation of adenylate cyclase. The receptor was obtained from solubilized turkey erythrocytes that were heated to inactivate the guanine nucleotide regulatory protein and the catalytic unit. The guanine nucleotide regulatory protein was resolved from the receptors by GTP affinity chromatography. These resolved components were reconstituted into phospholipid vesicles and treated with isoproterenol and Gpp(NH)p. This procedure could result in Gpp(NH)p binding to the guanine nucleotide regulatory protein only if the receptors were able to bind isoproterenol and interact normally with the guanine nucleotide regulatory protein. The proteins associated with the phospholipid vesicles were separated from the incubation mixture by centrifugation and fused with S49 lymphoma *cyc⁻* membranes, which provided the catalytic unit. Adenylate cyclase activity, assayed without added effectors, was reconstituted, suggesting that the Gpp(NH)p-loaded guanine nucleotide regulatory protein formed the requisite association with the *cyc⁻* catalytic unit. Similar approaches with increasingly purified components should lead to a better understanding of the individual functions of each unit and of the environment required for their interaction.

VI. A MODEL FOR ACTIVATION OF ADENYLATE CYCLASE BY β-ADRENERGIC HORMONES

Early models for the activation of adenylate cyclase by hormones considered the receptor to be an integral part or allosteric site of the enzyme (Robison *et al.*, 1966). Somewhat later, a "floating receptor" model that included the receptor and enzyme as individual components was introduced to explain the differences in agonist-binding properties from those predicted by simple mass action law (Boeynaems and Dumont, 1975; Jacobs and Cuatrecasas, 1976). This model suggested the concept that the mobility of individual proteins in the membrane was important to receptor–effector coupling. Derived from detailed kinetic analysis of adenylate cyclase activation, the "collision coupling" model described the rate-limiting step in enzyme activation as the diffusion-controlled, transient collision of mobile receptors and enzyme units (Tolkovsky and Levitzki, 1978). Neither model includes the more recently described guanine nucleotide regulatory component and its interactions with both receptor and adenylate cyclase.

A model that combines the interactions of receptor, guanine nucleotide regulatory protein, and catalytic unit described in previous
sections is shown in Fig. 4 (Stadel *et al.*, 1982). Binding of hormone (H)
to the receptor (R) promotes an interaction with the GDP-liganded
guanine nucleotide regulatory protein (N), resulting in formation of a
stable ternary complex HRN. This step is consistent with predictions
from computer modeling of agonist–receptor binding interactions
(Kent *et al.*, 1980; De Lean *et al.*, 1980) and biochemical evidence that
the agonist-promoted increase in receptor size results from binding to
the guanine nucleotide regulatory protein (Limbird and Lefkowitz,
1980). These interactions promote the release of GDP, allow GTP to
bind to N, and destabilize the ternary complex. In essence, the primary

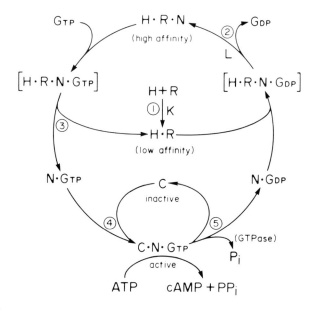

Fig. 4. Proposed mechanism of activation of adenylate cyclase by hormones and
guanine nucleotides. H, Hormone; R, receptor; N, guanine nucleotide regulatory protein;
C, catalytic unit of adenylate cyclase. Taken from Stadel *et al.* (1982).

role of the hormone receptor may be to facilitate the removal of GDP from N and the introduction of GTP into this site.

The next step would be for the guanine nucleotide regulatory protein bound with a guanosine nucleotide triphosphate (N-GTP) to associate with the catalytic unit of the enzyme. Stable association of N and C has been demonstrated by sucrose density gradient centrifugation studies (Pfeuffer, 1979; Guillon et al., 1979) and by reconstitutions (Sternweis and Gilman, 1979). Other reconstitution studies indicate that activation of N and subsequent activation of C by N are indeed discrete steps that can be separated in time and place (Citri and Schramm, 1980; Stadel et al., 1981b). Activation of adenylate cyclase also causes activation of a GTPase activity associated with N, leading to hydrolysis of bound GTP to GDP and reversion of the enzyme to the inactive state (Cassel and Selinger, 1976, 1977b).

A number of details of this process remain to be elucidated. For example, determination of the rate-limiting step in the activation of adenylate cyclase is still a matter of considerable controversy that may only be satisfactorily resolved when very precise kinetics of hormone binding, GDP release, and GTP binding are worked out, perhaps using stopped-flow techniques. Another question, whether any vital components remain to be identified, is now being approached by reconstitution studies using increasingly pure components. It will also be of interest to discover what role the organization of the membrane environment may play in transmitting information across the membrane. More recently there have been intriguing suggestions that adenylate cyclase may be associated with cytoskeletal elements (Simantov et al., 1980; Sahyoun et al., 1981) and that components of the adenylate cyclase system are organized in specific domains of the membrane (Levitzki and Helmreich, 1979) or in large aggregates that modulate enzyme activity (Rodbell, 1980). The information being obtained on a molecular scale can now begin to be assembled to describe the activation of adenylate cyclase as a transmembrane process.

REFERENCES

Alexander, R. W., Williams, L. T., and Lefkowitz, R. J. (1975). Identification of cardiac beta-adrenergic receptors by (−)[^{3}H]alprenolol binding. *Proc. Natl. Acad. Sci. U.S.A.* **72,** 1564–1568.

Anderson, W. B., and Jaworski, C. J. (1979). Isoproterenol-induced desensitization of adenylate cyclase responsiveness in a cell free system. *J. Biol. Chem.* **254,** 4596–4601.

Atlas, D., and Levitzki, A. (1978). Tentative identification of beta-adrenoreceptor subunits. *Nature (London)* **272,** 370–371.

Aurbach, G. D., Sedak, S. A., Woodard, C. J., Palmer, J. S., Hauser, D., and Troxler, F. (1974). Beta-adrenergic receptor: Stereospecific interaction of iodinated beta-blocking agent with high affinity site. *Science* **186**, 1223–1224.

Bakardjieva, A., Galla, H. J., and Helmreich, E. J. M. (1979). Modulation of the beta-receptor adenylate cyclase interactions in cultured Chang liver cells by phospholipid enrichment. *Biochemistry* **18**, 3016–3023.

Boeynaems, J. M., and Dumont, J. E. (1975). Quantitative analysis of the binding of ligands to their receptors. *J. Cyclic Nucleotide Res.* **1**, 123–142.

Briggs, M. M., and Lefkowitz, R. J. (1980). Parallel modulation of catecholamine activation of adenylate cyclase and formation of the high-affinity agonist-receptor complex in turkey erythrocyte membranes by temperature and cic-vaccenic acid. *Biochemistry* **19**, 4461–4466.

Bürgisser, E., Hancock, A. A., Lefkowitz, R. J., and De Lean, A. (1981). Anomalous equilibrium binding properties of high-affinity racemic radioligands. *Mol. Pharmacol.* **19**, 205–216.

Caron, M. G., and Lefkowitz, R. J. (1976). Solubilization and characterization of the beta-adrenergic receptor binding sites of frog erythrocytes. *J. Biol. Chem.* **251**, 2374–2384.

Cassel, D., and Pfeuffer, T. (1978). Mechanism of cholera toxin action: Covalent modification of the guanyl nucleotide-binding protein of the adenylate cyclase system. *Proc. Natl. Acad. Sci. U.S.A.* **75**, 2669–2673.

Cassel, D., and Selinger, Z. (1976). Catecholamine stimulated GTPase activity in turkey erythrocyte membranes. *Biochim. Biophys. Acta* **452**, 538–551.

Cassel, D., and Selinger, Z. (1977a). Catecholamine-induced release of Gpp(NH)p from turkey erythrocyte adenylate cyclase. *J. Cyclic Nucleotide Res.* **3**, 11–22.

Cassel, D., and Selinger, Z. (1977b). Mechanism of adenylate cyclase activation by cholera toxin. Inhibition of GTP hydrolysis at the regulatory site. *Proc. Natl. Acad. Sci. U.S.A.* **74**, 3307–3311.

Cassel, D., and Selinger, Z. (1978). Mechanism of adenylate cyclase activation through the beta-adrenergic receptor: Catecholamine-induced displacement of bound GDP by GTP. *Proc. Natl. Acad. Sci. U.S.A.* **75**, 4155–4159.

Chuang, D. M., and Costa, E. (1979). Evidence for internalization of the recognition site of beta-adrenergic receptors during receptor subsensitivity induced by $(^-)$isoproterenol. *Proc. Natl. Acad. Sci. U.S.A.* **76**, 3024–3028.

Citri, Y., and Schramm, M. (1980). Resolution, reconstitution, and kinetics of the primary action of a hormone receptor. *Nature (London)* **287**, 297–300.

Clark, R. B., and Butcher, R. W. (1979). Desensitization of adenylate cyclase in cultured fibroblasts with prostaglandin E_1 and epinephrine. *J. Biol. Chem.* **254**, 9373–9378.

Conti, M., Harwood, J. P., Dufau, M. L., and Catt, K. J. (1977). Regulation of luteinizing hormone receptors and adenylate cyclase activity by gonadotrophin in the rat ovary. *Mol. Pharmacol.* **13**, 1024–1032.

Cooper, D. M. F., Jagus, R., Somers, R. S., and Rodbell, M. (1981). Cholera toxin modifies diverse GTP-modulated regulatory proteins. *Biochem. Biophys. Res. Commun.* **101**, 1179–1185.

De Lean, A., Stadel, J. M., and Lefkowitz, R. J. (1980). A ternary complex model explains the agonist-specific binding properties of the adenylate-cyclase coupled beta-adrenergic receptor. *J. Biol. Chem.* **255**, 7108–7117.

De Lean, A., Hancock, A. A., and Lefkowitz, R. J. (1982). Validation and statistical analysis of a computer modeling method for quantitative analysis of radioligand binding data for mixtures of pharmacological receptor subtypes. *Mol. Pharmacol.*, **21**, 5–16.

Downs, R. W., Jr., Spiegel, A. M., Singer, M., Reen, J., and Aurbach, G. D. (1980). Fluoride stimulation of adenylate cyclase is dependent on the guanine nucleotide regulatory protein. *J. Biol. Chem.* **255**, 949–954.

Drummond, G. I., Sano, M., and Nambi, P. (1980). Skeletal muscle adenylate cyclase: Reconstitution of fluoride and guanylnucleotide sensitivity. *Arch. Biochem. Biophys.* **201**, 286–295.

Eimerl, S., Neufeld, G., Korner, M., and Schramm, M. (1980). Functional implantation of a solubilized beta-adrenergic receptor in the membrane of a cell. *Proc. Natl. Acad. Sci. U.S.A.* **77**, 760–764.

Feldman, H. A. (1972). Mathematical theory of complex ligand-binding systems at equilibrium: Some methods for parameter fitting. *Anal. Biochem.* **48**, 317–338.

Fleming, J. W., and Ross, E. (1981). Reconstitution of beta-adrenergic receptors into phospholipid vesicles: Restoration of [^{125}I]iodohydroxybenzylpindolol binding to digitonin-solubilized receptors. *J. Cyclic Nucleotide Res.* **4**, 407–419.

Gill, D. M., and Meren, R. (1978). ADP-ribosylation of membrane proteins catalyzed by cholera toxin: Basis of the activation of adenylate cyclase. *Proc. Natl. Acad. Sci. U.S.A.* **75**, 3050–3054.

Green, D. A., and Clark, R. B. (1981). Adenylate cyclase coupling proteins are not essential for agonist-specific desensitization of lymphoma cells. *J. Biol. Chem.* **256**, 2105–2108.

Guillon, G., Couraud, P. O., and Roy, C. (1979). Conversion of basal 6.0S adenylate cyclase into 7.4S by guanyl nucleotide treatment of membrane bound enzyme. *Biochem. Biophys. Res. Commun.* **87**, 855–861.

Haga, T., Haga, K., and Gilman, A. G. (1977). Hydrodynamic properties of the beta-adrenergic receptor and adenylate cyclase from wild type and variant S49 lymphoma cells. *J. Biol. Chem.* **252**, 5776–5782.

Hancock, A. A., De Lean, A. L., and Lefkowitz, R. J. (1979). Quantitative resolution of beta-adrenergic receptor subtypes by selective ligand binding: Application of a computerized model fitting technique. *Mol. Pharmacol.* **16**, 1–9.

Harden, T. K., Cotton, C. U., Waldo, G. L., Lutton, J. K., and Perkins, J. P. (1980). Catecholamine-induced alterations in sedimentation behavior of membrane-bound beta-adrenergic receptors. *Science* **210**, 441–443.

Hebdon, G. M., Le Vine, H., III, Minard, R. B., Sahyoun, N. E., Schmitges, C. J., and Cuatrecasas, P. (1979). Incorporation of rat brain adenylate cyclase into artificial phospholipid vescles. *J. Biol. Chem.* **254**, 10459–10465.

Hoffman, B. B., Mullikin-Kilpatrick, D., and Lefkowitz, R. J. (1979). Desensitization of beta-adrenergic stimulated adenylate cyclase in turkey erythrocytes. *J. Cyclic Nucleotide Res.* **5**, 355–366.

Hoffman, B. B., Mullikin-Kilpatrick, D., and Lefkowitz, R. J. (1980). Heterogeneity of radioligand binding to alpha-adrenergic receptors. *J. Biol. Chem.* **255**, 4645–4652.

Hoffman, F. M. (1979). Solubilization and reconstitution of dopamine-sensitive adenylate cyclase from bovine caudate nucleus. *J. Biol. Chem.* **254**, 255–258.

Howlett, A. C., and Gilman, A. G. (1980). Hydrodynamic properties of the regulatory component of adenylate cyclase. *J. Biol. Chem.* **255**, 2861–2866.

Hudson, T. H., and Johnson, G. L. (1980). Peptide mapping of adenylate cyclase regulatory proteins that are cholera toxin substrates. *J. Biol. Chem.* **255**, 7480–7486.

Iyengar, R., Bhat, M. K., Riser, M. E., and Birnbaumer, L. (1981). Receptor-specific desensitization of the S49 lymphoma cell adenylate cyclase. *J. Biol. Chem.* **256**, 4810–4815.

Jacobs, S., and Cuatrecasas, P. (1976). The mobile receptor hypothesis and "cooperativity" of hormone binding: Application to insulin. *Biochim. Biophys. Acta* **433**, 482–495.

Johnson, G. L., Kaslow, H. R., and Bourne, H. R. (1978a). Genetic evidence that cholera toxin substrates are regulatory components of adenylate cyclase. *J. Biol. Chem.* **253**, 7120–7123.

Johnson, G. L., Kaslow, H. R., and Bourne, H. R. (1978b). Reconstitution of cholera toxin-activated adenylate cyclase. *Proc. Natl. Acad. Sci. U.S.A.* **75**, 3113–3117.

Johnson, G. L., Wolfe, B. B., Harden, T. K., Molinoff, P. B., and Perkins, J. P. (1978c). Role of beta-adrenergic receptors in catecholamine-induced desensitization of adenylate cyclase in human astrocytoma cells. *J. Biol. Chem.* **253**, 1472–1480.

Kaslow, H. R., Farfel, Z., Johnson, G. L., and Bourne, H. R. (1979). Adenylate cyclase assembled *in vitro:* Cholera toxin substrates determine different patterns of regulation by isoproterenol and guanosine 5′triphosphate. *Mol. Pharmacol.* **15**, 472–483.

Kent, R. S., De Lean, A., and Lefkowitz, R. J. (1980). A quantitative analysis of beta-adrenergic receptor interactions: Resolution of high and low affinity states of the receptor by computer modeling of ligand binding data. *Mol. Pharmacol.* **17**, 14–23.

Kimura, N., and Shimada, N. (1980). Glucagon-stimulated GTP hydrolysis in rat liver plasma membranes. *FEBS Lett.* **117**, 172–174.

Laburthe, M., Rosselin, G., Rousset, M., Zweibaum, A., Korner, M., Selinger, Z., and Schramm, M. (1979). Transfer of the hormone receptor for vaso-intestinal peptide to an adenylate cyclase system in another cell. *FEBS Lett.* **98**, 41–43.

Lambert, M., Svoboda, M., and Christophe, J. (1979). Hormone-stimulated GTPase activity in rat pancreatic plasma membranes. *FEBS Lett.* **99**, 303–307.

Lands, A. M., Arnold, A., McAuliff, J. P., Luduena, F. P., and Brown, T. G. (1967). Differentiation of receptor systems activated by sympathomimetric amines. *Nature (London)* **214**, 597–598.

Lavin, T. N., Heald, S. L., Jeffs, P. W., Shorr, R. G. L., Lefkowitz, R. J., and Caron, M. G. (1981). Photoaffinity labeling of the beta-adrenergic receptor. *J. Biol. Chem.* **256**, 11944–11950.

Lefkowitz, R. J., and Caron, M. G. (1975). Characteristics of 5′-guanylyl imidodiphosphate-activated adenylate cyclase. *J. Biol. Chem.* **250**, 4418–4422.

Lefkowitz, R. J., and Williams, L. T. (1977). Catecholamine binding to the beta-adrenergic receptor. *Proc. Natl. Acad. Sci. U.S.A.* **74**, 515–519.

Lefkowitz, R. J., Mukherjee, C., Coverstone, M., and Caron, M. G. (1974). Stereospecific [^{3}H](−)alprenolol binding sites, beta-adrenergic receptors, and adenylate cyclase. *Biochem. Biophys. Res. Commun.* **60**, 703–710.

Lefkowitz, R. J., Wessels, M. R., and Stadel, J. M. (1980). Hormones, receptors, and cAMP: Their role in target cell refractoriness. *Curr. Top. Cell. Regul.* **17**, 205–230.

Levitzki, A., and Helmreich, E. J. M. (1979). Hormone-receptor-adenylate cyclase interactions. *FEBS Lett.* **101**, 213–219.

Limbird, L. E., and Lefkowitz, R. J. (1976). Adenylate cyclase-coupled beta-adrenergic receptors: Effect of membrane lipid perturbing agents on receptor binding and enzyme stimulation by catecholamines. *Mol. Pharmacol.* **12**, 559–567.

Limbird, L. E., and Lefkowitz, R. J. (1977). Resolution of beta-adrenergic receptor binding and adenylate cyclase activity by gel exclusion chromatography. *J. Biol. Chem.* **252**, 799–802.

Limbird, L. E., and Lefkowitz, R. J. (1978). Agonist-induced increase in apparent beta-adrenergic receptor size. *Proc. Natl. Acad. Sci. U.S.A.* **75**, 228–232.

Limbird, L. E., Gill, D. M., and Lefkowitz, R. J. (1980). Agonist-promoted coupling of the beta-adrenergic receptor with the guanine nucleotide regulatory protein of the adenylate cyclase system. *Proc. Natl. Acad. Sci. U.S.A.* **77**, 775–779.

Maguire, M. E., Wiklund, R. A., Anderson, H. J., and Gilman, A. G. (1976). Binding of [125I]iodohydroxybenzylpindolol to putative beta-adrenergic receptors of rat glioma cells and other cell clones. *J. Biol. Chem.* **251**, 1221–1231.

Mukherjee, C., Caron, M. G., and Lefkowitz, R. J. (1975). Catecholamine induced subsensitivity of adenylate cyclase associated with loss of beta-adrenergic receptor binding sites. *Proc. Natl. Acad. Sci. USA* **72**, 1945–1949.

Neer, E. J. (1974). The size of adenylate cyclase. *J. Biol. Chem.* **249**, 6527–6531.

Neer, E. J. (1976). Two soluble forms of guanosine 5'-(beta, gamma-imino)triphosphate and fluoride-activated adenylate cyclase. *J. Biol. Chem.* **251**, 5831–5834.

Neer, E. J., Echeverria, P., and Knox, S. (1980). Increase in the size of soluble brain adenylate cyclase with activation by guanosine 5'(beta, gamma-Imino)triphosphate. *J. Biol Chem.* **255**, 9782–9789.

Nielsen, T. B., Downs, R. W., and Spiegel, A. M. (1980). Restoration of guanine nucleotide- and fluoride-stimulated activity to an adenylate cyclase-deficient cell line with affinity-purified guanine nucleotide regulatory protein. *Biochem. J.* **190**, 439–443.

Northup, J. K., Sternweis, P. C., Smigel, M. D., Schleifer, L. S., Ross, E. M., and Gilman, A. G. (1980). Purification of the regulatory component of adenylate cyclase. *Proc. Natl. Acad. Sci. U.S.A.* **77**, 6516–6520.

Orly, J., and Schramm, M. (1975). Fatty acids as modulators of membrane functions: Catecholamine-activated adenylate cyclase of the turkey erythrocyte. *Proc. Natl. Acad. Sci. U.S.A.* **72**, 3433–3437.

Orly, J., and Schramm, M. (1976). Coupling of catecholamine receptor from one cell with adenylate cyclase from another cell by cell fusion. *Proc. Natl. Acad. Sci. U.S.A.* **73**, 4410–4414.

Pfeuffer, T. (1977). GTP-binding proteins in membranes and the control of adenylate cyclase activity. *J. Biol. Chem.* **252**, 7224–7234.

Pfeuffer, T. (1979). Guanine nucleotide controlled interactions between components of adenylate cyclase. *FEBS Lett.* **101**, 85–89.

Pike, L. J., and Lefkowitz, R. J. (1980a). Use of cell fusion techniques to probe the catecholamine-induced desensitization of adenylate cyclase in frog erythrocytes. *Biochim. Biophys. Acta* **632**, 354–365.

Pike, L. J., and Lefkowitz, R. J. (1980b). Activation and desensitization of beta-adrenergic receptor-coupled GTPase and adenylate cyclase of frog and turkey erythrocyte membranes. *J. Biol. Chem.* **255**, 6860–6867.

Pike, L. J., and Lefkowitz, R. J. (1981). Correlation of beta-adrenergic receptor-stimulated [3H]GDP release and adenylate cyclase activation. *J. Biol. Chem.* **256**, 2207–2212.

Pike, L. J., Limbird, L. E., and Lefkowitz, R. J. (1979). Beta-adrenoreceptors determine affinity but not intrinsic activity of adenylate cyclase stimulants. *Nature (London)* **280**, 502–504.

Pitha, J., Zjawiony, J., Nasrin, N., Lefkowitz, R. J., and Caron, M. G. (1980). Potent beta-adrenergic analog possessing chemically reactive group. *Life Sci.* **27**, 1791–1798.

Plas, C., and Nunez, J. (1975). Glycogenolytic response to glucagon of cultured fetal hepatocytes. *J. Biol. Chem.* **250**, 5304–5311.

Pohl, S. L., Krans, H. M. J., Kozyreff, V., Birnbaumer, L., and Rodbell, M. (1971). The glucagon-sensitive adenylate cyclase system in plasma membranes of rat liver. Evidence for a role of membrane lipids. *J. Biol. Chem.* **246**, 4447–4454.

Puchwein, G., Pfeuffer, T., and Helmreich, E. J. M. (1974). Uncoupling of catecholamine activation of pigeon erythrocyte membrane adenylate cyclase by filipin. *J. Biol. Chem.* **249**, 3232–3240.

Rashidbaigi, A., and Ruoho, A. (1981). Iodoazidobenzylpindolol, a photoaffinity probe for the beta-adrenergic receptor. *Proc. Natl. Acad. Sci. U.S.A.* **78**, 1609–1613.

Renart, M. F., Ayanoglu, G., Mansour, J. M., and Mansour, T. E. (1979). Fluoride and guanosine nucleotide activated adenylate cyclase from *Fasciola Hepatica:* Reconstitution after inactivation. *Biochem. Biophys. Res. Commun.* **89**, 1146–1153.

Rethy, A., Tomasi, V., Revisan, A., and Barabei, O. (1972). The role of phosphatidylserine in the hormonal control of adenylate cyclase of rat liver plasma membranes. *Biochim. Biophys. Acta* **290**, 58–69.

Robison, G. A., Butcher, R. W., and Sutherland, E. W. (1966). Adenylate cyclase as an adrenergic receptor. *Ann. N. Y. Acad. Sci.* **139**, 107–118.

Rodbell, M. (1980). The role of hormone receptors and GTP-regulatory proteins in membrane transduction. *Nature* **284**, 17–22.

Rodbell, M., Birnbaumer, L., Pohl, S. L., and Krans, M. J. (1971a). The glucagon-sensitive adenylate cyclase system in plasma membranes of rat liver. Obligatory role of guanyl nucleotides in glucagon action. *J. Biol. Chem.* **246**, 1877–1882.

Rodbell, M., Krans, M. J., Pohl, S. L., and Birnbaumer, L. (1971b). The glucagon-sensitive adenylate cyclase system in plasma membranes of rat liver. Effects of guanyl nucleotides on binding of ^{125}I-glucgon. *J. Biol. Chem.* **246**, 1872–1876.

Ross, E. M. (1981). Physical separation of the catalytic and regulatory proteins of hepatic adenylate cyclase. *J. Biol. Chem.* **256**, 1949–1953.

Ross, E. M., and Gilman, A. G. (1977). Reconstitution of catecholamine-sensitive adenylate cyclase activity: Interaction of solubilized components with receptor-replete membranes. *Proc. Natl. Acad. Sci. U.S.A.* **74**, 3715–3719.

Ross, E. M., Maguire, M. E., Sturgill, T. W., Biltonen, R. L., and Gilman, A. G. (1977). Relationship between the beta-adrenergic receptor and adenylate cyclase. *J. Biol. Chem.* **252**, 5761–5775.

Ross, E. M., Howlett, A. C., Ferguson, K. M., and Gilman, A. G. (1978). Reconstitution of hormone-sensitive adenylate cyclase activity with resolved components of the enzyme. *J. Biol. Chem.* **253**, 6401–6412.

Sahyoun, N. E., Le Vine H., III, Hebdon, G. M., Henadah, R., and Cuatrecasas, P. (1981). Specific binding of solubilized adenylate cyclase to the erthrocyte cytoskeleton. *Proc. Natl. Acad. Sci. U.S.A.* **78**, 2359–2362.

Scatchard, G. (1949). The attractions of proteins for small molecules and ions. *Ann. N.Y. Acad. Sci.* **51**, 660–672.

Schramm, M. (1979). Transfer of glucagon receptor from liver membranes to a foreign adenylate cyclase by a membrane fusion procedure. *Proc. Natl. Acad. Sci. U.S.A.* **76**, 1174–1178.

Schramm, M., Orly, J., Eimerl, S., and Korner, M. (1977). Coupling of hormone receptors to adenylate cyclase of different cells by cell fusion. *Nature (London)* **268**, 310–313.

Shear, M., Insel, P. A., Melmon, K. L., and Coffino, P. (1976). Agonist-specific refractoriness induced by isoproterenol. *J. Biol. Chem.* **251**, 7572–7576.

Shing, Y. W., Abramson, S. N., and Ruoho, A. E. (1980). Large scale purification of the beta-adrenergic receptor from duck erythrocytes. *Fed. Proc., Fed. Am. Soc. Exp. Biol.* **39**, 1616.

Shorr, R. G. L., Lefkowitz, R. J., and Caron, M. G. (1981). Purification of the beta-adrenergic receptor. Identification of the hormone binding subunit. *J. Biol. Chem.* **256**, 5820–5826.

Simantov, R., Shkolnik, T., and Sachs, L. (1980). Desensitization of enucleated cells to hormones and role of cytoskeleton in control of normal hormonal response. *Proc. Natl. Acad. Sci. U.S.A.* **77**, 4798–4802.

Simpson, I. A., and Pfeuffer, T. (1980). Functional desensitization of beta-adrenergic receptors of avian erythrocytes by catecholamines and adenosine 3', 5'-phosphate. *Eur. J. Biochem.* **111**, 111–116.

Soiefer, A. I., and Venter, J. C. (1980). Mammalian lung beta-adrenergic receptor purification utilizing an affinity reagent. *Fed. Proc., Fed. Am. Soc. Exp. Biol.* **39**, 313.

Spiegel, A. M., Downs, R. W., Jr., and Aurbach, G. D. (1979). Separation of a guanine nucleotide regulatory unit from the adenylate cyclase complex with GTP affinity chromatography. *J. Cyclic Nucleotide Res.* **5**, 3–17.

Stadel, J. M., DeLean, A., and Lefkowitz, R. J. (1980). A high affinity agonist beta-adrenergic receptor complex is an intermediate for catecholamine stimulation of adenylate cyclase in turkey and frog erythrocyte membranes. *J. Biol. Chem.* **255**, 1436–1441.

Stadel, J. M., De Lean, A., Mullikin-Kilpatrick, D., Sawyer, D. D., and Lefkowitz, R. J. (1981a). Catecholamine-induced densensitization in turkey erythrocytes: cAMP mediated impairment of high affinity agonist binding without alteration in receptor number. *J. Cyclic Nucleotide Res.* **7**, 37–47.

Stadel, J. M., Shorr, R. G. L., Limbird, L. E., and Lefkowitz, R. J. (1981b). Evidence that a beta-adrenergic receptor-assocated guanine nucleotide regulatory protein conveys guanosine 5'-0-(3'thiotriphosphate)-dependent adenylate cyclase activity. *J. Biol. Chem.* **256**, 8718–8723.

Stadel, J. M., De Lean, A., and Lefkowitz, R. J. (1982). Molecular mechanisms of coupling in hormone receptor-adenylate cyclase systems. *Adv. Enzymol.* **53**, 1–43..

Sternweis, P. C., and Gilman, A. G. (1979). Reconstitution of catecholamine-sensitive adenylate cyclase. *J. Biol. Chem.* **254**, 3333–3340.

Sternweis, P., Northup, J. K., Hanski, E., Schleifer, L. S., Smigel, M. D., and Gilman, A. G. (1981). Purification and properties of the regulatory component (G/F) of adenylate cyclase. *Adv. Cyclic Nucleotide Res.* **14**, 23–35.

Strittmatter, S., and Neer, E. J. (1980). Properties of the separated catalytic and regulatory units of brain adenylate cyclase. *Proc. Natl. Acad. Sci. U.S.A.* **77**, 6344–6348.

Su, Y. F., Cubeddu, X., and Perkins, J. P. (1976). Regulation of adenosine 3':5'-monophosphate contents of human astrocytoma cells: Desensitization to catecholamines and prostaglandins. *J. Cyclic Nucleotide. Res.* **2**, 257–270.

Su, K.-F., Harden, T. K., and Perkins, J. P. (1980). Catecholamine-specific desensitization of adenylate cyclase. *J. Biol. Chem.* **255**, 7410–4719.

Sutherland, E. W., and Robison, G. A. (1966). The role of cyclic-3', 5'-AMP in responses to catecholamines and other hormones. *Pharmacol. Rev.* **18**, 145–161.

Sutherland, E. W., Rall, T. W., and Menon, T. (1962). Adenylate cyclase. Distribution, preparation, and properties. *J. Biol. Chem.* **237**, 1220–1232.

Terasaki, W. L., Brooker, G., de Vellis, J., Inglish, D., Hsu, C. Y., and Moylan, R. D. (1978). Involvement of cyclic AMP and protein synthesis in catecholamine refractoriness. *Adv. Cyclic Nucleotide Res.* **9**, 33–52.

Tolkovsky, A. M., and Levitski, A. (1978). Mode of coupling between the beta-adrenergic receptor and adenylate cyclase in turkey erythrocytes. *Biochemistry* **17**, 3795–3810.

Vauquelin, G., Geynet, P., Hanoune, J., and Strosberg, A. D. (1977). Isolation of adenylate cyclase-free, beta-adrenergic receptor from turkey erythrocyte membranes by
   affinity chromatography. *Proc. Natl. Acad. Sci. U.S.A.* **74**, 3710–3714.
Voeikov, V., and Lefkowitz, R. J. (1979). Effects of local anesthetics on guanyl nucleotide
   modulation of the catecholamine-sensitive adenylate cyclase system and on beta-
   adrenergic receptors. *Biochim. Biophys. Acta.* **629**, 266–281.
Welton, A. F., Lad, P. M., Newby, A. C., Yamamura, H., Nicosia, S., and Rodbell, M.
   (1978). The characteristics of Lubrol-solubilized adenylate cyclase from rat liver
   plasma membranes. *Biophys. Biochim. Acta.* **522**, 625–642.
Williams, L. T., Jarett, L., and Lefkowitz, R. J. (1975). Adipocyte beta-adrenergic receptors. *J. Biol. Chem.* **251**, 3096–3104.
Williams, L. T., and Lefkowitz, R. J. (1977). Slowly reversible binding of catecholamine
   to a nucleotide-sensitive state of the beta-adrenergic receptor. *J. Biol. Chem.* **252**,
   7207–7213.

PART II
EARLY RESPONSES OF SECRETORY CELLS

3

Roles of Phospholipid Metabolism in Secretory Cells

SUZANNE G. LAYCHOCK AND JAMES W. PUTNEY, JR.

I. INTRODUCTION

The phenomenon of stimulus–secretion coupling in cells has come to be associated with secretagogue-induced changes in the phospholipid composition of membranes, enzyme activation and/or inhibition, altered ionic exchange mechanisms, and structural changes in the cell matrix. These alterations in cell composition or kinetic activity are often interrelated and are each integral to the secretory event. Alterations in phospholipid biosynthesis and/or turnover in cell membranes occupy an especially important place in the list of cell secretory events because they directly affect the fusogenic properties of membranes, the

53

activity of membrane-associated enzymes (also active in promoting secretion), and ionic exchange mechanisms including membrane transport, gating, and binding phenomena. In addition, the components of phospholipids (polar head groups, fatty acids, and diacylglycerol) may play individual roles in cation binding and release, in enhanced oxidative metabolism or metabolism to compounds active in mediating secretion, or in resynthesis of new phospholipids.

Any discussion of the importance of phospholipids to stimulus-evoked secretion needs to examine the relationship of receptor occupation to enzymes responsible for phospholipid metabolism/catabolism i.e., the phospholipases. The relationship of phospholipase C (PLC) and A (PLA) activites to stimulus–secretion coupling will be emphasized in this treatise. The ability of receptors to affect these enzyme activities and of the phospholipases to catalyze changes in the cell phospholipid profile to effect alterations in cation availability, enzyme activation, fatty acid metabolism, and secretion will be examined in a variety of secretory tissues.

II. FATTY ACIDS AND PHOSPHOLIPIDS AFFECT SECRETION

Most of the lipid in cell membranes is found in the phospholipid fraction, with phosphatidylcholine (PC), phosphatidylethanolamine (PE), phosphatidylserine (PS), and phosphatidylinositol (PI) being the major phospholipids in descending order of percentage of total lipid phosphate. Neutral lipids, triglycerides, cholesterol, and free fatty acids constitute the majority of the remaining lipid components. Although phosphatidic acid (PA), polyphosphoinositides, and the lyso-phosphatides are not major components of membranes on a percentage of total lipid basis, they are substances that are rapidly turning over and as such may represent acute regulatory intermediates in various membrane functions. In addition, the fatty acid moieties of phospholipids may play important roles in membrane and cell function because they too may be turning over as dictated by the activity of phospholipases.

A variety of phospholipases are found in cells, and each has either a specificity for hydrolyzing the phospholipid fatty acid ester bond at the 1-acyl (PLA_1) or 2-acyl (PLA_2) position, or for hydrolyzing the phospholipid base group (PLD) or the polar head group (PLC) (Fig. 1). A soluble group of phospholipases exists only in lysosomes; these enzymes have an acid pH optimum and generally are not dependent upon

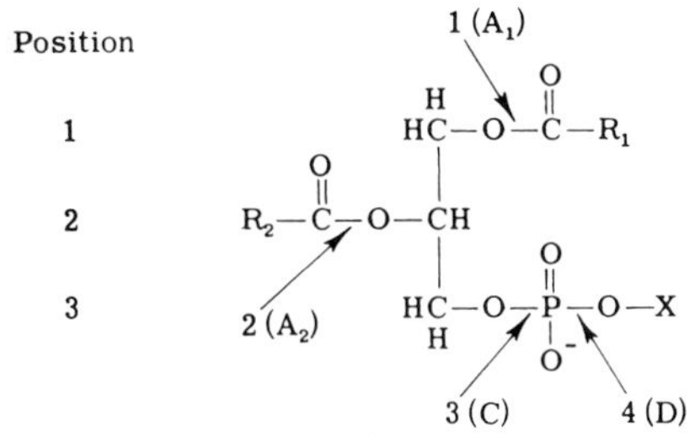

Position

Fig. 1.   Sites of hydrolysis of phospholipids by phospholipases A_1, A_2, C, and D.

calcium for their activity. On the other hand, numerous phospholipases exist in the cell with pH optima closer to neutrality than the lysosomal enzyme, and many of these enzymes can be activated by calcium ions. They have been localized to both soluble and particulate fractions of the cell, the latter including mitochondria, endoplasmic reticulum, and plasma membrane. The acyl groups of phospholipids appear to turn over independently as a result of PLA_1 and PLA_2 activity, forming 1-acyl and 2-acyl glyceryl phospholipids known as lysophospholipids. Phospholipids may be lost when the lysophospholipids are removed by endogenous lysophospholipase. In addition to phospholipases, microsomes and mitochondria possess acyl transferases that preferentially incorporate an acyl derivative into the 1 or 2 position of monoacylglyceryl phospholipids (Newkirk and Waite, 1971). Together, the acylating enzymes and phospholipases in cell organelles generate monoacyl-diacyl-phosphoglyceride cycles in the cell that play an important role in determining the nature of fatty acids in membrane phospholipids. The incorporation of acyl derivatives of different chain length and saturation into phospholipids will determine the physical nature and structure of membranes and regulate the functions of membranes important in the secretory process.

   Phospholipids and their molecular components affect cation transport and availability in secretory and nonsecretory cell types in various ways. Phospholipids, especially those containing unsaturated fatty acids, potentiate many membrane-bound enzyme activities, including β-hydroxybutyrate dehydrogenase, adenylate cyclase, glucose-6-phosphatase, and Ca^{2+}-ATPase (Coleman, 1973; Sandermann, 1978). Delipidation of muscle sarcoplasmic reticulum Ca^{2+}-ATPase, with subsequent readdition of PE or PC, results initially in loss of enzyme activity followed by restoration of phosphorylation and Ca^{2+} translocating ability (Knowles et al., 1976). The readdition of unsaturated fatty acids such as oleic or arachidonic acids to membranes previously treated with PLA to abolish ATP-driven Ca^{2+} storage will also restore ATPase activity (Martonosi et al., 1968; Fiehn and Hasselbach, 1970; Meissner and Fleischer, 1972). Ca^{2+}-ATPase activity is also important to cation transport in secretory cells; and phospholipids and their hydrolysis products (unsaturated fatty acids and lysophospholipids) may modulate this enzyme activity in secretory tissue. Phospholipids and lysophospholipids also mediate the transmembrane transport of amino acids, nucleotides, sugars, and metabolites as well as cations or anions across biological membranes (Green et al., 1980) and may participate as ionophores (Tyson et al., 1976). In low concentrations, the less saturated fatty acids of shorter chain length, such as oleic acid, also modify membranes so as to decrease Ca^{2+} permeability and efflux and thus improve the cation concentrating ability of microsomal vesicles (Seiler and Hasselbach, 1971; Katz et al., 1981).

Another component of phospholipids (the strongly ionic polar head groups) probably also participates in the regulation of cation availability. Thus, Ca^{2+} binding may be related to the levels of anionic di- and triphosphoinositides synthesized by specific kinases in membranes (Buckley and Hawthorne, 1972). The regulation of membrane-bound Ca^{2+} levels may participate in the regulation of various Ca^{2+}-dependent enzymes, including PLA_2. Because secretory events are generally accompanied by Ca^{2+} redistribution, binding, and permeability changes within the cells (Rubin, 1974), it is reasonable to assume that the activity of phospholipases and subsequent changes in membrane phospholipids and fatty acid composition and phosphorylation may mediate these changes.

Membrane fusion phenomena are central to the physical event of exocytosis of secretory granules. A role for phospholipids in this process has been postulated to include the formation of lysophospholipids in membranes along with their inherent lytic propensity for bestowing disorder among membrane lipid molecules (Poste and Allison, 1973). Lysophosphatidylcholine (LPC) may decrease the thermodynamic stability of the membrane bilayer and induce membrane fusion (Lucy, 1974). Fusogenic unsaturated fatty acids such as capric, oleic, or linoleic acids will induce physical changes in membrane lamellae and enhance membrane fluidity, which may also account for reduced stability and enhanced fusion processes (Lucy, 1974). In contrast, saturated palmitic or stearic acids are inactive in initiating membrane fusion. Fusogenic lipids appear to condense with PC, PS, or sphingomyelin, and fusion may entail an intermingling of the lipid molecules of two adjacent membranes in protein-free areas of the lipid bilayer. Because ionophore-induced Ca^{2+} movement through membranes may induce membrane fusion (Ahkong *et al.*, 1975), Ca^{2+}-activated PLA may be responsible for increasing lysophospholipid levels and promoting fusion events. Alternatively, Ca^{2+} may generate membrane instabilities prompting lipids to adopt nonbilayer phases that promote fusion reactions (Cullis *et al.*, 1980).

Apart from the involvement of phospholipids and fatty acids in regulating membrane phenomena involved with secretion, the fatty acids released from phospholipids as a result of PLA activity may also be free to interact intracellularly with other enzyme systems or to be metabolized as an energy source during secretion (Malaisse and Malaisse-Lagae, 1968). Arachidonic acid will act as a substrate for prostaglandin cyclooxygenase or lipoxygenase and be metabolized to other reactive lipid compounds with proposed roles in secretory phenomena (Rubin and Laychock, 1978). In addition, fatty acids may modulate the activities of enzymes such as guanylate cyclase or adenylate cyclase and thereby influence many intracellular events associated with stimulus–secretion coupling.

III. PHOSPHOLIPASE C, PHOSPHOINOSITIDES, AND Ca^{2+} MOBILIZATION

A. Historical Perspective and Development of a Model

Hokin and Hokin (1953) first demonstrated that acetylcholine stimulated the incorporation of radioactive phosphate into phospholipids of the exocrine pancreas incubated *in vitro* (Hokin and Hokin, 1953). Subsequent studies demonstrated that primarily PI and PA showed increased labeling (Hokin and Hokin, 1955). Because the main response of the exocrine pancreas to acetylcholine is an increase in enzyme secretion, a logical hypothesis was that the turnover of these phospholipids was in some manner involved in the mechanism of exocytotic discharge of zymogens (Hokin and Hokin, 1956). Subsequent findings, however, suggested that this was not the case. Specifically, it was found that (1) the omission of external Ca^{2+} blocked the secretory response to acetylcholine but did not prevent the labeling of PI (Hokin, 1966); (2) the concentration–effect relationships for acetylcholine stimulation of secretion and PI labeling did not coincide, i.e., higher concentrations of acetylcholine were required to stimulate phospholipid turnover than to stimulate secretion (Hokin and Hokin, 1954); (3) when the subcellular locus of the PI effect was investigated, most of the label was localized to the rough endoplasmic reticulum

(Redman and Hokin, 1959; Hokin and Heubner, 1967); and (4) in the parotid gland, activation of β-adrenoceptors stimulates exocytotic secretion to an extent substantially greater than that obtained through the α-adrenoceptors (Schramm and Selinger, 1975; Butcher and Putney, 1980). It is only through the latter pathway, however, that PI turnover is stimulated (Oron et al., 1973, 1975).

Other suggested roles for enhanced phosphoinositide turnover, including a role in regulating the Na^+-K^+ pump, have similarly been ruled out by careful experimental investigation (Putney, 1981). It now seems clear that in many tissues PI turnover does not necessarily reflect biochemical events associated with the final response or function of the tissue. Rather, as discussed later, PI labeling may reflect mechanisms involved in the initial transduction of an external stimulus into a series of biochemical reactions that can ultimately lead to a wide variety of final responses, depending on the nature of the cell and function of the tissue. This concept was originated by Michell in his 1975 review (Michell, 1975). He suggested that the apparent common denominator among systems showing enhanced PI turnover, or the PI effect, was not the final response of the tissue, but rather the second messenger involved in the response: calcium. Michell's original survey of the literature (Michell, 1975) and considerable additional research published since then have borne out this consistent association of PI labeling with receptors that activate cellular responses by mobilization of Ca^{2+}. Included in such a list of Ca^{2+}-mobilizing receptors that are associated with PI labeling would be the α-adrenergic, muscarinic cholinergic, substance P, cholecystokinin, serotonin, angiotension II, vasopressin, and thrombin receptors (cf. Michell, 1975, 1979; Berridge, 1980). Significantly, however, PI labeling does not (generally) appear to be a *consequence* of Ca^{2+} mobilization. As already mentioned for the case of the exocrine pancreas, in most secretory and other tissues, the PI turnover response is not substantially inhibited by cellular Ca^{2+} depletion or, at least, it is substantially less sensitive to Ca^{2+} depletion than the known Ca^{2+}-mediated responses (Michell, 1975, 1979; Putney, 1981). Furthermore, divalent cation ionophores such as A23187 and ionomycin do not stimulate PI turnover (measured as $^{32}PO_4$ incorporation) but do stimulate the various tissue responses believed to be Ca^{2+} dependent (Rossignol et al., 1974; Billah and Michell, 1979; Fain and Berridge, 1979a; Poggioli et al., 1982).

Thus, the observation that the PI effect is apparently associated with receptors that mobilize Ca^{2+}, but is not itself a response to Ca^{2+} mobilization, led to the suggestion (Michell, 1975, 1979) that the reaction was indicative of a biochemical mechanism through which receptor activation was coupled to Ca^{2+} mobilization:

Receptor activation $\rightarrow$ PI turnover $\rightarrow$ Ca^{2+} mobilization

The assignment of PI labeling as an early event following receptor activation was also consistent with the concentration–effect curve discrepancy for the pancreas (see earlier), as argued by Michell's group (Michell *et al.,* 1976). This hypothesis, coming some 20 years after the original observation of the Hokins, has substantially stimulated interest in studying this phenomenon. More recent findings on PI turnover and its role in receptor activation of some model secretory systems will be discussed later. First, however, some brief consideration of the biochemical pathways involved in the PI effect is necessary.

Figure 2 illustrates the generally accepted pathways for the PI effect discussed in this section. According to this scheme, the combination of an agonist with its receptor in some manner activates the degradation of PI by a PLC reaction that yields inositol phosphates and diacylglycerol. Presumably, rapid phosphorylation of diacylglycerol from radioactive ATP by diacylglycerol kinase follows, which results in the synthesis of PA. Subsequent reactions (Fig. 2) lead to resynthesis of PI, retaining the radioactive phosphorus from the PA. This is the pathway originally proposed by Hokin and Hokin (1964) for the case of the avian salt gland and generalized by Michell (1975) for a variety of other systems. The pathway is consistent with three general phenomena that collectively constitute the "PI effect" (Putney, 1981): (1)

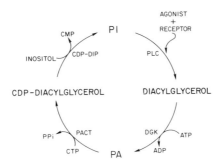

Fig. 2. Cyclic metabolism of PI. Agonist–receptor stimulation of PLC converts PI to diacylglycerol, which becomes PA by the action of diacylglycerol kinase (DGK) in the presence of ATP. PA is converted first to CDP-diacylglycerol by the action of PA:CTP-cytidyltransferase (PACT), and ultimately to PI through CDP-diacylglycerol inositol phosphatidyltransferase (CDP-DIP). Reprinted with permission, see Putney (1981).

an increased labeling by $^{32}PO_4$ of PI and PA, (2) a net breakdown of PI, and (3) a net biosynthesis of PA. It is important for a given system that, at least initially, all three of these phenomena be demonstrated before invoking hypotheses about the PI effect as shown in Fig. 2. For example, generation of diglyceride by PLC attack of phospholipids other than PI may result in (1) and (3), but not (2). Breakdown of PI by PLA_2 would result in (2), but not in (1) or (3). Examples of experimental results possibly misinterpreted in this way will be discussed later.

The scheme in Fig. 2 has gained general acceptance largely as a result of conceptual fit to the three aforementioned phenomena. Beyond this, there is little direct evidence to support this specific pathway. This is due to the failure of investigators to demonstrate any reproducible effects of receptor activation on phospholipid metabolism in broken cell preparations. All of the enzymes in Fig. 2 have been demonstrated in cells that show a PI turnover effect, but that these are the precise pathways activated on stimulation is difficult to prove.

A further complication in understanding the pathways of the PI effect concerns the subcellular locus of each of the enzymes and reactions. As mentioned earlier, most of the increase in radioactive PI appears to be localized to the rough endoplasmic reticulum. This is consistent with the generally held belief that the enzymes involved in the synthesis of PI and PA are also largely in the endoplasmic reticulum (Bell and Coleman, 1980). The locus of the initial steps, the breakdown of PI and synthesis of PA, are less certain. In the absence of any known intermediates linking receptors to PI breakdown, it seems reasonable that the initial event would be at the plasma membrane, although no definitive evidence for this exists. For the case of the platelet, as discussed later, there is some evidence that PI breakdown is mediated by a soluble PLC. Such an enzyme could attack PI at a number of intracellular sites. Some specificity for PI at the plasma membrane would be obtained if the receptor acted directly on plasma membrane PI molecules, increasing their vulnerability to hydrolysis.

There is some indirect evidence that PA synthesis may take place at the plasma membrane. This is based on a comparison of the relative labeling of PA and PI in the avian salt gland as compared to mammalian exocrine glands. In the latter systems, there is a considerable excess of membrane associated with endoplasmic reticulum as compared to the plasmalemma; for the avian salt gland, the opposite is true (see, for example, electron micrographs in the monograph by Berridge and Oschman, 1972). After stimulation of the exocrine glands, PI labeling generally exceeds PA labeling. In the avian salt gland, however, PA labeling greatly exceeds PI labeling (Hokin and Hokin, 1964,

1967). These observations are consistent with the idea that PA synthesis occurs in the plasma membrane, whereas resynthesis of PI takes place at the endoplasmic reticulum.

If this general scheme is correct—that PI breakdown and PA synthesis occur at the plasma membrane, whereas the resynthesis of PI and PA occurs at the endoplasmic reticulum—then it is necessary to have some functional connection between phospholipid pools at these two loci in order to account for the cyclic nature of the process indicated in Fig. 2. This connection can be readily accounted for by the existence of a family of phospholipid transfer proteins that catalyze the exchange or net transport of phospholipids (including PI and PA) from one membrane to another (Wirtz and Zilversmit, 1969; Demel *et al.*, 1977; Brophy *et al.*, 1978; DiCorleto *et al.*, 1979; Stukne-Sekalec and Stanacev, 1980).

Kirk *et al.* (1981), using isolated hepatocytes, have obtained experimental findings that may suggest a more complex series of reactions than those illustrated in Fig. 2. They investigated the effects of receptor activation on phosphatidylinositol 4-phosphate (PIP) and phosphatidylinositol 4,5-bisphosphate (PIP_2). These inositol phospholipids, collectively referred to as polyphosphoinositides, are generally present in mammalian cells in much lower concentrations than PI. They, and PI, are believed to be rapidly interconverted by addition and/or removal of one or two monoester phosphates to the inositol ring by the action of specific kinases and monoesterases (Michell, 1975). There is evidence that these minor inositides, as well as the enzymes responsible for their synthesis, are localized in the plasma membrane (Michell, 1975).

In a variety of systems, including iris smooth muscle, synaptosomes, and erythrocytes, the breakdown of polyphosphoinositides appears to be a Ca^{2+}-mediated event (Michell, 1975; Ahktar and Abdel-Latif, 1978; Putney, 1978). This has led to the formulation of hypotheses according to which the control of polyphosphoinositide metabolism and its role in cell function are distinct from that of PI breakdown, the latter being a Ca^{2+}-independent phenomenon (Putney, 1978). In hepatocytes, however, Kirk *et al.* (1981) found that stimulated PIP_2 breakdown was relatively Ca^{2+} independent. Also, the calcium ionophore A23187 failed to provoke PIP_2 breakdown. On the basis of these results, Kirk *et al.* (1981) suggest that there is no apparent difference with respect to Ca^{2+} dependence of PIP_2 and PI breakdown; and as the two compounds may be linked by rapid interconversion, the breakdown of either could represent the initial receptor-regulated event, the other phospholipid falling by a mass-action effect. Definitive evidence as to which molecule breaks down first is not available, but Kirk *et al.* (1981) point out that the rate and extent (expressed as percentage) of PIP_2 breakdown is considerably greater than for PI breakdown. Obviously, continued experimentation is needed in a variety of tissues in order to properly assess the relative roles of PIP_2 and PI breakdown in basic receptor mechanisms.

Despite considerable recent conjecture, little is known about the precise manner by which alterations in PI metabolism could lead to Ca^{2+} mobilization. For many of the systems studied, the mechanism of Ca^{2+} mobilization involves both an increase in membrane permeability to Ca^{2+} and a release of Ca^{2+} from either the plasma membrane or some intracellular organelle (Putney, 1978; Putney *et al.*, 1981b). A logical candidate for the Ca^{2+} release mechanism would be the breakdown of PIP_2 because this phospholipid is known to bind Ca^{2+} tightly (Dawson and Hauser, 1970). It has been suggested that the membrane permeability component of the response might result from the synthesis of PA in the plasma membrane, with the PA acting as a Ca^{2+} ionophore (Salmon and Honeyman, 1979, 1980; Putney *et al.*, 1980). The evidence for this is the ability of PA to mimic the effects of receptor activation in some (but not all) systems (Salmon and Honeyman, 1980; Putney *et al.*, 1980; Harris *et al.*, 1981; exceptions, see Putney, 1981; Gomperts, 1981). In addition, PA will function as a Ca^{2+} ionophore in artificial membrane systems (Tyson *et al.*, 1976; Serhan *et al.*, 1981). Finally, in one system that shows the PI effect (the rat parotid gland), drugs that act as Ca^{2+} antagonists also block Ca^{2+} binding to PA, and with similar orders of potency (Putney *et al.*, 1980). There have been objections raised to this hypothesis, however (Gomperts, 1981). It will obviously be necessary to await the outcome of continuing research in this area to resolve this rather controversial point.

As discussed later in more detail, phosphatidylinositol is particularly enriched in position 2 with arachidonic acid. As this is the rate-limiting substrate for synthesis of prostaglandins, leukotrienes, and the like, it would not be unreasonable to propose that perturbation of PI metabolism might ultimately lead to the production of such substances, which in turn could mediate or modify the appropriate end response of the tissue. In fact, there is good evidence for such an hypothesis for the mouse pancreas (Marshall *et al.*, 1980, 1981, 1982). However, for a number of other tissues that show the PI effect, involvement of prostaglandin-like substances as obligatory intermediates in stimulus–response coupling has been effectively ruled out (Chauvelot *et al.*, 1979; Lapetina and Cuatrecasas, 1979; Putney *et al.*, 1981a;

Putney, 1981). This does not indicate that PLA_2 and possibly prostaglandin synthesis do not play a major role in stimulus–secretion coupling in a variety of tissues (see Section IV). It does indicate, however, that the specific phenomenon characterized in this section as the PI effect probably plays some functional role in Ca^{2+} gating other than the generation of arachidonate residues for prostanoid synthesis.

B. Phosphatidylinositol and Ca^{2+} Mobilization in Specific Systems

1. The Exocrine Glands

It was in the exocrine pancreas that the PI effect was initially observed (Hokin and Hokin, 1953). The exocrine pancreas was also the first system for which experimental evidence suggested that PI labeling was not Ca^{2+} dependent (Hokin, 1966). In a more recent study, the turnover of PI was measured as incorporation of [^{3}H]acetate into PI (Calderon et al., 1980). Consistent with the proposed PI–Ca^{2+} gating hypothesis was the finding that agonists that stimulated amylase secretion by Ca^{2+}-dependent mechanisms (carbachol, bombesin, pancreozymin) also stimulated PI turnover, whereas those that acted through cyclic AMP (secretin, vasoactive intestinal peptide) did not (Calderon et al., 1980). These investigators were also able to block almost completely the secretory response to carbachol and pancreozymin by substitution of D_2O for 90% of the H_2O in the medium. This procedure, however, had no significant effect on the PI turnover responses to these agonists. In addition, they found that A23187 efficiently stimulated amylase secretion from pancreatic fragments, but that the ionophore caused only a modest increase in PI labeling, which was not significant prior to 60 minutes of incubation (Calderon et al., 1980). The conclusion drawn from this study, therefore, was that PI turnover was an intermediate reaction in the Ca^{2+}-dependent pathway (but not in the cAMP pathway) for amylase secretion and that the reaction probably occurred somewhere between receptor activation and Ca^{2+} mobilization (Calderon et al., 1980).

In another report, Farese et al. (1980) found that A23187 provoked a substantial decrease (30–40%) in pancreatic PI, an effect that required the presence of external Ca^{2+}. Farese and co-workers (1980) point out that these data are in conflict with the purported Ca^{2+} independence of PI breakdown that is integral to the Ca^{2+} gating hypothesis. However, it is important to remember that the PI effect as it pertains to Ca^{2+} gating refers specifically to the pathways shown in Fig. 2. As discussed earlier, evidence that this particular cycle has been activated would require demonstration of an enhanced incorporation of $^{32}PO_4$ into PI and PA, a net breakdown of PI, and a net synthesis of PA. In the report by Farese et al. (1980), no labeling data are given; PA levels, however, are reported to fall on stimulation by A23187, by more than 50%. Clearly this indicates that in these experiments, pathways other than those shown in Fig. 2 have been activated. Without data on precursor labeling, it is difficult to say what those pathways might be. It is noteworthy, however, that the concentration of A23187 used by Farese et al. (1980) (20 μM) is in the range shown by others to cause Ca^{2+}-dependent lysis of the pancreatic acinar cell (Chandler and Williams, 1977; Williams, 1978). Thus, it is possible that the sizable breakdown of PI and PA due to high concentrations of A23187 might result from activation of lysosomal phospholipases, perhaps of the A_2 variety.

The PI effect has also been extensively studied in the rat parotid salivary gland. It is one of the few times where all three components of the PI effect have been demonstrated: labeling of PI, breakdown of PI, and synthesis of PA (Oron et al., 1973; Jones and Michell, 1974; Putney et al., 1980). The parotid gland is a useful preparation for such studies, as cellular activation occurs by any of four different receptor pathways; one pathway utilizes as second messenger cAMP (β-adrenoceptor) and the other three utilize Ca^{2+} (α-adrenoceptor, muscarinic, and substance P receptors) (Butcher and Putney, 1980). The cAMP pathway is considerably more efficient than the Ca^{2+} pathway in activating amylase secretion, whereas the Ca^{2+} pathway, but not the cAMP pathway, activates membrane permeabilities to Na^+ and K^+ that may be important in generating transepithelial water flow (Schramm and Selinger, 1975; Putney, 1978). Thus, when it was disclosed that the PI effect was an α-adrenergic and not a β-adrenergic response (Hokin and Sherwin, 1957; Oron et al., 1973; Michell and Jones, 1974), a clear *dissociation* between PI turnover and exocytotic secretion was established. The other receptor pathways (muscarinic, substance P), pathways that utilize Ca^{2+} as second messenger, also stimulate PI labeling and breakdown (Jones and Michell, 1974, 1978). The effect, whether measured as labeling or breakdown, is clearly independent of Ca^{2+} (Oron et al., 1975; Jones and Michell, 1975) or, for that matter, any other electrolyte in the incubation medium (Jones and Michell, 1976; but see Keryer et al., 1979, for conflicting results and Putney, 1981, for discussion of the discrepancy).

The calcium ionophores A23187 and ionomycin will faithfully mimic the effects of activation of Ca^{2+}-mobilizing receptors, including K^+

release, Na^+ uptake, and limited protein secretion (Schramm and Selinger, 1975; Butcher, 1975; Poggioli et al., 1982). Neither of the Ca^{2+} ionophores, however, activates PI turnover (Rossignol et al., 1974; Jones and Michell, 1975; Oron et al., 1975; Poggioli et al., 1982). The parotid gland is thus one tissue for which the dissociation of the PI effect from Ca^{2+}-mediated responses is absolute. This is not meant to imply, however, that one or more of the enzymes involved in the PI cycle might not be Ca^{2+} dependent. The possibility of association of small quantities of Ca^{2+} with cell membranes or enzymes cannot be excluded. What these observations do show is that in the parotid, the effect is not Ca^{2+} mediated. This distinction between being Ca^{2+} mediated and Ca^{2+} dependent is an important one, as emphasized by Michell and Kirk (1981), and may serve to explain some puzzling contradictions obtained in other secretory systems discussed later.

Weiss and Putney (1981) examined the relationship of parotid receptors to one another with respect to their ability to activate PI labeling. Previous studies showed that the three Ca^{2+}-mobilizing receptors (muscarinic, α-adrenergic, and substance P) all activate the same population of Ca^{2+} channels and release Ca^{2+} intracellularly from a common Ca^{2+} pool (Putney, 1977; Marier et al., 1978). When agonists were tested for their abilities to stimulate PI labeling when applied in combination, it was found that the combination of any two of the three agonists studied (methacholine, epinephrine, and substance P) failed to activate PI labeling to an extent greater than the more efficacious of the two given alone (Weiss and Putney, 1981). This was true even for the combination of epinephrine and substance P, neither of which is capable of provoking a maximal (equal to methacholine) response, thus showing that the failure to summate was not due to saturation of some intermediate step in the PI labeling cycle (Weiss and Putney, 1981).

The aforementioned result indicate that although PLC cleavage of PI is in all likelihood a very early step in the stimulus–response sequence in the parotid, it is apparently not a reaction intrinsic to each separate receptor activation mechanism, i.e., it is unlikely that the receptor is itself a PLC. Further support for this concept was obtained from analysis of the dose–response relationship for PI labeling attributable to methacholine. In the parotid gland, the dose–response relationship for methacholine receptor occupation lies about one order of magnitude to the right of that for Ca^{2+}-dependent K^+ efflux (an index of Ca^{2+} gating) (Putney and Van DeWalle, 1980). This is presumably due to the presence of an approximate 10-fold excess of muscarinic receptors relative to the number required to open all of the available Ca^{2+} channels (Putney and Van DeWalle, 1980; Butcher and Putney, 1980). Thus, the location of the PI labeling curve would give some indication as to whether this reaction was quantitatively associated with the number of receptors occupied or with the extent of Ca^{2+} channel activation. The experimental results suggested the latter alternative: The dose–response curve for PI labeling lay about one order of magnitude to the left (lower concentrations) of the receptor occupancy curve and corresponded well with the dose–response relationship for Ca^{2+}-dependent K^+ efflux (Weiss and Putney, 1981). Again, as for the summation experiments, this suggests a quantitative relationship between PI turnover and Ca^{2+} mobilization. This result is consistent with (but by no means a strong point of evidence for) the hypothesis discussed earlier relating Ca^{2+} gating to PA synthesis.

2. Calliphora Salivary Gland

The isolated salivary gland of the blowfly (*Calliphora erythrocephala*) has proved to be an extremely useful preparation for studies of basic secretory mechanisms. The glands are tubular structures composed of a single layer of homogeneous epithelial cells that secrete fluid and digestive enzymes in response to 5-hydroxytryptamine (5-HT) (Berridge, 1977, 1980; Hansen-Bay, 1978). Evidence suggests that both cyclic AMP and Ca^{2+} are involved as second messengers in the secretory response (Berridge, 1977). Probably, as for the adrenergic receptors, separate 5-HT receptors regulate cAMP and Ca^{2+} metabolism.

It is possible with the isolated fly glands to continuously monitor Ca^{2+} gating concomitantly with fluid secretion. By including $^{45}Ca^{2+}$ in the fluid bathing the basolateral surface of the gland, the rate of emergence of $^{45}Ca^{2+}$ in the saliva can be assumed to reflect the permeability of the basolateral membranes to Ca^{2+} (Berridge and Lipke, 1979). Furthermore, if glands are preincubated in medium containing [^{3}H]inositol, the label is rapidly accumulated into PI (Fain and Berridge, 1979a). On stimulation with 5-HT, PI breakdown occurs, resulting in a substantial release of [^{3}H]inositol into the incubation medium. It is possible, therefore, to continually monitor the rate of PI breakdown by measurement of the rate of release of [^{3}H]inositol into the incubation medium (Fain and Berridge, 1979a). Notably, most of the radioactivity was released into the bathing medium rather than into the saliva, despite the fact that the apical surface area of these cells is considerably larger than the basolateral surface (Fain and Berridge, 1979a). This rather strongly suggests that PI hydrolysis probably occurs in the basolateral membranes where the 5-HT receptors are presumably located.

Berridge and Fain, therefore, utilized this experimental model to investigate the relationship between PI hydrolysis and Ca^{2+} gating (Fain and Berridge, 1979a,b; Berridge and Fain, 1979). Many of their findings were similar to those discussed earlier for exocrine glands. For one, PI hydrolysis bore no apparent relationship to the cAMP pathway. Release of [^{3}H]inositol was not stimulated by cAMP; fluid secretion was; but PI breakdown was not potentiated by phosphodiesterase inhibition (Fain and Berridge, 1979a). Also, secretion due to 5-HT eventually fails if extracellular Ca^{2+} is chelated with EGTA, but under these conditions PI breakdown continues at a substantially elevated rate (Fain and Berridge, 1979a). Finally, A23187 was capable of stimulating secretion and $^{45}Ca^{2+}$ flux but did not increase the rate of [^{3}H]inositol release (Fain and Berridge, 1979a). Collectively, these results suggest that the fly gland is similar in many ways to the parotid. It is apparently the Ca^{2+} pathway rather than the cAMP pathway with which the PI effect is associated, but the experiments with EGTA and A23187 clearly indicate that PI hydrolysis is not a response mediated by Ca^{2+} mobilization. Again, the circumstantial evidence would suggest that the PI turnover might, as Michell suggests, mediate Ca^{2+} gating.

Other studies of Fain and Berridge provide additional support for a cause–effect relationship between PI breakdown and Ca^{2+} gating (Berridge and Fain, 1979; Fain and Berridge, 1979b). These investigators exploited the fact that in the fly gland stimulation by large concentrations of 5-HT in the presence of Ca^{2+} not only stimulates PI hydrolysis but also inhibits PI synthesis. Thus, the activation of Ca^{2+} gating by high concentrations of 5-HT declines on prolonged exposure, and Berridge and Fain (1979) suggest that this inactivation may be secondary to the depletion of a critical pool of cellular PI. In support of this, these investigators found that including 2 mM inositol in the incubation medium substantially reduced the rate of inactivation. Furthermore, inositol, but not choline or ethanolamine, hastened the recovery of the Ca^{2+}-gating response to 5-HT after inactivation (Berridge and Fain, 1979; Fain and Berridge, 1979b). Studies on the tissue content of PI and the rate of resynthesis indicate that the critical pool of PI may be only a few percent of the total PI of the cell (Fain and Berridge, 1979b).

These findings suggest that in the fly salivary gland, breakdown of PI is associated with the opening of surface membrane Ca^{2+} gates but that depletion of PI results in Ca^{2+} gates in the closed configuration. Thus, a role for PI as simply an occluding or inhibitory molecule is not readily reconciled with these findings. Several alternative hypotheses can be constructed, however. Berridge and Fain (1979) have suggested that a physical association of PI with a Ca^{2+}-gate molecule (presumably a membrane protein) is necessary to impart hormone or receptor sensitivity to the gate. The actual hydrolysis reaction could, they suggest, provide impetus for either opening or closing the channel. In the former case, the channel would presumably close spontaneously and remain hormone insensitive until a new PI molecule is associated. A schematic depiction of this model is given in a publication by Berridge and Fain (1979). These experimental findings are also consistent with the hypothesis discussed earlier, according to which PI breakdown leads to PA synthesis, the latter molecule acting as a Ca^{2+} gate. Thus, depletion of PI would be seen as depletion of the precursor molecule for synthesis of the Ca^{2+} gate molecule (PA).

3.   The Liver

For the liver, PI turnover is associated with metabolic (glucose mobilizing) responses rather than true secretory responses, but it will be considered as a model system here because it is one of the better-characterized systems with regard to the PI effect. Like the parotid, the liver contains receptors that produce their characteristic cellular effects through either cAMP (glucagon, β-adrenergic) or Ca^{2+} (vasopressin, angiotensin II, α-adrenergic) pathways (Exton, 1981). Thus, an association of the PI effect with Ca^{2+} mobilization in the liver is evident from the findings of Kirk et al. (1977), who reported that vasopressin and epinephrine, but not glucagon, stimulated the incorporation of radioactive phosphate into phosphatidylinositol in isolated hepatocytes. The effects of epinephrine, but not vasopressin, were completely blocked by the α-adrenergic blocking drug dihydroergotamine. Billah and Michell (1979) demonstrated that angiotensin II also stimulated PI labeling and also that angiotensin II and vasopressin each caused a small (3–5%), but statistically significant, net breakdown of phosphatidylinositol. The role of calcium in the PI effect of the hepatocyte was also investigated by Billah and Michell (1979). The results of their experiments suggest that Ca^{2+} may play a role in one or more steps in the PI cycle but do not suggest that PI turnover follows or results from Ca^{2+} mobilization during stimulus–response coupling. First, removal of external Ca^{2+} substantially inhibited (by more than 50%) the PI labeling response to angiotensin II, vasopressin, or epinephrine, but did not completely block the effect. A23187, on the other hand, failed to markedly stimulate PI labeling or to cause PI breakdown when applied in concentrations known to activate glycogenolysis. In addition, the ionophore failed to potentiate the PI labeling response to agonists. These results show that the PI response of the hepatocyte is not a consequence of the increase in cytosolic Ca^{2+}, but unlike the situation for the parotid gland, for example, some Ca^{2+} is apparently required for optimal stimulation.

A similar situation was obtained in the study of PIP_2 breakdown in hepatocytes already discussed in a preceding section (Kirk *et al.*, 1981). Thus, vasopressin (0.23 μ*M*) caused rapid breakdown of about 30% of the hepatocyte content of PIP_2. Removal of external Ca^{2+} for 15 minutes prior to addition of the hormone reduced the breakdown to about 10%, although the effect was still statistically significant. A23187, in a relatively high concentration (10 μ*M*), had no discernible effect on PIP_2 content. Again, as for PI breakdown and turnover, these results are consistent with a requirement for Ca^{2+} for optimum PIP_2 breakdown, but they also suggest that PIP_2 breakdown is not a consequence of hormone-induced Ca^{2+} mobilization.

4. The Platelet

The involvement of lipids and phospholipids in the aggregation and secretory responses of platelets has been extensively studied. There is considerable data on the possible role of PLA_2 and possibly arachidonic acid metabolites, which will be considered in a later section. The combination of a receptor-activated PI cycle together in the same cell with an active Ca^{2+}-mediated series of reactions, possibly acting on the same molecules, has understandably generated some confusion.

To varying degrees, depending on the agonist, platelet activation is associated with PLC degradation of PI, synthesis of PA, PLA_2 attack of PI, PA, and PC, arachidonic acid release, and synthesis of prostaglandins, thromboxanes, and lipoxygenase products (Feinstein *et al.*, 1981; Gerrard *et al.*, 1981; Lapetina, 1982). Separating early receptor-regulated events from later reactions associated with secretion and/or prostanoid synthesis has not been easily accomplished, and, indeed, all of the several pathways may to varying degrees be interrelated.

Dissociation of arachidonate metabolism from the PI cycle and thrombin-induced secretion was achieved by Lapetina and Cuatrecasas (1979) by using the arachidonic acid analog eicosatetraynoic acid (ETYA). In the presence of ETYA, arachidonate metabolism by both the cyclooxygenase and lipoxygenase pathways was completely inhibited whereas thrombin-induced 5-HT secretion continued unimpaired. ETYA did not block the thrombin-induced synthesis of PA, which Lapetina and Cuatrecasas (1979) found to be elevated within 2–5 seconds and which preceded the release (presumably by PLA_2) of arachidonic acid. A23187 was compared to thrombin with respect to PA synthesis, the two drugs being employed in concentrations essentially equipotent for stimulating 5-HT secretion. The ionophore caused a slight but statistically significant labeling of PA; the effect of thrombin was substantially greater (Lapetina and Cuatrecasas, 1979). Applied together, the effects of thrombin and A23187 were additive (Lapetina *et al.*, 1981a).

These observations, together with earlier findings suggesting that PA synthesis derives primarily from PI breakdown (Michell, 1975), indicate that thrombin activates the PI cycle shown in Fig. 2 and that the primary effect of receptor activation is, in all likelihood, activation of a PI-directed PLC. Data on the actions of cyclic AMP in platelets provide the first indictment of a specific enzyme activity in the PI cycle. It is well known that phosphodiesterase inhibitors and cyclic AMP inhibit the various responses of platelets to agonists such as thrombin (Feinstein *et al.*, 1981). Lapetina and Cuatrecasas (1979) observed that stimulation of PA synthesis due to thrombin was almost completely blocked by incubation of the platelets with 0.1 mM dibutyryl cAMP or with a combination of 2.5 mM aminophylline and 0.22 mM methylisobutylxanthine. Also, this same group (Billah *et al.*, 1979) found that on treatment of platelets with deoxycholate (a detergent), a PLC activity is unmasked that specifically degrades PI to 1,2-diacylglycerol. More significantly, pretreatment of intact platelets with phosphodiesterase inhibitors or with dibutyryl cAMP substantially reduced the PLC activity subsequently assayed in the deoxycholate-solubilized preparation (Billah *et al.*, 1979). Other data have shown that cAMP has other significant effects on phospholipid metabolism in the platelet (Lapetina *et al.*, 1981b). The significance of the action of cAMP on the PLC is that it provides a cause–effect relationship between an enzyme that can be assayed in broken cells and a phospholipid turnover and secretory response measured in intact cells. It is also of notable significance that the PLC was primarily localized in the soluble rather than in the particulate fraction of the cell (Billah *et al.*, 1980). This could indicate that the primary action of the receptor is to modify the substrate (PI), perhaps by orientation in the membrane, rather than the enzyme itself.

The rapidity with which PA is synthesized following a thrombin stimulus has led Lapetina and Billah (1982; Lapetina, 1982) to conclude that PA synthesis may represent the primary receptor-activated stimulus in the platelet. If PA subsequently mobilizes Ca^{2+} or permits Ca^{2+} entry (possibly by acting as a Ca^{2+} ionophore; Gerrard *et al.*, 1978a, 1981; Lapetina, 1982), the increase in intracellular Ca^{2+} could trigger other alterations in phospholipid metabolism, specifically PLA_2 reactions leading to arachidonate liberation and possibly generation of fusogenic lyso compounds (see Section IV,A). As for most secretory systems, there is little direct evidence for PA functioning as a Ca^{2+} ionophore in the platelet; PA will induce Ca^{2+} release from platelet membranes but does not have agonist activity in intact platelets (Gerrard et al., 1978a). As discussed earlier, the failure of PA to act as an ionophore when applied exogenously can be readily rationalized, but not conclusively reconciled.

5. The Neutrophil

Neutrophils can be stimulated by receptor-specific peptides to respond both by chemotaxis and secretion of lysosomal enzymes (Becker, 1977). Evidence strongly suggests that Ca^{2+} is second messenger in these responses (Putney, 1978). It is not surprising, therefore, that on stimulation of neutrophils with the chemoattractant–secretagogue peptide formylmethionylleucylphenylalanine (fMet-Leu-Phe), there is net breakdown of PI, net synthesis of PA (both occurring within seconds), and increased labeling of PI with $^{32}PO_4$ (Bennett et al., 1980; Cockcroft et al., 1980a,b). However, in direct opposition to results discussed earlier for other secretory systems, all of these effects require the presence of external Ca^{2+} and can be mimicked by the Ca^{2+} ionophore ionomycin (Cockcroft et al., 1980a,b). On omission of external Ca^{2+}, enzyme secretion due to fMet-Leu-Phe is only partially inhibited, presumably due to an internal Ca^{2+}-release component of the response; a similar treatment results in total abolition of the PI effect (Cockcroft et al., 1980b).

These results would tend to exclude any role for PI turnover in Ca^{2+} gating in the neutrophil. It is possible to rationalize the Ca^{2+} dependency by assuming that the PLC or receptor may require Ca^{2+}, although the linkage between the two may still be direct. It is not so easy, however, to explain the observed effect of ionomycin in activating PI breakdown and PA synthesis in a Ca^{2+}-dependent manner. A more reasonable interpretation of these data is simply that no Ca^{2+}-independent PI effect occurs in the neutrophil and, therefore, that some completely different mechanism exists for coupling receptor activation to Ca^{2+} mobilization. It is important to point out, however, that these results have no immediately obvious bearing on theories developed for a number of secretory systems (discussed earlier) for which Ca^{2+} independence of the PI effect can be clearly demonstrated.

IV. PHOSPHOLIPASE A, PHOSPHOLIPIDS, AND SECRETION

A. Regulation of Phospholipase A

As noted in Section II, the activity of phospholipase A is dependent upon Ca^{2+}. This property of the enzyme has spawned numerous studies designed to elucidate the nature of the interaction between cation and enzyme. The platelet as a secretory organ proved very early on to be a convenient model upon which to draw for phospholipase–Ca^{2+} secretion coupling information. Knapp *et al.* (1977) suggested a major role for Ca^{2+} in stimulating prostaglandin and thromboxane biosynthesis in platelets based upon their findings that divalent cation ionophores, such as A23187 or X537A, stimulated production of these compounds as well as the platelet release response and aggregation. In the same year, Pickett and co-workers (1977) showed that phospholipase A_2 activity in platelets could be induced by A23187.

Thus, a sequential event in the platelet, and presumably other secretory systems (which will be discussed in Section IV,D), for prostaglandin synthesis is fatty acid liberation by a phospholipase A_2 stimulated by increased Ca^{2+} availability. The ubiquitous Ca^{2+}-binding protein calmodulin has been invoked as a possible mediator of Ca^{2+}-activated phospholipase A_2 activity in platelets (Wong and Cheung, 1979). As with other enzymes, calmodulin may titrate the availability of Ca^{2+} for phospholipase activation.

B. Pharmacological Modulation of Phospholipase A_2 Activity

In order to investigate the role of phospholipase activity in secretion, as well as the molecular requirements for induction of activity, a number of methods and pharmacological agents have proved useful. Inhibition of PLA_2 is achieved with *p*-bromophenacyl bromide, which alkylates the His-48 active center residue and distorts the binding of the cofactor Ca^{2+} (Verheij *et al.*, 1980). Use of this agent in studies linking PLA_2 activity and steroidogenesis have shown that inhibition of the enzyme is accompanied by inhibition of arachidonate turnover in phospholipids as well as depressed steroid secretion (Schrey and Rubin, 1979). Other agents that have been shown to specifically inhibit PLA_2 in platelets and leukocytes are indomethacin and other nonsteroidal antiinflammatory agents (Kaplan *et al.*, 1978; Jesse and Franson, 1979). These agents were formerly believed to inhibit prostaglandin biosynthesis by an action on cyclooxygenase; however, that inhibition is now expanded to include inhibition of PLA_2 and arachidonate release. The mechanism of this inhibition is due to competitive Ca^{2+} antagonism (Franson et al., 1980). However, various phospholipases A_2 have different sensitivities to the nonsteroidal antiinflammatory drugs, with some agents inhibitory at as low a concentration as 1 μM (Kaplan et al., 1978).

As a result of the importance of Ca^{2+} in phospholipase activity, agents that alter Ca^{2+} binding in membranes are effective modulators of enzyme activity because they displace Ca^{2+} from biological membranes (Scarpa and Azzi, 1968). In early studies, it was reported that local anesthetics inhibited prostaglandin biosynthesis either by a direct action on prostaglandin synthetase (benzocaine) or by inhibition of PLA_2 activity (tetracaine) (Kunze et al., 1974). This inhibition of phospholipase activity was thought to be due to interference with Ca^{2+} binding. Later studies showed that local anesthetics can interact directly with the enzyme rather than by antagonism of Ca^{2+} binding to the enzyme (Hendrickson and Van Dam-Mieras, 1976). In addition, local anesthetics may interact with the substrate rather than with the enzyme (Scherphof et al., 1972; Scherphof and Westenberg, 1975). The theory that anesthetic molecules produce a physiochemical effect by insertion into membrane phospholipid densities, thus perhaps altering the orientation of the phospholipid substrate so as to enhance phospholipase activity, may explain the stimulatory effect of low anesthetic concentrations on hydrolysis of phospholipids. An inhibitory effect at high concentrations of local anesthetic may be due to disorientation of the phospholipid substrate–phospholipase binding complex and/or to alteration of Ca^{2+} binding. Some investigators have found the inhibition due to local anesthetics of phospholipid hydrolysis by PLA_2 to be competitive with respect to Ca^{2+}, whereas stimulation of PLA_2 is independent of Ca^{2+} (Kunze et al., 1976). Therefore, stimulation or inhibition of phospholipase activities may depend upon whether the enzyme or substrate is predominantly affected by the anesthetic agent.

Glucocorticoids are another interesting group of compounds that have been known for many years to inhibit prostaglandin release from leukocytes and to act as antiinflammatory agents. Originally, the glucocorticoids were believed to act on the cell membrane and to antagonize the release of arachidonate for prostaglandin biosynthesis. More recently, however, studies have shown that glucocorticoids stimulate the biosynthesis and release of a polypeptide from leukocytes and neutrophils that inhibits PLA_2 (Blackwell et al., 1980; Flower, 1981). This inhibitory peptide, dubbed "macrocortin," may eventually prove useful as a modulator of PLA_2 in studies attempting to define the role of PLA_2 in secretory processes.

C. Phospholipases, Prostaglandins, Cyclic Nucleotides, and Secretion

Prostaglandins have been described as defensive agents, tending to protect the homeostasis of the *milieu interieur* of cells challenged by various agents (McGiff, 1981). This interpretation of the action of prostaglandins in cell function is novel and departs from the more widely held view that these long-chain, unsaturated fatty acids actively participate in some way in promoting the effects of cellular stimulating agents. The latter hypothesis is commonly based upon the observation that mammalian cells biosynthesize *de novo* and release prostaglandins in response to many physiological, pharmacological, or pathological stimuli (Piper and Vane, 1971). Prostaglandin biosynthesis in secretory organs in response to various stimuli has been amply documented and will be discussed with regard to specialized secretory models in later sections.

Arachidonate release from phospholipids has a direct relationship to prostaglandin biosynthesis (Flower and Blackwell, 1976). However, it has been hypothesized that more than one deacylation mechanism exists in cells, with one reaction providing substrate for prostaglandin biosynthesis, whereas another deacylation process(es) releases fatty acid for other nonspecified roles (Isakson *et al.,* 1977). The hypothesis arises from the observation that hormonal stimulation releases arachidonate in excess of that utilizable by the cyclooxygenase pathway. The thesis—that prostaglandin biosynthesis is dependent upon PLA_2 activity in tissues—is founded upon studies showing that prostaglandin release from tissues induced by exogenous arachidonate is Ca^{2+} independent, whereas Ca^{2+} is required for prostaglandin release induced by membrane active agents such as adrenergic receptor agonists, hormones, or A23187 (Forstermann and Hertting, 1979).

Prostaglandins have been investigated for many years with regard to their potential for regulating calcium availability in cells. Because this cation is of supreme importance as a modulator of secretion, prostaglandins might play important regulatory roles as participants in a stimulus–secretion sequence. Prostaglandins (PGE, PGA, PGB) release Ca^{2+} from mitochondria (Malmstrom and Carafoli, 1975). Weissmann *et al.* (1980) demonstrated similarity between stable prostaglandin free radical derivatives and A23187 in their abilities to translocate divalent cations across multi- and unilamellar liposomal membranes; naturally occurring prostaglandins were not active in this system, however. In certain secretory systems, the hypothesis of prostaglandins behaving as ionophores is supported. For instance, in membrane fractions from platelets, the prostaglandin endoperoxides PGG_2 and PGH_2 promote Ca^{2+} release, an action that may promote platelet activation and secretion of granule contents under *in vivo* conditions (Gerrard *et al.*, 1978b). In neutrophils, hydroxyacid arachidonate metabolites (HETE and leukotrienes), which are related to the prostaglandins but are synthesized via the lipoxygenase pathway, appear to enhance the permeability of neutrophil plasma membranes to calcium (Volpi *et al.*, 1980; Naccache *et al.*, 1981). Such an action may play a role in enhancing secretory events in neutrophils.

The mechanism(s) by which prostaglandins or their derivatives enhance the translocation of calcium across membranes is not completely understood. Prostaglandins may exert their effects by forming lipid-soluble cation complexes in an ionophoretic fashion (Eagling *et al.*, 1972) and/or by displacing Ca^{2+} from membrane binding sites (Ramwell and Shaw, 1970; Silver and Smith, 1975). The ability of HETE compounds to be incorporated into phospholipids (Stenson and Parker, 1979b) may be related to changes in calcium translocation properties of membranes with subsequent alterations in PLA and other membrane-associated Ca^{2+}-dependent and/or Ca^{2+}-regulatory enzymes. The interaction of prostaglandins, as unsaturated fatty acids, with Ca^{2+}-dependent ATPase (Seiler and Hasselbach, 1971; Meissner and Fleisher, 1972) would be another mechanism for regulating cell calcium availability.

Prostaglandins do not behave strictly as ionophores in all biological systems studied. In the anterior pituitary, for instance, PGE_2 and the ionophores A23187 and X537A promote growth hormone release; however, their mechanisms of action differ (Hertelendy *et al.*, 1978). PGE in this system results in secretion as a result of generation of the second messenger cAMP as well as elevation of cytoplasmic Ca^{2+}; the ionophores bypass the mediation by cyclic nucleotides and directly increase cytoplasmic Ca^{2+} levels, which stimulate hormone secretion. In addition, prostaglandin I_2 (prostacyclin) has even been described as an inhibitor of intracellular calcium release (Ally *et al.*, 1978), although other investigators have provided evidence that PGI_2 mobilizes calcium from intracellular pools (Rubin *et al.*, 1980). PGI_2 in many tissues appears to act through the stimulation of adenylate cyclase, and it may be the resultant increase in the levels of cyclic AMP that alters calcium homeostasis and cell response (Laychock and Walker, 1979; Rubin *et al.*, 1980; Holzmann *et al.*, 1980). The ratio among different prostaglandins may also be important in regulation of cellular calcium homeostasis.

Prostaglandin and cyclic nucleotide production in cells appear to have a close interregulatory relationship. Cyclic AMP has been shown to inhibit prostaglandin biosynthesis in a number of cell types, including cervical ganglia (Webb *et al.*, 1978), renal medullary interstitial cells (Kalisker and Dyer, 1972), and platelets, where cAMP inhibits endogenous PLA_2 (Minkes *et al.*, 1977; Gerrard *et al.*, 1977; Salzman *et al.*, 1978). Not only does cAMP impair phospholipid metabolism in platelets and thus inhibit prostaglandin formation, but even prostacyclin inhibits prostaglandin biosynthesis by stimulation of platelet adenylate cyclase (Lapetina *et al.*, 1977). Similarly, in macrophages, an ionophore-induced increase in cellular Ca^{2+} stimulates prostaglandin formation, which in turn mediates increases in cAMP (Gemsa *et al.*, 1979). Thus, a mechanism would appear to exist whereby certain prostaglandins can feed back upon a modulatory pathway and thus regulate further prostaglandin biosynthesis. In addition, dibutyryl cAMP inhibits PI-directed PLC in platelets (discussed earlier) and probably also inhibits PLC in fibroblasts (Hoffman *et al.*, 1974). As a consequence, the synthesis of PI may be inhibited along with the release of fatty acids that is attributable to PI-specific PLA_2 activity.

Perhaps an acceptable hypothesis accounting for the inhibitory action of cAMP on arachidonate mobilization and prostaglandin biosynthesis is that intracellular levels of ionized "free" calcium are reduced or made unavailable by active uptake and sequestration in cell organelles, thus inhibiting Ca^{2+} dependent PLA_2 and cyclooxygenase activity. A decrease in available calcium would also inhibit contractile proteins and other organelles involved in the secretory process. Conversely, prostaglandins or hydroxyacids may mobilize Ca^{2+} from cell depots, and this rise in Ca^{2+} levels can in turn inhibit adenylate cyclase and cAMP formation. The applicability of each possibility is ultimately dependent upon the cell type under investigation.

The activity of adenylate cyclase is also affected by membrane phospholipid composition and phospholipase activity. In fibroblasts, basal, fluoride-, and prostaglandin-stimulated adenylate cyclase activities are adversely affected by both increased primary amino groups in phospholipid polar head groups and the degree of fatty acid unsaturation (Gidwitz *et al.*, 1980). Adenylate cyclase activity has also been shown to be dependent upon an optimal phospholipid milieu, and phospholipase A, C, or D digestion of myocardial membranes, for instance, reduces cyclase activity (Lefkowitz, 1975). Although the aforementioned studies were not conducted in secretory cell systems, regulation of adenylate cyclase activity by membrane-active agents in secretory cells may be achieved by alterations in the phospholipid composition as a result of changes in phospholipase activity. In addition, alterations in membrane phospholipids due to PLA activity can affect receptor binding and coupled adenylate cyclase (Lad *et al.*, 1979), whereas PLC causes altered cyclase activity as a result of modification of a guanyl nucleotide regulatory process (Rubalcava and Rodbell, 1973).

In addition to cAMP, cGMP levels in cells may also be regulated by prostaglandins and other fatty acid derivatives. Guanylate cyclase, the enzyme responsible for cGMP biosynthesis, is activated by prostaglandin endoperoxides, hydroperoxy fatty acids, and arachidonic acid and other unsaturated fatty acids (Wallach and Pastan, 1976; Goldberg *et al.*, 1978; Cantieri *et al.*, 1980). In platelets, prostaglandin endoperoxides increase the level of cGMP and induce aggregation (Glass *et al.*, 1977). Of course, Ca^{2+} may directly modulate guanylate cyclase activity (Chrisman *et al.*, 1975; Garbers *et al.*, 1975). Because the local anesthetic tetracaine can antagonize the stimulation of cellular guanylate cyclase by membrane-active agents (DeRubertis and Craven, 1976), perhaps enhancement of phospholipase activity with resultant alterations in fatty acid release, arachidonate metabolism, and Ca^{2+} mobilization participate in regulation of guanylate cyclase. PLA_2, added to tissue homogenates containing guanylate cyclase or to partially purified soluble guanylate cyclase from several tissues, will activate the enzyme (Gruetter and Ignarro, 1979; Vesely, 1981). PLA_2-induced physicochemical alterations in the phospholipid–protein matrix associated with guanylate cyclase may facilitate interaction of the enzyme with cofactors and/or substrate.

Guanylate cyclase, unlike adenylate cyclase, however, has the potential for activation by a specialized mechanism of solubilization. Guanylate cyclase exists in both a particulate and soluble form in mammalian cells, and when the enzyme is solubilized it becomes more active than the particulate form of the enzyme (Chrisman *et al.*, 1975). The particulate enzyme can be activated by perturbation of the membrane architecture, and PLA is particularly effective in this capacity (Fujimoto and Okabayashi, 1975; Rillema and Linebaugh, 1978). In addition to PLA, the product of PLA activity (lysophospholipids) are effective activators of this cyclase. In the adrenal medulla and cortex, lysophosphatidylcholine (LPC), in contrast to other lysophospholipids, stimulates particulate guanylate cyclase activity several fold. Because soluble guanylate cyclase is many times more active than the particulate form of the enzyme in mammalian tissues, it has been suggested that the detergent properties of lysophospholipids are responsible for their activating properties (Shier *et al.*, 1976; Aunis *et al.*, 1978a,b; Struck and Glossmann, 1978). In contrast, adenylate cyclase in these studies was inhibited by LPC. Thus, lysophospholipids generated in response to PLA activation may modulate adenylate and guanylate cyclase activities in a reciprocal manner.

In addition to guanyl nucleotide cyclase activation by LPC and fatty acids, cyclic nucleotide phosphodiesterase is activated by PI or LPC as well as certain fatty acids (Wolff and Brostrom, 1976). Obviously, the regulation of the metabolism of cyclic nucleotides by alteration in phospholipid metabolism represents another important mechanism for control of cyclic nucleotide levels and their resultant actions in cells.

D.   Models of Phospholipid Metabolism and Secretion

1.   The Platelet

Platelets have proved to be a rich source of information for investigators unraveling the interdependencies of phospholipid metabolism and other cellular phenomena involved in secretion. Investigations in platelets demonstrated that PLA_2 was an endoenzyme (Derksen and Cohen, 1975), being mostly membrane bound in platelet subcellular fractions (Trugnan *et al.*, 1979). At about the same time, labeled arachidonic acid was found to be esterified in platelet PC, PI, PE, and PS, and stimulation by thrombin released arachidonate mostly from PC and PI (Bills *et al.*, 1976). Besides thrombin, collagen and A23187 stimulated PLA_2 activity and mobilized arachidonate for synthesis of prostaglandin endoperoxides, thromboxanes, and hydroxyeicosatetraenoic acids (Vanderhoek and Feinstein, 1979).

Evidence favoring a role of arachidonate metabolites in the platelet release reaction was afforded by findings that the prostaglandin endoperoxides and thromboxane A_2 are positive mediators, although perhaps not initiators, in platelet aggregation and secretion of ADP and serotonin from granules (Smith *et al.*, 1974; Hamberg *et al.*, 1975; Needleman *et al.*, 1976). These mediators appear to act by mobilizing calcium sequestered in the platelet dense tubular network (Gorman, 1979). Local anesthetics, mepacrine, papaverine, chlorpromazine, and propranolol, and the PLA_2 alkylating agent *p*-bromophenacyl bromide inhibit the hydrolysis of platelet phospholipids induced by thrombin in blocking the activation of PLA_2, which in turn inhibits the production of oxygenated products from arachidonic acid and inhibits secretion (Vallee *et al.*, 1979; Vanderhoek and Feinstein, 1979). However, multiple pharmacological effects of local anesthetics are expressed in the platelet, including the antagonism of Ca^{2+}-dependent membrane adhesion and fusion processes, interference with intracellular Ca^{2+} mobilization, and disruption of cytoskeletal organization; thus, local anesthetics have also been shown to block aggregation induced by exogenous thromboxane A_2 (Vanderhoek and Feinstein, 1979).

In addition to the cyclooxygenase and lipoxygenase products active in promoting platelet secretory phenomena secondary to PLA_2 activation, the direct products of phospholipid hydrolysis (lysophospholipids) have also been shown to be potent aggregatory agents (Benveniste et al., 1977), perhaps as a result of their effects on calcium mobilization in the platelet membrane (Gerrard et al., 1978b, 1979).

In addition to PLA_2, however, recent evidence has shown that PLC plays an important role in phospholipid turnover (see Section III), with subsequent arachidonic acid release for support of platelet secretion. Several studies have pointed out the importance of platelet PI as a source of much of the arachidonic acid released during stimulation (Bills et al., 1976; Bell and Majerus, 1980; Prescott and Majerus, 1981). The sequence of events between stimulation with thrombin and secretion involves initially the activation of PLC, which in platelets has a specificity for PI as substrate, and the appearance of 1,2-diacylglycerol as the product of the PI breakdown (Billah et al., 1979; Rittenhouse-Simmons, 1979). The diacylglycerol may then be metabolized in two different ways by the platelet, and both biochemical conversions will result in the liberation of arachidonic acid. First, upon platelet stimulation, a large increase in PA turnover occurs largely as a result of the phosphorylation of diacylglycerol by a kinase dependent upon ATP and Mg^{2+} (Billah et al., 1979; Lapetina and Cuatrecasas, 1979). The resultant PA may directly activate PLA_2 and cause the release of arachidonic acid from phospholipids. PA may release its own arachidonate through the action of PA-specific PLA_2 (Billah et al., 1981), and in addition, PA or the lyso-PA derivative may have an ionophoretic action in the platelet membrane. Alternatively, the arachidonic acid in PA may be exchanged by an acyltransferase reaction with fatty acids in other phospholipids that are subsequently hydrolyzed by PLA_2. Last, PA can mobilize Ca^{2+} for activation of PLA_2 and release of arachidonate from phospholipids other than PI (Rittenhouse-Simmons and Deykin, 1978; Lapetina and Cuatrecasas, 1979; Billah et al., 1980). The second pathway through which diacylglycerol can yield free arachidonic acid depends upon diglyceride lipase, which cleaves the fatty acid ester bond at sn-1 and produces a 2-arachidonyl monoglyceride, which releases free fatty acid (preferentially arachidonic acid) upon hydrolysis at sn-2 by monoglyceride lipase (Bell et al., 1979; Broekman *et al.*, 1980; Chau and Tai, 1981). The diglyceride kinase pathway, however, is more active than the diglyceride lipase pathway. Because PLC is activated prior to PLA_2 and arachidonic acid liberation (Lapetina and Cuatrecasas, 1979), it would appear that the production of PA is a very important link between secretagogue activity and PLA_2 activation. A membrane-active agent such as thrombin may induce a conformational change in the membrane such as to allow exposure of PI to the cytosolic enzyme PLC, for eventual production of PA and arachidonate release (Billah *et al.*, 1980).

However, the production of PA by the platelet, as well as the release reaction and aggregation, are not dependent upon the activity of either PLA_2, cyclooxygenase, or lipoxygenase (Lapetina *et al.*, 1978; Lapetina and Cuatrecasas, 1979). The generation of PA and/or diacylglycerol is sufficient to affect membrane properties relating to shape changes, fusogenesis, or aggregation. Subsequent to changes in PA levels and Ca^{2+} availability induced by thrombin, there is an activation of PLA_2 and biosynthesis of prostaglandin and hydroxyacid, all of which could augment Ca^{2+} availability, the release reaction, and aggregation.

Another element in the regulation of platelet secretion and aggregation is cAMP. Increases in the level of this nucleotide are antiaggregatory, and there are accompanying decreases in arachidonate release and prostaglandin synthesis (Rittenhouse-Simmons and Deykin, 1978). Because cAMP has no direct effect on PLA_2 from disrupted platelets (Rittenhouse-Simmons and Deykin, 1978; Kannagi and Koizumi, 1979), it was assumed to act indirectly to modulate PLA_2 activity through Ca^{2+} availability or by inducing changes in the conformation of phospholipids. Because A23187 with Ca^{2+} can overcome the nucleotide-induced inhibition of PLA_2 (Rittenhouse-Simmons and Deykin, 1978), it would seem that the restriction of cation availability plays an important part in the inhibition. Consistent with this idea is the finding that cAMP enhances the cellular sequestration of Ca^{2+} (Kaser-Glanzman *et al.*, 1977). Restriction of Ca^{2+} stores may also inhibit a Ca^{2+}-dependent cyclooxygenase (Gorman *et al.*, 1979) and decrease the steady-state levels of PA (Lapetina *et al.*, 1981b). In addition, cAMP could enhance the inhibitory phosphorylation of PLA_2. Perhaps more importantly, however, cAMP inhibits the conversion of PI to diacylglycerol and thus may act primarily to inhibit PLC activation and PA formation and secondarily to inhibit PLA_2 and prostaglandin formation (Billah *et al.*, 1979). In keeping with this hypothesis, PGI_2 supplied to the platelet from endothelial tissue would stimulate cAMP formation through adenylate cyclase activation and thus promote calcium sequestration and the other associated phenomena previously discussed, and inhibit secretion (Gorman, 1979). Although the action of cAMP on PI turnover appears to be inhibitory, it has been proposed that cAMP also enhances the activity of PA:CTP-cytidyl-transferase (Fig. 2), which converts phosphatidic acid to CDP-di-acylglycerol in the PI cycle. This ultimately decreases the steady-state level of phosphatidate and inhibits all of the resultant consequences of elevated phosphatidate levels (Lapetina et al., 1981b).

2. The Neutrophil

The release of lysosomal enzymes from granules in neutrophils constitutes a secretory response to various chemotactic agents. A review of the events in this stimulus–secretion coupled reaction has been presented (Smolen and Weissmann, 1980). Within the realm of phospholipid participation in neutrophil secretion, several cellular phenomena are of particular interest. Secretion can be induced by increasing cellular Ca^{2+} levels, either by use of ionophores, such as A23187 or valinomycin, or by high Ca^{2+} concentrations. Additionally, chemotactic agents elevate levels of cAMP and cGMP, the kinetic response of which parallels that of Ca^{2+} accumulation. Finally, arachidonic acid metabolism is increased by secretagogues, and arachidonate metabolites stimulate secretion.

Studies by Rubin and co-workers (1979, 1981a,b) have confirmed that arachidonyl-PI turnover in rabbit neutrophils is stimulated by A23187, presumably through activation of PLA_2. Chemotactic peptide stimulates not only lysosomal enzyme release but also arachidonate turnover in PI, suggesting that surface receptors activate a Ca^{2+}-dependent PLA_2 in addition to PLC in rabbit neutrophils as a mechanism for inducing perturbations in cell membrane morphology during accelerated secretory activity (Cockcroft et al., 1980b; Rubin et al., 1981a,b). Because there does not appear to be any PLC activation or diacylglycerol formation in the human neutrophil upon stimulation to release arachidonic acid, PLA_2 hydrolysis of PI and PC would seem to be mainly responsible for free fatty acid mobilization (Walsh et al., 1981). Moreover, in the leukocyte, chemoattractants stimulate the release of arachidonate from PC by PLA_2 activation, and local anesthetics, hydrocortisone, and β-bromophenacyl bromide inhibit the enzyme's activity and lysosomal enzyme release (Hirata et al., 1979; Elferink, 1979; Smolen and Weissmann, 1980).

In addition to PI and PC involvement in arachidonate mobilization, arachidonic acid demonstrates a rapid deacylation–reacylation mechanism for arachidonate turnover in neutrophils. Perhaps PA participates in a transesterification reaction in which arachidonic acid is transferred from PA to other phospholipids for eventual hydrolysis by PLA_2 (Lapetina et al., 1980). Alternatively, PA may also serve as a substrate for PLA_2. It has been argued, however, that PI turnover in rabbit neutrophils does not participate in cellular calcium mobilization in the neutrophil during secretion (Cockcroft et al., 1980b).

The importance of arachidonic acid metabolism in neutrophil function is supported by the finding that the addition of arachidonic acid to neutrophils results in several cellular changes characteristic of activation. Arachidonic acid mimics the effects of chemotactic factors such as C5a or synthetic oligopeptides in inducing the aggregation response and stimulating carrier-mediated hexose transport in neutrophils; in addition, inhibition of arachidonate metabolism by eicosatetraynoic acid or nonsteroidal antiinflammatory drugs inhibits the effects of arachidonate as well as the chemotactic factors in inducing chemotaxis (O'Flaherty et al., 1979; Bass et al., 1980). Thus, arachidonic acid metabolites would appear to play an important role in certain aspects of neutrophil physiology.

Analysis of the routes of metabolism of arachidonic acid released from neutrophil phospholipids by PLA_2 has shown the fatty acid to be metabolized to cyclooxygenase-derived prostaglandins and lipoxygenase-derived hydroxyeicosatetraenoic acids (HETE and leukotrienes) (Stenson and Parker, 1979a; Borgeat and Samuelsson, 1979; Siegel et al., 1981; Walsh et al., 1981). Both cyclooxygenase and lipoxygenase activities in the leukocyte are calcium dependent, stimulated by A23187, and responsive to chemotactic peptides that enhance the biosynthesis of $PGF_{2\alpha}$, PGE_2, thromboxane B_2, and 5-HETE by specific receptor stimulation (Bokoch and Reed, 1980).

In the neutrophil, the status of lipoxygenase products as important mediators or even second messengers of activation has been avidly promoted and supported. The inhibition of HETE and leukotriene B_4 biosynthesis by nordihydroguaiaretic acid inhibits Ca^{2+}-dependent and -independent lysosomal enzyme release, whereas exposure of cells to HETE, and leukotriene B_4 especially, induces the chemotactic response and a modest degree of degranulation (Showell et al., 1980; Bokoch and Reed, 1981). Human neutrophils treated with exogenous HETE compounds fail to release lysosomal enzymes, and HETE does not generate superoxide as does IgG receptor stimulation (Goetzl et al., 1980). Thus, there may be a selective activation by hydroxyacids in promoting chemotaxis rather than degranulation. In addition, intracellular levels of the arachidonate metabolites elicited by receptor stimulation may affect the release response differently from exogenous agents. In support of the latter hypothesis, when prostaglandin synthesis alone is inhibited by cyclooxygenase inhibitors, lysosomal enzyme release still occurs in response to stimuli, presumably as a result of the persistence of lipoxygenase activity (Smolen and Weissmann, 1980).

The fate and possible mechanism of action of the lipoxygenase-derived arachidonate metabolites appear to be intimately involved with Ca^{2+} availability in the neutrophil. It has been determined that 5-HETE can be esterified into phospholipids of neutrophils (Stenson and Parker, 1979b; Walsh et al., 1981). This esterification could result in alterations in membrane characteristics, ultimately affecting cation permeability. Arachidonic acid metabolites of lipoxygenase release Ca^{2+} from intracellular pools, whereas chemotactic peptides release in addition Ca^{2+} from a separate, perhaps ligand receptor-linked, pool (Sha'afi et al., 1981). In addition, the HETE and leukotriene compounds enhance Ca^{2+} uptake by neutrophils, and leukotriene B_4 displaces intracellular Ca^{2+}. However, leukotriene B_4, unlike HETE, achieves this effect at physiological concentrations (Naccache et al., 1981).

A model for phospholipid mediation of neutrophil secretion in response to ligand–receptor stimulation might include (1) the mobilization and/or rearrangement of membrane-bound Ca^{2+} upon receptor occupancy, with (2) resultant PLA_2 and PLC stimulation and arachidonate release from phospholipids, followed (3) by prostaglandin and HETE/leukotriene biosynthesis and, further, (4) increases in intracellular Ca^{2+} levels due to transport or displacement of bound Ca^{2+} from cellular pools, with (5) subsequent changes in microtubule assembly, cyclic nucleotide biosynthesis, and membrane fusion phenomena associated with exocytosis.

3. The Mast Cell

The involvement of phospholipids in histamine release has been examined in comprehensive reviews (Bach, 1974; Foreman, 1981). In the mast cell, stimulation of secretion and phospholipase activation produces lysophosphatides and fatty acids, while inhibiting adenylate cyclase and Ca^{2+}-dependent ATPase activities. Consequent changes in the Ca^{2+} equilibrium of the cell apparently reduces the rigidity of the microfilament system that facilitates basophil granule movement, and the lysophosphatides may promote fusion of granule and plasma membranes. More specifically, PS or LPS together with concanavalin A elicit histamine release at low concentrations, whereas other lysophospholipids such as LPC or LPE potentiate histamine release only at high, perhaps cytolytic, concentrations (Sydbom and Uvnas, 1976; Whelan, 1978; Martin and Lagunoff, 1979). These phospholipids may be important for regulation of ion transport mechanisms, Ca^{2+} binding in membranes, and adenylate cyclase activity (Wheeler and Whittman, 1970; Mongar and Svec, 1972).

Arachidonic acid released from mast cell phospholipids is converted to leukotrienes by a lipoxygenase pathway or to prostaglandins and thromboxanes by cyclooxygenase (Foreman, 1981). The leukotrienes or slow reacting substances (SRS) are recognized mediators of release in these cells, and a selective antagonist of SRS (FPL 55712) antagonizes release (Augstein et al., 1973). Eicosatetraynoic acid also inhibits histamine secretion as a result of inhibition of lipoxygenase rather than of inhibition of cyclooxygenase (Sullivan and Parker, 1979). Evidence that prostaglandins are not the preferred mediators of release derives from studies showing that inhibition of cyclooxygenase with the non-steroidal antiinflammatory drugs indomethacin, meclofenamic acid, or aspirin can enhance antigen-induced histamine release as a result of the increased availability of arachidonic acid to the lipoxygenase pathway. The enhanced HETE formation can antagonize inhibition of release caused by PGE_2 (Marone et al., 1979). In addition, exogenous arachidonic acid is channeled to prostaglandin biosynthesis and antagonizes the release of histamine in response to agents such as concanavalin A; prostaglandin synthetase inhibitors block this inhibition (Sullivan and Parker, 1979). Thus, prostaglandins appear to be negative modulators of release in basophilic mast cells, and, in fact, the addition of PGE_2 will inhibit histamine release in response to IgE (Lichtenstein et al., 1972). However, the enhancement of HETE production by the addition of arachidonic acid to mast cells is not a sufficient stimulus for secretion. This suggests that arachidonic metabolites are most likely secondary modulators of the receptor-mediated stimulus–secretion coupling mechanism in mast cells.

The stimulus–secretion coupling mechanism in mast cells has been postulated to be negatively modulated by elevations in cell cAMP levels as well as by prostaglandins (Foreman, 1981). In many cells, prostaglandins activate adenylate cyclase and increase cAMP levels (Robison et al., 1971), but because nonsteroidal antiinflammatory drugs that block prostaglandin production in mast cells do not alter the increases in cell cAMP levels as a result of β-adrenergic or H_2 receptor stimulation, it appears unlikely that prostaglandins modulate adenylate cyclase activity in this cell type (Marone et al., 1979). However, indomethacin will reverse the inhibition of histamine release caused by agents that activate adenylate cyclase (Marone et al., 1979), suggesting that prostaglandins participate in the inhibition of release during an important step distal to the formation of cAMP.

However, several reports indicate that cyclic nucleotides are not regulators of histamine release, and caution has been advised regarding the interpretation of pharmacological effects of cyclic nucleotides on secretion (Sydbom *et al.*, 1981). Obviously, reservations regarding the role of cyclic nucleotides in secretion should prompt investigators to examine closely the mechanism(s) whereby prostaglandins might adversely affect secretion.

Thus, it appears that homeostatic mechanisms in the mast cell are mediated by the steady-state levels of prostaglandins and hydroxyacids and that enhanced levels of prostaglandins would return the cell and its secretory mechanisms to a basal resting state. Cellular mechanisms responsible for the differential regulation of cyclooxygenase and lipoxygenase activity have yet to be determined.

4. The Adrenal Cortex

The adrenal cortex has been thoroughly investigated with regard to the relationships between phospholipids and secretion. Studies *in vivo* have shown that adrenocorticotropin (ACTH) increases the phospholipid content of adrenal glands (Ichii *et al.*, 1971, 1972). *In vitro*, in response to ACTH, adrenal cortical cells not only biosynthesize increased amounts of PI and PA, but there is also enhanced turnover of arachidonic acid in PI (Schrey and Rubin, 1979; Farese *et al.*, 1981). The turnover of arachidonate in PI is believed to be in part due to ACTH-stimulated PLA_2 activity (Laychock *et al.*, 1977b). Characteristically, adrenal cortical PLA_2 is calcium dependent and can be stimulated by A23187 (Schrey and Rubin, 1979). Inhibition of PLA_2 by *p*-bromophenacyl bromide also blocks steroidogenesis, suggesting that PLA_2 plays an important role in steroidogenesis and/or secretion. Thus, adrenocortical PLA_2 results in production of arachidonic acid and lysophospholipids for eventual participation in prostaglandin biosynthesis, enzyme activation, or membrane biophysical events.

A role for prostaglandins in steroidogenesis has been earnestly sought. Prostaglandins stimulate adrenal cortical steroidogenesis (Flack *et al.*, 1969) as well as the hydrolysis of cholesterol esters (Hodges *et al.*, 1978), and the biosynthesis of these compounds is increased in adrenal cortical cells exposed to ACTH (Laychock and Rubin, 1976a; Chanderbhan *et al.*, 1979). However, inhibition of prostaglandin biosynthesis with indomethacin and eicosatetraynoic acid is associated with only moderate decreases in steroidogenesis, suggesting that prostaglandins are not obligatory intermediates in the secretory response (Honn and Chavin, 1976; Laychock and Rubin, 1976b; Laychock et al., 1977a).

Prostaglandins may be positive modulators of ACTH-induced steroidogenesis because they increase levels of steroidogenic cyclic AMP (Hodges et al., 1978; Shima et al., 1980) and also mobilize cellular calcium (Rubin et al., 1980). In addition, cyclic AMP stimulates prostaglandin biosynthesis (Laychock et al., 1977a). This latter stimulation is not entirely dependent upon extracellular calcium, even though ACTH-induced prostaglandin biosynthesis is Ca^{2+} dependent. Thus, cAMP may mobilize intracellular pools of calcium to sustain arachidonic acid metabolism. Thus, in the adrenal cortex, both cyclic AMP and prostaglandins may modulate the ACTH response in an interdependent manner.

5. Islets of Langerhans

Evidence for the involvement of phospholipid turnover in endocrine secretion from pancreatic islets has been accumulating for the past decade. The glucose-stimulated turnover of $^{32}PO_4$ in islet phospholipids attributable to enhanced PLC activity or de novo synthesis has been well documented (Freinkel and Cohanim, 1972; Freinkel et al., 1975; Berne, 1975; Clements and Rhoten, 1976). An effect of glucose on PLA_2 in islets has been less vigorously tested. Indirect evidence provided from studies using tetracaine, showing that the local anesthetic inhibits insulin secretion even though phospholipid synthesis occurs, suggests that the inhibition of phospholipid catabolism may be integral to inhibition of secretion (Freinkel et al., 1975).

Whether or not the fatty acids released as a consequence of phospholipid catabolism are a key element in the inhibition of secretion attributable to local anesthetics is open to question. But, it is known that fatty acids play a number of roles in secretion of hormones from pancreatic islets. Fatty acids, such as palmitic acid, and unsaturated fatty acids not only turn over in phospholipids more rapidly upon glucose stimulation, but they are also utilized as fuel in oxidative metabolism (Malaisse and Malaisse-Lagae, 1968; Berne, 1975; Montague and Parkin, 1980). Phospholipid fatty acid turnover and release may be part of the glucose signal for insulin release. Fatty acids, whether through pathways of oxidative metabolism or cyclooxygenase/lipoxygenase metabolism may affect islet calcium mobilization. The enhancement of Ca^{2+}–calmodulin complexation could alter microtubule assembly (see chapters 6 and 7), adenylate cyclase activity, protein phosphorylation, and other enzyme activities that affect secretion. Although fatty acid release from specific phospholipids in islet membranes has not been reported, evidence that glucose stimulates PLA$_2$ has been presented (Laychock, 1981). Moreover, islets possess cyclooxygenase and lipoxygenase activities for synthesizing several prostaglandins and hydroxyacids from arachidonic acid substrate (Kelly and Laychock, 1981).

What role do arachidonate metabolites have in insulin secretion? The effects of prostaglandins on insulin secretion have been described as inhibitory (Robertson, 1979), without effect (Landgraf and Landgraf-Leurs, 1979), or stimulatory (Pek *et al.*, 1978, 1980), depending upon the specific prostaglandin, route of administration, or the islet/pancreas preparation used in the study. On the other hand, arachidonic acid stimulates glucagon release from guinea pig islets. This stimulus is presumably mediated by prostaglandin biosynthesis because indomethacin blocks the response (Luyckx and Lefebvre, 1980). Prostaglandins E$_2$ and F$_{2\alpha}$ also stimulate the release of glucagon (Pek *et al.*, 1978), and PGE$_2$ enhances the release of somatostatin-like immunoreactive products from pancreatic islet delta cells (Schusdziarra *et al.*, 1981). Prostaglandins may participate in secretion through activation of adenylate cyclase in islets (Sharp, 1979). However, a role for endogenous prostaglandins or lipoxygenase products in islet secretory mechanisms has yet to be demonstrated.

Glucose also stimulates the turnover of unsaturated fatty acids in islet phospholipids (Montague and Parkin, 1980) and decreases the viscosity of islet cell membranes (DeLeers *et al.*, 1981). Through these actions, glucose may affect the fusogenic properties and fluidity of membranes and/or secretory granules and influence secretion. Changes in membrane unsaturation properties also alter cation transport (Hirata and Axelrod, 1980), which may mediate the secretory response to secretagogues in islets.

6. The Thyroid Gland

Stimulation of the thyroid gland by thyrotropin is accompanied by changes in the activities of PLC (Scott *et al.*, 1968) and PLA$_2$ (Haye *et al.*, 1973, 1976). Altered PLC activity results in enhanced levels of 1,2-diacylglycerol, which may act as precursors for phospholipid biosynthesis. Thyroidal diacylglycerols are especially enriched in arachidonic acid and can result in the biosynthesis of arachidonate-enriched PI (Haye and Jacquemin, 1974). The importance of PI turnover specifically, in contrast to other phospholipids, is underscored by the enhanced uptake into PI of not only radiolabeled fatty acids such as arachidonate, oleate, and palmitate, but also labeled glucose and glycerol (Scott *et al.*, 1968; Haye and Jacquemin, 1977). Thus, there appears to be recycling of thyroidal diacylglycerol moieties as well as *de novo* biosynthesis of PI.

Studies have also demonstrated the release of arachidonic acid from PI upon stimulation of the thyroid gland with thyrotropin, presumably through the activation of a calcium-dependent PLA_2 (Haye *et al.*, 1973, 1976). However, another study ascribed the fatty acid releasing effects of thyrotropin to an artifactual phenomenon of serum albumin, while supporting the evidence of enhanced diacylglycerol and phosphoinositol formation (Irvine *et al.*, 1980). The latter report contends that fatty acids are released through diacylglycerol lipase activity. A hormone-stimulatable lipase also appears to be important in the metabolism of triacylglycerols, which constitute 96% of the neutral lipids of the thyroid and contain 4% of the arachidonic acid (Haye *et al.*, 1976; Haye and Jacquemin, 1977). Low concentrations of thyrotropin apparently stimulate the release of arachidonate from the triacylglycerol pool by cAMP-dependent lipolysis (Haye *et al.*, 1973, 1976). Thus, there appear to be at least two pools of arachidonic acid in the thyroid: a diacylglycerol pool that releases fatty acids upon metabolism by PLA_2 and/or diglyceride lipase and a triacylglycerol pool that releases fatty acids upon lipolysis.

The arachidonate released from thyroid phospholipid or neutral lipid reservoirs participates in the biosynthesis of prostaglandins E_2, $F_{2\alpha}$, thromboxane B_2, and prostacyclin (Boeynaems *et al.*, 1979; Takasu *et al.*, 1981). Thyrotropin elevates the levels of prostaglandins in thyroid cells (Yu *et al.*, 1972), and carbamylcholine and epinephrine enhance the release of prostaglandins from dog thyroid slices through muscarinic and α-adrenergic receptor activation, respectively (Boeynaems *et al.*, 1979). Exogenous calcium is required for the stimulation of prostaglandin formation by the aforementioned agents, and A23187 mimics the stimulation caused by receptor agonists. Of course, calcium may regulate fatty acid mobilization by phospholipases as discussed in previous sections.

Several possible roles for prostaglandins in the thyroid gland have been proposed. They may affect guanylate cyclase activity, which increases during stimulation with carbamylcholine, although no effect of arachidonic acid vis-à-vis prostaglandin E_2 or $F_{2\alpha}$ was seen on dog thyroid cGMP levels (Boeynaems *et al.*, 1980). In the latter study, however, arachidonate inhibited the accumulation of cAMP in response to TSH, presumably by a mechanism independent of prostaglandin production and also inhibited the effects of low concentrations of thyrotropin on secretion. An action of the fatty acid on unidentified membrane properties may be responsible for the inhibitory effects. It has been proposed that some prostaglandins in the thyroid gland stimulate adenylate cyclase and secretion, whereas others inhibit the enzyme (Burke, 1974; Boeynaems *et al.*, 1979; Takasu *et al.*, 1981). In addition, approximately 35% of the cAMP generated in response to thyrotropin may be due to the nonobligatory participation of prostaglandins in adenylate cyclase activation (Haye *et al.*, 1976). Prostaglandin antagonists have been shown to inhibit PGE_1- or thyrotropin- stimulated cAMP formation as well as thyroid hormone release (Burke, 1974). Perhaps excessive levels of exogenous arachidonate nonspecifically inhibit adenylate cyclase activity, whereas endogenous prostaglandins serve as specific modulators in the precarious balance of cellular equilibrium. And, perhaps one of the novel roles for arachidonic acid metabolites in the thyroid gland is proposed by Boeynaems and co-workers (1980) as being the involvement of thyroid lipoxygenase products in protein iodination in this gland.

V.   CONCLUSIONS

This chapter has attempted to deal with possible roles of phospholipid metabolism in the stimulus–secretion coupling pathway. We have emphasized the roles of PLC and PLA; other possibly important reactions that we have not covered in detail would include phospholipid methylation covered in some detail in recent reviews (Hirata and Axelrod, 1980; and Chapter 7 in this volume). It is clear that specific systems may differ in the relative significance of the various reactions discussed here. A few fairly general patterns emerge, however.

In many systems, the initial effects of receptor activation may involve activation of a PI- (or perhaps PIP_2-) directed PLC. In some manner, perhaps through subsequent synthesis of PA, this reaction provokes Ca^{2+} mobilization (influx, release, or both), which leads to an increase in the concentration of ionized Ca^{2+} in the cytoplasm. The increase in "available" Ca^{2+} appears to activate PLA_2 and/or diglyceride lipase, the result of which is the production of lysophospholipids and free fatty acids. These products may participate in the secretory process directly (for example, the lysolipids may act as fusigens) or be metabolized to other biologically active substances. Notable in this latter regard is the fate of released arachidonic acid, which can be metabolized by cyclooxygenase to prostaglandins and thromboxanes or by lipoxygenase to leukotrienes and hydroxy fatty acids. These arachidonate metabolites may play a number of important roles in the stim-

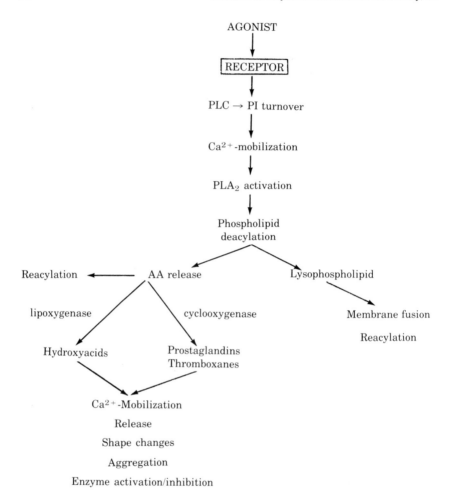

Fig. 3. Schematic relationship of receptor stimulation, PI turnover, fatty acid turnover, and stimulus–secretion coupling. Following receptor stimulation by an agonist, PLC is activated, promoting PI turnover, PA formation, and Ca^{2+} mobilization. The available Ca^{2+} activates PLA_2, with consequent phospholipid hydrolysis, fatty acid (arachidonic acid, AA) release, and lysophospholipid formation. AA is either reacylated into phospholipids or metabolized to products of lipoxygenase or cyclooxygenase, which may participate in secretion by alteration of the cellular processes listed. Lysophospholipids may also be reacylated back to phospholipids or promote secretion by promoting membrane fusion.

ulus–secretion pathway, the nature of importance of which apparently varies from tissue to tissue.

A summary of these primary conclusions is depicted in Fig. 3. Clearly regulation of phospholipid metabolism plays a central role in the stimulus–secretion coupling process. As research continues in this area, we hope that more precise molecular mechanisms will be formulated for each of these various steps and that a clearer understanding will evolve as to the precise role of these reactions in the secretory process.

ACKNOWLEDGMENTS

Work from the authors' laboratories described in this chapter was supported by grants from the NIH: R23 AM25705 (SGL); De-05764 and EY-03533 (JWP).

REFERENCES

Ahkong, Q. F., Tampion, W., and Lucy, J. A. (1975). Promotion of cell fusion by divalent cation ionophore. *Nature (London)* **256**, 208–209.

Ahktar, R. A., and Abdel-Latif, A. A. (1978). Calcium ion requirement for acetylcholine-stimulated breakdown of triphosphoinositide in rabbit iris smooth muscle. *J. Pharmacol. Exp. Ther.* **204**, 655–668.

Ally, A. I., Barrette, W. E., Cunnane, S., Horrobin, D. F., Karmali, R. A., Karmazyn, M., Manku, M. S., Morgan, R. O., and Nicolaou, K. C. (1978). Prostaglandin I_2 (prostacyclin) inhibits intracellular calcium release. *J. Physiol. (London)* **276**, 40P–41P.

Augstein, A., Farmer, J. F., Lee, T. B., Sheard, P., and Tattersall, M. L. (1973). Selective inhibitor of slow reacting substance of anaphylaxis. *Nature (London), New Biol.* **245**, 215–217.

Aunis, D., Pescheloche, M., and Zwiller, J. (1978a). Guanylate Cyclase from bovine adrenal medulla: Subcellular distribution and studies on the effect of lysolecithin on enzyme activity. *Neuroscience* **3**, 83–93.

Aunis, D., Pescheloche, M., Zwiller, J., and Mandel, P. (1978b). Effect of lysolecithin on adenylate cyclase and guanylate cyclase activities in bovine adrenal medullary plasma membranes. *J. Neurochem.* **31**, 355–357.

Bach, M. K. (1974). A molecular theory to explain the mechanisms of allergic histamine release. *J. Theor. Biol.* **45**, 131–151.

Bass, D. A., O'Flaherty, J. T., Szejda, P., DeChatelet, L. R., and McCall, C. E. (1980). Role of arachidonic acid in stimulation of hexose transport by human polymorphonuclear leukocytes. *Proc. Natl. Acad. Sci. U.S.A.* **77**, 5125–5129.

Becker, E. L. (1977). Stimulated neutrophil locomotion. *Arch. Pathol. Lab. Med.* **101**, 509–513.

Bell, R. M., and Coleman, R. A. (1980). Enzymes of glycerolipid synthesis of eukaryotes. *Annu. Rev. Biochem.* **49**, 459–487.

Bell, R. L., and Majerus, P. W. (1980). Thrombin-induced hydrolysis of phosphatidylinositol in human platelets. *J. Biol. Chem.* **255**, 1790–1792.

Bell, R. L., Kennerly, D. A., Stanford, N. and Majerus, P. W. (1979). Diglyceride lipase: A pathway for arachidonate release from human platelets. *Proc. Natl. Acad. Sci.* **76,** 3238–3241.

Bennett, J. P., Cockcroft, S., and Gomperts, B. D. (1980). Use of cytochalasin B to distinguish between early and late events in neutrophil activation. *Biochim. Biophys. Acta* **601,** 584–591.

Benveniste, S., LeCouedic, J. P., Polonsky, J., and Tence, M. (1977). Structural analysis of purified platelet-activating factor by lipases. *Nature (London)* **269,** 170–71.

Berne, C. (1975). The metabolism of lipids in mouse pancreatic islets. *Biochem. J.* **152,** 667–673.

Berridge, M. J. (1977). Cyclic AMP, calcium, and fluid secretion. *In* "Transport of Ions and Water in Animals" (B. L. Gupta, R. B. Moreton, J. L. Oschman, and B. J. Wall, eds.), pp. 225–238. Academic Press, New York.

Berridge, M. J. (1980). Receptors and calcium signalling. *Trends Pharmacol. Sci.* **1,** 419–424.

Berridge, M. J., and Fain, J. N. (1979). Inhibition of phosphatidylinositol synthesis and the inactivation of calcium entry after prolonged exposure of the blowfly salivary gland to 5-hydroxytryptamine. *Biochem. J.* **17,** 59–69.

Berridge, M. J., and Lipke, H. (1979). Changes in calcium transport across *Calliphora* salivary gland induced by 5-hydroxytryptamine and cyclic AMP. *J. Exp. Biol.* **78,** 137–148.

Berridge, M. J., and Oschman, J. L. (1972). "Transporting Epithelia." Academic Press, New York.

Billah, M. M., and Michell, R. H. (1979). Phosphatidylinositol metabolism in rat hepatocytes stimulated by glycogenolytic hormones. Effects of angiotensin, vasopressin, adrenaline, ionophore A23187 and calcium-ion deprivation. *Biochem. J.* **182,** 661–668.

Billah, M. M., Lapetina, E. G., and Cuatrecasas, P. (1979). Phosphatidylinositol-specific phospholipase-C of platelets: Association with 1,2-diacylglycerol-kinase and inhibition by cyclic AMP. *Biochem. Biophys. Res. Comm.* **90,** 92–98.

Billah, M. M., Lapetina, E. G., and Cuatrecasas, P. (1980). Phospholipase A_2 and phospholipase C activities of platelets. Differential substrate specificity, Ca^{2+} requirement, pH dependence, and cellular localization. *J. Biol. Chem.* **255,** 10227–10231.

Billah, M. M., Lapetina, E. G., and Cuatrecasas, P. (1981). Phospholipase A_2 activity specific for phosphatidic acid. *J. Biol. Chem.* **256,** 5399–5403.

Bills, T. K., Smith, J. B., and Silver, M. J. (1976). Metabolism of [^{14}C] arachidonic acid by human platelets. *Biochim. Biophys. Acta* **424,** 303–314.

Blackwell, C. J., Carnuccio, R., DiRosa, M., Flower, R. J., Parente, L., and Persico, P. (1980). Macrocortin: A polypeptide causing the anti-phospholipase effects of glucocorticoids. *Nature (London)* **287,** 147–149.

Boeynaems, J. M., Waelbroeck, M., and Dumont, J. E. (1979). Cholinergic and α-adrenergic stimulation of prostaglandin release by dog thyroid *in vitro*. *Endocrinology (Baltimore)* **105,** 988–995.

Boeynaems, J. M., Van Sande, J., Decoster, C., and Dumont, J. E. (1980). *In vitro* effects of arachidonic acid and of inhibitors of its metabolism on the dog thyroid gland. *Prostaglandins* **19,** 537–550.

Bokoch, G., and Reed, P. W. (1980). Stimulation of arachidonic acid metabolism in the polymorphonuclear leukocyte by an N-formylated peptide. *J. Biol. Chem.* **255,** 10223–10226.

Bokoch, G. M., and Reed, P. W. (1981). Effect of various lipoxygenase metabolites of arachidonic acid on degranulation of polymorphonuclear leukocytes. *J. Biol. Chem.* **256,** 5317–5320.

Borgeat, P., and Samuelsson, B. (1979). Arachidonic acid metabolism in polymorphonuclear leukocytes: Effects of ionophore A23187. *Proc. Natl. Acad. Sci. U.S.A.* **76,** 2148–2152.

Broekman, M. J., Ward, J. W. and Marcus, A. J. (1980). Phospholipid metabolism in stimulated human platelets. Changes in phosphatidylinositol, phosphatidic acid, and lysophospholipids. *J. Clin. Invest.* **66,** 275–283.

Brophy, P. J., Burbach, P., Nelemans, S. A., Westerman, J., Wirtz, K. W. A., and Van Deenen, L. L. M. (1978). The distribution of phosphatidylinositol in microsomal membranes from rat liver after biosynthesis *de novo*. Evidence for the existence of different pools of phosphatidylinositol by the use of phosphatidylinositol-exchange protein. *Biochem. J.* **174,** 413–420.

Buckley, J. T., and Hawthorne, J. N. (1972). Erythrocyte membrane polyphosphoinositide metabolism and the regulation of calcium binding. *J. Biol. Chem.* **247,** 7218–7223.

Burke, G. (1974). Effects of prostaglandin antagonists on the induction of cyclic 3',5'-adenosine monophosphate formation and thyroid hormone secretion *in vitro*. *Endocrinology (Baltimore)* **94,** 91–96.

Butcher, F. R. (1975). The role of calcium and cyclic nucleotides in α-amylase release from slices of rat parotid: Studies with the divalent cation inophore A23187. *Metabolism* **24,** 409–418.

Butcher, F. R., and Putney, J. W., Jr. (1980). Regulation of parotid gland function by cyclic nucleotides and calcium. *Adv. Cyclic Nucleotide Res.* **13,** 215–249.

Calderon, P., Furnelle, J.,and Christophe, J. (1980). Phosphatidylinositol turnover and calcium movement in the rat pancreas. *Am. J. Physiol.* **238,** G247–G254.

Cantieri, J. S., Graff, G., and Goldberg, N. D. (1980). Increased activity and stimulability of psoriatic epidermal soluble guanylate cyclase by arachidonic acid and 12-hydroxy-5,8,10,14-eicosatetraenoic acid. *Adv. Cyclic Nucleotide Res.* **12,** 139–145.

Chanderbhan, R., Hodges, V. A., Treadwell, C. R., and Vahouny, G. V. (1979). Prostaglandin synthesis in rat adrenocortical cells. *J. Lipid Res.* **20,** 116–123.

Chandler, D. E., and Williams, J. A. (1977). Intracellular uptake and α-amylase and lactate dehydrogenase releasing actions of the divalent cation ionophore A23187 in dissociated pancreatic acinar cells. *J. Membr. Biol.* **32,** 201–230.

Chau, L.-Y. and Tai, H.-H. (1981). Release of arachidonate from diglyceride in human platelets requires the sequential action of a diglyceride lipase and a monoglyceride lipase. *Biochem. Biophys. Res. Comm.* **100,** 1688– 1695.

Chauvelot, L., Heisler, S., Huot, J., and Gagnon, D. (1979). Prostaglandins and enzyme secretion from dispersed rat pancreatic acinar cells. *Life Sci.* **25,** 913–920.

Chrisman, T. D., Garbers, D. L., Parks, M. A., and Hardman, J. G. (1975). Characterization of particulate and soluble guanylate cyclases from rat lung. *J. Biol. Chem.* **250,** 374–381.

Clements, R. S., Jr., and Rhoten, W. B. (1976). Phosphoinositide metabolism and insulin secretion from isolated rat pancreatic islets. *J. Clin. Invest.* **57,** 684–691.

Cockcroft, S., Bennett, J. P., and Gomperts, B. D. (1980a). Stimulus secretion coupling in rabbit neutrophils is not mediated by phosphatidylinositol breakdown. *Nature (London)* **288,** 275–277.

Cockcroft, S., Bennett, J. P., and Gomperts, B. D. (1980b). F-Met-Leu-Phe-Induced phosphatidylinositol turnover in rabbit neutrophils is dependent on extracellular calcium. *FEBS Lett.* **110,** 115–118.

Coleman, R. (1973). Membrane-bound enzymes and membrane ultrastructure. *Biochim. Biophys. Acta* **300**, 1–30.

Cullis, P. R., DeKruijff, B., Hope, M. J., Nayar, R., and Schmid, S. L. (1980). Phospholipids and membrane transport. *Can.J. Biochem.* **58**, 1091–1100.

Dawson, R. M. C., and Hauser, H. (1970). Binding of calcium to phospholipids. *In* "Calcium and Cellular Function" (A. W. Cuthbert, ed.), pp. 17–41. Macmillan, London.

DeLeers, M., Ruysschaert, J. M., and Malaisse, W. J. (1981). Glucose induces membrane changes detected by fluorescence polarization in endocrine pancreatic cells. *Biochem. Biophys. Res. Commun.* **98**, 255–260.

Demel, R. A., Kalsbeek, R., Wirtz, K. W. A., and VanDeenen, L. L. M. (1977). The protein-mediated net transfer of phosphatidylinositol in model systems. *Biochim. Biophys. Acta* **466**, 10–22.

Derksen, A., and Cohen, P. (1975). Patterns of fatty acid release from endogenous substrates by human platelet homogenates and membranes. *J. Biol. Chem.* **250**, 9342–9347.

DeRubertis, F. R. and Craven, P. A. (1976). Calcium-independent modulation of cyclic GMP and activation of guanylate cyclase by nitrosamines. *Science* **193**, 897–899.

DiCorleto, P. E., Waroch, J. B., and Zilversmit, D. B. (1979). Purification and characterization of two phospholipid exchange proteins from bovine heart. *J. Biol. Chem.* **254**, 7795–7802.

Eagling, E. M., Lovell, H. G., and Pickles, V. R. (1972). Interactions of prostaglandin El and calcium in the guinea-pig myometrium. *Br. J. Pharmacol.* **44**, 510–516.

Elferink, J. G. R. (1979). Chlorpromazine inhibits phagocytosis and exocytosis in rabbit polymorphonuclear leukocytes. *Biochem. Pharmacol.* **28**, 965–968.

Exton, J. H. (1981). Mechanisms involved in α-adrenergic effects of catecholamines. *In* "Adrenoceptors and Catecholamine Action, Part A (G. Kunos, ed.), pp. 117–129. Wiley (Interscience), New York.

Fain, J. N., and Berridge, M. J. (1979a). Relationship between hormonal activation of phosphatidylinositol, hydrolysis, fluid secretions, and calcium flux in the blowfly salivary gland. *Biochem. J.* **178**, 45–58.

Fain, J. N., and Berridge, M. J. (1979b). Relationship between phosphatidylinositol synthesis and recovery of 5-hydroxytryptamine-responsive Ca^{2+} flux in blowfly salivary glands. *Biochem. J.* **180**, 655–661.

Farese, R. V., Larson, R. E., and Sabir, M. A. (1980). Effects of Ca^{2+} ionophore A23187 and Ca^{2+} deficiency on pancreatic phospholipids and amylase release *in vitro. Biochim. Biophys. Acta* **633**, 479–484.

Farese, R. V., Sabir, M. A., and Larson, R. E. (1981). A23187 inhibits adrenal protein synthesis and the effects of adrenocorticotropin (ACTH) on steroidogenesis and phospholipid metabolism in rat adrenal cells *in vitro:* Further evidence implicating phospholipids in the steroidogenic action of ACTH. *Endocrinology (Baltimore)* **108**, 1243–1245.

Feinstein, M. B., Rodan, G. A., and Cutler, L. S. (1981). Cyclic AMP and calcium in platelet function. *In* "Platelets in Biology and Pathology" (J. L. Gordon, ed.), Vol. 2, pp. 437–472. Elsevier/North-Holland, Amsterdam.

Fiehn, W., and Hasselbach, W. (1970). The effect of phospholipase A on the calcium transport and the role of unsaturated fatty acids in ATPase activity of sarcoplasmic vesicles. *Eur. J. Biochem.* **13**, 510–518.

Flack, J. D., Jessup, R., and Ramwell, P. W. (1969). Prostaglandin stimulation of rat corticosteroidogenesis. *Science* **163**, 691–692.

Flower, R. J. (1981). Glucocorticoids, phospholipase A_2 and inflammation. *Trends Pharmacol. Sci.* **2**, 186–189.

Flower, R. J., and Blackwell, G. J. (1976). The importance of phospholipase-A_2 in prostaglandin biosynthesis. *Biochem. Pharmacol.* **25**, 285–291.

Foreman, J. C. (1981). The pharmacological control of immediate hypersensitivity. *Annu. Rev. Pharmacol. Toxicol.* **21**, 63–81.

Forstermann, U., and Hertting, G. (1979). The importance of Ca^{2+} mediated phospholipase A_2 activation for stimulus-evoked PGE_2-release from rabbit splenic capsular strips. *N-S Arch. Pharmacol.* **307**, 243–249.

Franson, R. C., Eisen, D., Jesse, R., and Lanni, C. (1980). Inhibition of highly purified mammalian phospholipase A_2 by non-steroidal anti-inflammatory agents. *Biochem. J.* **186**, 633–636.

Freinkel, N., and Cohanim, N. (1972). Islet phospholipogenesis and glucose-stimulated insulin secretion. *J. Clin. Invest.* **51**, 33a.

Freinkel, N., El Younsi, C., and Dawson, R. M. (1975). Inter-relations between the phospholipids of rat pancreatic islets during glucose stimulation and their response to medium inositol and tetracaine. *Eur. J. Biochem.* **59**, 245–252.

Fujimoto, J., and Okabayashi, T. (1975). Proposed mechanisms of stimulation and inhibition of guanylate cyclase with reference to the actions of chlorpromazine, phospholipases, and triton X-100. *Biochem. Biophys. Res. Commun.* **67**, 1332–1336.

Garbers, D. L., Dyer, E. L., and Hardman, J. G. (1975). Effects of cations on guanylate cyclase of sea urchin sperm. *J. Biol. Chem.* **250**, 382–387.

Gemsa, D., Seitz, M., Kramer, W., Grimm, W., Till, G., and Resch, K. (1979). Ionophore A23187 raises cyclic AMP levels in macrophages by stimulating prostaglandin E formation. *Exp. Cell Res.* **118**, 55–62.

Gerrard, J. M., Poller, J. D., Krick, T. P., and White, J. G. (1977). Cyclic AMP and platelet prostaglandin synthesis. *Prostaglandins* **14**, 39–50.

Gerrard, J. M., Butler, A. M., Peterson, D. A., and White, J. G. (1978a). Phosphatidic acid releases calcium from a platelet membrane fraction *in vitro*. *Prostaglandins Med.* **1**, 387–396.

Gerrard, J. M., Butler, A. M., Graff, G., Stoddard, S. F., and White, J. G. (1978b). Prostaglandin endoperoxides promote calcium release from platelet membrane reaction *in vitro*. *Prostaglandins Med.* **1**, 373–385.

Gerrard, J. M., Kindom, S. E., Peterson, D. A., and White, J. G. (1979). Lysophosphatidic Acids II: Interaction of the effects of ADP and lysophosphatidic acids in dog, rabbit, and human platelets. *Am. J. Pathol.* **97**, 531–548.

Gerrard, J. M., Peterson, D. A., and White, J. G. (1981). Calcium mobilization. *In* "Platelets in Biology and Pathology" (J. L. Gordon, ed.), Vol. 2, pp. 407–436. Elsevier/North-Holland, Amsterdam.

Gidwitz, S., Pessin, J. E., Weber, M. J., Glaser, M., and Storm, D. R. (1980). Effect of membrane phospholipid composition changes on adenylate cyclase activity in normal and Rous-Sarcoma-transformed chicken embryo fibroblasts. *Biochim. Biophys. Acta* **628**, 263–276.

Glass, D. B., Gerrard, J. M., Townsend, D., Carr, D. W., White, J. G., and Goldberg, N. D. (1977). The involvement of prostaglandin endoperoxide formation in the elevation of cyclic GMP levels during platelet aggregation. *J. Cyclic Nucleotide Res.* **3**, 37–44.

Goetzl, E. J., Brash, A. R., Tauber, A. I., Oates, J. A., and Hubbard, W. C. (1980). Modulation of human neutrophil function by monohydroxy-eicosatetraenoic acids. *Immunology* **39**, 491–501.

Goldberg, N. D., Graff, G., Haddox, M. K., Stephenson, J. H., Glass, D. B., and Moser, M. E. (1978). Redox modulation of splenic cell soluble guanylate cyclase activity: Activation by hydrophilic and hydrophobic acids, fatty acid hydroperoxides, and prostaglandin endoperoxides. *Adv. Cyclic Nucleotide Res.* **9**, 101–130.

Gomperts, B. D. (1981). Discussion following: Putney, J. W., Jr., Poggioli, J., and Weiss, S. J. Receptor regulation of calcium release and calcium permeability in parotid gland cells. *Phil Trans. R. Soc. London, Ser. B*, **296**, 37–45.

Gorman, R. R. (1979). Modulation of human platelet function by prostacyclin and thromboxane A_2. *Fed. Proc., Fed. Am. Soc. Exp. Biol.* **38**, 83–88.

Gorman, R. R., Wierenga, W., and Miller, O. V. (1979). Independence of the cyclic AMP-lowering activity of thromboxane A_2 from the platelet release reaction. *Biochim. Biophys. Acta* **572**, 95–104.

Green, D. E., Fry, M., and Blondin, G. A. (1980). Phospholipids as the molecular instruments of ion and solute transport in biological membranes. *Proc. Natl. Acad. Sci. U.S.A.* **77**, 257–261.

Gruetter, D. Y., and Ignarro, L. J. (1979). Arachidonic acid activation of guinea pig lung guanylate cyclase by two independent mechanisms. *Prostaglandins* **18**, 541–556.

Hamberg, M., Svensson, J., and Samuelsson, B. (1975). Thromboxanes: A new group of biologically active compounds derived from prostaglandin endoperoxides. *Proc. Natl. Acad. Sci. U.S.A.* **72**, 2994–2998.

Hansen-Bay, C. M. (1978). The control of enzyme secretion from fly salivary glands. *J. Physiol. (London)* **274**, 421–435.

Harris, R. A., Schmidt, J., Hitzemann, B. A., and Hitzemann, R. J. (1981). Phosphatidate as a molecular link between depolarization and neurotransmitter release in brain. *Science* **212**, 1290–1291.

Haye, B., and Jacquemin, C. (1974). Stimulation par la thyréostimuline de la production de l'inositol 1-2 phosphate cyclique. *Biochimie* **56**, 1283–1285.

Haye, B., and Jacquemin, C. (1977). Incorporation of [^{14}C] arachidonate in pig thyroid lipids and prostaglandins. *Biochim. Biophys. Acta* **487**, 231–242.

Haye, B., Champion, S., and Jacquemin, C. (1973). Control by TSH of a phospholipase A_2 activity, a limiting factor in the biosynthesis of prostaglandins in the thyroid. *FEBS Lett.* **30**, 253–260.

Haye, B., Champion, S., and Jacquemin, C. (1976). Stimulation by TSH of prostaglandin synthesis in pig thyroid. *Adv. Prostaglandin Thromboxane Res.* **1**, 29–34.

Hendrickson, H. S., and Van Dam-Mieras, M. C. E. (1976). Local anesthetic inhibition of pancreatic phospholipase A_2 action on lecithin monolayers. *J. Lipid Res.* **17**, 399–405.

Hertelendy, F., Todd, H., and Narconis, R. F., Jr. (1978). Studies on growth hormone secretion. IX. Prostaglandins do not act like ionophores. *Prostaglandins* **15**, 575–590.

Hirata, F., and Axelrod, J. (1980). Phospholipid methylation and biological signal transmission. *Science* **209**, 1082–1090.

Hirata, F., Corcoran, B. A., Venkatsubramanian, K., Schiffmann, E., and Axelrod, J. (1979). Chemoattractants stimulate degradation of methylated phospholipids and release of arachidonic acid in rabbit leukocytes. *Proc. Natl. Acad. Sci. U.S.A.* **76**, 2640–2643.

Hodges, V. A., Treadwell, C. T., and Vahouny, G. V. (1978). Prostaglandin E_2-induced hydrolysis of cholesterol esters in rat adrenocortical cells. *J. Steroid Biochem.* **9**, 1111–1118.

Hoffmann, R., Ristow, H. J., Pachowsky, H., and Frank, W. (1974). Phospholipid metabolism in embryonic rat fibroblasts following stimulation by a combination of the serum proteins S_1 and S_2. *Eur. J. Biochem.* **49**, 317–324.

Hokin, L. E. (1966). Effects of calcium omission on acetylcholine-stimulated amylase secretion and phospholipid synthesis in pigeon pancreas slices. *Biochim. Biophys. Acta* **115**, 219–221.

Hokin, L. E., and Heubner, D. (1967). Radioautographic localization of the increased synthesis of phosphatidylinositol in response to pancreozymin or acetylcholine in guinea pig pancreas slices. *J. Cell Biol.* **33**, 521–530.

Hokin, L. E., and Hokin, M. R. (1955). Effects of acetylcholine on the turnover of phosphoryl units in individual phospholipids of pancreas slices and brain cortex slices. *Biochim. Biophys. Acta* **18**, 102–110.

Hokin, L. E., and Hokin, M. R. (1956). The actions of pancreozymin in pancreas slices and the role of phospholipids in enzyme secretion. *J. Physiol. (London)* **132**, 442–453.

Hokin, L. E., and Sherwin, A. L. (1957). Protein secretion and phosphate turnover in the phospholipids in salivary glands *in vitro*. *J. Physiol. (London)* **135**, 18–29.

Hokin, M. R., and Hokin, L. E. (1953). Enzyme secretion and the incorporation of P^{32} into phospholipides of pancreas slices. *J. Biol. Chem.* **203**, 967–977.

Hokin, M. R., and Hokin, L. E. (1954). Effects of acetylcholine on phospholipids in the pancreas. *J. Biol. Chem.* **209**, 549–558.

Hokin, M. R., and Hokin, L. E. (1964). Interconversions of phosphatidylinositol and phosphatidic acid involved in the response of acetylcholine in the salt gland. *In* "Metabolism and Physiological Significance of Lipids" (R. M. C. Dawson and D. N. Rhodes, eds.), pp. 423–434. Wiley, New York.

Hokin, M. R., and Hokin, L. E. (1967). The formation and continuous turnover of a fraction of phosphatidic acid on stimulation of NaCl secretion by acetylcholine in the salt gland. *J. Gen. Physiol.* **50**, 793–811.

Holzmann, S., Kukovetz, W. R., and Schmidt, K. (1980). Mode of action of coronary arterial relaxation by prostacyclin. *J. Cyclic Nucleotide Res.* **6**, 451–460.

Honn, K. V., and Chavin, W. (1976). Role of prostaglandins in aldosterone production by the human adrenal. *Biochem. Biophys. Res. Commun.* **72**, 1319–1326.

Ichii, S., Ikeda, A., Izawa, M., and Ohta, A. (1971). Effect of ACTH on turnover of phospholipids in rat adrenal glands. *Endocrinol. Jpn.* **18**, 169–173.

Ichii, S., Ikeda, A., Ohta, A., and Izawa, M. (1972). Effect of cortocotrophin on protein and phospholipid metabolism in subcellular fractions of adrenal glands. *J. Biochem. (Tokyo)* **71**, 615–623.

Irvine, R. F., Letcher, A. J., and Dawson, R. M. C. (1980). Thyrotropin-stimulated phosphatidylinositol-specific phospholipase A_2 in pig thyroid, a re-examination. *FEBS Lett.* **119**, 287–289.

Isakson, P. C., Raz, A., Denny, S. E., and Wyche, A. (1977). Hormonal stimulation of arachidonate release from isolated perfused organs. Relationship to prostaglandin biosynthesis. *Prostaglandins* **14**, 853–871.

Jesse, R. L., and Franson, R. C. (1979). Modulation of purified phospholipase A_2 activity from human platelets by calcium and indomethacin. *Biochim. Biophys. Acta* **575**, 467–470.

Jones, L. M., and Michell, R. H. (1974). Breakdown of phosphatidylinositol provoked by muscarinic cholinergic stimulation of rat parotid gland fragments. *Biochem. J.* **142**, 583–590.

Jones, L. M., and Michell, R. H. (1975). The relationship of calcium to receptor-controlled stimulation of phosphatidylinositol turnover. Effects of acetylcholine, adrenaline, calcium ions, cinchocaine, and a bivalent cation ionophore on rat parotid-gland fragments. *Biochem. J.* **148**, 479–485.

Jones, L. M., and Michell, R. H. (1976). Cholinergically stimulated phosphatidylinositol breakdown in parotid gland fragments is independent of the ionic environment. *Biochem J.* **158**, 505–507.

Jones, L. M., and Michell, R. H. (1978). Enhanced phosphatidylinositol breakdown as a calcium-independent response of rat parotid fragments to substance P. *Biochem. Soc. Trans.* **6**, 1035–1037.

Kalisker, A., and Dyer, D. C. (1972). *In vitro* release of prostaglandins from the renal medulla. *Eur. J. Pharmacol.* **19**, 305–309.

Kannagi, R., and Koizumi, K. (1979). Phospholipid-deacylating enzymes of rabbit platelets. *Arch. Biochem. Biophys.* **196**, 534–542.

Kaplan, L., Weiss, J., and Elsback, P. (1978). Low concentrations of indomethacin inhibit phospholipase A_2 of rabbit polymorphonuclear leukocytes. *Proc. Natl. Acad. Sci. U.S.A.* **75**, 2955–2958.

Käser-Glanzmann, R., Jakabova, M., George, J. N., and Lüscher, E. F. (1977). Stimulation of calcium uptake in platelet membrane vesicles by adenosine 3′,5′-cyclic monophosphate and protein kinase. *Biochim. Biophys. Acta* **446**, 429–440.

Katz, A. M., Messineo, F., Miceli, J., and Nash-Adler, P. A. (1981). Low concentrations of fatty acids can inhibit calcium efflux from sarcoplasmic reticulum. *Life Sci.* **28**, 1103–1107.

Kelly, K. L., and Laychock, S. G. (1981). Prostaglandin synthesis and metabolism in isolated pancreatic islets of the rat. *Prostaglandins* **21**, 759–769.

Keryer, G., Herman, G., and Rossignol, B. (1979). Sodium requirement in secretory processes regulated through muscarinic receptors in rat parotid glands: Its effect on amylase secretion and phosphatidylinositol labelling. *FEBS Lett.* **102**, 4–8.

Kirk, C. J., Verrinder, T. R., and Hems, D. A. (1977). Rapid stimulation by vasopressin and adrenaline of inorganic phosphate incorporation into phosphatidylinositol in isolated hepatocytes. *FEBS Lett.* **83**, 267–271.

Kirk, C. J., Creba, J. A., Downes, C. P., and Michell, R. H. (1981). Hormone-stimulated metabolism of inositol lipids and its relationship to hepatic receptor function. *Biochem. Soc. Trans.* **9**, 377–379.

Knapp, H. R., Oelz, O., Roberts, L. J., Sweetman, B. J., Oates, J. A., and Reed, P. W. (1977). Ionophores stimulate prostaglandin and thromboxane biosynthesis. *Proc. Natl. Acad. Sci. U.S.A.* **74**, 4251–4255.

Knowles, A. F., Eytan, E., and Racker, E. (1976). Phospholipid-protein interactions in the Ca^{2+} adenosine triphosphatase of sarcoplasmic reticulum. *J. Biol. Chem.* **251**, 5161–5165.

Kunze, H., Bohn, E., and Vogt, W. (1974). Effects of local anesthetics on prostaglandin biosynthesis *in vitro*. *Biochim. Biophys. Acta* **360**, 260–269.

Kunze, H., Nahas, N., Traynor, J. R., and Wurl, M. (1976). Effects of local anesthetics on phospholipases. *Biochim. Biophys Acta* **441**, 93–102.

Lad, P. M., Preston, M. S., Welton, A. F., Nielsen, T. B., and Rodbell,M. (1979). Effects of phospholipase A_2 and filipin on the activation of adenylate cyclase. *Biochim. Biophys. Acta* **551**, 368–381.

Landgraf, R., and Landgraf-Leurs, M. M. (1979). The prostaglandin system and insulin release. Studies with the isolated perfused rat pancreas. *Prostaglandins* **17**, 599–613.

Lapetina, E. G. (1982). Regulation of arachidonic acid production: Role of phospholipases C and A_2. *Trends Pharmacol. Sci.*, **3**, 115–118.

Lapetina, E. G., and Billah, M. M. (1982). The inositol lipids metabolism and the release of arachidonic acid as a fundamental mechanism for platelet activation. *INSERM Symp.,* in press.

Lapetina, E. G., and Cuatrecasas, P. (1979). Stimulation of phosphatidic acid production in platelets precedes the formation of arachidonate and parallels the release of serotonin. *Biochim. Biophys. Acta* **573**, 394–402.

Lapetina, E. G., Schmitges, C. J., Chandrabose, K., and Cuatrecasas, P. (1977). Cyclic adenosine 3',5'-monophosphate and prostacyclin inhibit membrane phospholipase activity in platelets. *Biochem. Biophys. Res. Commun.* **76**, 828–835.

Lapetina, E. G., Chandrabose, K. A., and Cuatrecasas, P. (1978). Ionophore A23187 and thrombin-induced platelet aggregation: Independence from cyclooxygenase products. *Proc. Natl. Acad. Sci. U.S.A.* **75**, 818–822.

Lapetina, E. G., Billah, M. M., and Cuatrecasas, P. (1980). Rapid acylation and deacylation of arachidonic acid into phosphatidic acid of horse neutrophils. *J. Biol. Chem.* **255**, 10966–10970.

Lapetina, E. G., Billah, M. M., and Cuatrecasas, P. (1981a). The initial action of thrombin on platelets. Conversion of phosphatidylinositol to phosphatidic acid preceding the production of arachidonic acid. *J. Biol. Chem.* **256**, 5037–5040.

Lapetina, E. G., Billah, M. M., and Cuatrecasas, P. (1981b). The phosphatidylinositol cycle and the regulation of arachidonic acid production. *Nature (London)* **292**, 367–369.

Laychock, S. G. (1981). Pancreatic islet phospholipase is stimulated by glucose. *Fed. Proc., Fed. Am. Soc. Exp. Biol.* **40**, 458.

Laychock, S. G., and Rubin, R. P. (1976a). Radioimmunoassay measurement of ACTH-facilitated PGE_2 and $PGF_{2\alpha}$ release from isolated cat adrenocortical cells. *Prostaglandins* **11**, 753–767.

Laychock, S. G., and Rubin, R. P. (1976b). Indomethacin induced alterations in corticosteroid and prostaglandin release by isolated adrenocortical cells of the cat. *Br. J. Pharmacol.* **57**, 273–278.

Laychock, S. G., and Walker, L. (1979). Evidence for 6-keto-$PGF_{1\alpha}$ in adrenal cortex of the rat and effects of 6-keto-$PGF_{1\alpha}$ and PGI_2 on adrenal cAMP levels and steroidogenesis. *Prostaglandins* **18**, 793–811.

Laychock, S. G., Warner, W., and Rubin, R. P. (1977a). Further studies on the mechanisms controlling prostaglandin biosynthesis in the cat adrenal cortex: The role of calcium and cyclic AMP. *Endocrinology (Baltimore)* **100**, 74–81.

Laychock, S. G., Franson, R. C., Weglicki, W. B., and Rubin, R. P. (1977b). Identification and partial characterization of phospholipases in isolated adrenocortical cells. *Biochem. J.* **164**, 753–756.

Lefkowitz, R. J. (1975). Catecholamine stimulated myocardial adenylate cyclase: Effects of phospholipase digestion and the role of membrane lipids. *J. Mol. Cell. Cardiol.* **7**, 27–37.

Lichtenstein, L. M., Gillespie, E., Bourne, H. R., and Henney, C. S. (1972). The effects of a series of prostaglandins on *in vitro* models of the allergic response and cellular immunity. *Prostaglandins* **2**, 519–528.

Lucy, J. A. (1974). Lipids and membranes. *FEBS Lett.* **40**, 5105–5111.

Luyckx, A. S., and Lefebvre, P. J. (1980). Further studies on the role of prostaglandins in glucagon secretion. *In* "Current Views on Hypoglycemia and Glucagon" (D. Andreani, P. J. Lefebvre, and V. Marks, eds.), pp. 47–56. Academic Press, New York.

McGiff, J. C. (1981). Prostaglandins, prostacyclin, and thromboxanes. *Annu. Rev. Pharmacol. Toxicol.* **21**, 479–509.

Malaisse, W. J., and Malaisse-Lagae, F. (1968). Stimulation of insulin secretion by noncarbohydrate metabolites. *J. Lab. Clin. Med.* **72**, 438–448.

Malmstrom, K., and Carafoli, E. (1975). Effects of prostaglandins on the interaction of Ca^{++} with mitochondria. *Arch. Biochem. Biophys.* **171**, 418–423.

Marier, S. H., Putney, J. W., Jr., and Van De Walle, C. M. (1978). Control of calcium channels by membrane receptors in the rat parotid gland. *J. Physiol. (London)* **279**, 141–151.

Marone, G., Sobotka, A. K., and Lichtenstein, L. M. (1979). Effects of arachidonic acid and its metabolites on antigen-induced histamine release from human basophils *in vitro*. *J. Immunol.* **123**, 1669–1677.

Marshall, P. J., Dixon, J. F., and Hokin, L. E. (1980). Evidence for a role in stimulus-secretion coupling of prostaglandins derived from release of arachidonyl residues, as a result of phosphatidylinositol breakdown. *Proc. Natl. Acad. Sci. U.S.A.* **77**, 3292–3296.

Marshall, P. J., Boatman, D. E., and Hokin, L. E. (1981). Direct demonstration of the formation of prostaglandin E_2 due to phosphatidylinositol breakdown associated with stimulation of enzyme secretion in the pancreas. *J. Biol. Chem.* **256**, 844–847.

Marshall, P. J., Dixon, J. F., and Hokin, L. E. (1982). Prostaglandin derived from phosphatidylinositol breakdown in the exocrine pancreas facilitates secretion by an action on the ducts. *J. Pharmacol. Exp. Ther.* **221**, 645–649.

Martin, T. W., and Lagunoff, D. (1979). Interactions of lysophospholipids and mast cells. *Nature (London)* **279**, 250–252.

Martonosi, A., Donley, J., and Halpin, R. A. (1968). Sarcoplasmic reticulum. III. The role of phospholipids in the adenosine triphosphatase activity and Ca^{++} transport. *J. Biol. Chem.* **243**, 61–70.

Meissner, G., and Fleischer, S. (1972). The role of phospholipid in Ca^{2+}-stimulated ATPase activity of sarcoplasmic reticulum. *Biochim. Biophys. Acta* **255**, 19–33.

Michell, R. H. (1975). Inositol phospholipids and cell surface receptor function. *Biochim. Biophys. Acta* **415**, 81–147.

Michell, R. H. (1979). Inositol phospholipids in membrane function. *Trends Biochem. Sci.* **4**, 128–131.

Michell, R. H., and Jones, L. M. (1974). Enhanced phosphotidylinositol labelling in rat parotid fragments exposed to α-adrenergic stimulation. *Biochem. J.* **138**, 47–52.

Michell, R. H., and Kirk, C. J. (1981). Why is phosphotidylinositol degraded in response to stimulation of certain receptors? *Trends Pharmacol. Sci.* **2**, 86–89.

Michell, R. H., Jafferji, S., and Jones, L. M. (1976). Receptor occupancy dose-response curve suggests that phosphatidylinositol breakdown may be intrinsic to the mechanism of the muscarinic cholinergic receptor. *FEBS Lett.* **69**, 1–5.

Minkes, M., Stanford, N., Cli, M. M., Gerald, R. J., Amiran, R., Needham, P., and Majerus, P. W. (1977). Cyclic adenosine 3',5'-monophosphate inhibits the availability of arachidonate to prostaglandin synthase in human platelet suspensions. *J. Clin. Invest.* **59**, 449–454.

Mongar, J. L., and Svec, P. (1972). The effects of phospholipids on anaphylatic histamine release. *Br. J. Pharmacol.* **46**, 741–752.

Montague, W., and Parkin, E. N. (1980). Changes in membrane lipids of the B-cell during insulin secretion. *Horm. Metab. Res., Suppl. Ser.* **10**, 153–157.

Naccache, P. H., Sha'afi, R. I., Borgeat, P., and Goetzl, E. J. (1981). Mono-and dihydroxyeicosatetraenoic acids alter calcium homeostasis in rabbit neutrophils. *J. Clin. Invest.* **67**, 1584–1587.

Needleman, P., Minkes, M., and Raz, A. (1976). Thromboxanes: Selective biosynthesis and distinct biological properties. *Science* **193**, 163–165.

Newkirk, J. D., and Waite, M. (1971). Identification of a phospholipase A_1 in plasma membranes of rat liver. *Biochim. Biophys. Acta* **225**, 224–233.

O'Flaherty, J. T., Showell, H. J., Ward, P. A., and Becker, E. L. (1979). A possible role of arachidonic acid in human neutrophil aggregation and degranulation. *Am. J. Pathol.* **96**, 799–809.

Oron, Y., Lowe, M., and Selinger, Z. (1973). Involvement of the α-adrenergic receptor in the phospholipid effect in rat parotid. *FEBS Lett.* **34**, 198–200.

Oron, Y., Lowe, M., and Selinger, Z. (1975). Incorporation of inorganic [^{32}P] phosphate into rat parotid phosphatidylinositol. Induction through activation of alpha-adrenergic and cholinergic receptors ptors and relation to K^+ release. *Mol. Pharmacol.* **11**, 79–86.

Pek, S., Tai, T. Y., and Elster, A. (1978). Stimulatory effects of prostaglandins E_1, E_2, and $F_{2\alpha}$ on glucagon and insulin release *in vitro*. *Diabetes* **27**, 801–809.

Pek, S., Lands, W. E. M., Akpan, J., and Hurley, M. (1980). Effects of prostaglandins H_2, D_2, I_2 and thromboxane on *in vitro* secretion of glucagon and insulin. *Adv. Prostaglandin Thromboxane Res.* **8**, 1295–1298.

Pickett, W. C., Jesse, R. L., and Cohen, P. (1977). Initiation of phospholipase A_2 activity in human platelets by the calcium ion ionophore A23187. *Biochim. Biophys. Acta* **486**, 209–213.

Piper, P., and Vane, J. (1971). The release of prostaglandins from lung and other tissues. *Ann. N. Y. Acad. Sci.* **180**, 363–385.

Poggioli, J., Leslie, B. A., McKinney, J. S., Weiss, S. J., and Putney, J. W., Jr. (1982). Actions of ionomycin in rat parotid gland. *J. Pharmacol. Exp. Ther.* **221**, 247–253.

Poste, G., and Allison, A. C. (1973). Membrane fusion. *Biochim. Biophys. Acta* **300**, 421–465.

Prescott, S. M., and Majerus, P. W. (1981). The fatty acid composition of phosphatidylinositol from thrombin-stimulated human platelets. *J. Biol. Chem.* **256**, 579–582.

Putney, J. W., Jr. (1977). Muscarinic, α-adrenergic, and peptide receptors regulate the same calcium influx sites in the parotid gland. *J. Physiol (London)* **268**, 139–149.

Putney, J. W., Jr. (1978). Stimulus permeability coupling: Role of calcium in the receptor regulation of membrane permeability. *Pharmacol. Rev.* **30**, 209–245.

Putney, J. W., Jr. (1981). Recent hypotheses regarding the phosphatidylinositol effect. *Life Sci.* **29**, 1183–1194.

Putney, J. W., Jr., and Van DeWalle, C. M. (1980). The relationship between muscarinic receptor binding and ion movements in the rat parotid gland. *J. Physiol. (London)* **299**, 521–531.

Putney, J. W., Jr., Weiss, S. J., Van DeWalle, C. M., and Haddas, R. A. (1980). Is phosphatidic acid a calcium ionophore under neurohumoral control? *Nature (London)* **284**, 345–347.

Putney, J. W., Jr., DeWitt, L. M., Hoyle, P. C., and McKinney, J. S. (1981a). Calcium, prostaglandins and the phosphatidylinositol effect in exocrine gland cells. *Cell Calcium* **2**, 561–571.

Putney, J. W., Jr., Poggioli, J., and Weiss, S. J. (1981b). Receptor regulation of calcium release and calcium permeability in parotid gland cells. *Phil. Tran. R. Soc. London, Ser. B* **296**, 37–45.

Ramwell, P. W., and Shaw, J. E. (1970). Biological significance of the prostaglandins. *Rec. Prog. Horm. Res.* **26**, 139–187.

Redman, C. M., and Hokin, L. E. (1959). Phospholipid turnover in microsomal membranes of the pancreas during enzyme secretion. *J. Biophys. Biochem. Cytol.* **6,** 207–214.

Rillema, J. A., and Linebaugh, B. E. (1978). Effects of phospholipase A and triton X-100 on guanylate cyclase activity in mammary gland homogenates from mice. *Horm. Metab. Res.* **10,** 331–336.

Rittenhouse-Simmons, S. (1979). Production of diglyceride from phosphatidylinositol in activated human platelets. *J. Clin. Invest.* **63,** 580–587.

Rittenhouse-Simmons, S., and Deykin, D. (1978). The activation by Ca^{2+} of platelet phospholipase A_2: Effects of dibutyrylcyclic adenosine monophosphate and 8-(N,N-diethylamino)-octyl-3,4,5-trimethoxy benzoate. *Biochim. Biophys. Acta* **543,** 409–422.

Robertson, R. P. (1979). Prostaglandins as modulators of pancreatic islet function. *Diabetes* **28,** 943–948.

Robison, G. A., Butcher, R. W., and Sutherland, E. W. (1971). "Cyclic AMP." Academic Press, New York.

Rossignol, B., Herman, G., Chambaut, A. M., and Keryer, G. (1974). The calcium ionophore A23187 as a probe for studying the role of Ca^{2+} ions in the mediation of carbachol effects on rat salivary glands: Protein secretion and metabolism of phospholipids and glycogen. *FEBS Lett.* **43,** 241–246.

Rubalcava, B., and Rodbell, M. (1973). The role of acidic phospholipids in glucagon action on rat liver adenylate cyclase. *J. Biol. Chem.* **248,** 3831–3837.

Rubin, R. P. (1974). "Calcium and the Secretory Process." Plenum, New York.

Rubin, R. P., and Laychock, S. G. (1978). Prostaglandins and calcium-membrane interactions in secretory glands. *Ann. N. Y. Acad. Sci.* **307,** 377–390.

Rubin, R. P., Sink, L. E., Schrey, M. P., Day, A. R., Liao, C. S., and Freer, R. J. (1979). Secretagogues for lysosomal enzyme release as stimulants of arachidonyl phosphatidylinositol turnover in rabbit neutrophils. *Biochem. Biophys. Res. Commun.* **90,** 1364–1370.

Rubin, R. P., Shen, J. C., and Laychock, S. G. (1980). Evidence for the mobilization of cellular calcium by prostacyclin in cat adrenocortical cells: The effect of TMB-8. *Cell Calcium* **1,** 391–400.

Rubin, R. P., Sink, L. E., and Freer, R. J. (1981a). On the relationship between formylmethionyl-leucyl-phenylalanine stimulation of arachidonyl phosphatidylinositol turnover and lysosomal enzyme secretion by rabbit neutrophils. *Mol. Pharmacol.* **19,** 31–37.

Rubin, R. P., Sink, L. E., and Freer, R. J. (1981b). Activation of (arachidonyl) phosphatidylinositol turnover in rabbit neutrophils by the calcium ionophore A23187. *Biochem. J.* **194,** 497–505.

Salmon, D. M., and Honeyman, T. W. (1979). Increased phosphatidate accumulation during single contractions of isolated smooth muscle cells. *Biochem. Soc. Trans.* **7,** 986–988.

Salmon, D. M., and Honeyman, T. W. (1980). Proposed mechanism of cholinergic action in smooth muscle. *Nature (London)* **284,** 344–345.

Salzman, E. W., MacIntyre, D. E., Steer, M. L., and Gordon, J. L. (1978). Effect on platelet activity of inhibition of adenylate cyclase. *Thrombos. Res.* **13,** 1089–1101.

Sandermann, H., Jr. (1978). Regulation of membrane enzymes by lipids. *Biochim. Biophys. Acta* **515,** 209–237.

Scarpa, A., and Azzi, A. (1968). Cation binding to submitochondrial particles. *Biochim. Biophys. Acta* **150,** 473–481.

Scherphof, G., and Westenberg, H. (1975). Stimulation and inhibition of pancreatic phospholipase A_2 by local anesthetics as a result of their interaction with the substrate. *Biochim. Biophys. Acta* **398,** 442–451.

Scherphof, G. L., Scarpa, A., and Van Toorenenbergen, A. (1972). The effects of local anesthetics on the hydrolysis of free and membrane bound phospholipids catalyzed by various phospholipases. *Biochim. Biophys. Acta* **270,** 226–240.

Schramm, M., and Selinger, Z. (1975). The functions of cyclic AMP and calcium as alternative second messengers in parotid gland and pancreas. *J. Cyclic Nucleotide Res.* **1,** 181–192.

Schrey, M. P., and Rubin, R. P. (1979). Characterization of a calcium mediated activation of arachidonic acid turnover in adrenal phospholipids by corticotropin. *J. Biol. Chem.* **254,** 11234–11241.

Schusdziarra, V., Rouiller, D., Harris, V., Wasada, T., and Unger, R. H. (1981). Effect of prostaglandin E_2 upon release of pancreatic somatostatin-like immunoreactivity. *Life Sci.* **28,** 2099–2102.

Scott, T. W., Mills, S. C., and Freinkel, N. (1968). The mechanism of thyrotropin action in relation to lipid metabolism in thyroid tissue. *Biochem. J.* **109,** 325–332.

Seiler, D., and Hasselbach, W. (1971). Essential fatty acid deficiency and the activity of the sarcoplasmic calcium pump. *Eur. J. Biochem.* **21,** 385–387.

Serhan, C., Anderson, P., Goodman, E., Dunham, P., and Weissmann, G. (1981). Phosphatidate and oxidized fatty acids are calcium ionophores: Studies employing arsenazo III in liposomes. *J. Biol. Chem.* **256,** 2736–2741.

Sha'afi, R. I., Naccache, P. H., Alobaidi, T., Molski, T. F. P., and Volpi, M. (1981). Effect of arachidonic acid and the chemotactic factor F-Met-Leu-Phe on cation transport in rabbit neutrophils. *J. Cell. Physiol.* **106,** 215–223.

Sharp, G. W. G. (1979). The adenylate cyclase-cyclic AMP system in islets of Langerhans and its role in the control of insulin release. *Diabetologia* **16,** 287–296.

Shier, W. T., Baldwin, J. H., Nilsen-Hamilton, M., Hamilton, R. T., and Thanassi, N. M. (1976). Regulation of guanylate and adenylate cyclase activities by lysolecithin. *Proc. Natl. Acad. Sci. U.S.A.* **73,** 1586–1590.

Shima, S., Kawashima, Y., Hirai, M., and Asakura, M. (1980). Studies on cyclic nucleotides in the adrenal gland. X. Effects of adrenocorticotropin and prostaglandin on adenylate cyclase activity in the adrenal cortex. *Endocrinology (Baltimore)* **106,** 948–951.

Showell, H. J., Naccache, P. H., Sha'afi, R. I., and Becker, E. L. (1980). Inhibition of rabbit neutrophil lysosomal enzyme secretion, non-stimulated and chemotactic factor stimulated locomotion by nordihydroguaiaretic acid. *Life Sci.* **27,** 421–426.

Siegel, M. I., McConnell, R. T., Bonser, R. W., and Cuatrecasas, P. (1981). The production of 5-HETE and leukotriene B in rat neutrophils from carrageenan pleural exudates. *Prostaglandins* **21,** 123–132.

Silver, M. J., and Smith, J. B. (1975). Prostaglandins as intracellular messengers. *Life Sci.* **16,** 1635–1648.

Smith, J. B., Ingerman, C., Kolis, J. J., and Silver, M. J. (1974). Formation of an intermediate in prostaglandin biosynthesis and its association with platelet release reaction. *J. Clin. Invest.* **53,** 1468–1472.

Smolen, J. E., and Weissmann, G. (1980). Effects of indomethacin, 5,8,11,14-eicosatetraynoid acid, and p-bromophenacyl bromide on lysosomal enzyme release and superoxide anion generation by human polymorphonuclear leukocytes. *Biochem. Pharmacol.* **29,** 533–538.

Stenson, W. F., and Parker, C. W. (1979a). Metabolism of arachidonic acid in ionophore-stimulated neutrophils. *J. Clin. Invest.* **64**, 1457–1465.

Stenson, W. F., and Parker, C. W. (1979b). 12-L-hydroxy-5,8,10,14-eicosatetraenoic acid, a chemotactic fatty acid, is incorporated into neutrophil phospholipids and triglycerides. *Prostaglandins* **18**, 285–292.

Struck, C.-J., and Glossmann, H. (1978). Soluble bovine adrenal cortex guanylate cyclase: Effect of sodium nitroprusside, nitrosamines, and hydrophobic ligands on activity, substrate specificity and cation requirement. *N-S Arch. Pharmacol.* **304**, 51–61.

Stukne-Sekalec, L., and Stanacev, N. F. (1980). Mitochondrial importation of lipids and liponucleotides from microsomes independent of and facilitated by cytosol proteins. *Can. J. Biochem.* **58**, 1082–1090.

Sullivan, T. J., and Parker, C. W. (1979). Possible role of arachidonic acid and its metabolites in mediator release from rat mast cells. *J. Immunol.* **122**, 431–436.

Sydbom, A., and Uvnäs, B. (1976). Potentiation of anaphylactic histamine release from isolated rat pleural mast cells by rat serum phospholipids. *Acta Physiol. Scand.* **97**, 222–232.

Sydbom, A., Fredholm, B., and Uvnäs, B. (1981). Evidence against a role of cyclic nucleotides in the regulation of anaphylactic histamine release in isolated rat mast cells. *Acta Physiol. Scand.* **112**, 47–56.

Takasu, N., Yamada, T., and Shimizu, Y. (1981). An important role of prostacyclin in porcine thyroid cells in culture. *FEBS Lett.* **129**, 83–88.

Trugnan, G., Bereziat, G., Manier, M.-C., and Polonovski, J. (1979). Phospholipase activities in subcellular fractions of human platelets. *Biochim. Biophys. Acta* **573**, 61–72.

Tyson, C. A., Zande, H. V., and Green, D. E. (1976). Phospholipids as ionophores. *J. Biol. Chem.* **251**, 1326–1332.

Vallee, E., Gougat, J., Navarro, J., and Delahayes, J. F. (1979). Anti-inflammatory and platelet anti-aggregant activity of phospholipase A_2 inhibitors. *J. Pharm. Pharmacol.* **31**, 588–592.

Vanderhoek, J. Y., and Feinstein, M. B. (1979). Local anesthetics, chlorpromazine, and propranolol inhibit stimulus-activation of phospholipase A_2 in human platelets. *Mol. Pharmacol.* **16**, 171–180.

Verheij, H. M., Volwerk, J. J., Jansen, E. H. J. M., Puyk, W. C., Dijkstra, B. W., Drenth, J., and deHaas, G. H. (1980). Methylation of histidine-48 in pancreatic phospholipase A_2. Role of histidine and calcium ion in the catalytic mechanism. *Biochemistry* **9**, 743–750.

Vesely, D. L. (1981). Bee venom enhances guanylate cyclase activity. *Science* **213**, 359–360.

Volpi, M., Naccache, P. H., and Sha'afi, R. I. (1980). Arachidonate metabolite(s) increase the permeability of the plasma membrane of the neutrophils to calcium. *Biochem. Biophys. Res. Commun.* **92**, 1231–1237.

Wallach, D., and Pastan, I. (1976). Stimulation of guanylate cyclase of fibroblasts by free fatty acids. *J. Biol. Chem.* **251**, 5802–5809.

Walsh, C. E., Waite, B. M., Thomas, M. J., and DeChatelet, L. R. (1981). Release and metabolism of arachidonic acid in human neutrophils. *J. Biol. Chem.* **256**, 7228–7234.

Webb, J. G., Saelens, D. A., and Halushka, P. V. (1978). Biosynthesis of prostaglandin E by rat superior cervical ganglia. *J. Neurochem.* **31**, 13–19.

Weiss, S. J., and Putney, J. W., Jr. (1981). The relationship of phosphatidylinositol turnover to receptors and calcium channels in rat parotid acinar cells. *Biochem. J.* **194,** 463–468.

Weissmann, G., Anderson, P., Serhan, C., Samuelsson, E., and Goodman, E. (1980). A general method, employing arsenazo III in liposomes, for study of calcium ionophores: Results with A23187 and prostaglandins. *Proc. Natl. Acad. Sci. U.S.A.* **77,** 1506–1510.

Wheeler, K. P., and Whittman, R. (1970). The involvement of phosphatidylserine in adenosine triphosphatase activity of the sodium pump. *J. Physiol.* **207,** 303–328.

Whelan, C. J. (1978). Histamine release from rat peritoneal mast cells by phospholipase A. The activation of phospholipase A by phospholipids. *Biochem. Pharmacol.* **27,** 2115–2118.

Williams, J. A. (1978). The effect of the ionophore A23187 on amylase release, cellular integrity and ultrastructure of mouse pancreatic acini. *Cell Tissue Res.* **186,** 287–295.

Wirtz, K. W. A., and Zilversmit, D. B. (1969). Participation of soluble liver proteins in the exchange of membrane phospholipids. *Biochim. Biophys. Acta* **193,** 105–116.

Wolff, D. J. and Brostrom, C. O. (1976). Calcium-dependent cyclic nucleotide phosphodiesterase from brain: identification of phospholipids as calcium-independent activators. *Archiv. Biochem. Biophys.* **173,** 720–731.

Wong, P. Y. K., and Cheung, W. Y. (1979). Calmodulin stimulates human platelet phospholipase A_2. *Biochem. Biophys. Res. Commun.* **90,** 473–480.

Yu, S. C., Chang, L., and Burke, G. (1972). Thyrotropin increases prostaglandin levels in isolated thyroid cells. *J. Clin. Invest.* **51,** 1038.

4

Electrophysiological Correlates of Secretion in Endocrine Cells

JEAN-DIDIER VINCENT AND BERNARD DUFY

I. ENDOCRINE CELLS VERSUS NEURONS

Neuroendocrinologists are generally familiar with semantic problems because their discipline floats over the uncertain boundaries separating the endocrine and nervous systems (Fig. 1). On the one hand, the term endocrine (*endon,* within; *kreinen,* to separate), which designates secretion into the bloodstream, was first extended to the nervous system through the concept of neurosecretion. Although the neurosecretory cell is clearly neuronal, it also synthetizes and secretes peptides that are released into the blood system in a manner similar to that of endocrine cells in general. On the other hand, the term "hormone" signifies a substance that is secreted at one place and is transported to another, where it acts. This term is now also commonly applied to the nervous system (Barker and Smith, 1977). A major

107

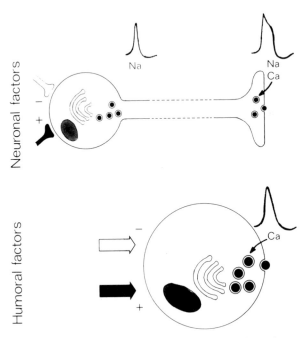

Fig. 1. Comparison of some features of endocrine cells and neurons.

difference between neurons and endocrine cells is the regenerative voltage-dependent conductance changes (action potentials) observed in the former and the passive membrane characteristics of the latter. In nerve terminals, including neurosecretory endings, action potentials provoke the release of secretory products by the opening of voltage-dependent Ca^{2+} channels (Douglas, 1974). However, in endocrine cells, the increase of intracellular Ca^{2+} concentration which accompanies hormone release, has for a long time not been associated with any change in membrane electrical properties (Lundberg, 1958). This basic difference in the release mechanism of excitable nerve cells and nonexcitable gland cells is no longer tenable.

Data that challenge this classical division between neurons and endocrine cells have accumulated. An increasing number of exceptions have been found, including cells of the pancreas (Matthews and Sakamoto, 1975a), adrenal chromaffin cells (Biales *et al.*, 1976; Brandt *et al.*, 1976), pituitary cells (Taraskevitch and Douglas, 1977; Douglas and Taraskevitch, 1978), and different neoplastic cell types of endocrine origin (Kidokoro, 1975; Tischler *et al.*, 1976; Biales *et al.*, 1977;

Dufy *et al.*, 1979a). It has been claimed that these excitable endocrine cells may belong to Pearse's APUD (amine precursor uptake decarboxylase) series and thus may share common physiological properties that include secretion of low-weight polypeptide hormones and a common parentage from neuroectoderm (Pearse, 1969; Takor-Takor and Pearse, 1975). Even though one may question the application of this concept to endocrine cells of the gut and the pancreas (Fontaine and Le Douarin, 1977), it may still be relevant to adenohypophyseal cells because they differentiate from the hypophyseal placode and so share a common ectodermal origin with neural crest derivatives (Le Douarin, 1978).

In this chapter we will focus our attention mainly on electrically excitable endocrine and neuroendocrine cells, i.e., hypothalamic neurosecretory cells, adrenal chromaffin cells, adenohypophyseal cells, and β cells of the pancreas, which share the common properties of synthetizing and releasing low-weight peptide substances. Other endocrine cells will not be considered here because their electrophysiological properties have not been studied or exhibit unclear physiological implications.

II. PASSIVE MEMBRANE PROPERTIES

Like all living cells, endocrine cells have a membrane potential that depends upon ionic gradients of Na^+ and K^+, maintained by a NA^+, K^+ pump, and upon their relative conductances. Other ions, such as Cl^-, which is generally passively distributed according to the membrane potential, and Ca^{2+}, may also be directly or indirectly involved in the resting properties of endocrine cells (Fig. 2). It has been suggested that endocrine cells have smaller membrane potentials than muscle or nerve cells (Matthews, 1974). As pointed out by Andersen (1980), this is mainly due to the influence of leakage artifacts on the findings in earlier reports. The small size of such cells makes impalement difficult and the recordings unstable. The leakage of ions from the interior of the micropipet into the relatively small intracellular volume may also modify the normal ionic gradient. Reported values of the resting membrane potential are increasing as progress is made in glass microelectrode recording techniques. The introduction of the voltage clamp technique in the field of endocrine electrophysiology has enabled direct measurement of membrane current and thereby calculation of membrane ionic conductance, which is related to membrane

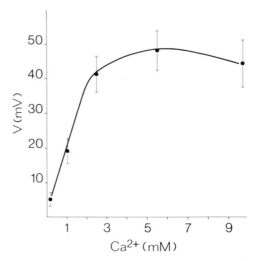

Fig. 2.   Effect of modifying the extracellular concentration of Ca^{2+} on the membrane resting potential (V) of GH3/B6 pituitary cells.

permeability (Smith *et al.*, 1981). Another interesting recent technique is the membrane noise analysis, which allows one to estimate the ionic currents carried by individual channels (Lecar and Sachs, 1981).

A.   Resting Membrane Potential and Resistance

1.   *Hypothalamic Neurosecretory Neurons*

Few successful intracellular recordings from magnocellular neu-roendocrine cells have been made. The first measurement of mem-brane constants, made in goldfish hypothalamic neuroendocrine cells, indicated that these cells have a resting potential of -50 mV and an input resistance of 33 MΩ; they seem, therefore, to have electrical membrane properties similar to those of other central neurons (Kan-del, 1964). Analogous observations were made by Koizumi and Yama-shita (1972) in magnocellular neurons of rats. The technical difficul-ties of making intracellular recordings *in vivo* have prompted the recent development of *in vitro* methods using hypothalamic slices con-taining magnocellular nuclei (Dudek *et al.*, 1980; Mason, 1980), organ-cultured explants of the supraoptic nucleus (Sakai *et al.*, 1974; Gäh-wiler and Dreifuss, 1979), or primary cultures of dispersed neurons from fetal mouse hypothalamus (Legendre *et al.*, 1981). The values of the resting membrane properties from neurons obtained by these different methods were similar to values observed *in vivo,* indicating the viability and, hence, the potential usefulness of such *in vitro* preparations.

Legendre *et al.* (1981) have measured the input resistance of the membrane in cultured hypothalamic neurons (identified as peptidergic from their morphology and their immunoreactivity) by injecting intracellular current of different amplitudes. The afferent input resistance, determined by the slope of the linear portion of the intensity–voltage curve, ranged between 90 and 200 MΩ. Such neurons are characterized mainly by their active electrical properties and by their ability to show all-or-none plateau depolarizations in response to spontaneous synaptic bombardment or to brief depolarizing pulses (Section III,A,1).

2. Adrenal Chromaffin Cells

These cells can be considered to be modified postsynaptic neurons. In their study of the electrical properties of rat adrenal chromaffin cells in culture, Brandt *et al.* (1976) recorded a resting potential that generally exceeded 50 mV and an average value of the input resistance close to 400 MΩ. For hyperpolarizing currents, the relationship between intensity and potential displacement was linear. The shift of the curve for depolarizing currents indicated an outward rectification and was related to the electrical excitability of these "paraneurons."

3. β Cells of the Pancreas

Several investigators have measured membrane potentials from pancreatic islet β cells (Dean and Matthews, 1968, 1970a,b; Pace and Price, 1972; Meissner and Schmelz, 1974). In other experiments, Atwater *et al.* (1978) injected current pulses through the recording electrode and were able to measure the input resistance of the membrane. They were able to follow the changes in ionic permeability induced by the presence of glucose in the medium. Under the resting conditions (i.e., in the absence of glucose), the resting potential had an average value of 48.5 mV and a total membrane resistance of 86 MΩ ($\pm$ 42). This membrane potential was dependent upon external K^+ concentration. Introduction of glucose (11.1 mM) in the medium induced a progressive depolarization of the membrane potential that was accompanied by an elevation of the input membrane resistance. After reaching a threshold, this slow depolarization was followed by the typical pattern of spike bursting activity (Section III,B,3), characterized by the succession of silent and active phases. The resistance was found to oscillate between a basal value (120 MΩ) before each burst and a lower value

(90 MΩ) at the end of the burst. This oscillation of the membrane resistance will be considered in detail later. What should be noted at this point is that the progressive depolarization that led to the electrical activity induced by glucose depended upon an increase in resistance, which was shown to be due to a decrease in K^+ permeability (Henquin, 1977, 1978a).

4. Anterior Pituitary Cells

   Different values of the mean resting membrane potential of anterior pituitary cells have been reported, varying with the cell type and the technical conditions. *In vitro* measurements of membrane potentials recorded from superficial cells of a halved anterior pituitary gave a mean value of 49.3 ± 2.6 mV (Poulsen and Williams, 1976). Using slices of rat pituitary gland, Osawa and Sand (1978) found resting potentials ranging from -20 to -65 mV. In the rat pituitary pars intermedia, the cells that yielded action potentials in response to depolarization had a resting potential of -66 ± 2.8 mV. Cells with lower resting potentials had probably been damaged by electrode penetration because spikes either failed to appear or could be evoked only by terminating the hyperpolarizing pulse (Douglas and Taraskevich, 1978). A large range of values of mean resting potential have also been obtained from pituitary cell tumors. In early studies of GH3 cells (a prolactin-secreting clonal cell line), Kidokoro (1975) found a value of -41 ± 4 mV, which was lower than the -57 ± 3.1 mV obtained by Taraskevich and Douglas (1980) and by Biales *et al.* (1977). Using GH4/C1 cells, a subclone of GH3, Taraskevich and Douglas (1980) obtained a mean value of -40 ± 2 mV, which is close to the Kidokoro values. In our studies of GH3/B6, another subclone of GH3, we found different values of resting potentials in successive experiments (-49 ± 8 mV, Dufy *et al.*, 1979a; -45 ± 3 mV, Dufy *et al.*, 1979b; -40 ± 5 mV, Vincent *et al.*, 1980a; -44 ± 3 mV, Vincent *et al.*, 1980b). Furthermore we observed that the excitable cells had a mean resting potential (-50 ± 2 mV) that was significantly higher than that of the nonexcitable cells (-31 ± 6 mV, Israël *et al.*, 1981). The lower values may be due to damage of the cell membrane. Because impalement of small cells usually causes more damage, the size of the cells may be a significant factor. The type of electrode may also influence the value of the resting potential; in GH3/B6, the membrane was more polarized when using K_2SO_4 pipets than with KCl pipets (-55 ± 1.8 mV versus -45 ± 2 mV). Nevertheless, it cannot be excluded that differences in resting potentials reflect variations in the culture of the cells that were used,

including differences between subclones (GH3/B6, GH4/C1) or variations within the same subclone.

The reported input resistance of pituitary cells that have been studied exhibited such large discrepancies that they can hardly be compared: 42 ± 15 MΩ in rat adenohypophysis *in vivo* (York *et al.*, 1971)
versus 112 ± 456 MΩ in rat pituitary slices *in vitro* (Ozawa and Sand,
1978), or 118 MΩ for cells recorded from a halved anterior pituitary *in
vitro* (Poulsen and Williams, 1976). Differences were also observed
among tumor cells. Taraskevich and Douglas (1980) found an input
resistance ranging from 69 to 480 MΩ for GH4/C1 cells, and from 320
to 880 MΩ for GH3. These last values are within the range observed by
others (Kidokoro, 1975; Biales *et al.*, 1977) in GH3 but are higher than
those we usually observe in GH3/B6: 169 ± 58 MΩ (Dufy *et al.*, 1979a).
Furthermore, the excitable cells had a mean value that was significantly higher than those of nonexcitable cells (280 ± 80 MΩ versus 115
± 35 MΩ, Israël *et al.*, 1981). It is difficult to assign a functional
significance to such discrepancies, because technical conditions may
play an important role in determining the value of the input resistance. Conditions can vary between normal pituitary cells and tumor-derived cells; they can also vary from one culture to another. Even
in the same culture, differences can be due to asynchronism of mitosis
in the cell population (Vincent *et al.*, 1980a).

The current voltage relation has been established for both normal
pituitary cells *in vitro* (Ozawa and Sand, 1978) and GH3/B6 cells (Vincent *et al.*, 1980b). In both cases, anterior pituitary cells have the
property of outward rectification seen in most excitable cells.

There is little data relating the resting membrane properties of anterior pituitary cells to cell type. With the exception of recordings from
dissociated rat pituitary cells (Taraskevitch and Douglas, 1979) or
from slices of rat adenohypophysis (Ozawa and Sand, 1978) (in which
the cell type could not be determined), most of the experiments have
been done on prolactin-secreting cells. Using hemi-pituitaries from
ovariectomized rats, Poulsen and Williams (1976) made the assumption that they recorded from gonadotropic cells. More recently, the
electrophysiological properties of a clonal mouse pituitary cell line
secreting ACTH and endorphins have been studied (Adler *et al.*, 1980).
These cells exhibited a low resting potential (-33 ± 22 mV) that did
not seem to be linked with cellular injury. We have studied the electrophysiological properties of cells cultured from four types of human
adenoma (Dufy *et al.*, 1981). The mean resting potential was usually
low and differed only slightly from one type of pituitary tumor to the

other. Cells secreting prolactin and those derived from tumors secreting ACTH were less polarized (-26 ± 7 mV, with a resistance of 66 ± 44 MΩ for PRL; -22 ± 5 mV, with a resistance of 63 ± 30 MΩ for ACTH) than those recorded from tumors that released growth hormone (-35 ± 8 mV; 78 ± 41 MΩ). The most polarized cells (-40 ± 10 mV), which also had a higher resistance (82 ± 70 MΩ) were those cultured from a patient with a "nonfunctioning" pituitary tumor and with no detectable elevated hormone secretion. It is not possible to determine whether the differences in passive membrane characteristics reflect an *in vivo* function of the cells or a difference in response of the cells to particular culture conditions.

B. Basal Currents under Voltage Clamp Conditions

A more reliable understanding of the excitability of endocrine cells may be obtained from voltage clamp studies of the plasma membrane. Despite the relatively small size of pituitary GH3 cells (15–20 μm diameter), recordings lasting from 30 minutes to 1 hour were obtained routinely under voltage clamp conditions (Dufy and Barker, 1982).

Until now, no attempt has been made to study inward ionic currents and only outward currents have been analyzed. During depolarization, outward current rose to a peak and then declined over several seconds to a steady-state value. The peak component of outward current became more pronounced as the membrane potential was clamped to more positive values. The outward current was associated with a corresponding voltage-dependent increase in membrane fluctuations (Fig. 3). Tetraethylammonium ion (TEA), which blocks a variety of voltage-dependent and chemically activated K^+ conductances in other excitable membranes (Meech and Standen, 1975), depolarized the cells and rectified much of the nonlinearity observed in steady-state membrane properties. TEA also eliminated the transient peak in outward current and reduced membrane current fluctuations. This K^+ conductance actively sets the level of the resting membrane potential. The GH3/B6 resting membrane properties, like those of cultured sensory neurons, are altered by both Co^{2+} and D600, suggesting that steady-state K^+ conductance probably involves Ca^{2+}. A variety of K^+ conductance mechanisms in other excitable membranes are activated by Ca^{2+}, including those recorded in molluscan ganglia neurons (Meech and Standen, 1975; Thompson, 1977), pancreatic cells (Atwater *et al.*, 1981), and chromaffin cells of the adrenal medulla (Marty, 1981). The GH3/B6 cells have a resting membrane potential of less than -10 mV

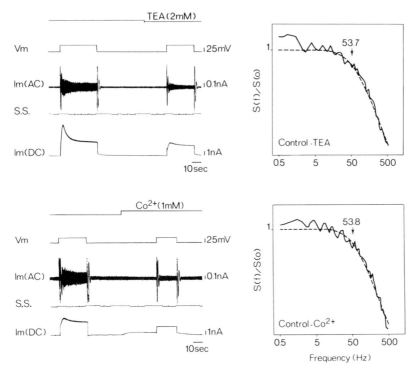

Fig. 3. Basic electrophysiological properties of GH3/B6 under voltage clamp. Vm represents membrane voltage; Im (DC), membrane current; Im (AC), a high-gain AC recording of Im (DC) filtered at 0.5–500 Hz. S.S. represents the time at which samples were acquired by the computer for spectral analysis. The figure shows membrane current responses of two GH3/B6 cells (varying from -45 to -15 mV) during control conditions and under TEA (2 mM) and Co^{2+} (1 mM). Difference spectra (right) were obtained by subtracting the spectra calculated in the presence of TEA or Ca^{2+} from that derived from membrane current fluctuations under control conditions. Half-power frequencies obtained in a population of channels sensitive to TEA (53.7 Hz) do not differ from those obtained under Co^{2+} (53.8 Hz). The Co^{2+} application induces a steady 0.2-nA outward current. From Dufy and Barker (1982).

in the absence of extracellular Ca^{2+}, again indicating that Ca^{2+} is important in setting resting membrane properties.

Special analysis of membrane current fluctuations show well-developed Lorentzian spectra at depolarized levels (Fig. 3). If we assume a relatively simple model of channel operation, the Lorentzian character of the spectra suggests the presence of a single population of two-state ion channels. The cutoff frequency is close to 50 Hz, which gives an average duration of putative K^+ channels estimated at about 3 milliseconds (Dufy and Barker, 1982). Another important conclusion to be drawn from this study with GH3 pituitary cells is that it is not possible to distinguish between Co^{2+}-sensitive and TEA-sensitive ion channels on the basis of their kinetics (Fig. 3).

As already pointed out, using patch clamp techniques in chromaffin cells, Marty (1981) showed Ca^{2+}-activated K^+ channels of large unitary conductance ($\sim$ 180 pS), which is more than 10 times higher than the value calculated from the variance of membrane fluctuations of pituitary GH3 cells. $[Ca^{2+}]_i$ increases the average number of open channels and modifies the conductance of K^+ channels. Considerable variability in the pattern of outward currents was observed in different types of identified cells (for review, see Adams et al., 1980). A large part of this variability results from differences in the relative contribution of voltage-dependent K^+ conductance and Ca^{2+}-activated K^+ conductance to the total outward current. In the endocrine cells so far studied (chromaffin cells and GH3 clonal pituitary cells), Ca^{2+} ions appear to play an important role in the K^+ conductance that sets membrane resting properties and excitability.

III. ACTIVE MEMBRANE PROPERTIES

A number of endocrine cells have been shown to be electrically excitable in that they respond to a sudden depolarization by a regenerative phenomenon. This consists of changes in ionic conductances that are voltage sensitive and time dependent; they vary from single action potentials to plateau depolarizations. In many cases they occur spontaneously and can be modified by physiological stimulants (Section III,B).

A. Electrical Activity of Neuroendocrine and Endocrine Cells

Regenerative phenomena have been observed not only in all neuroendocrine cells but also in a number of endocrine cells, including cells from the adrenal medulla, pancreatic islets, anterior pituitary and various other tumor-derived cells. In contrast to these cells, which secrete protein hormones via exocytosis, cells secreting steroid hormones seem to be electrically inexcitable. In the latter, which appear to release lipophilic hormones by simple diffusion across the membrane, release is not accompanied by any detectable electrical changes.

The only exception appears to be the spiking activity induced by ACTH in adrenal cortex cells maintained in K^+-free medium (Matthews and Saffran, 1973).

1. Neurosecretory Cells

Numerous observations of the electrical activity of neurosecretory cells in invertebrates have been reported (for review, see Cooke, 1977). In contrast, there are few reports of successful intracellular recordings from hypothalamic neurosecretory neurons in mammals. Action potentials of the latter do not differ greatly from those observed in nonendocrine elements in the central nervous system (Koizumi and Yamashita, 1972). However, the action potentials recorded intracellularly in mammalian neurosecretory cells seem to be of long duration (lasting up to 5 mseconds), as in other neurosecretory systems (Yagi and Iwasaki, 1977; Cooke, 1977). The cells also show postsynaptic excitatory or inhibitory potentials, providing electrophysiological confirmation of ultrastructural evidence that the activity of magnocellular cells can be modulated by synaptic input (Leranth *et al.*, 1975). Most of the electrophysiological data concerning neuroendocrine cells are derived, in fact, from extracellular recordings. The technique of antidromic stimulation has been particularly useful in studying the electrical properties of these neurons. The waveform of antidromic potential has been analyzed in some detail (Novin *et al.*, 1970; Yamashita *et al.*, 1970). In many instances, antidromic potentials show an inflection of their positive phase. During fast stimulation, the potential can be divided into two separate components—A and B. By analogy with other neurons (Coombs *et al.*, 1957), the A wave could represent the spikes of the initial segment and B the soma invasion. It may indicate that the axon possesses *in vivo* a zone of spike initiation separate from the soma, which is of interest when compared to our observations *in vitro* (Legendre *et al.*, 1981).

Electrical activity has been recorded from neurons that have differentiated in cultures of dispersed fetal mouse hypothalami. After 5 weeks in culture, a distinct morphological type of neuron is recognizable. It has a relatively large soma (15–20 μm), two or three stout dentritic-like processes possessing numerous spines, and a long, thin, axon-like process bearing dilatations. Such cells, which resemble magnocellular neurons *in vivo,* represent 15% of the total neuronal population in the culture. With the electron microscope, it is possible to see that such neurons exhibit many features typical of neurosecretory cells, including dense-cored secretory granules that occur in small numbers in perikarya and more frequently in processes and dilatations. During intracellular recordings, the neurons exhibit spontaneous postsynaptic potentials (psps) and overshooting impulses (action potentials). The electrical activity of these neurons is characterized by two types of regenerative phenomena of long duration: (1) slow potentials and (2) plateau potentials. The *slow potentials* (1) consist of regenerative responses to depolarization (psps or applied current), reaching an absolute potential of -30 mV in about 50 mseconds, then repolarizing over 0.2 to 2 seconds. The *plateau potentials* (2) are observed from more than one-half of the neurons showing slow potentials. They occur spontaneously (in response to psps) or after a depolarizing pulse. They arise from the falling phase of an action potential. Depolarization to an absolute potential of -20 mV requires 50 to 100 mseconds and is then sustained from 0.5 to 2 minutes. During the plateau, cell input resistance (80–150 MΩ) is decreased by 85%. Repolarization occurs after a slight hyperpolarizing drift with a rapid and slow phase requiring 0.5 minute or more. Both slow and plateau potentials involve conductance increases to Ca^{2+}. Both are reversibly blocked by Co^{2+} or Cd^{2+}. They are not blocked by tetrodotoxin (TTX). Brief application of TEA prolongs the plateau by several minutes (Fig. 4). A plateau is followed by a refractory period. With strong spontaneous synaptic bombardment or repeated current pulses, the occurrence of the plateau responses becomes periodic. This periodicity and the duration of the plateau response (and their variability) resemble the periodicity and the duration of extracellularly recorded impulse bursts of vasopressin secretory neurons *in vivo* (Section III,B,1). Preliminary observations associating neurons having plateau potentials with neurons immunoreactive to sera against vasopressin suggest that these unusual, presumably endogenous, responses may reflect unique membrane properties developed by adult hypothalamic neurosecretory cells secreting vasopressin (Theodosis *et al.*, 1981; Legendre *et al.*, 1981). The plateau potential is, indeed, of appropriate form and magnitude to serve as a driver potential supplying depolarizing current to an axonal impulse-initiating zone, as has been seen to occur in certain crustacean neurons (Tasaki and Cooke, 1979). This plateau also evokes the phasic activity of β cells of the pancreas, where they are stimulated by glucose (Section III,B,3).

2. Adrenal Chromaffin Cells

In his original study, Douglas (1968) stated that chromaffin cells did not display action potentials; a voltage-dependent Ca^{2+} influx was, however, of primary importance for release of catecholamines from the cells. Today, it has been clearly established that the chromaffin cells do indeed behave as nerve cells; which is not surprising, considering that they can be regarded as modified postsynaptic neurons in sympathetic

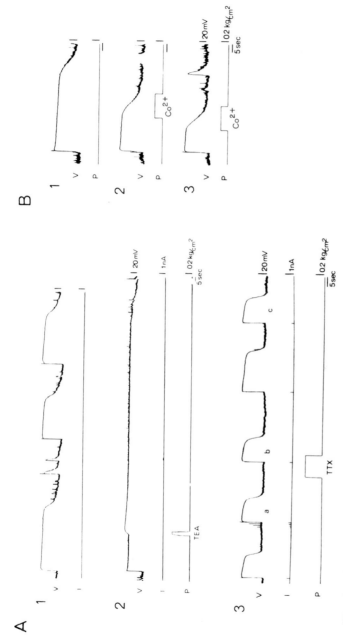

Fig. 4. (A) (1) Examples of slow potentials and plateau potentials recorded from a neuron differentiated in a culture from dispersed, 14-day-old fetal mouse hypothalamus. (2) Effects of tetraethylammonium (TEA) on the plateau potentials. Pressure ejection of TEA (1 mM in the milieu) from a delivery pipet near the soma induces an immediate, 10-mV increase in plateau depolarization, an increase of plateau duration, and inhibits the rapid phase of repolarization. (3) Resistance of plateau potentials to tetrodotoxin (TTX). (B) Ca²⁺ dependence of plateau potentials. Effects of pressure ejection of Co²⁺ (10 mM in the milieu) from a delivery pipet placed close to the soma are shown: (1) control; (2) and (3) Co²⁺ application prematurely terminates the plateau.

ganglia. Brandt *et al.* (1976) showed that chromaffin cells produce overshoot action potentials spontaneously or in response to depolarizing current pulses. These spikes are considerably reduced after replacing extracellular Na^+ by Tris buffer or completely abolished by tetrodotoxin (Biales *et al.*, 1976). Besides the major Na^+ component of the action potential, a small Ca^{2+}-dependent component can also be demonstrated (Brandt *et al.*, 1976). The increase in catecholamine secretion in a Ca^{2+}-dependent manner observed after a depolarization induced by K^+ also confirms the original assumption by Douglas (1968) that voltage-dependent Ca^{2+} channels are present in the membrane of adrenal chromaffin cells. Correlative measurements of both $^{45}Ca^{2+}$ and $^{22}Na^+$ influxes and of catecholamine release have been possible in a chromaffin-derived clonal cell line (Stallcup, 1979). Spontaneous action potentials also have been recorded extracellularly, using suction microelectrodes, from isolated chromaffin cells. Depolarization of the cell by application of current through the recording electrodes increased the frequency of the spike proportionally with the amount of stimulus current (Brandt *et al.*, 1976).

3. β *Cell of the Pancreas*

In the absence of, or in low concentrations of glucose, β cells of the pancreas are spontaneously silent. By injecting depolarizing current through the intracellular microelectrodes, it is possible to evoke a spike potential in only 10% of the cell population impaled (Matthews and Sakamoto, 1975a). It is difficult to assess whether this loss of signal occurs as a consequence of cell injury or whether it represents a functional loss of excitability of the cells in the absence of glucose. It has to be noted that, if the majority of the inexcitable cells have a low resting potential (< -30 mV), that is not the case for some of them having a resting potential in excess of -50 mV (Matthews and Sakamoto, 1975a). These observations have to be compared with our observations of pituitary cells in which 50% of the cell population was inexcitable without any clear-cut difference in their resting potentials (Section II,A,4a).

The spikes observed in β cells are of long duration (25 mseconds) but of small amplitude (10 to 30 mV) without overshooting. Removal of Ca^{2+} from the recording medium depolarizes the cells and suppresses their excitability; depolarizing current fails to evoke a spike event with a conditioning hyperpolarization. D600, a Ca^{2+} channel blocker, has no effect on the resting membrane potential of β cells, yet blocks the spiking response to depolarizing currents. All these data clearly indicate that the action potential of the β cell is Ca^{2+}-dependent.

When glucose at physiological concentrations is added to the medium, electrical properties of the β cell change dramatically. They will be described in Section III,B,3.

4. Anterior Pituitary Cells

Regenerative voltage-dependent conductance changes have been described in different types of anterior pituitary cells. They consist of all-or-none, high-amplitude phenomena (action potentials) and low-amplitude potential fluctuations.

   a. Action Potentials.   Several groups have reported the occurrence of action potentials in normal pituitary cells and in cells derived from tumors. Normal hypophyseal cells (pars distalis), derived from adult rat tissue and maintained in culture, showed an electrical activity consisting of large-amplitude spikes (Taraskevich and Douglas, 1977). Action potentials recorded extracellularly occurred spontaneously or were initiated by depolarization. Because spiking persisted in the presence of TTX and in the absence of Na^+, but was inhibited by Ca^{2+} blockers, such action potentials appeared to be Ca^{2+} spikes; contributions to spiking by other ions could not be excluded. The fact that only approximately one in three of the cells displayed spontaneous or evoked action potentials does not mean that electrical activity and excitability is a property of only some categories of adenohypophyseal cells; others may have lost excitability as a result of dissociation procedures, e.g., trypsinization or other conditions of culture. By intracellular recording from slices of nondissociated pituitary glands of normal rats, Ozawa and Sand (1978) were able to demonstrate that most cells were electrically excitable either during an outward current pulse or at the cessation of an inward current pulse, but they never observed any spontaneous spiking activity. After studying the electrical activity of the pituitary cells in Na^+- and Ca^{2+}-free solutions, they concluded that the membrane of most adenyhypophyseal cells is able to generate Ca^{2+}-dependent regenerative responses and that some cells have a Na^+ component in addition. On the other hand, in cells of rat pituitary pars intermedia, the major portion of the action potential was Na^+ dependent, and there was only a small Ca^{2+} component (Douglas and Taraskevitch, 1978). Nevertheless, the Ca^{2+} component appeared to give a more important contribution to spiking activity in cells of the pars intermedia of the lizard (Taraskevitch and Douglas, 1979) and in prolactin-secreting cells of the pars distalis in the fish (Taraskevich and Douglas, 1978).

   The electrical behavior of anterior pituitary cells from tumors has now been extensively studied. In rat tumor anterior pituitary cells of the GH3 line, which secrete prolactin spontaneously, Kidokoro (1975) observed spontaneously occurring spikes and concluded that the inward action current was exclusively carried by Ca^{2+}. This was later confirmed by Dufy et al. (1979a,b) and by Taraskevich and Douglas (1980). Biales et al. (1977) have also reported that GH3 cells generate action potentials that are Ca^{2+}-dependent but with an additional Na^+ component.

Using GH3/B6, a subclone of the GH3 rat prolactin cell line, Dufy et al. (1979a) demonstrated that 50% of the cells were electrically excitable, i.e., they display action potentials during a depolarizing intracellular current injection. Spikes were also obtained during depolarization induced by application close to the cell of KCl using a pneumatic ejection system. Twenty-eight percent of all cells were spontaneously active, with a firing rate that never exceeded 2 Hz. The observation that only half of the cells were excitable is puzzling. The possibility that the membrane of the nonexcitable cells was damaged cannot be excluded, but it is also possible that the difference was due to asynchronism of mitosis in the cell population. The all-or-none action potentials had a positive overshoot and a prominent after potential. (Figs. 5 and 6). Furthermore, they were reduced or totally abolished by D600 (Fig. 5). They were also inhibited by replacing Ca^{2+} by Mn^{2+} in the bathing solution or by directly applying Co^{2+} close to the cell (Fig. 5). Addition of TEA prolonged the duration of the regenerative Ca^{2+} potential. This result is in agreement with the delayed rectification that can be observed in GH3 cells. Exposure to TTX ($2 \times 10^{-6}\ M$) or replacement of Na^+ in the bathing solution with choline chloride did not suppress the action potentials but decreased their amplitude by preventing the overshoot (Fig. 6). These findings clearly indicate that opening of potential-dependent Ca^{2+} channels is responsible for a major part of the action potentials.

At present, most of the observations from pituitary tumor cells concern prolactin-secreting cells. In a preliminary report, Adler et al. (1980) have described a rhythmic electrical activity in an anterior pituitary cell line secreting ACTH and endorphins. Single events consisted of several brief Na^+ spikes superimposed on the rising phase of a slow Ca^{2+}-dependent spike; such events occurred periodically with a frequency varying from 2 to 8 Hz.

Cells cultured from human prolactinomas and from ACTH-secreting tumors were rarely excitable and did not show any spontaneous activity (Dufy et al., 1981). Conversely, a majority of cells recorded from growth hormone-secreting and "nonfunctioning" pituitary tumors

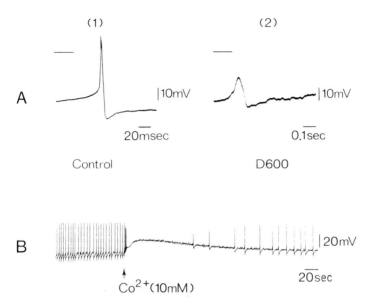

Fig. 5. Action potentials in GH3/B6 pituitary cells. (A) Effect of D600 (10^{-4} M): (1) control; (2) 2 minutes after application of D600. (B) Effect of Co^{2+}. (10 mM) on action potential firing. The cell depolarizes and action potentials are temporarily blocked.

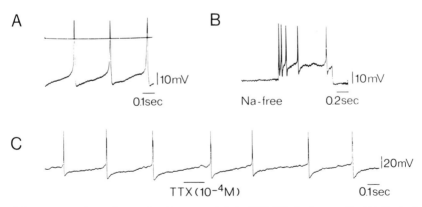

Fig. 6. Na^+ dependence of action potentials in GH3/B6 pituitary cells. (A) Control. (B) Action potentials recorded in a sodium-free medium of the following composition (in mM): choline chloride, 142.6; KCl, 5.6; $CaCl_2$, 10; glucose, 5; HEPES buffer, 5; pH 7.4. (C) Lack of effect of tetrodotoxin (TTX; 10^{-4} M) on action potential firing in GH3/B6 cells.

were excitable and were spontaneously active. The action potentials were Ca^{2+}-dependent because they were observed in Na^+-free medium and were completely blocked by Co^{2+}.

   b.   **Fluctuations of the Membrane Potential.**   In normal rat pituitary cells from slice preparations, Ozawa and Sand (1978) described spontaneous depolarizing potentials of less than 5-mV amplitude. In GH3 cells, prominent fluctuations of the membrane potential of approximately 4-mV amplitude were observed (Kidokoro, 1975). These fluctuations appeared as an increase in the baseline noise (Taraskevich and Douglas, 1980) and occasionally initiated action potentials. In human pituitary adenomas, all recorded cells showed important fluctuations of membrane potentials. These fluctuations ranged from 1 to 6 mV and were voltage dependent, because they increased with the level of depolarization. This voltage-dependent increase of membrane fluctuations was not due to a nonspecific increase in K^+ permeability because they occurred at membrane potential values for which the voltage–current relationship was linear and the membrane input resistance was not affected by depolarization. Moreover, these fluctuations involved a calcium component because their amplitude was greatly reduced by Co^{2+}. Cells derived from prolactinomas or ACTH-secreting tumors that were not spontaneously spiking displayed only this type of Ca^{2+}-dependent active process. Because these cells release large amounts of hormone spontaneously in the recording medium, it is tempting to speculate that spontaneous Ca^{2+}-dependent potential fluctuations are involved in the secretory process.

   To summarize, these results demonstrate that normal and tumor-derived pituitary cells are able to generate active electrical membrane phenomena that consist of action potentials and/or low-amplitude potential fluctuations; both phenomena are at least partially Ca^{2+} dependent. Because Ca^{2+} is intimately involved with release mechanisms in secretion, it is worthwhile to examine whether factors that influence secretion also have an effect on the Ca^{2+}-dependent electrical activity of the pituitary cells.

B.   Effects of Substances that Influence Hormonal Secretion

1.   Neuroendocrine Cells

   In all mammalian species so far studied, there are separate magnocellular neurosecretory cells secreting either vasopressin or oxytocin

(Swaab *et al.*, 1975; Vandesande and Diericks, 1975). The two types of neurons exist in equal proportions in both the supraoptic and the paraventricular nuclei of the hypothalamus and can be distinguished electrophysiologically by their responses to various stimuli, leading to the release of the hormones.

   a.   **Electrical Activity in Response to Various Stimuli.**   Oxytocin neurons were the first neurosecretory cells to be identified by electrophysiological means because a specific stimulus exists for their activation. In the lactating rat, suckling induces intermittent milk ejections that occur every 5 to 15 minutes and are caused by pulses of 0.5 to 1 mU of oxytocin. As has been shown by the work of Wakerley and Lincoln (1973), before each milk ejection there is a high-frequency discharge of action potentials, usually followed by a few seconds of inhibition. This pattern of discharge is observed in about half the population of neurosecretory cells in the supraoptic and paraventricular nuclei (Fig. 7).

   The lack of a specific stimulus (under experimental conditions) for vasopressin release has, for a long time, prevented the identification of vasopressin neurons *in vivo*. About half of the magnocellular neurons of the supraoptic and paraventricular nuclei do not react to suckling and this proportion correlates well with the percentage of magnocellular neurons that react with a specific antibody against vasopressin. Under normal conditions, the majority of the neurons showing no response to suckling have a slow irregular pattern of electrical activity (<3 spikes/second) similar to the background activity of oxytocin neurons. During hemorrhage or intraperitoneal injection of hypertonic saline, the same neuron that did not react to suckling showed a progressive increase in firing rate and the appearance of a bursting pattern of activity. This bursting pattern could not be induced in oxytocin neurons. The bursting pattern described in the rat (Wakerley and Lincoln, 1971), sheep (Haskings *et al.*, 1975), and monkey (Arnauld *et al.*, 1975) consists of periodic bursts of action potentials followed by a period of quiescence (Fig. 7). Several stimuli are capable of eliciting this bursting pattern in vasopressin neurons: intracarotid injection, slow intravenous infusion, intraperitoneal injections of hypertonic saline, and also, dehydration by water deprivation, hemorrhage, and carotid occlusion. However, the reaction of vasopressin neurons is dependent upon the intensity of the stimulus (review in Vincent *et al.*, 1980). In the monkey, during progressive dehydration by water deprivation, the number of bursting neurons increases progressively as plasma osmolality rises. In the lactating rat, after 12 hours of dehydration, 80 to

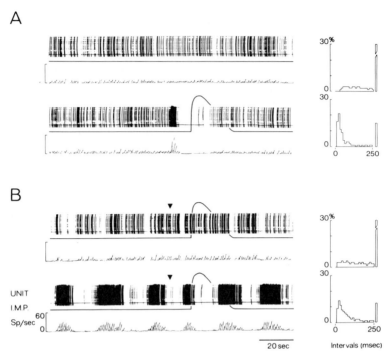

Fig. 7. Patterns of electrical activity of oxytocin and VP neurons. Antidromically identified neurosecretory cells were recorded in the supraoptic nucleus of anesthetized lactating rats during suckling. On these polygraph records, action potentials represented by the polygraph pen deflections (UNIT) are drawn alongside the rate meter output (spike/sec) and the intramammary pressure recording (I.M.P.) from a cannulated mammary gland. (A) Oxytocin neuron. Top: Background activity during suckling (note the flat intramammary pressure recording). Bottom: The same oxytocin neuron at the time of a milk ejection. The rise in intramammary pressure corresponds to 20 mm Hg, equivalent to the response elicited by iv injection of 1 mU oxytocin. Note the brief high-frequency discharge of action potentials occurring 14 seconds before milk ejection (peak firing rate over a 0.5-second period, 65 spikes/sec). Interspike interval histograms (Bin width: 10 msec) have been drawn for the background activity (top) and for periods of 15 seconds around the high-frequency discharges (bottom: pooled data from eight consecutive milk ejections). (B) VP neurons. Examples of one VP neuron displaying a bursting mode of firing (bottom). In the few seconds preceding the milk ejection induced by suckling, no high-frequency discharges occurred (arrowheads). Note the similarity between the slow irregular activity of the oxytocin neuron outside the period of milk ejection and of the first VP neuron; in both cases, interspike interval histograms are flat. Despite the striking difference between the high-frequency discharge of the oxytocin neuron and the bursting pattern of the VP neuron, these enhanced activities result in a shift of their interspike interval toward short intervals. From Vincent *et al.* (1980c).

100% of the vasopressin neurons display this mode of firing (Wakerley *et al.*, 1978). As the mean firing rate of vasopressin neurons increases, one can also observe an increase in the frequency of action potentials inside the bursts and in the duration of these bursts.

The mechanism underlying the phasic pattern of vasopressin neurons is unknown. On the one hand, the possibility remains that this particular property of the vasopressin neurons is synaptically driven even though bursting activity has been recorded in supraoptic neurons in cultured explants (Gähwiler and Dreifuss, 1979, 1980). That it may result from the activity of an intranuclear neuronal network is supported by anatomical studies showing that two-thirds of the synaptic boutons impinging on supraoptic neurons have an intranuclear origin (Leranth *et al.*, 1975). On the other hand, recent evidence has been obtained *in vitro* and supports the alternative hypothesis of an endogenous property of vasopressin neurons to generate the bursting pattern of spike activity (Legendre *et al.*, 1981; and Section III,B,3).

Another unanswered question concerns the mechanisms by which the total population of oxytocin neurons responds to the continuous suckling stimulus by an intermittent synchronous discharge. Despite the striking difference between the high-frequency discharge of oxytocin neurons and the bursting pattern of vasopressin neurons, these enhanced activities both result in a shift of their interspike intervals toward short intervals, an observation that may be relevant in terms of functional significance.

b. **Functional Significance of the Electrical Activity.** Since the original work of Haterius and Fergusson (1928), many studies have confirmed that the release of neurohypophyseal hormones can be evoked by electrical stimulation of the hypophyseal tract (see Vincent *et al.*, 1980c). Douglas (1963) observed that depolarization of the neurosecretory axons by an excess of K^+ in the bathing medium causes hormone liberation from isolated neurohypophysis. He further demonstrated that the presence of Ca^{2+} was necessary in the medium and that hormone release increased when the external Ca^{2+} was raised. Douglas proposed that hormone release was initiated on arrival of impulses that, by depolarizing the axon endings, promote Ca^{2+} influx. The amount of hormone released and the influx of $^{45}Ca^{2+}$ are both stimulated by increasing K^+ depolarization, although prolonged K^+ depolarization leads to a decline in hormonal output by inactivation of Ca^{2+} entry (Nordmann, 1976). Subsequent reactivation of Ca^{2+} entry by veratridine is able to restart hormone release (Dyball and Nordmann, 1977). Further information showing the importance of Ca^{2+}

has been obtained from studies with the squid giant synapse preparation. Using the voltage clamp technique, it was found that an inward Ca^{2+} current in the presynaptic fiber preceded the excitatory postsynaptic potential (Llinas, 1977). The Ca^{2+} current evoked by depolarization is slow in onset, rapidly decaying with hyperpolarization and does not appear to inactivate. There is a linear relationship between peak Ca^{2+} current and the amplitude of the postsynaptic potential, i.e., the amount of transmitter released.

Ca^{2+} activation and the resulting hormone release in neurosecretory presynaptic terminals are not exclusively dependent on the action potential per se (Katz and Miledi, 1967). TTX did not inhibit hormonal release induced by K^+ depolarization (Dreifuss et al., 1971). When the neurosecretory endings are directly stimulated by current pulses (2-msecond duration) in Na^+-free Locke solution (which precludes action potential generation), a clearcut dependence of hormone release on frequency of stimulation can be observed (Nordmann and Dreifuss, 1972); an identical number of pulses will release more hormone when delivered at a higher frequency. Thus, from these *in vitro* experiments it can be concluded that hormone release depends both on the amplitude of the depolarization and on the frequency of the depolarizing pulses. The action potential per se, however, does play a role in the mechanisms underlying hormone release. When the isolated neurohypophysis is stimulated in normal Locke solution (Dreifuss et al., 1971)—such that depolarization is generated in the endings by action potentials—the results are different from those obtained in Na^+-free Locke solution. With a frequency of stimulation below 35 Hz, hormone release was found to depend on the total number of stimuli applied as well as on the frequency of stimulation. Above 35 Hz, an identical number of stimuli were progressively less effective as the frequency of stimulation was increased. The inefficiency of a long train of high-frequency stimulations is probably due to the inability of the fibers to conduct action potentials at a frequency higher than 35 Hz. Gainer (1978) has pointed out that the frequency potentiation of hormone release for frequencies under 35 Hz is considerably greater than that already observed in the absence of action potentials. This observation suggests that the frequency potentiation of hormone release may depend upon frequency per se and, in addition, upon a frequency-dependent property of the spike.

As already discussed, numerous *in vivo* studies have demonstrated a correlation between the extent of phasic activity in the magnocellular neurons and their secretory activity. The only direct evidence that the bursting pattern is highly efficient in stimulating hormone release has been obtained by stalk stimulation of an isolated neurohypophysis (Dyball and Thomson, 1977). Clustering stimulus pulses with an overall frequency of 5.5 Hz released the same amount of hormone as a regular stimulation at 20 Hz. In a further experiment, action potentials of phasically firing units recorded *in vivo* were used to trigger pulses delivered to neurohypophysis *in vitro* (Dutton *et al.*, 1978); more vasopressin was released by pulses driven from phasic neurons than by regularly spaced pulses at the same overall frequency. Moreover, the amount of hormone released correlated with the number of short interspike intervals (<100 mseconds) within the bursts. Under physiological conditions, the phasic pattern may represent the most economical way of obtaining short interspike intervals and thus producing frequency potentiation of hormone release.

The mechanism of potentiation is not clear. It has been shown by voltage-clamp experiments in invertebrate neurosecretory cells that the repolarization of action potentials is regulated by their frequency of discharge (Barker and Smith, 1977). The higher the frequency, the more rapid and thorough is the depression of the repolarization. This leads to a progressive augmentation of the duration of action potentials during the burst. Because Ca^{2+} entry is directly related to depolarization with a slow onset and without inactivation, the slower the repolarization and the longer the spike duration, the greater is the entry of Ca^{2+} into the cell body. Finally, if we assume that action potentials recorded at the cell body are conducted unaltered down to the axon endings and that the membrane of the terminals has the same properties as that of the cell body, then the bursting pattern would facilitate Ca^{2+} entry, thereby facilitating neurohormone release.

2. Adrenal Chromaffin Cells

In their early studies on chromaffin cells, Douglas (1968) showed that acetylcholine (ACh) induced a parallel depolarization of the cell membrane and release of catecholamines. They therefore suggested that ACh-induced depolarization was responsible for the voltage-dependent Ca^{2+} influx which, in turn, was the determining event in the stimulus–secretion sequence coupling. More recently, Brandt *et al.* (1976) and Biales *et al.* (1976) have shown that iontophoretic application of ACh on isolated chromaffin cells resulted in a depolarization that was associated with action potentials. Despite the fact that the major component of the action potential is Na^+ dependent, a minor

Ca^{2+} component exists that may account for the ACh-induced secretion of catecholamines. In that sense, chromaffin cells would not behave differently from typical nerve or neurosecretory cells.

3. β Cell of the Pancreas

Dean and Matthews (1968, 1970a) first reported that β cells of the pancreas exhibit electrical activity when stimulated with glucose or other insulin-releasing agents. Meissner and Schmelz (1974), using microelectrode recording from single β cells of isolated and continuously perfused mouse islets, have given a description of this typical burst-patterned activity (Fig. 8). Each burst is preceded by a slow depolarization (A) of the resting membrane potential. After reaching a threshold level (B), there is a rapid depolarization to a plateau potential upon which fast spikes are superimposed (C). Within a few seconds, the spiking activity stops and the membrane repolarizes to a level slightly more polarized than at the beginning of the plateau (D). During the burst, the frequency of the spikes decreases from the beginning to the end. The amplitude of the spikes is variable from 5 to 30 mV with no overshoot. At the end of the repolarization, a new progressive depolarization brings the membrane potential to the plateau threshold and a new burst occurs (Fig. 8). This phase bursting activity

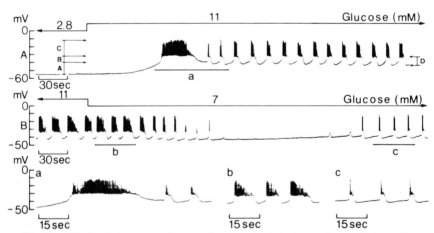

Fig. 8. Effects of glucose on the membrane potential of a single β cell. Record B is the continuation of record A after an interval of 9 minutes. Letters A, B, C, and D in trace A refer to the different phases described in the text. The records a, b, c show, on an expanded time scale and sometimes with a higher voltage gain, the sections marked by bars in the slower traces. From Meissner *et al.* (1980).

is observed as long as the glucose concentration is maintained in the perfusing medium. After removal of glucose, the membrane potential returns to its initial hyperpolarized level.

It must be pointed out that this glucose-induced electrical activity occurs only at glucose concentrations that also stimulate insulin release (>5 mM). The plateau threshold and its level of depolarization remain remarkably constant, independently of the glucose concentration. On the other hand, the duration of the burst increases, whereas that of the silent phase decreases, in relation to the glucose concentration. When the glucose concentration is higher than 15 mM, the β cell remains permanently depolarized with a continuous spiking activity. Therefore, a correlation exists between the duration of the burst, the spike frequency, and the glucose concentration. These dose–response curves strongly resemble the sigmoidal relationship between insulin release and glucose concentration (Meissner, 1976). Furthermore, by comparing the dynamics of insulin secretion with the kinetics of the electrical activity in response to a sudden and sustained stimulation with glucose, it is possible to establish a direct correlation between these two phenomena (Meissner and Atwater, 1976). The electrical activity shows a biphasic time course that evokes the biphasic release obtained from the whole pancreas.

Different ionic mechanisms have been proposed to explain the electrical response of β cells to glucose. K^+ and Ca^{2+} seem to be the major ions affected by change in the membrane properties. The depolarization that leads to the plateau threshold corresponds to an increase in the apparent input resistance (Atwater et al., 1978). Henquin (1978a) has clearly demonstrated, using isotopic measurement, that it is due to a decrease in K^+ conductance. The cyclic decrease in K^+ permeability, which periodically depolarizes the membrane to the level of plateau threshold, is directly induced by glucose but is independent of insulin secretion. It still appears at glucose concentrations (3–5 mM) insufficient to stimulate insulin secretion and it persists in the presence of Co^{2+} (Henquin and Lambert, 1975) or in the absence of extracellular Ca^{2+} (Grodski and Bennet, 1966; Henquin, 1978b), which block both bursting activity and insulin secretion. Unlike the initial depolarization, the plateau and the spike are suppressed in Ca^{2+}-free medium (Matthews and Sakamoto, 1975b; Atwater and Beigelman, 1976) or when Ca^{2+} influx is blocked by Co^{2+} or D600. This clearly indicates that bursting activity is mainly Ca^{2+} dependent. Nevertheless, as has been described for similar phenomena (Section III,A,1), the cessation of bursting and the repolarizing phase appear to be related to an increase in K^+ conductance. This K^+ conductance is probably activated by an increase of intracellular Ca^{2+}. Quinine, which may inhibit specifically the Ca^{2+} activation of K^+ channels (Armando-Hardy et al., 1975) suppresses the repolarizing phase of electrical activity stimulated by glucose and augments insulin secretion.

The mechanism by which the metabolism of glucose interacts with the ionic permeability of the β cell membrane is still very hypothetical and will not be discussed here (see Malaisse et al., 1979).

To summarize, a model can be proposed for the control of insulin release by glucose (Henquin, 1980): Glucose metabolism in β cells decreases the K^+ permeability of the plasma membrane; this leads to a progressive depolarization from the resting membrane potential. When the concentration of glucose reaches 5–6 mM, the fall in K^+ permeability is sufficient to depolarize β cells to a threshold potential, at which point Ca^{2+} channels are activated. The resulting Ca^{2+} influx is accompanied by a further depolarization with Ca^{2+}-dependent spiking activity that then triggers the exocytosis of insulin granules. However, the rise in cytoplasmic Ca^{2+} also activates K^+ channels; the ensuing increase in K^+ permeability tends to repolarize β cells and to inactivate Ca^{2+} channels. As the influx of Ca^{2+} stops, the level of free Ca^{2+} falls and the K^+ permeability of the membrane decreases again. A new depolarization follows, which then triggers a new influx of Ca^{2+}. This simple model may explain the oscillations of the membrane potential during stimulation of insulin release by intermediate concentrations of glucose (6–15 mM). When the glucose concentration is higher (> 15 mM), K^+ channels can no longer be activated by intracellular Ca^{2+}, the membrane remains depolarized and exhibits a continuous electrical activity, and the secretion of insulin increases.

4. Anterior Pituitary Cells

Secretory activity of the anterior pituitary gland is regulated by the brain through stimulatory and inhibitory substances released from nerve endings in the median eminence of the hypothalamus and carried by the adenohypophyseal portal blood system to their respective target cells. On the other hand, the peripheral hormones exert feedback influences on pituitary cells. Very little data exists concerning the effect of these different factors on the electrical activity of the pituitary cells: Prolactin-secreting cells have been frequently studied. We shall describe the effects of the major substances known to affect prolactin secretion.

a. Thyroid-Stimulating Hormone-Releasing Hormone (TRH). Kidokoro (1975) found that the mean rate of action potential firing in a population of GH3 cells exposed to 30 nM TRH was higher than when

TRH was absent. Taraskevitch and Douglas (1980) confirmed that application of TRH (10–100 nM) close to the membrane increases the frequency of extracellularly recorded action potentials within a few seconds. On the other hand, TRH failed to increase action potential activity in GH4/C1 cells, a clonal line that has lost their TRH receptors.

We have studied the effect of TRH on GH3/B6 cells by recording their electrical activity (Dufy *et al.,* 1979a). TRH (25–125 nM), added to the bathing solution, increased the percentage of cells displaying action potentials, as previously shown by extracellular recording of GH3 (Kidokoro, 1975) and of normal rat anterior pituitary cells (Taraskevich and Douglas, 1977). Application of TRH (50 nM, 2 nl) close to the cell evoked a train of action potentials within 1 minute (Fig. 9). The spike discharge was preceded by a progressive increase of the input resistance without any detectable change in the resting membrane polarization apart from an early hyperpolarization. This early TRH-induced hyperpolarization has been shown to be due to an increase in the membrane permeability to K^+ (Ozawa and Kimura, 1979). This transient phenomenon appeared less consistently in our preparations and did not seem to be directly involved in the spiking activity. Furthermore, because this early phenomenon was not affected by Co^{2+}, which blocked both spiking activity and hormone release, it did not appear to be closely related to the TRH-stimulated hormone release. The TRH-induced spiking activity was also accompanied by an increase in the membrane noise. After 1 to 10 minutes, the cells stopped firing as the resistance and the membrane noise re-

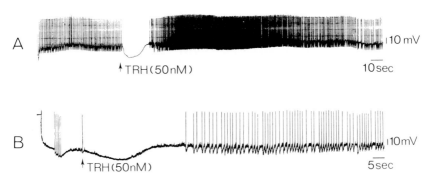

Fig. 9. Effect of TRH (50 nM) on two GH3/B6 pituitary cells. The neuropeptide induces a hyperpolarization, followed by generation of action potentials. (A) TRH increases the rate of firing of a spontaneously firing cell. (B) TRH induces action potentials in a silent cell; excitability of the cell has been tested prior to administration of TRH by depolarizing pulses.

turned to the resting level. Repeated administration of TRH at less than 10-minute intervals showed a desensitization of the response. The electrical response was reduced or totally abolished by D600 and by introduction of Co^{2+} into the medium.

The fact that TRH induces a change in membrane resistance without a corresponding change in membrane potential remains puzzling. This observation has been confirmed by Ozawa and Kimura (1979), who showed that (1) the enhancement of spike generation was not due to a membrane depolarization, (2) the response also occurred in Na^+-free solution, which indicated that a change in Na^+ conductance was not indispensable for the initiation of spike facilitation, and (3) the input resistance increased during the facilitatory period. The mechanism by which TRH induces spiking without changing the resting potential remains to be determined. TRH may increase the excitability by lowering the spike threshold after having modified the voltage at which activation of the Ca^{2+} conductance underlying spikes occurs. Such a direct effect of a peptide in changing the action potential threshold and hence the excitability has already been observed in spinal cord neurons (Barker *et al.*, 1978). Other examples of the action of peptides on voltage-dependent conductances have also been described for invertebrate neuronal systems (Barker and Smith, 1977). Using a Cl^--free propionate saline recording medium, Ozawa (1981) has observed late depolarization of the resting membrane potential in response to TRH, which supports the spiking activity and which may be due to a decrease in K^+ conductance.

Besides the increase in the frequency of Ca^{2+}-dependent action potentials, another electrophysiological mechanism by which TRH may affect the entry of Ca^{2+} into the cell has been described (Sand *et al.*, 1980). Intracellular recordings from the same GH3 cell before and during TRH stimulation showed this peptide to prolong the duration of the action potentials. We have not, however, been able to observe any effect of TRH on spike duration in our GH3/B6 preparations.

TRH, which is remarkably effective in causing growth hormone release in acromegalic patients, has been also applied to cells cultured from pituitary fragments of an acromegalic patient (Dufy *et al.*, 1981). Cells responded to TRH by a depolarization accompanied by an increase in the size of membrane fluctuations. Some of the cells, in addition, showed a prolonged burst of action potentials during the depolarization. Because TRH was highly effective in augmenting growth hormone secretion, these observations suggest that not only action potentials but also membrane fluctuations may be involved in the secretory process.

b. Estrogen. When 17β-estradiol (17β-E) was added to the bathing solution (50 pg/ml) of GH3/B6 cells, the percentage of spontaneously firing cells was greater than in a nontreated control group. Furthermore, ejection of 17β-E (10^{-10}–10^{-8} M) in the close vicinity of the cell elicited two different effects (Fig. 10). The first one, observed in all of the excitable cells, consisted of a brief depolarization triggering a burst of action potentials. This effect could be repeated several times on the same cell. It did not appear to be Ca^{2+} dependent because administration of Co^{2+} did not significantly modify the depolarization. This transient response, which never exceeded 20 seconds duration, was followed 1 minute later by a second effect, which was a prolonged discharge of action potentials accompanied by an increase of the membrane resistance without any change in the membrane potential. The spiking activity lasted 3 to 30 minutes after application of 17β-E and was reduced or almost totally suppressed by application of D600. The discharge of spikes in response to 17β-E was only observed in about 30% of the excitable cells. Furthermore, when one application of 17β-E was successful in eliciting spikes, a subsequent ejection was totally

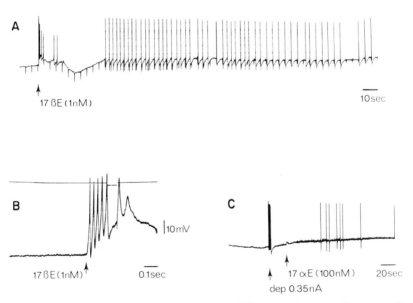

Fig. 10. Effect of 17β-estradiol and 17α-estradiol on membrane resting properties and action potential generation of GH3/B6 pituitary cells. (A) Effect of 17β-estradiol (10^{-9} M). (B) Precocious effect of 17β-E expanded from A. (C) Effect of 17α-estradiol (10^{-7} M) on a GH3/B6 cell; excitability of this cell has been tested prior to administration of 17α-E by a depolarizing pulse.

ineffective, although the cell remained excitable. 17α-E had a much weaker effect even at higher doses but prevented the effect of 17β-E. Progesterone and testosterone were not able to induce spiking activity. This indicates a high degree of stereospecificity for the effects of estrogen on the electrical activity of pituitary cells (Dufy et al., 1979a). The spiking effect of 17β-E was similar in time course, passive membrane property changes, and Ca^{2+} dependence to that induced by TRH. The rapid and specific effect of 17β-E on membrane properties implies recognition sites for the steroid at the membrane surface and most probably reflects conformational changes in membrane components. The physiological implication of such early effects of estrogen on the membrane properties of GH3/B6 remains unclear. It has been demonstrated that prolactin release is stimulated within minutes after 17β-E ejection, which is consistent with the Ca^{2+}-dependent electrical effect of 17β-E (Zyzek et al., 1981). It is also possible that Ca^{2+} is required to initiate the long-term effect of 17β-E in prolactin synthesis. Finally, the changes in ionic permeability may also initiate other unknown intracellular processes triggered by the steroid.

c. **Catecholamines.** Douglas and Taraskevitch (1978) have demonstrated that the action potentials in the pars intermedia cells were suppressed by dopamine (DA) and noradrenaline (NA), both of which are inhibitors of secretion of the pars intermedia in the rat (Tilders and Smelik, 1977). A similar inhibitory action of catecholamines on electrical activity has been directly recorded from the frog neurointermediate lobe (Davis and Hadley, 1978). DA and NA have also been noted to inhibit electrical activity of cultured prolactin cells obtained from the fish pars distalis (Taraskevitch and Douglas, 1979). In our studies of GH3/B6, we have observed that the firing of 40% of the spontaneously active cells was inhibited by an application of DA close to the cells (Dufy et al., 1979b). This inhibition was concomitant with a rapid decrease of the input resistance without any detectable change in the resting membrane polarization (Fig. 11). In addition, DA inhibited the TRH-induced action potentials. The DA agonist RU24213 (Roussel-UCLAF) mimicked the effect of DA. Conversely, the DA antagonists haloperidol and chlorpromazine suppressed the inhibitory effect of DA on action potentials. We observed also that the inhibitory effect of DA on prolactin secretory cells was modulated by estrogen. The percentage of cells inhibited by DA was different according to the presence or absence of estrogen in the medium in which the cells were grown: When the cells were grown for at least 24 hours in an estrogen-de-

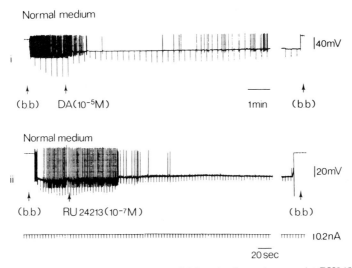

Fig. 11. Effect of dopamine (DA) (10^{-5} M) and a dopamine agonist RU24213 (from Roussel-UCLAF) on membrane resting properties and action potential firing of two GH3/B6 pituitary cells. Membrane resistance was monitored by applying hyperpolarizing current pulses. b.b. indicates balance of the bridge amplifier. DA and RU induced a decrease in membrane resistance and cessation of firing of action potentials. From Dufy *et al.* (1979b).

pleted medium, the percentage of DA-inhibited cells reached 80% instead of the 40% observed in normal medium.

We have also tested the effects of DA on growth hormone secretion from human tumor cells. When RU24213 was applied close to the cell, it induced a hyperpolarization, with a decrease in the input resistance of the membrane; a reduction or a cessation of spiking activity accompanied the hyperpolarization. In parallel, it was possible to demonstrate that RU24213 inhibits the release of GH in the same preparation.

Finally, the fact that DA inhibits firing and hormone release (Meites, 1977) once again supports the hypothesis that Ca^{2+}-dependent electrical activity is involved in the mechanism of release of anterior pituitary hormones.

d. **γ-Aminobutyric Acid (GABA).** Local application of this amino acid was able to alter the electrophysiological properties of GH3/B6 (Israël *et al.*, 1981). The effects of GABA on these cells were (1) decrease in membrane conductance; (2) hyperpolarization of 5–10 mV, and (3) inhibition or suppression of the spontaneous spiking activity. GABAergic receptor antagonists such as picrotoxin and bicuculline prevented the effects of GABA, whereas dopaminergic receptor antagonists such as haloperidol had no effect. A partial inhibition of prolactin release by GABA has been observed in a GH3/B6 cells (D. Gourdji, unpublished data). It is possible to conclude, therefore, that the inhibitory effect of GABA on electrical activity of prolactin cells may correspond to an inhibitory effect of this substance on prolactin secretion (Enjalbert et al., 1979).

IV.   FUNCTIONAL SIGNIFICANCE OF ELECTRICAL EVENTS

Endocrine cells store their hormones in essentially two ways: in a precursor form free in the cytoplasm or in membrane-bounded vesicles or granules. Because of their lipophilic nature, steroids can readily diffuse across the plasma membrane; cells producing such substances, therefore, do not accumulate large amounts of the final hormone, but only its precursor. These cells have not been reported to be excitable. Other cells, such as those of the glands presented in this chapter, store large amounts of their hormones in secretory granules. There is now sufficient biochemical and morphological evidence to demonstrate that, even though these cells are stimulated by different external factors and secrete different macromolecules, they release their products in a similar manner, i.e., by exocytosis.

The final common pathway leading to the process of exocytosis requires Ca^{2+} ions. Indeed, it is now thought that an accumulation of Ca^{2+} ions at the inner surface of the cell membrane tirggers exocytosis of the secretory granules. Because release is a rapid phenomenon, modification of the concentration of Ca^{2+} in the cytoplasm is the result of a dynamic balance between the processes that supply the ion and those that remove it. Alteration of the concentration of intracellular Ca^{2+} is possible in three ways: (1) increasing the influx of extracellular Ca^{2+} by augmenting the permeability of the membrane to Ca^{2+}; (2) mobilizing Ca^{2+} from intracellular Ca^{2+} stores; and (3) decreasing the efflux of intracellular Ca^{2+} either by a $Ca^{2+}-Na^{+}$ exchange or by an alteration of an ATP Ca^{2+} pump. All three ways have been identified in neuroendocrine and endocrine cells. They come into play to a different extent according to the type of cell or the stimulus used. On the other hand, their contribution to the electrophysiological phenomena occurring during release appears to vary.

It is well known that in many tissues cAMP plays a role in modulating Ca^{2+} homeostasis and may contribute to the mobilization of intracellular sequestered Ca^{2+}. In recent experiments (J.-D. Vincent and B. Dufy, unpublished observations), we have observed that substances known to activate the cAMP-producing system did not modify the electrophysiological properties of prolactin-secreting cells in culture although some of these substances, such as VIP, were very active on release. Therefore, in our opinion, mobilization of intracellular Ca^{2+} by activation of cAMP cannot account for the electrical events reported earlier, at least for pituitary cells.

In many secretory tissues, the process of release depends on energy metabolism. However, it is not known whether the energy is required for maintaining general cell function or whether it is needed at some step in the stimulus–secretion coupling (Trifaro, 1977). The electrophysiological observations reported in this chapter cannot answer this question, because it is known that energy processes involved in the restoration of ionic gradients do not interfer either with the maintenance of the passive properties of the membrane or with the generation of action potentials.

One means of increasing intracellular Ca^{2+} is by stimulating the influx of extracellular Ca^{2+}. There is general agreement that K^+, which passively depolarizes membranes, stimulates the release of secretory products; this depolarization then opens the voltage-dependent Ca^{2+} channels. Indeed, high extracellular concentrations of K^+ have been shown to stimulate the uptake of $^{45}Ca^{2+}$ in various endocrine tissues (Milligan and Kraicer, 1973; Zyzek et al., 1982). The increased concentration of intracellular Ca^{2+} would then trigger the process of exocytosis by a series of steps not yet completely characterized.

In contrast to this unspecific process, a number of external factors stimulate or inhibit hormonal release by interacting with specific receptor sites and then by altering the electrical properties of the cells so as to lead to stimulation or inhibition of Ca^{2+}-dependent action potentials. Calcium ions that enter the cells as a result of action potentials may then provide the ionized calcium required for the process of exocytosis. Regenerative phenomena such as Ca^{2+}-dependent spikes and plateau potentials would represent a discrete but effectual way to modulate physiologically the entry of Ca^{2+} into the cell.

However, as previously pointed out, there are other ways to alter the intracellular concentration of Ca^{2+}. Ca^{2+} action potentials, although they may be involved, may not be the unequivocal means by which external stimuli provide endocrine cells with the Ca^{2+} required for the release process.

ACKNOWLEDGMENTS

We thank D. Theodosis for her help with the manuscript. This work has been supported by grants from INSERM (CRL 78.1.2656-PRC 120052), DGRST, the University of Bordeaux II, and CNRS (ERA 493-ATP 4081).

REFERENCES

Adams, D. J., Smith, S. J., and Thompson, S. H. (1980). Ionic currents in molluscan soma. *Annu. Rev. Neurosci.* **3,** 141–167.

Adler, M., Busis, N., Higashida, H., Sabol, B., Rotter, A., and Nirenberg, M. (1980). Modulation of rhythmic electrical activity in an anterior pituitary cell line. *10th Neurosci. Meet., Abstr.* **6,** 107–111.

Andersen, O. H. (1980). "The Electrophysiology of Gland Cells." Academic Press, New York.

Armando-Hardy, M., Ellory, J. C., Ferreira, H. G., Fleminger, S., and Lew, V. L. (1975). Inhibition of the calcium-induced increase in the potassium permeability of human red cells by quinine. *J. Physiol. (London)* **250,** 32P–33P.

Arnauld, E., Dufy, B., and Vincent, J. D. (1975). Hypothalamic supraoptic neurones: Rates and patterns of action potential firing during water deprivation in the unanaesthetized monkey. *Brain Res.* **100,** 315–325.

Atwater, I., and Beigelman, P. (1976). Dynamic characteristics of electrical activity in pancreatic β cells. Effects of calcium and magnesium removal. *J. Physiol. (Paris)* **72,** 769–786.

Atwater, I., Ribalet, B., and Rojas, E. (1978). Cyclic changes in potential and resistance of the β cell membrane induced by glucose in islets of langerhans from mouse. *J. Physiol. (London)* **278,** 117–139.

Atwater, I., Dawson, C. M., Eddlestone, G. T., and Rojas, E. (1981). Voltage noise measurements across the pancreatic β cell membrane calcium channel characteristics. *J. Physiol. (London)* **314,** 195–212.

Barker, J. L., and Smith, T. G. (1977). Peptides as neurohormones. *Soc. Neurosci. Symp.* **2,** 340–373.

Barker, J. L., Gruol, D. L., Huang, M. L., Neale, J. H., and Smith, T. G. (1978). Enkephalin: Pharmacologic evidence for diverse functional roles in the neurons system using primary cultures of dissociated spinal neurons. *In* "Characteristics and Functions of opioids" (L. Terenius, ed.), pp. 87–98. Elsevier/North-Holland, Amsterdam.

Biales, B., Dichter, M. S., and Tischler, A. (1976). Electrical excitability of cultured adrenal chromaffin cells. *J. Physiol. (London)* **262,** 743–753.

Biales, B., Dichter, M. S., and Tischler, A. (1977). Sodium and calcium action potential in pituitary cells. *Nature (London)* **267,** 172–174.

Brandt, B. L., Hagiwara, S., Kidokoro, Y., and Miyazaki, S. (1976). Action potentials in the rat chromaffin cell and effects of acetylcholine. *J. Physiol. (London)* **263,** 417–439.

Cooke, I. M. (1977). Electrical activity of neurosecretory terminals and control of peptide hormone release. *In* "Peptides in Neurobiology" (H. Gainer, ed.), pp. 345–374. Plenum, New York.

Coombs, J. S., Curtis, D. R., and Eccles, J. C. (1957). The generation of impulses in motoneurones. *J. Physiol. (London)* **139**, 232–249.

Davis, M. D., and Haddley, M. E. (1976). Spontaneous electrical potentials and pituitary hormone secretion. *Nature (London)* **261**, 422–423.

Dean, P. M., and Matthews, E. K. (1968). Electrical activity in pancreatic islet cells. *Nature (London)* **219**, 389–390.

Dean, P. M., and Matthews, E. K. (1970a). Glucose induced electrical activity in pancreatic islet cells. *J. Physiol. (London)* **210**, 255–264.

Dean, P. M., and Matthews, E. K. (1970b). Electrical activity in pancreatic islet cells: Effect of ions. *J. Physiol. (London)* **210**, 265–275.

Douglas, W. W. (1963). A possible mechanism of neurosecretion: Release of vasopressin by depolarization and its dependence on calcium. *Nature (London)* **197**, 81–84.

Douglas, W. W. (1968). Stimulus-secretion coupling: The concept and clues from chromaffin and other cells. *Br. J. Pharmacol.* **34**, 451–474.

Douglas, W. W. (1974). Mechanism of release of neurohypophysial hormones: Stimulus-secretion coupling. *Handb. Physiol., Sect. 7: Endocrinol. 1972–1976* **4**, Part 1, 191–224.

Douglas, W. W., and Taraskevich, P. S. (1978). Action potentials in gland cells of rat pituitary pars intermedia: Inhibition by dopamine, an inhibitor of MSH secretion. *J. Physiol. (London)* **285**, 171–184.

Dreifuss, J. J., Kalnins, I., Kelly, J. S., and Ruf, K. B. (1971). Action potentials and release of neurohypophyseal hormones *in vitro*. *J. Physiol. (London)* **215**, 805–817.

Dudek, F. E., Hatton, G. I., and Mac Vicar, B. A. (1980). Intracellular recordings from the paraventricular nucleus in slices of rat hypothalamus. *J. Physiol. (London)* **301**, 101–114.

Dufy, B., and Barker, J. L. (1981). *Life Sci.* **30**, 1933–1941.

Dufy, B., and Vincent, J. D. (1980). Effects of sex steroids on cell membrane excitability: A new concept for the action of steroids on the brain. *In* "Hormones and the Brain" (D. De Wied and P. A. Van Keep, eds.), pp. 29–42. M.T.P. Press, Lancaster.

Dufy, B., Vincent, J. D., Fleury, H., Du Pasquier, P., Gourdji, D., and Tixier-Vidal, A. (1979a). Membrane effects of thyrotropin-releasing hormone and estrogen shown by intracellular recording from pituitary cells. *Science* **204**, 509–511.

Dufy, B., Vincent, J. D., Fleury, H., Du Pasquier, P., Gourdji, D., and Tixier-Vidal, A. (1979b). Dopamine inhibition of action potentials in a prolactin secreting cell line is modulated by estrogen. *Nature (London)* **282**, 855–857.

Dufy, B., Israël, J. M., Guerin, J., Dufy-Barbe, L., Zyzek, E., Fleury, H., and Vincent, J. D. (1981). Electrophysiological properties of human pituitary cells in culture. *Endocr. Soc. Annu. Meet., Cincinnati, June 17–19, 1981,* Ost. 560.

Dutton, A., Dyball, R. E. J., Poulain, D. A., and Wakerley, J. B. (1978). The importance of short interspike intervals in determining vasopressin release from isolated neurohypophysis. *J. Physiol. (London)* **280**, 23P.

Dyball, R. E. J., and Nordmann, J. J. (1977). Reactivation by veratridine of hormone release from the K^+-depolarized rat neurohypophysis. *J. Physiol. (London)* **269**, 65P.

Dyball, R. E. J., and Thomson, R. E. (1977). Augmentation of vasopressin release from the electrically stimulated rat neurohypophysis by clustering of stimulus pulses. *J. Physiol. (London)* **271**, 13P.

Enjalbert, A., Ruberg, M., Arancibia, S., Fivre, L., Priam, M., and Kordon, C. (1979). Independent inhibition of prolactin secretion by dopamine and γ-aminobutyric acid *in vitro. Endocrinology (Baltimore)* **105**, 823–826.

Fontaine, J., and Le Douarin, N. (1977). Analysis of endoderm formation in the avian blastoderm by the use of the quail-chick chimeras. The problem of the neuroectodermal origin of the cells of the APUD serie. *J. Embryol. Exp. Morphol.* **41,** 209–222.

Gähwiler, B. H., and Dreifuss, J. J. (1979). Phasically firing neurons in long term cultures of the rat hypothalamus supraoptic area: Pacemaker and follower cells. *Brain Res.* **177,** 95–103.

Gähwiler, B. H., and Dreifuss, J. J. (1980). Transition from random to phasic firing induced in neurones cultured from the hypothalamic supraoptic area. *Brain Res.* **193,** 415–425.

Gainer, H. (1978). Input-output relations of neurosecretory cells. *Comp. Endocrinol., Proc. Int. Symp., 8th, 1978* pp. 293–304.

Grodski, G. M., and Bennet, L. L. (1966). Cation requirements for insulin secretion in the isolated perfused pancreas. *Diabetes* **15,** 910–913.

Haskins, J. T., Jennings, D. P., and Rogers, J. M. (1975). Response of neuroendocrine cell firing pattern types to measured changes in plasma osmolality. *Physiologist (London* **18,** 240.

Haterius, H. O., and Fergusson, J. K. W. (1938). Evidence for the hormonal nature of the oxytocic principle of the hypophysis. *Am. J. Physiol.* **124,** 314–321.

Henquin, J. C. (1977). Tetraethylammonium potentiation of insuline release and inhibition of rubidium efflux in pancreatic islets. *Biochem. Biophys. Res. Commun.* **77,** 551–556.

Henquin, J. C. (1978a). D.-glucose inhibits potassium efflux from pancreatic islet cells. *Nature (London)* **271,** 271–273.

Henquin, J. C. (1978b). Relative importance of extracellular and intracellular calcium for the two phases of glucose stimulated insuline release: Studies with theophylline. *Endocrinology (Baltimore)* **102,** 723.

Henquin, J. C. (1980). Regulation de la sécrétion d'insuline par les changements de perméabilité au potassium des cellules β. Thèse d'agrégation, Université Catholique de Louvain.

Henquin, J. C., and Lambert, A. E. (1975). Cobalt inhibition of insulin secretion and calcium uptake by isolated rat islets. *Am. of Physiol.* **228,** 1669–1677.

Israël, J. M., Dufy, B., Gourdji, D., and Vincent, J. D. (1981). Effect of Gaba on electrical properties of cultured rat pituitary tumor cells: An intracellular recording study. *Life Sci.* **29,** 351–359.

Kandel, E. R. (1964). Electrical activity of hypothalamic neuroendocrine cells. *J. Gen. Physiol.* **47,** 691–717.

Katz, B., and Miledi, R. (1967). A study of synaptic transmission in the absence of nerve impulses. *J. Physiol. (London)* **192,** 407–436.

Kidokoro, Y. (1975). Spontaneous calcium action potentials in a clonal pituitary cell line and their relationship to prolactin secretion. *Nature (London)* **258,** 741–742.

Koizumi, K., and Yamashita, H. (1972). Studies of antidromically identified neurosecretory cells of the hypothalamus by intracellular and extracellular recordings. *J. Physiol. (London)* **221,** 683–705.

Lecar, H., and Sachs, F. (1981). Membrane noise analysis. *In* "Excitable Cells in Tissue Culture" (P. G. Nelson and M. Lieberman, eds.), pp. 137–172. Academic Press, New York.

Le Douarin, N. (1978). The embryological origin of the endocrine cells associated with the digestive tract. *In* "Gut Hormones" (S. R. Bloom, ed.), pp. 49–56. Livingstone, Edinburgh.

Legendre, P., Cooke, I. M., and Vincent, J. D. (1981). Electrophysiology of cultured hypothalamic neurons: Ca dependent plateau potentials. *11th Annu. Neurosci. Meet., Abstr.* p. 225.

Leranth, Cs., Zaborsky, L., Marton, J., and Palkovits, M. (1975). Quantitative studies on the supraoptic nucleus in the rat. I. Synaptic organization. *Exp. Brain Res.* **22,** 509–523.

Llinas, R. R. (1977). Calcium and transmitter release in squid synapse. *In* "Approaches to Cell Biology of Neurons" (W. M. Cowan and J. A. Ferrendelli, eds.), pp. 139–155. Society for Neuroscience, Bethesda, Maryland.

Lundberg, A. (1958). Electrophysiology of salivary gland. *Physiol. Rev.* **38,** 21–40.

Malaisse, W. J., Hutton, J. C., Kawazu, S., Herchuelz, A., Valverde, I., and Sener, A. (1979). The stimulus secretion coupling of glucose-induced insuline release. The links between metabolic and cationic events. *Diabetologia* **16,** 331–341.

Marty, A. (1981). Ca dependent K channels with large unitary conductance in chromaffin cell membranes. *Nature (London)* **291,** 497–500.

Mason, W. T. (1980). Supraoptic neurons of rat hypothalamus are osmosensitive. *Nature (London)* **287,** 154–157.

Matthews, E. K. (1974). Bioelectrical properties of secretory cells. *In* "Secretory Mechanisms of Exocrine Glands" (N. A. Thorn and O. H. Petersen, eds.), pp. 185–198. Munksgaard, Copenhagen.

Matthews, E. K., and Saffran, M. (1973). Ionic dependence of adrenal steroidogenesis and ACTH-induced changes in the membrane potential of adrenocortical cells. *J. Physiol. (London)* **234,** 43–64.

Matthews, E. K., and Sakamoto, Y. (1975a). Electrical characteristics of pancreatic islet cells. *J. Physiol. (London)* **246,** 421–437.

Matthews, E. K., and Sakamoto, Y. (1975b). Pancreatic islet cells: Electrogenic and electrodiffusional control of membrane potential. *J. Physiol. (London)* **246,** 439–457.

Meech, R. W., and Standen, N. B. (1975). Potassium activation in Helix neurons under voltage clamp: A component mediated by calcium influx. *J. Physiol. (London)* **249,** 211–239.

Meissner, H. P. (1976). Electrical characteristics of the beta cells in pancreatic islets. *J. Physiol. (Paris)* **72,** 757–767.

Meissner, H. P., and Atwater, I. J. (1976). The kinetics of electrical activity of beta cells in response to a square wave stimulation with glucose or glibenclamide. *Horm. Met. Res.* **351,** 195–206.

Meissner, H. P., and Schmelz, H. (1974). Membrane potential of beta cells in pancreatic islets. *Pfuegers Arch.* **351,** 195–206.

Meissner, H. P., Preissler, M., and Henquin, J. C. (1980). Possible ionic mechanisms of the electrical activity induced by glucose and tolbutamide in pancreatic beta cells. *Proc. 10th Congr. Int. Diabetis Fed.* pp. 166–171.

Meites, J. (1977). Catecholamines and prolactin secretion. *Adv. Biochem. Psychopharmacol.* **16,** 139–146.

Milligan, J. V., and Kraicer, J. (1973). Physical characteristics of the Ca^{++} compartments associated with *in vitro* ACTH release. *Endocrinology (Baltimore)* **94,** 435–443.

Nordmann, J. J. (1976). Evidence for calcium inactivation during hormone release in the rat neurohypophyses. *J. Exp. Biol.* **65,** 669–695.

Nordmann, J. J., and Dreifuss, J. J. (1972). Hormone release evoked by electrical stimulation of rat neurohypophysis in the absence of action potentials. *Brain Res.* **45,** 604–607.

Novin, D., Sundsten, J. W., and Cross, B. A. (1970). Some properties of antidromically activated units in the paraventricular nucleus of the hypothalamus. *Exp. Neurol.* **26**, 330–341.

Ozawa, S. (1981). Biphasic effect of thyrotropin-releasing hormone on membrane K^+ permeability in clonal pituitary cells. *Brain Res.* **209**, 240–244.

Ozawa, S., and Kimura, N. (1979). Membrane potential changes caused by thyrotropin-releasing hormone in the clonal GH3 cell and their relationship to secretion of pituitary hormone. *Proc. Natl. Acad. Sci. U.S.A.* **76**, 6017–6020.

Ozawa, S., and Sand, O. (1978). Electrical activity of rat anterior pituitary cells *in vitro*. *Acta Physiol. Scand.* **102**, 330–341.

Pace, C. S., and Price, S. (1972). Electrical responses of pancreatic islet cell to secretory stimuli. *Biochem. Biophys. Res. Commun.* **46**, 1557–1563.

Pearse, A. G. E. (1969). The cytochemistry and ultrastructure of polypeptide hormone-producing cells of the APUD series and the embryologic, physiologic, and pathologic implications of the concept. *J. Histochem. Cytochem.* **17**, 303–313.

Poulsen, J. H., and Williams, J. A. (1976). Spontaneous repetitive hyperpolarisations from cells in the rat adenohypophysus. *Nature (London)* **263**, 156–158.

Sakai, K. K., Marks, B. H., George, J.M., and Koestner, A. (1974). The isolated organ-cultured supraoptic nucleus as a neuropharmacological test system. *J. Pharmacol. Exp. Ther.* **190**, 482–491.

Sand, O., Haug, E., and Gautvik, K. M. (1980). Effects of thyroliberin and 4-amino-pyridine on action potentials and prolactin release and synthesis in rat pituitary cells in culture. *Acta Physiol. Scand.* **108**, 247–252.

Smith, T. G., Jr., Barker, J. L., Smith, B. M., and Colburn, T. R. (1981). Voltage clamp techniques applied to cultured skeletal muscle and spinal neurons. *In* "Excitable Cells in Tissue Culture" (P. G. Nelson and M. Lieberman, eds.), pp. 111–136. Academic Press, New York.

Stallcup, W. B. (1979). Sodium and calcium fluxes in a clonal nerve cell line. *J. Physiol. (London)* **286**, 525–540.

Swaab, D. F., Nihveledt, F., and Pool, C. W. (1975). Distribution of oxytocin and vasopressin in the rat supraoptic and paraventricular nucleus. *J. Endocrinol.* **67**, 461–462.

Takor-Takor, T., and Pearse, A. G. E. (1975). Neurectodermal origin of avian hypo-thalamo-hypophyseal complex: The role of the ventral neural ridge. *J. Embryol. Exp. Morphol.* **31**, 311–325.

Taraskevitch, P. S., and Douglas, W. W. (1977). Action potentials occur in cells of the normal anterior pituitary gland and are stimulated by the hypophysiotropic peptide thyrotropin-releasing hormone. *Proc. Natl. Acad. Sci. U.S.A.* **74**, 4064–4067.

Taraskevitch, P. S., and Douglas, W. W. (1978). Catecholamines of supposed inhibitory hypophysiotropic function supress action potentials in prolactin cells. *Nature (London)* **276**, 831–834.

Taraskevitch, P. S., and Douglas, W. W. (1979). Stimulant effect of 5-hydroxytryptamine on action potential activity in pars intermedia cells of the lizard, *Anolis car-olineuris:* Contrasting effects in pars intermedia of rat and rostral pars distalis of fish (*Alosa pseudoharengus*). *Brain Res.* **178**, 584–588.

Taraskevitch, P. S., and Douglas, W. W. (1980). Electrical behavior in a line of anterior pituitary cells (GH cells) and the influence of the hypothalamic peptide, thy-rotropin releasing factor. *Neuroscience* **5**, 421–431.

Tasaki, K., and Cooke, I. M. (1979). Spontaneous electrical activity and interaction of large and small cells in cardiac ganglion of the crab, *Portunus sanguinolentus*. *J. Neurophysiol.* **42**, 975–999.

Theodosis, D., Legendre, P., and Vincent, J. D. (1981). Evidence for vasopressin like neurons in primary cultures of dissociated fetal mouse hypothalamus. *11th Annu. Neurosci. Meet., Abstr.* pp. 150.

Thompson, S. (1977). Three pharmacologically distinct potassium channels in molluscam neurones. *J. Physiol. (London)* **265**, 465–488.

Tilders, F. J. H., and Smelik, P. G. (1977). Direct neural control of MSH secretion in mammals: The involvement of dopaminergic tubero-hypophyseal neurons. *Front. Horm. Res.* **4**, 80–93.

Tischler, A. S., Dichter, M. A., Biales, B., Delellis, R. A., and Wolfe, H. (1976). Neural properties of cultured human endocrine tumors of proposed neural crest origin. *Science* **192**, 902–904.

Trifaro, J. M. (1977). Common mechanisms of hormone secretion. *Am. Rev. Pharmacol. Toxicol.* **17**, 27–47.

Vandesande, F., and Diericks, K. (1975). Identification of the vasopressin producing and of the oxytocin producing neurons in the hypothalamic magnocellular neurosecretory system of the rat. *Cell Tissue Res.* **164**, 153–162.

Vincent, J. D., Dufy, B., Israel, J. M., Zyzek, E., Dufy-Barbe, L., Guerin, J., Gourdji, D., and Tixier-Vidal, A. (1980a). Neurohormonal communication: An electrophysiological study of the membrane properties of anterior pituitary cells. *In* "Progress in Psychoneuroendocrinology" (F. Brambilla, G. Racagni, and D. De Wied, eds.), pp. 25–37. Elsevier, Amsterdam.

Vincent, J. D., Dufy, B., Gourdji, D., and Tixier-Vidal, A. (1980b). Electrical correlates of prolactin secretion in cloned pituitary cells. *In* "Central and Peripheral Regulation of Prolactin Function" (R. M. MacLeod and V. Scapagnini, eds.), pp. 141–157. Raven, New York.

Vincent, J. D., Poulain, D., and Arnauld, E. (1980c). Electrophysiology of magnocellular neuroendocrine cells. *In* "The Role of Peptides in Neuronal Function" (J. L. Barker, and T. G. Smith, Jr., eds.), pp. 230–272. Dekker, New York.

Wakerley, J. B., and Lincoln, D. W. (1971). Phasic discharge of antidromically identified units in the paraventricular nucleus of the hypothalamus. *Brain Res.* **25**, 192–194.

Wakerley, J. B., and Lincoln, D. W. (1973). The milk ejection reflex of the rat: A 20 to 40 fold acceleration in the firing of paraventricular neurones during oxytocin release. *J. Endocrinol.* **57**, 477–493.

Wakerley, J. B., Poulain, D. A. and Brown, D. (1978). Comparison of firing patterns in oxytocin- and vasopressin-releasing neurones during progressive dehydration. *Brain Res.* **148**, 425–440.

Yagi, K., and Iwasaki, S. (1977). Electrophysiology of the neurosecretory cell. *Int. Rev. Cytol.* **48**, 141–186.

Yamashita, H., Koizumi, K., and Brooks, C., McC. (1970). Electrophysiological studies of neurosecretory cells in the cat hypothalamus. *Brain Res.* **20**, 462–466.

York, D. H., Baker, F. L. and Kraicer, J. (1971). Electrical properties of cells in the adenohypophysis. An in vivo study. *Neuroendocrinology* **8**, 10–16.

Zyzek, E., Dufy-Barbe, L., Dufy, B., and Vincent, J. D. (1981). Short-term effect of estrogen release of prolactin by pituitary cells in culture. *Biochem. Biophys. Res. Commun.* **102**, 1151–1152.

Zyzek, E., Dufy, B., Fleury, H., and Vincent, J. D. (1982). Flux de ^{45}Ca dans des cellules hypophysaires en culture. Effet du Potassium et du TRH. *C. R. Soc. Biol. Ses. Fil.* in press.

5

Protein-Carboxyl Methylation: Putative Role in Exocytosis and in the Cellular Regulation of Secretion and Chemotaxis

EMANUEL J. DILIBERTO, JR.

I. INTRODUCTION

Protein structure is primarily determined by the amino acid sequence of the polypeptide that is genetically expressed during transla-

147

tion. Additional changes in protein structure can occur posttranslationally through modifications of amino acid side chains. Reactions such as hydroxylation, acetylation, thiolation, adenylation, glycosylation, phosphorylation, and methylation are well recognized as contributors to the final structure of many proteins.

In recent years, the modification of proteins by methylation has been studied extensively and shown to be a widely occurring reaction in both eukaryotes and prokaryotes. Protein methylation may occur at several different amino acid residues and involves specific enzymes. Three different enzymes are involved in N-methylation of lysyl, arginyl, and histidyl residues, with S-adenosyl-L-methionine as the methyl donor (Paik and Kim, 1975).

One additional protein methylase that has received considerable attention catalyzes the O-methylation of free carboxyl groups of proteins. Protein-carboxyl methylase (S-adenosylmethionine:protein-carboxyl methyltransferase, EC 2.1.1.24; protein carboxymethylase; protein methylase II) transfers a methyl group from S-adenosyl-L-methionine to glutamyl or aspartyl residues in the formation of protein-carboxyl methyl esters (Liss *et al.,* 1969; Kim and Paik, 1970; Diliberto and Axelrod, 1974). Thus, at physiological pH, protein-carboxyl methylation results in the neutralization of negative charges on proteins. In contrast to other protein methylation reactions, the protein-carboxyl methyl ester product is labile, suggesting that this enzyme system functions to induce rapid and reversible changes in the conformation of proteins (Diliberto and Axelrod, 1976). It is tempting to speculate that this type of system may be involved in the activation or inactivation of enzymes, protein hormones, or other biologically active proteins. This chapter examines the evidence for an alternative function for protein-carboxyl methylation, i.e., the neutralization of negative charges on intracellular membranes, promoting fusion of different membranes such as occurs in the secretory process. This chapter also explores the possible participation of protein-carboxyl methylation in the processing of exportable products and describes its known function in bacterial chemotaxis.

II. PROTEIN-CARBOXYL METHYLASE

A. History

In a study of the distribution of phenylethanolamine-N-methyltransferase in various tissues, Axelrod and Daly (1965) observed that, upon incubation of pituitary extracts with S-adenosyl-L-[*methyl*-^{14}C]methionine, a radioactive product was formed that was volatile and extractable with organic solvents. The volatile product was identified as methanol, which was concomitantly formed with S-adenosyl-L-homocysteine (the second product of the enzymatic reaction). The enzyme responsible for this reaction was thus called the "methanol-forming" enzyme. Independently, Liss and Edelstein (1967) observed a puromycin-insensitive incorporation of L-[*methyl*-^{14}C]methionine into proteins in rat skin extracts. Because L-[*methyl*-^{14}C]methionine and ATP could be replaced by S-adenosyl-L-[*methyl*-^{14}C]methionine and because the product of hydrolysis of the protein in alkali was [^{14}C]methanol, the reaction was thought to involve methylation of proteins, possibly at free carboxyl groups of protein (Liss *et al.*, 1969). Subsequently, Kim and Paik (1970) partially purified a protein methylase from calf thymus that transferred labile methyl groups to proteins with S-adenosyl-L-methionine as the methyl donor. Again, the product of hydrolysis was identified as methanol and the reaction was proposed to involve an ester linkage. Within 8 years of the initial observations by Axelrod and Daly (1965), Morin and Liss (1973) and Kim (1973) established that the "methanol-forming" enzyme was a protein-carboxyl methylase. Under the assay conditions (mild alkaline extraction) of Axelrod and Daly (1965), the enzymatically formed protein-carboxyl methyl esters were hydrolyzed to liberate methanol. Consequently, methanol was thought to be the final product of the reaction.

B.   Enzymology

1.   *Site of Methylation*

Early studies on the site of methylation by protein-carboxyl methylase suggested free carboxyl groups of substrate proteins (see Section II,A). Additional evidence for the formation of an ester linkage at free carboxyl groups of proteins was provided in a study where a parallel decrease in methyl-acceptor activity was observed when free carboxyl groups on the substrate protein were progressively blocked by conversion to glycine methyl ester amides (Kim and Paik, 1971a). Methyl-acceptor activity was recovered upon hydrolysis of the ester bond of the modified protein.

Evidence suggesting that free carboxyl groups on side chains and not the C-terminal carboxyl group were the sites of methylation was provided in a study where the protein substrate (oxidized ribonuclease) was partially digested with trypsin and/or chymotrypsin. Because the number of methyl groups transferred per unit weight of protein was not changed by this treatment, the C-terminal carboxyl group was probably not a methyl-acceptor site (Kim and Paik, 1971a). Moreover, chemical reduction of enzymatically methylated proteins with lithium borohydride followed by hydrolysis in 6 N HCl yielded two new hydroxyamino acids: δ-hydroxy-α-aminovaleric acid and γ-hydroxy-α-aminobutyric acid (Paik and Kim, 1975), indicating that the free carboxyl groups of glutamic and aspartic acids (respectively) were the likely sites of methylation. Direct evidence that glutamyl and/or aspartyl residues were indeed the methylation sites was first provided in bacteria. Bacterial protein-carboxyl methylase was shown to catalyze the formation of a γ-glutamyl methyl ester in membrane proteins of *Salmonella typhimurium* (Van Der Werf and Koshland, 1977) and *Escherichia coli* (Kleene *et al.*, 1977). Mammalian protein-carboxyl methylase yields a product with much greater instability than that of the bacterial product; thus, until recently, direct evidence that glutamyl and/or aspartyl residues were involved in this system was lacking. Janson and Clarke (1980) identified aspartic acid β-methyl ester in proteolytic digests of *in vivo* and *in vitro* methylated plasma membrane proteins from human erythrocytes. Because glutamic acid γ-methyl ester was not detected, they suggested that aspartic acid residues were the methylation sites in human red blood cells. This difference in the site of methylation between prokaryotic and eukaryotic cells may explain the greater lability of methylated eukaryotic proteins (Bernhard *et al.*, 1962). Whether glutamyl residues are also methylation sites for eukaryotic protein is unclear; however, indirect evidence suggesting the formation of a glutamic acid γ-methyl ester of α_s-ACTH has been reported (Kim and Li, 1979a; see also Paik and Kim, 1975). Thus, the product of protein-carboxyl methylation is indeed protein-carboxyl methyl esters at glutamyl and/or aspartyl residues of proteins.

In characterizing the product of the reaction as protein-carboxyl methyl ester, it was important to eliminate the possibility that other reactions such as cleavage of peptide bonds might be occurring in addition to transmethylation. Several studies with the bovine pituitary enzyme and a number of purified protein substrates showed that after incubation with S-adenosyl-L-[*methyl*-^{14}C]methionine single radioactive peaks were isolated by gel filtration chromatography and coeluted with single protein peaks (E. J. Diliberto, Jr. and J. Axelrod, unpublished observations). These results have now been repeated by other laboratories (see Section II,D); thus, peptide cleavage is not catalyzed by this enzyme.

Protein-carboxyl methylase is highly specific for S-adenosyl-L-methionine as the methyl donor. The specificity for polypeptide and protein substrates will be discussed in a separate section on methyl-acceptor proteins (Section II,D).

2. Physical Properties

Protein-carboxyl methylase has been purified from various sources, such as calf spleen (Liss *et al.*, 1969), calf thymus (Kim and Paik, 1970; Kim, 1973), bovine pituitary (Diliberto and Axelrod, 1974, 1976), equine erythrocytes (Polastro *et al.*, 1978), rat erythrocytes (Kim, 1974), and calf brain (Kim *et al.*, 1978).

The mammalian enzyme has an apparent molecular mass of 25,000 daltons in most tissues examined (Kim, 1974; Kim *et al.*, 1978; Polastro *et al.*, 1978). Although it has been proposed that the enzyme exists in various molecular forms, with a subunit molecular weight of 8000 (Paik and Kim, 1975), studies by Polastro *et al.* (1978) show that the enzyme is a single polypeptide chain with a molecular weight of 25,000. Purified protein-carboxyl methylase from calf thymus was reported to have an isoelectric point of 4.95 (Kim and Paik, 1978), whereas multiple peaks of enzyme activity were observed during electrofocusing of partially purified rat erythrocyte enzyme (Kim, 1974). However, highly purified equine erythrocyte enzyme gives only a single peak of activity, with an isoelectric point of 5.6 (Polastro *et al.*, 1978). Equine erythrocyte protein-carboxyl methylase is a glycoprotein containing 2% neutral hexose. A protein-carboxyl methylase from *Salmonella typhimurium* has also been purified and shown to have a M_r of approximately 38,000 (Springer and Koshland, 1977; Clarke *et al.*, 1980).

3. Catalytic Properties

The pH optimum for protein-carboxyl methylase varies with the protein substrate. The bovine pituitary enzyme has a narrow pH optimum at pH 5.5, with luteinizing hormone as the protein substrate (Diliberto and Axelrod, 1974). Protein substrates from various sources showed different pH optima: 6.0 for histone and fibrinogen; 6.5 for γ-globulin; and 7.4 for gelatin (Kim and Paik, 1970, 1971a; Kim, 1974). Membrane-bound and soluble proteins from adrenal chromaffin vesicles had a pH optimum of approximately 6.0 to 6.5 (Gagnon *et al.*, 1978a; E. J. Diliberto, Jr. and O. H. Viveros, unpublished observations). This variability of pH optimum probably reflects the fact that the dissociated carboxyl group is the chemical species being methylated. The enzyme appears to be stable at alkaline pH values up to approximately 10 (Kim, 1973).

The kinetics for protein-carboxyl methylation were first studied with the bovine pituitary enzyme and luteinizing hormone as the protein substrate (Diliberto and Axelrod, 1974). A sequential mechanism (Cleland, 1970) was shown, indicating that S-adenosyl-L-methionine and luteinizing hormone combined with the enzyme to form a ternary complex before product formation. In this study, a limiting K_m of 1.47 μM was calculated for S-adenosyl-L-methionine (Diliberto and Axelrod, 1974). The kinetic parameters, however, were shown to vary greatly, depending on the polypeptide or protein substrate (Jamaluddin et al., 1976). Also, a discrepancy in the apparent K_m for S-adenosyl-L-methionine with luteinizing hormone as the protein substrate suggests a difference between bovine pituitary (Diliberto and Axelrod, 1974) and calf thymus (Jamaluddin et al., 1976) protein-carboxyl methylases. Further studies on the kinetic mechanism were performed with the product inhibitor S-adenosyl-L-homocysteine. The results of these experiments indicate a rapid equilibrium, random Bi–Bi mechanism, where the rate-limiting step may be in the interconversion of the central ternary complexes (Jamaluddin et al., 1975).

Although the bacterial enzyme appears to be similar to the mammalian enzyme with respect to molecular weight and pH optimum, the apparent K_m (10 μM) with respect to S-adenosyl-L-methionine is 5- to 10-fold greater than the mammalian system (Springer and Koshland, 1977).

4. Activators and Inhibitors

Protein-carboxyl methylase isolated from various sources does not require a metal cofactor. Ions such as Ca^{2+}, Mn^{2+}, Cu^{2+}, Zn^{2+}, Co^{2+}, Fe^{2+}, Fe^{3+}, and Mg^{2+} at 2 mM had no effect on the enzyme activity (Kim and Paik, 1970). Also, the divalent cations Ca^{2+} and Mg^{2+} did not alter the in vitro rate of methylation of membrane fractions of the adrenal medulla (Diliberto et al., 1979). With regard to potential activators of this enzyme, postmicrosomal supernatant fractions of the bovine adrenal medulla exhibited a positive cooperativity with increasing concentrations of this fraction, suggesting the presence of soluble activators in this tissue (E. J. Diliberto, Jr., and O. H. Viveros, unpublished observations).

More recently, the bacterial protein-carboxyl methylase was shown to be competitively inhibited by Ca^{2+}, with a K_i of approximately 80 nM (Ullah and Ordal, 1981). This exquisite sensitivity to Ca^{2+} may represent an additional difference between the bacterial and mammalian enzymes.

Protein-carboxyl methylase, like other methyltransferases, is inhibited by S-adenosyl-L-homocysteine, a product of the transmethylation reaction (Zappia et al., 1969; Deguchi and Barchas, 1971; Kim, 1974). In addition, analogs of S-adenosyl-L-homocysteine with greater inhibitory potency (including the antifungal antibiotics sinefungin and A9145C) have been described (Borchardt, 1980; O'Dea et al., 1981).

C. Functional Significance of the Reaction

In Section I, I alluded to the consequences of methylation of free carboxyl groups with regard to the neutralization of negative charges on proteins. Theoretical considerations, based on the increase in the hydrophobic character of proteins by the addition of a nonpolar methyl group as well as the neutralization of a negative charge on proteins, would suggest major conformational changes arising from protein-carboxyl methylation (Tanford, 1962). The effect of chemical modification of carboxyl side chains on the three-dimensional structure of proteins has been intensely studied in recent years. In one study, a derivative of hemoglobin was prepared by reduction of some glutamyl and aspartyl residues to their corresponding alcohols by diborane. Substantial conformational changes were observed in the modified protein (Atassi and Nakhleh, 1975). Coupling the glutamyl residues 83 and 85 of myoglobin with glycine methyl ester, after carbodiimide activation, showed gross conformational changes. On the other hand, when myoglobin was coupled with histidine methyl ester, no conformational changes were observed; thus, the loss in the hydrophilic character of the carboxyl group with the glycine methyl ester appears to be the major force involved in refolding of the protein (Atassi and Singhal, 1972). These results indicate that as a consequence of protein-carboxyl methylation gross changes would occur in the structure of proteins. The tendency toward a more hydrophobic character suggests that greater changes may occur upon methylation of membrane protein. Protein-carboxyl methylation of membrane proteins may increase the interaction between the protein and the lipid layer of the membrane, allowing for partial internalization of the protein. It should be apparent from the aforementioned data that protein-carboxyl methylation has the potential to cause specific functional modifications of biologically active proteins.

D. Methyl-Acceptor Proteins

A systematic approach to the investigation of the biological function(s) of mammalian protein-carboxyl methylase has been hampered by the unstable nature of the product. This fact is best exemplified by a comparison of the bacterial and mammalian systems. The much greater stability of bacterial protein-carboxyl methyl esters has enabled the identification of specific natural substrates that play a key role in chemotaxis (Springer and Koshland, 1977; Van Der Werf and Koshland, 1977; Goy *et al.*, 1977; Springer *et al.*, 1979). The presence and participation of a protein-carboxyl methylase in bacterial chemotaxis (Springer and Koshland, 1977) followed the earlier identification of specific proteins (Kort *et al.*, 1975) that were methylated in response to the chemotactic stimulus. Isolation of such products from mammalian cells was not possible until recently, presumably as a result of their lability. Thus, although the presence of the enzyme in mammalian cells has been recognized for many years, the physiological role(s) of this enzyme remains unknown. This prompted investigators to concentrate on the identification of those proteins that may be physiological substrates for this enzyme.

1. Structural Requirements

The three-dimensional structure of the protein substrate is an important factor influencing its ability to accept a methyl group from *S*-adenosyl-L-methionine (Paik and Kim, 1975). With pancreatic ribonuclease, Kim and Paik (1971a) showed that denaturation of the protein by oxidation or reduction resulted in an increase in the rate of methylation when compared to the native protein. They postulated that denaturation of ribonuclease made the reactive carboxyl groups more easily accessible to protein-carboxyl methylase. Furthermore, partial digestion of oxidized ribonuclease did not alter the methyl-acceptor capacity of the substrate protein. More complete digestion with Pronase, however, destroyed the ability of oxidized ribonuclease to serve as substrate. Thus, it would appear that a minimum peptide chain sequence is necessary for substrate activity (Kim and Paik, 1971a). It should be pointed out that although the ribonuclease fragments can function as methyl-acceptor proteins, they have a much lower apparent K_m for protein-carboxyl methylase than native proteins (Jamaluddin *et al.*, 1976).

2. Ligand-Induced Changes in Substrate Activity

Ligand-mediated changes in the conformation of specific proteins have been shown to affect the rate of methylation. The posterior pituitary hormone-binding proteins (neurophysins) are effective methyl acceptors for protein-carboxyl methylase whereas the posterior pituitary hormones oxytocin and vasopressin did not serve as substrates (see

Section II,D,3). An increase in the rate of neurophysin II methylation was observed with both oxytocin and the hormone-related tripeptide ligand methionyltyrosylphenylalaninamide. This ligand-induced response did not occur with either native neurophysin I or disulfide-scrambled neurophysin II (Diliberto et al., 1976a). The greater affinity of neurophysin for the enzyme by ligand binding suggests that the tertiary and/or quaternary structure of the protein substrate is important in the formation of the enzyme–substrate complex. Similar results were obtained with neurophysin I and the ligand arginine-vasopressin, although the ligand-induced increase in the rate of methylation appeared to be due to an increase in the maximum velocity, with no change in the apparent K_m (Edgar and Hope, 1976). Finally, an increase in the rate of methylation of α^{7-38}-ACTH was observed after prolonged incubation with α^{1-17}-ACTH. Because α^{1-17}-ACTH did not serve as a methyl acceptor, an induced conformational change probably occurred in the α^{7-38}-ACTH fragment (Kim and Li, 1979b).

3. Substrate Specificity

When a number of soluble and membrane-bound proteins were tested as substrates on the bacterial protein-carboxyl methylase system, only the 56,000- to 65,000-dalton proteins of bacterial membranes could serve as methyl acceptors in vitro (Stock and Koshland, 1978; Springer et al., 1979; Panasenko and Koshland, 1979). Unlike the bacterial system, the substrate specificity of the mammalian enzyme is quite broad (Kim and Paik, 1970; Diliberto and Axelrod, 1974). One of the first studies designed to probe the function of protein-carboxyl methylase through an examination of its substrate specificity was conducted by Diliberto and Axelrod (1974). In a search for possible endogenous substrates for this enzyme, the ability of protein pituitary hormones to serve as methyl acceptors was examined. The most active substrates were the anterior pituitary hormone, luteinizing hormone, and the posterior pituitary carrier proteins (neurophysins) (Diliberto and Axelrod, 1974; Axelrod and Diliberto, 1975; Diliberto et al., 1976a). In fact, all anterior pituitary hormones were found to be effective methyl acceptors. The posterior pituitary hormones oxytocin and vasopressin, poly-L-aspartic acid, and poly-L-glutamic acid were not substrates for this enzyme. In addition, the calcium-binding protein calmodulin was also shown to be an especially active methyl-acceptor protein (Gagnon et al., 1981).

Concurrent with investigations uncovering the role of protein-carboxyl methylase in bacterial chemotaxis involving methylation of specific cytoplasmic membrane proteins, the participation of the mammalian enzyme in adrenomedullary secretion was under investigation. In the course of these experiments, the ability of membrane proteins to function as methyl acceptors for protein-carboxyl methylase was demonstrated (Diliberto et al., 1976b). The selective methylation of two groups of chromaffin vesicle membrane polypeptides was the first demonstration of specificity for this enzyme (Gagnon et al., 1978a). Subsequently, a number of mammalian systems have been examined, and the specific protein-carboxyl methylation of certain membrane proteins was observed. One system worthy of mention at this point is the erythrocyte, which has enzyme predominantly in the cytosol (Kim et al., 1975a; O'Dea et al., 1978a), whereas methyl-acceptor proteins are exclusively associated with the plasma membrane (O'Dea et al., 1978a). Galletti et al. (1978) demonstrated the selective methyl esterification of erythrocyte membrane proteins with apparent molecular weights of 97,000, 75,000, and 48,000. Subsequently, the high-molecular-weight methylated polypeptides (97,000) were partially characterized and one component was identified as glycophorin A (Galletti et al., 1979). The [³H]methyl incorporation into membrane proteins in vivo was observed when human erythrocytes were incubated with L-[methyl-³H]methionine (Kim et al., 1980). Analysis of the methylated proteins by gel electrophoresis revealed two major radioactive peaks, tentatively identified as glycophorin A and "band 4.5" (similar to the in vitro methylation pattern). The selective methylation of membrane proteins in human erythrocytes also has been studied with a pH 2.4 sodium dodecyl sulfate gel electrophoretic system (Fairbanks and Avruch, 1972), which minimizes hydrolysis of the protein-carboxyl methyl esters (Terwilliger and Clarke, 1981). The in vitro incubation of lysed erythrocytes in the presence of S-adenosyl-L-[methyl-[³H]methionine resulted in the specific incorporation of labile methyl groups into polypeptides with M_r = 96,000, 44,000, and 27,000. The radioactive peak at 96,000 comigrated with the Coomassie blue staining in the "band 3" region, wheras the 44,000 peak comigrated only with the periodic acid-Schiff reagent-1-stained polypeptide. The radioactive peak at 27,000 was not associated with any major stained peaks. With lithium diiodosalicylate pretreatment, it was shown that no extrinsic membrane proteins are methylated in this system. Further analysis showed that the band 3 anion transport protein and the major sialoglycoprotein (glycophorin) are specifically methylated. In addition, two minor unidentified intrinsic membrane proteins are methylated in vitro; one peptide comigrates with the band 3 anion transport protein (M_r = 96,000) and the other migrates as a polypeptide of M_r = 23,000 (Terwilliger and Clarke, 1981). Experiments with intact

human erythrocytes incubated with L-[*methyl*-³H]methionine showed
that at least 90% of the methyl groups incorporated were base labile.
The major methylated species include the cytoskeletal polypeptides
"band 2.1" (ankyrin) and "band 4.1" as well as the band 3 anion transport protein; the major sialoglycoprotein was not methylated (Freitag
and Clarke, 1981). These studies illustrate the necessity for *in vivo*
studies for two reasons: (1) the patterns of methylated proteins obtained from *in vitro* versus *in vivo* labeling experiments showed at
least one common labeled polypeptide (band 3 anion transport protein),
but also showed major differences; and (2) the *in vivo* experiments
uncovered a selective methylation of the cytoskeletal polypeptides,
suggesting a different specificity for protein-carboxyl methylation *in
vivo*. Finally, the *in vivo* rate of turnover of the various methylated
proteins was shown to vary markedly, with half-lives ranging from
less than 2 to 29 hours (Freitag and Clarke, 1981). The hydrolysis of
these protein-carboxyl methyl esters *in vivo* can result from enzymatic
and nonenzymatic reactions (see Section II,D,4). This suggests that
demethylation is probably a component of the protein-carboxyl methylase system and may constitute an additional factor involved in the
participation of methylation in the regulation of cell functions.

   In this section, we were able to explore in some detail the question of
whether the broad substrate specificity of the mammalian enzyme
found *in vitro* might be restricted to a much greater specificity *in vivo*.
The broad substrate specificity of this enzyme *in vitro* might be explained by a high degree of conformational mobility (Jarabak and
Westley, 1974; see Section III,B,2).

4. Stability of Protein-Carboxyl Methyl Esters

   Early studies on protein-carboxyl methylation clearly showed that
the product of this reaction was base labile (Liss *et al.*, 1969; Kim and
Paik, 1970; Diliberto and Axelrod, 1974). However, the functional significance of spontaneous hydrolysis in terms of the physiological role
for protein-carboxyl methylation was more recently examined. Enzymatically prepared methyl esters of ovalbumin were shown to undergo rapid spontaneous hydrolysis; at physiological pH and temperature,
less than 25% of the methyl ester remained after 1 hour (Diliberto and
Axelrod, 1976). A similar half-life of hydrolysis was obtained for
ribonuclease-carboxyl methyl ester (Kim and Paik, 1976; Galletti *et
al.*, 1978). In the course of experiments studying enzymatic methylation of chromaffin vesicle membrane proteins, a much greater rate of
hydrolysis was observed with these membrane protein methyl esters
(Gagnon *et al.*, 1978a). In fact, this *in vitro* rate of demethylation is

more rapid than the shortest half-life observed in human erythrocytes *in vivo* (Freitag and Clarke, 1981). Nonetheless, preliminary experiments did suggest that *in vivo* demethylation was more rapid than the spontaneous hydrolysis rate (Viveros *et al.*, 1977). It was not until recently, however, that this process was considered to be enzymatic in eukaryotes. The presence of such an esterase in mammalian tissue was first reported by Gagnon (1979) in a variety of organs, with the highest specific activity present in the kidney.

E.   The Protein-Carboxyl Methylesterase

Because the bacterial protein-carboxyl methylase system generates a product with much greater stability, it is not surprising that the existence of a protein methylesterase was first discovered in bacteria. Protein-carboxyl methylation is essential for bacterial chemotaxis; and in nonchemotactic mutants, protein-carboxyl methylase or its methyl-accepting chemotaxis proteins are lacking (Van Der Werf and Koshland, 1977; Springer and Koshland, 1977; Goy *et al.*, 1977; Springer *et al.*, 1979). Motile bacteria also contain a protein methylesterase that catalyzes the deesterification of the methylated chemotaxis proteins, thus influencing the steady-state levels of carboxyl-methylated proteins (Stock and Koshland, 1978, 1979; Toews and Adler, 1979). Because of the greater stability of bacterial protein-carboxyl methyl esters, a protein methylesterase is needed for the rapid and reversible changes in protein-carboxyl methylation that are required for this system to be an effective transducer in stimulus– response coupling.

In mammals, protein-carboxyl methylesterase is associated with both soluble and membrane-bound fractions in several tissues (Gagnon, 1979). In rabbit neutrophils, the methylesterase is mainly localized in the cytosolic fraction, although a substantial enzyme activity was found in the microsomal fraction (Venkatasubramanian *et al.*, 1980). In addition, methylation and demethylation of nuclear proteins at carboxyl groups has been described. The methylation of non-histone chromosomal proteins was investigated *in vitro* and *in vivo*. Specific chromosomal proteins were shown to be methylated in various tissues, and different patterns of protein methyl esters were obtained. The presence of a protein methylesterase possibly bound to chromatin was suggested in these studies (Quick *et al.*, 1981).

The protein methylesterase activity observed in various tissues may well represent the presence of an enzyme that specifically catalyzes the hydrolysis of protein-carboxyl methyl esters. On the other hand, this activity may be the result of previously reported carboxylesterases purified from the liver of several species (Inkerman *et al.*, 1975; Dudman and Zerner, 1975; Scott and Zerner, 1975). Purification and characterization of this protein methylesterase will be required to demonstrate whether this enzyme is unique to the protein-carboxyl methylation system.

F.   The Protein-Carboxyl Methylation System

It is now well recognized that eukaryotes and prokaryotes possess an enzyme system that catalyzes the specific methyl esterification of carboxyl side chains of proteins (Fig. 1). This enzyme, coupled to the recently demonstrated protein methylesterase activity, represents a readily reversible system for the neutralization of negative charges, which may produce conformational changes in proteins. Through charge neutralization and/or subsequent conformational change, the function of biologically active proteins is altered. This system has been implicated as an important regulator of a number of cellular events, including neurosecretion and chemotaxis (Fig. 1). The next section presents arguments in favor of the participation of this system in the secretory process.

III.   EXOCYTOTIC SECRETION AND PROTEIN-CARBOXYL METHYLATION

A.   Initial Studies on the Biological Functions of Protein-Carboxyl Methylation

1.   *Tissue Distribution of Protein-Carboxyl Methylase and Methyl-Acceptor Proteins*

Protein-carboxyl methylase is ubiquitously distributed in mammalian tissues. Initial studies on the tissue distribution in rats showed a high specific activity of the enzyme in testis and brain and low activity in liver (Kim and Paik, 1971b; Kim *et al.*, 1975a). As a result of the finding that the anterior pituitary hormones were very active as methyl-acceptor proteins (Diliberto and Axelrod, 1974), an extensive study of the enzyme activity as well as the presence of endogenous substrates in various rat tissues was undertaken (Diliberto and Axelrod, 1976). The various tissues and brain regions were assayed in the presence of added protein substrates (exogenous activity) as a measure of total enzyme activity or in the absence of added protein substrates

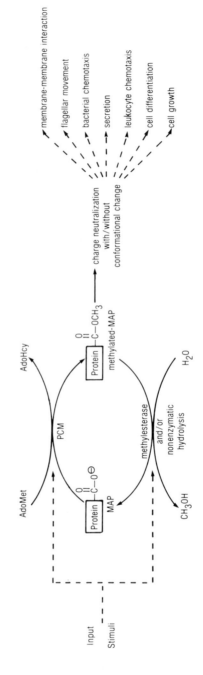

Fig. 1. A scheme representing the role of protein-carboxyl methylation and demethylation in the transduction of ligand–receptor interaction to cellular responses. PCM, Protein-carboxyl methylase; MAP, methyl-acceptor protein; AdoMet, S-adenosyl-L-methionine; AdoHcy, S-adenosyl-L-homocysteine.

(endogenous activity), which is a measure of the endogenous methyl-acceptor proteins undergoing enzymatic carboxyl methylation. The highest specific activity of any tissue examined was found in the brain, followed by the testis, pituitary, and heart. The activity of the posterior lobe of the pituitary was found to be twice that of the anterior lobe. The ratio of enzyme activities in the presence and absence of protein substrate was used to estimate the level of endogenous substrate(s) present in a given tissue: the lower the ratio, the greater the amount of endogenous substrate(s). The results showed that the pituitary gland has the greatest amount of endogenous protein substrate, with the two lobes being equal. This specific activity ratio varied from 2.0 for the pituitary gland to 35.2 for the testis. Secretory tissues, such as the adrenal and thyroid glands, and neural tissues had substantial enzyme activity and endogenous methyl-acceptor protein content (Diliberto and Axelrod, 1976). In the testis, approximately 70% of the enzyme activity was found in the seminiferous tubule (Sertoli cells) and the remainder in the interstitial (Leydig cells) compartment (Kim et al., 1975b). Testicular cells were dissociated with collagenase and trypsin and fractionated on an albumin gradient, and the highest specific activity was found in spermatids; the pachytene spermatocytes had about one-half the specific activity of the spermatids. The methyl-acceptor protein content was also highest in the spermatid fraction (Gagnon et al., 1979a).

Protein-carboxyl methylase was shown to be present in erythrocytes (Kim, 1974; O'Dea et al., 1978a), leukocytes (O'Dea et al., 1978b), and platelets (O'Dea et al., 1978a), although the enzyme activity was nearly absent from blood plasma (Kim, 1974). In human erythrocytes, the cytosol, which is where the enzyme is predominantly localized, was devoid of methyl-acceptor protein. On the other hand, the methyl-acceptor proteins were associated with the plasma membrane fraction (O'Dea et al., 1978a; see Section II,D,3).

Diliberto and Axelrod (1976) examined tissues with several different protein substrates to assess whether protein-carboxyl methylase from different tissues was the same enzyme. Because a nearly identical specific activity ratio for two different protein substrates was obtained in all tissues examined, one enzyme appears to be responsible for carboxyl methylase activity throughout different tissues. However, further analysis of this question requires purification of the enzyme from the various tissues, followed by determination of their physical and catalytic properties. More recent attempts have made major advances, but conflicting results have appeared (Kim, 1974; Paik and Kim, 1975; Kim and Paik, 1978; Polastro et al., 1978) and make a complete analysis difficult (see Section II,B,2). However, with the advent of better enzyme purification procedures, the answer to this question should be forthcoming in the near future.

2. Subcellular Distribution

The high specific activity of protein-carboxyl methylase in the brain (Kim et al., 1975a; Diliberto and Axelrod, 1976) prompted investigation of the subcellular localization of this enzyme in rat brain. The major portion of the enzyme is in the soluble fraction. Neither the washed nuclear nor the microsomal fractions contain much enzymatic activity, whereas a large amount of enzyme activity is present in the crude synaptosomal fraction, which is increased 3-fold by osmotic lysis. Purification of the synaptosomes increased further the specific activity of the lysed as compared to the unlysed synaptosomes (5-fold). Considerable activity was present in intact synaptosomes incubated with S-adenosyl-L-methionine, suggesting that the methyl donor was taken up into these particles; the enzyme does not appear to be membrane bound. These data indicate that protein-carboxyl methylase is present in "nerve terminals" (Diliberto and Axelrod, 1976).

The predominant localization of the enzyme in the cytosol has now been demonstrated in a number of tissues, such as rat liver (Kim and Paik, 1971b); bovine adrenal medulla (Diliberto et al., 1976b); human platelets and erythrocytes (O'Dea et al., 1978a); rabbit peritoneal neutrophils (O'Dea et al., 1978c); rat anterior, posterior, and intermediate pituitary (Gagnon and Axelrod, 1979); and rat pancreatic lobules (Povilaitis et al., 1981). In the adrenal medulla, the localization of the enzyme in the postmicrosomal supernatant fraction was similar for several species examined (E. J. Diliberto, Jr., and O. H. Viveros, unpublished observations). The bacterial enzyme was also found in the soluble fraction of extracts derived from E. coli and S. typhimurium cells (Panasenko and Koshland, 1979).

3. A Neuronal Role for Protein-Carboxyl Methylase

The primary localization of protein-carboxyl methylase in the cytosol of brain cells and in synaptosomes suggests a role for this enzyme at "nerve terminals." In support of this hypothesis, evidence for a slow rate of axonal transport was provided by studying the accumulation of the enzyme proximal to a ligation in rat sciatic nerve (Diliberto and Axelrod, 1976). Axonal transport of the enzyme in sympathetic nerves has been confirmed. One day after unilateral crushing of the external and internal carotid nerves (3–5 mm from the ganglion), enzyme activity in the proximal nerve stump increased, whereas protein-carboxyl methylase activity did not change in the superior cervical ganglion (Gilad et al., 1980). The results of these studies are compatible with a role for this enzyme in neuronal function, more specifically for an event at "nerve terminals."

The ontogenetic approach has been particularly fruitful in studying neuronal mechanisms. Early developmental studies on rat brain showed that protein-carboxyl methylase activity increases gradually during the first 10 days after birth; this period is followed by a rapid increase, nearly reaching adult levels at 40 days of age. By contrast, the specific activities of protein-N-arginyl- and protein-N-lysyl-methyltransferases are high in the fetal rat brain and decrease rapidly after birth (Paik et al., 1972; Paik and Kim, 1973). Neuronal ontogenesis was also studied in the rat cerebellum. Changes in the activities of several enzymes involved in neuronal proliferation and growth and neurotransmitter synthesis as well as protein-carboxyl methylase were examined. The activity of this methylase follows the same pattern as glutamic acid decarboxylase activity during cerebellar development. Because glutamic acid decarboxylase activity serves to indicate maturation of several GABAergic interneurons of the cerebellum (Curtis and Johnston, 1974), the parallel changes in methylase and decarboxylase activities probably reflect the overall cerebellar maturation (Gilad and Kopin, 1979). This ontogenetic change in protein-carboxyl methylation would be expected for an enzyme involved in neurotransmission.

In the peripheral nervous system, the developmental pattern for protein-carboxyl methylase activity in the rat superior cervical ganglion was similar to that described for the cerebellum. This enzyme increases and reaches adult levels later than tyrosine hydroxylase, which is an enzyme involved in neurotransmitter synthesis. The data for developmental changes in target tissues such as the iris is more complicated because the source of methylase activity is mainly in tissues other than sympathetic terminals (85 and 10% of the methylase and tyrosine hydroxylase activities, respectively, remain in the iris 10 days after ganglionectomy). Nonetheless, methylase activity increases 4-fold during development and appears to coincide with the maturation of tyrosine hydroxylase in the iris. These studies, as well as changes in methylase activity in response to axonal injury, support a role for protein-carboxyl methylase in neurotransmitter release (Gilad et al., 1980).

B. Putative Role for Protein-Carboxyl Methylase in Excitation–Secretion Coupling

The tissue and subcellular distributions suggest that protein-carboxyl methylase participates in the regulation of specific cell functions by changing the negative charge density and/or inducing conformational changes in proteins. The high specific activity in nervous and endocrine tissues, its presence in brain synaptosomes, and the evidence for its axonal transport (Diliberto and Axelrod, 1974, 1976) imply a role for this enzyme in synaptic function and merocrine secretion. One cellular function where charge neutralization may play a major role is the exocytotic secretion of exportable products contained in vesicles (Matthews *et al.*, 1972; Dean, 1975).

1. A Model of the Minimum Steps Required for Exocytosis

The minimum requirements for exocytosis, which mediates a direct discharge of vesicle content into the extracellular space, is depicted in Fig. 2. The resting state (I) in this model refers to a mature vesicle, with its final content, in close apposition to the plasma membrane. At this point, recognition sites on the vesicular and plasma membranes may be opposing at the active zone (Satir *et al.*, 1973). The cytoplasmic surfaces of the plasma and vesicle membranes have net negative charges (Meves, 1966; Matthews *et al.*, 1972; Van Der Kloot and Kita, 1973; Dean, 1975); thus, an electrostatic potential energy barrier exists and prevents contact and fusion of the two membranes. Exocytosis would require diminution of this barrier as a first step prior to membrane fusion (Matthews *et al.*, 1972; Dean, 1975; Fig. 2, II). Fusion of the membranes further requires removal of the intramembranous particles at the confronting cytoplasmic surfaces (Satir *et al.*, 1973; Ahkong *et al.*, 1975; Fig. 2, II and III). Following discharge of the vesicular content (Fig. 2, IV), reversal of the change in surface charge may contribute to the retrieval of the empty vesicle membrane (Fig. 2, V).

2. In Vitro Experiments on the Adrenal Medulla

The adrenal medulla has proved to be a useful model to study the process of exocytosis. Catecholamines are packaged in discrete vesicles and secretion from the adrenal medulla occurs by exocytosis (DeRobertis and Vaz Ferreira, 1957; Douglas and Poisner, 1966; Diner, 1967; Douglas, 1968; Kirshner and Viveros, 1972; Viveros, 1975). Because the negative surface potential of the catecholamine-containing chromaffin vesicle is mainly derived from carboxyl groups of constituent

I. RESTING STATE

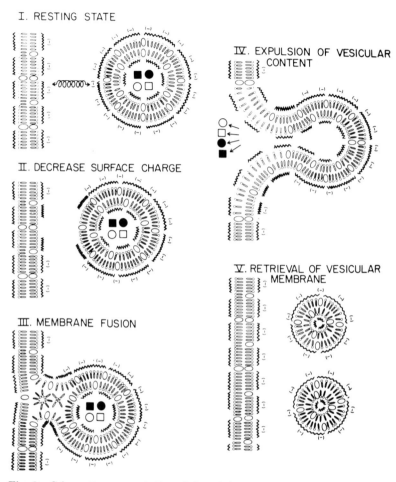

Fig. 2. Schematic representation of the minimum steps required for exocytosis.

proteins in the vesicle membrane (Matthews *et al.*, 1972), it was tempting to speculate that protein-carboxyl methylase might participate in exocytosis through the neutralization of negative charges on these proteins (Diliberto *et al.*, 1976b). Although charge neutralization and intramembrane particle migration can be obtained with Ca^{2+} *in vitro*, the concentrations required are several orders of magnitude greater than the physiological intracellular levels of Ca^{2+} (Matthews *et al.*, 1972; Schober *et al.*, 1977). Mg^{2+}, generally an inhibitor of cell secretion, will also neutralize the surface charge of chromaffin vesicles *in vitro* (Matthews *et al.*, 1972).

For protein-carboxyl methylase to function at this step in exocytosis, the protein(s) in the cytoplasmic surface of the plasma and/or chromaffin vesicle membrane should be exposed to, and be substrate(s) for, the enzyme. In the bovine adrenal medulla, the specific activity of protein-carboxyl methylase is three times higher than in the cortex. Furthermore, the endogenous enzyme activity, which is a function of the enzyme and substrate concentrations present in the tissue, is seven-fold greater in the medulla. In the adrenal medulla, greater than 90% of the enzyme is in the cytosol, whereas methyl-acceptor proteins are located in the membranes of all subcellular fractions as well as in the cytosol. Of the unlysed particulate fractions, the large-granule fraction had the lowest apparent K_m and the highest V_{max}. Separation of the various components of the large-granule fraction by continuous sucrose density centrifugation followed by incubation of the intact particles with purified protein-carboxyl methylase and S-adenosyl-L-[$methyl$-^{3}H]methionine revealed preferential methylation of the cytoplasmic surface proteins of chromaffin vesicles. Furthermore, incubation of the large-granule fraction under methylating conditions prior to separation of the particles on a sucrose gradient also indicated a specific methylation of the intact chromaffin vesicles (Diliberto et al., 1976b).

In another experiment, an entire incubation sample, after incubating the washed large-granule fraction with purified enzyme, was layered on a sucrose gradient. Surprisingly, a large amount of methylated protein was found in the upper portion of the gradient in the region of soluble proteins. Because methylation did not appear to alter the integrity of chromaffin vesicles as measured by the negligible percentage of catecholamines in the soluble fractions, the most likely source of the methylated proteins was the membranes of the particles. Subsequent experiments using intact particles and chromaffin vesicle membranes showed that carboxyl methylation of proteins on these membranes caused a release of about 67% of the methylated proteins (Diliberto et al., 1976b,c; Viveros et al., 1977). The question of whether the methyl-acceptor proteins are released following methylation has important physiological implications with regard to exocytosis. For this reason, Borchardt et al. (1978) and Eiden et al. (1979) have examined methyl-acceptor protein release as a function of chromaffin vesicle methylation in greater detail. Again, methylation of chromaffin vesicle membranes appeared to evoke a release of membrane proteins. If this observation could be extended to suggest methylation and subsequent release of specific chromaffin vesicle membrane protein, then carboxyl methylation would satisfy two steps in the process of exocytosis, i.e., charge neutralizations to reduce the energy barrier between the vesicle and plasma membranes and removal of some intramembranous proteins to allow for fusion of the membranes. On the other hand, if release of the specific membrane proteins did not occur, an alternative mechanism could be envisioned to describe the role of carboxyl methylation in exocytosis. Again, charge neutralization would participate in reducing the surface charge to increase the probability of collision of the vesicle with the plasma membrane (Dean, 1975). Protein-carboxyl methylation could also aid in the fusion process by esterifying the carboxyl group of a specific vesicular membrane protein. This event may be responsible for an increase in the hydrophobic character of the protein, enabling internalization of the methylated protein into the lipid structure of the membrane and exposing the lipid layers to facilitate fusion (see Section II,C). Fusion is followed by expulsion of the vesicular content and retrieval of the vesicular membrane.

The specificity for carboxyl methylation was examined with purified enzyme and vesicle membranes by using a modified polyacrylamide gel electrophoretic system run under acid conditions to prevent hydrolysis of the methyl esters. The radioactivity migrated with two minor protein bands with M_r of approximately 32,000 and 55,000. The high-molecular-weight methylated membrane protein did not correspond to the major protein band or radioactive peak found in the chromaffin vesicle lysate (which is chromagranin A) or the major protein component of vesicle membranes (dopamine-β-hydroxylase) (Gagnon et al., 1978a).

The characteristics of the protein-carboxyl methylase system (Section II,F) and the in vitro experiments described earlier support the concept that this enzyme participates in the process of exocytosis. There is, however, at least one serious limitation of the protein-carboxyl methylase system that should be considered. From data obtained with highly purified enzyme (homogeneous by several criteria) and the best known protein substrate for this enzyme, a turnover number of less than 1 can be calculated for this reaction in vitro. If Ca^{2+} entry is indeed the trigger for exocytosis, it has been estimated that only 200 μsec remain for the process of exocytosis, for transmitter diffusion across the cleft, and for depolarization of the postsynaptic membrane (Llinas, 1977). Obviously, even if the modification of a single carboxyl group was the only requirement for release from a single vesicle, the rate of catalysis of protein-carboxyl methylase is not fast enough to participate in this event. Enzyme turnover, however, describes the time required for the completion of a catalytic cycle that includes the time required for catalysis as well as reactivation of the enzyme. With an enzyme involved in macromolecular interactions where multifunctional groups may be important for binding, relaxation of the enzyme from a conformation induced during catalysis may represent the rate-limiting step in the overall enzymatic reaction. Such conformational changes in the enzyme induced by substrate binding are now well recognized in enzymology, and the phenomenon is often called enzyme memory (Jarabak and Westley, 1974; Katz and Westley, 1979; Neet and Ainslie, 1980). In fact, this phenomenon, which involves a high degree of conformational mobility, might explain the broad substrate specificity for this enzyme. By imposing this argument, protein-carboxyl methylation may still participate in exocytosis if product release were a very rapid process. Furthermore, the *in vivo* rate of methylation may be considerably greater than the rate of catalysis obtained with the purified enzyme. The presence of unknown endogenous factors may be required for the physiological activation of the enzyme.

3. Adrenomedullary Protein-Carboxyl Methylation in Vivo

So far, we have shown through tissue and cellular distribution studies that protein-carboxyl methylase is present in neuronal and secretory tissues and is localized in the appropriate compartment to be involved in the secretory process. Studies on axonal transport and neuronal development appeared to correlate this enzyme activity with neuronal function and, in particular, neurotransmission. Finally, we have provided *in vitro* evidence that suggests that this enzyme might represent an important step in the process of exocytosis. To explore this hypothesis, several *in vivo* models were examined.

The first *in vivo* model used to study the role of protein-carboxyl methylation in excitation–secretion coupling was the perfused bovine adrenal gland. In these studies, perfusion of the gland with L-[*methyl*-^{3}H]methionine followed by fractionation of the medulla indicated the presence of carboxyl-methylated proteins in chromaffin vesicle and postmicrosomal supernatant fractions (Viveros *et al.*, 1977). Also, S-adenosyl-L-homocysteine, an inhibitor of transmethylation (see Section II,B,5), inhibits acetylcholine-induced catecholamine release from the perfused cat adrenal gland (C. Gorman and O. H. Viveros, unpublished observation). A major objective of the *in vivo* experiments was to first demonstrate that physiological stimulation of the adrenal medulla produces catecholamine secretion with a parallel activation of the protein-carboxyl methylase system. Catecholamine secretion from the adrenal medulla is controlled *via* the splanchnic nerves, which pass through but do not synapse in the coeliac ganglia.

Splanchnic nerve stimulation can be evoked by insulin-induced hypoglycemia, thus producing reflex stimulation of the adrenal medulla.
Because protein-carboxyl methyl esters undergo rapid spontaneous hydrolysis to liberate methanol (Diliberto and Axelrod, 1976), both *in
vivo*-generated methanol and protein-carboxyl methyl ester content
were examined during infusion of L-[*methyl*-^{3}H]methionine into anesthetized rats (Fig. 3). The specific stimulation of epinephrine-contain-
ing chromaffin cells by insulin hypoglycemia produced a marked increase in protein-carboxyl methylation (Fig. 3; Viveros *et al.*, 1977).
This increase was observed in *in vivo*-generated [^{3}H]methanol and in
protein-carboxyl [^{3}H]methyl esters. In other experiments, when the
adrenal gland vasculature was extensively washed with normal saline
(pH 2.5) before removal of the gland, there was a decrease in the
content of *in vivo*-released [^{3}H]methanol in the cortex and the medulla,
resulting in a disappearance of the difference between control and

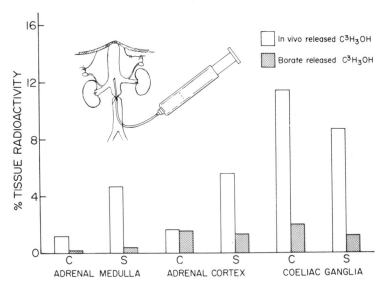

Fig. 3. Neurogenic stimulation of protein-carboxyl methylation. Osborne Mendel
white rats were anesthetized with urethane. The left splanchnic nerve was severed and
the right adrenal gland was stimulated reflexly by insulin hypoglycemia (10 μg/kg iv).
Five millicuries of L-[*methyl*-^{3}H]methionine (10 Ci/mmole) in 2.0 ml of saline was infused into the aorta in a 30-minute period. The tissues were homogenized in 1.0 ml of
cold 10% TCA and carboxyl methylation determined as previously described (O'Dea *et
al.*, 1978b). Paired tissues had no difference in total radioactivity. Total catecholamines
were 49 μg/mg protein (left medulla) and 25.2 μg/mg protein (right medulla). Reprinted
by permission of the publishers from Viveros and Diliberto (1979) and Diliberto *et al.*
(1979).

stimulated cortexes. The increase in *in vivo*-released [³H]methanol found in the cortex probably originates in the medulla and is the result of backflow through the portal circulation during removal and dissection of the gland (Viveros and Diliberto, 1979; Diliberto *et al.*, 1979). It would appear from these studies that selective stimulation of the adrenal medulla causes activation of protein-carboxyl methylation and catecholamine secretion.

Studies have established differences in the responsiveness of the sympathetic nervous system and the adrenal medulla to stress in different strains of rats. These strains also show differences in the regulation of catecholamine biosynthesis and metabolism. Despite higher activities of tyrosine hydroxylase and other catecholamine-synthesizing enzymes and higher catecholamine content in their adrenal medulla, Brown-Norway rats (less responsive strain) secrete a smaller amount of catecholamines under stress than do Wistar-Kyoto rats (greater responsive strain) (McCarty *et al.*, 1979). Protein-carboxyl methylase activity was measured in the adrenal medullas of these two strains and the only difference observed was in the endogenous enzyme activity (greater for the Brown-Norway strain). Endogenous enzyme activity, measured in the absence of added protein substrate or enzyme (Section III,A,1), is presumably a function of the enzyme and substrate concentrations present in the tissue. This strain difference in endogenous activity was attributed to a difference in the methyl-acceptor protein content of the large-granule fraction. Furthermore, reflex stimulation of the adrenal medulla by 2 hours of immobilization stress caused an increase in endogenous carboxyl methylase activity in Wistar-Kyoto rats although remaining unaltered in the less responsive Brown-Norway rats (Gilad *et al.*, 1979). Thus, a correlation exists between the greater release of catecholamines and the increase in endogenous enzyme activity in response to stress in the Wistar-Kyoto rats (the strain more responsive to stress). A strain difference in vesicle turnover may account for the difference in responsiveness.

4. Protein-Carboxyl Methylation in Other Secretory Cells

Secretion by exocytosis is not unique to the adrenal medulla; thus, other secretory tissues were investigated as potential models to be used in the study of the *in vivo* role of carboxyl methylation in secretion. Amylase secretion from the parotid gland is known to occur through a β-adrenergic receptor mechanism (Batzri *et al.*, 1971; Batzri and Selinger, 1973). Administration of isoproterenol (8 mg/kg ip), followed by removal and homogenization of the parotid gland at various times after injection, caused a rapid decrease in the amylase content of the gland; 82% of the total gland content was released in 30 minutes (Strittmatter *et al.*, 1978; Gagnon *et al.*, 1979b). Protein-carboxyl methylase activity increased rapidly for the first 10 minutes and continued to rise more slowly, with a peak at 30 minutes. This increase in enzymatic activity suggests receptor-mediated activation of protein-carboxyl methylase, because inhibition of protein synthesis by cycloheximide did not affect isoproterenol-induced amylase secretion or the concomitant increase in methylase activity. A rather surprising result was a similar increase in methyl-acceptor capacity of proteins, which again was not blocked by protein synthesis inhibition. Pharmacological studies using appropriate agonists and antagonists show that the increase in enzyme activity and methyl-acceptor capacity is indeed associated with β-adrenergic receptor stimulation. The isoproterenol-induced increase in methyl-acceptor capacity was analyzed by separation of the methylated proteins using polyacrylamide gel electrophoresis; there was a specific 2- to 3-fold increase in the carboxyl methylation of two peaks of low-molecular-weight proteins (less than 25,000) (Strittmatter *et al.*, 1978; Gagnon *et al.*, 1979b). Unfortunately, the subcellular localization of these carboxyl-methylated proteins was not determined. The time course for amylase secretion and protein-carboxyl methylase activation suggests a relationship between these events and the process of exocytosis.

The exocrine pancreas was also found to be a useful model to study the role of protein-carboxyl methylation in secretion. In these experiments, *in vivo* methylation was measured by incubation of the isolated lobules with L-[*methyl*-^{3}H]methionine (0.8 μM), and the formation of protein-carboxyl methyl esters was determined. In isolated pancreatic lobules, pancreozymin and carbachol caused a concentration-dependent stimulation in protein-carboxyl methylation and concomitant amylase secretion. The progress curves for secretagogue-induced amylase secretion and increase in carboxyl methylation were similar (Povilaitis *et al.*, 1981). Dibutyryl cGMP, an inhibitor of the pancreozymin-induced amylase secretion (Peikin *et al.*, 1979), completely blocked the pancreozymin-stimulated increase in carboxyl methylation and amylase secretion (Povilaitis *et al.*, 1981). Similarly, the effect of carbachol was completely blocked by the antimuscarinic agent atropine.

Incubation of cells with a combination of adenosine, homocysteine, *erythro*-9-[3-(2-hydroxynonyl)]adenine, and 3-deazaadenosine increases the intracellular levels of *S*-adenosyl-L-homocysteine, the product inhibitor of protein-carboxyl methylase and other methyltransferases (Pike *et al.*, 1978; Chiang *et al.*, 1979). Lobules pretreated for 1 hour in the presence of a combination of these methylation inhibitors showed a marked decrease in basal carboxyl methylation and prevented the pancreozymin-induced increase in methylation, yet basal or stimulated amylase release was not altered by this treatment (Povilaitis *et al.*, 1981). These results are not compatible with the participation of protein-carboxyl methylase in the process of exocytosis and require two possible considerations. First, the residual protein-carboxyl methylation, after exposure to the inhibitors, may be sufficient to drive exocytosis (Povilaitis *et al.*, 1981); or, second, several classes of protein-carboxyl methylases may exist (Janson and Clarke, 1980) with different sensitivities to inhibition by S-adenosyl-L-homocysteine or in a subcellular compartment protected from the action of the drugs or of the cytoplasmic increases in S-adenosyl-L-homocysteine.

Calcium entry into neurons can be correlated with transmitter release (Rubin, 1970; Llinas, 1977). Evidence that release is due to an elevation of intracellular calcium was provided by microinjection studies (Miledi, 1973). Moreover, the requirement for calcium in catecholamine secretion from the adrenal medulla (Douglas, 1966, 1968) and in enzyme secretion from the exocrine pancreas (Case, 1978) is also well established. The pancreozymin- and carbachol-stimulated increases in carboxyl methylation and amylase release were completely blocked in the absence of calcium and in the presence of EGTA (Povilaitis *et al.*, 1981). The actions of calcium are known to be distal to the agonist-receptor interaction; the preceding results indicate that increase in protein-carboxyl methylation induced by the secretagogues is distal to the calcium requirement in secretion. Neither calcium nor EGTA has an effect on methylase activity in adrenal medulla (Diliberto *et al.*, 1979) or pancreatic lobule (Povilaitis *et al.*, 1981) homogenates. Thus, it would appear that calcium entry into the cell is required to indirectly activate the protein-carboxyl methylase system.

Synaptosomes (isolated and resealed nerve endings) have been a useful model system in which to study the mechanism of neurotransmitter secretion. Elevated K^+ concentrations and veratridine cause membrane depolarization and calcium-dependent neurotransmitter release in brain synaptosomes (Levy *et al.*, 1974). In hypothalamic synaptosomes, stimulation of transmitter release by elevated K^+ or veratridine causes a decrease in the content of protein-carboxyl methyl ester after 30 minutes of incubation at 37°C (Eiden *et al.*, 1979). However, it is the rate of esterification rather than the steady-state levels of methyl esters that may be important in neurotransmitter secretion. For protein-carboxyl methylation to participate in exocytosis, an increase in the turnover of the methyl esters would be expected and static determinations of this process may reveal only decreases in the methyl ester content. These experiments also showed a calcium-dependency in the effect of high K^+ on protein-carboxyl methylation (Eiden *et al.*, 1979). Because removal of calcium abolishes depolarization-induced neurotransmitter release but does not affect membrane depolarization itself (Blaustein and Goldring, 1975), calcium entry is most likely the trigger for changes in the rate of protein-carboxyl methylation. Furthermore, these results support an involvement of methylation in neurosecretory activity, because persistent membrane depolarization in the absence of Ca^{2+}, which results in metabolic changes such as ATP depletion and ion movements, does not induce neurosecretion or activation of the protein-carboxyl methylase system.

In another experimental paradigm, ethionine ingestion reduced mouse protein-carboxyl methylase activity and increased pancreatic digestive enzyme content. Simultaneous choline deficiency potentiated the effects of ethionine ingestion. The inhibition of methylase activity by ethionine administration is presumably due to the accumulation of S-adenosyl-L-ethionine in the tissue; S-adenosyl-L-ethionine has been shown to be a competitive inhibitor of this enzyme (Gilliland *et al.*, 1981). Although protein-carboxyl methylase can function with S-adenosyl-L-ethionine as the ethyl donor, the activity is only 2.4% of the activity with S-adenosyl-L-methionine as substrate (Kim and Paik, 1978). These findings suggest that reduced protein-carboxyl methylase activity results in an impairment in the discharge of digestive enzymes from the pancreas (Gilliland *et al.*, 1981).

5. The Interaction of Ca^{2+}, Calmodulin, and Protein-Carboxyl Methylation

It is now known that most of the regulatory roles of Ca^{2+} are not attributable to free Ca^{2+} but rather to its association with the ubiquitous Ca^{2+}-binding protein calmodulin. For details regarding the role of calmodulin in excitation–secretion coupling, the reader should refer to Chapters 13 and 14 in this volume. A brief discussion, however, of how calmodulin and protein-carboxyl methylase might interact in the secretory process is necessary. Calmodulin exists as a monomer of $M_r = 17,000$ with four Ca^{2+}-binding sites (Dedman *et al.*, 1977). Binding of Ca^{2+} to any one of the four equivalent sites results in a conformational change. Another property of calmodulin, which is particularly important for our consideration here, is the high ratio of acidic to basic amino acid residues (2.7), accounting for the low isoelectric point (3.9) (Dedman *et al.*, 1977). Perhaps for this reason, calmodulin would be expected to be an exceptional substrate for protein-carboxyl methylase (Gagnon *et al.*, 1981). In that study, calmodulin was not only shown to be an excellent substrate for protein-carboxyl methylase, but also *in vivo* carboxyl methylation of calmodulin was shown to occur in ascitic Walker carcinoma cells. Because the calmodulin fraction was prepurified with a phenothiazine-Sepharose affinity column prior to gel electrophoresis, it is not possible to assess the proportion of carboxyl-methylated calmodulin to the total carboxyl-methylated proteins. *In vitro* methylation in the absence of Ca^{2+} reduced the ability of calmodulin to activate phosphodiesterase in the presence of Ca^{2+}. It was claimed that the reduction in calmodulin activity correlated with the extent of methylation, but the data was not presented. The mechanism by which methylation alters calmodulin function is not known. However, the carboxyl-methylated calmodulin was able to bind to a phenothiazine-Sepharose column in the presence of Ca^{2+} and was eluted with an EGTA-containing buffer (Gagnon *et al.*, 1981). Thus, it appears unlikely that methylation is altering the ability of calmodulin to bind Ca^{2+} (Weiss *et al.*, 1980), but carboxyl methylation of calmodulin may prevent the appropriate Ca^{2+}-induced conformational change to be biologically active. Moreover, methylation may inactivate the Ca^{2+}–calmodulin complex.

The Ca^{2+}–calmodulin complex has been proposed to regulate a number of cellular fractions, including secretion (Means and Dedman, 1980). Even though the binding of only one Ca^{2+} results in a conformational change, phosphodiesterase activation occurs maximally with only one Ca^{2+} bound and microtubule depolymerization requires all four Ca^{2+}-binding sites to be occupied. It is possible that the fractional occupancy of the Ca^{2+}-binding sites may determine the specificity of system activation. Ca^{2+}–calmodulin also activates the Ca^{2+}, Mg^{2+}-ATPase located on the plasma membrane, the endoplasmic reticulum, and the mitochondria. This enzyme is part of a Ca^{2+} active transport system that functions to reduce cytosolic Ca^{2+} concentrations (Pershadsingh *et al.*, 1980). Thus, calmodulin transduces the Ca^{2+} message during cell stimulation and subsequently activates a Ca^{2+} pump that provides a negative feedback control of Ca^{2+}.

In Section III,B,4, two *in vivo* model systems were examined. These models showed that the role of protein-carboxyl methylation is distal to the requirement of Ca^{2+} (Fig. 4). Accordingly, activation of carboxyl methylation may occur through the Ca^{2+}–calmodulin complex. Exocytosis may be a consequence of the effects of carboxyl methylation on the vesicular membrane methyl-acceptor proteins (Section III,B,2) and/or on the cytoskeletal plasma membrane proteins (Freitag and

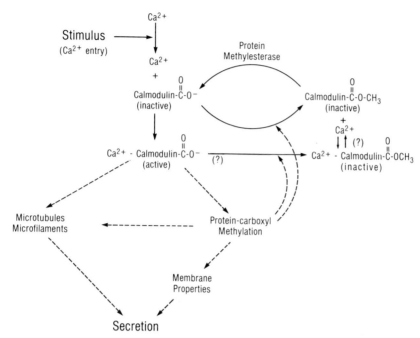

Fig. 4.　A schematic representation of the possible mechanism for the interaction of calmodulin and protein-carboxyl methylase in the primary secretory pathway and in the negative feedback regulatory pathway. The active form for calmodulin is the Ca^{2+}-calmodulin complex, which has direct actions on microtubular and microfilament structures and is proposed to be involved in the activation of protein-carboxyl methylase. Thus, the primary secretory pathway involves protein-carboxyl methylase-dependent steps (such as the primary effects of carboxyl methylation on vesicular membrane proteins) and independent steps. The model depicts several inactive forms of calmodulin: calmodulin-COO^-, calmodulin-$COOCH_3$, and Ca^{2+}-calmodulin-$COOCH_3$. The feedback inhibition of calmodulin functions may be mediated by the formation of the inactive form Ca^{2+}-calmodulin-$COOCH_3$, which may control the duration of a given secretory cycle or subsequent refractory period. Methylation of calmodulin-COO^- represents possible feedback control over the initiation of a subsequent secretory cycle.

Clarke, 1981; Section II,D,3) as well as of the effect of Ca^{2+}–calmodulin on microtubule depolymerization. The simultaneous participation of Ca^{2+}–calmodulin and carboxyl methylation in stimulus–secretion coupling may represent an amplification system for this event. Additionally, protein-carboxyl methylation may function in the inactivation of the calmodulin system. The preliminary results showing the effect of protein-carboxyl methylation on Ca^{2+}–calmodulin activation of phosphodiesterase (Gagnon *et al.*, 1981) presented earlier in this section need to be confirmed using other calmodulin-dependent systems. The model in Fig. 4 shows carboxyl methylation of calmodulin prior to and following its binding with Ca^{2+}. Thus, methylation may be an additional negative feedback system to terminate secretion in a given cycle and to control premature reactivation of the secretory process. Obviously, the data with regard to carboxyl methylation of calmodulin is not complete enough to judge the adequacy of this model; however, such speculation may provide a foundation for further investigations on this complex cellular process.

6. Final Comments on the Putative Role of Protein-Carboxyl Methylase in Exocytosis

We have presented a review of the evidence leading to the conclusion that protein-carboxyl methylation probably plays an important role in the process of secretion, perhaps at some step in the exocytotic mechanism. From a physicochemical standpoint, protein-carboxyl methylation is a unique posttranslational modifier of proteins and results in the rapid and reversible neutralization of negatively charged groups. Furthermore, because this enzyme seems to have a special affinity for proteins in membranes, the involvement of this enzyme in charge modification and/or subsequent changes in hydrophobicity of membrane proteins altering membrane–membrane interactions appears likely. Collectively, the biological data implicates this enzyme system in the secretory process and is generally compatible with its participation in exocytosis. However, in the absence of evidence for the specific *in vivo* methylation of proteins that function in the coupling of excitation to secretion, the role of protein-carboxyl methylase in this cellular event will remain a hypothesis. With the advent of new gel electrophoretic and high performance liquid chromatographic systems, experiments designed to identify the endogenous methyl-acceptor protein(s) putatively involved in exocytosis should be possible. As a note of caution, the protein-carboxyl methylation system probably involves enzymes responsible for both the esterification and deesterification of methyl-acceptor protein(s); thus, isolation of specific proteins that participate in exocytosis might require critical timing to capture the methylation process.

In recent years, our understanding of the mechanism of secretion has increased exponentially. The impetus behind our expanding knowledge of biological systems is the vision of scientists to speculate beyond current facts. In approaching an understanding of the role of protein-carboxyl methylation in the secretory process such vision is, indeed, required. Protein-carboxyl methylase and calmodulin, two ubiquitous intracellular proteins, apparently are involved in cellular secretion and may be part of a common pathway in this process. Protein-carboxyl methylation of calmodulin may represent an additional negative feedback control for the deactivation of calmodulin function. Inhibition of calmodulin action may occur as a mechanism to turn off secretion in a given cycle or to down regulate subsequent secretory cycles. Accordingly, inhibition of protein-carboxyl methylation might be expected to remove the negative feedback control and enhance secretion. Indeed, Rabe et al. (1980) showed that 3-deazaadenosine, a compound that causes inhibition of transmethylation reactions, enhanced norepinephrine release from pheochromocytoma cells (PC12) in response to nicotinic receptor stimulation. Also, this effect of 3-deazaadenosine was augmented by the addition of S-adenosyl-L-homocysteine, a result that is consistent with the hypothesis that the enhanced secretion is due to inhibition of transmethylation. Furthermore, the enhancement of release was shown to be Ca^{2+} dependent as well as dependent on the concentration of 3-deazaadenosine (Rabe et al., 1980).

In conclusion, inhibition of protein-carboxyl methylation might be expected to either inhibit or enhance the secretory process, depending on a balance between its action on the primary pathway leading to secretion or as a regulator of calmodulin function. Nonetheless, the present data does suggest a role for this enzyme, either as a participant in the exocytotic process or in some regulatory capacity.

IV. ALTERNATIVE SECRETORY FUNCTIONS FOR PROTEIN-CARBOXYL METHYLASE

A. Role in the Pituitary Gland

Protein-carboxyl methylase in the pituitary gland was first described as the "methanol-forming" enzyme by virtue of the high content of methyl-acceptor proteins in this tissue (Axelrod and Daly, 1965). Simultaneous with the discovery that the "methanol-forming" enzyme and protein-carboxyl methylase were the same enzyme, Diliberto and Axelrod (1974) purified the enzyme from the bovine pituitary and surveyed a number of biological proteins as potential substrates for the enzyme. As a result of these studies, the anterior pituitary hormones and the posterior pituitary carrier proteins (neurophysins) were shown to be effective methyl-acceptor proteins in vitro

(Diliberto and Axelrod, 1974; Axelrod and Diliberto, 1975; Section II,D,3). In view of results by Li and Fraenkel-Conrat (1947), which demonstrated that esterification of carboxyl groups of prolactin with methanol progressively lowered hormonal activity as more methyl groups were introduced into the molecule, it was proposed that protein-carboxyl methylase functions in the hypophysis to inactivate the anterior pituitary hormones (Diliberto and Axelrod, 1974).

The high specific activity of the enzyme and large content of methyl-acceptor proteins are unique features of the pituitary (Diliberto and Axelrod, 1976; Section III,A,1). It is perhaps for this reason that the pituitary gland has been under such intense investigation. Consistent with the findings that neurophysin is a substrate for protein-carboxyl methylase (Edgar and Hope, 1974; Axelrod and Diliberto, 1975) are the results obtained in organ cultures of guinea pig hypothalamo-neurohypophyseal explants (Kim et al., 1975c). Hypothalamic endogenous enzyme activity, which measures the enzyme and substrate protein concentration in vitro, increased progressively with time in culture, with a maximum at day 7; however, no change in activity was observed with added protein substrate. The changes in endogenous activity correlate with the biosynthesis of vasopressin and neurophysin in this system (Pearson et al., 1975). These results as well as gel electrophoretic studies (Gagnon and Axelrod, 1979) on posterior pituitary granule lysates strongly suggest that the neurophysins are the major methyl-acceptor proteins in this tissue when measured in vitro.

Insofar as neurophysins are active substrates for protein-carboxyl methylase and neurophysin-hormone binding activity appears to involve an ionic interaction between a side chain carboxyl group of neurophysin and the α-amino group of vasopressin or oxytocin (Walter and Hoffman, 1973), a role for carboxyl methylation in neurophysin–hormone binding must be considered. However, because neurophysin ligands do not inhibit but rather enhance methylation of neurophysin, hormone binding and carboxyl methylation probably occur at different sites (Diliberto et al., 1976a; Section II,D,2). Although these results do not support a role for this enzyme in the regulation of neurohypophyseal function through a disruption of the hormone–carrier complex, they are still consistent with the involvement of methylation in hormone–neurophysin function.

In the anterior, posterior, and intermediate lobes of the rat pituitary, protein-carboxyl methylase is found predominately in the cytosolic fraction, whereas the methyl-acceptor proteins are distributed mostly in the large-granule and cytosolic fractions. The high content of methyl-acceptor proteins in the cytosol may reflect some lysis of the granules during fractionation. In addition to the presence of this enzyme in the cytosol, a small portion was present in the large-granule fraction. After osmotic lysis of this fraction followed by separation of granular membrane and lysate fractions, methylase activity was found in both subfractions (Gagnon and Axelrod, 1979). Nonetheless, the predominant localization of the enzyme in the cytosol, a site that is inaccessible to methyl-acceptor proteins in the granules, suggests a role for this enzyme in the exocytotic process (Section III,B). In support of this notion, an increase in methylase activity (progressive increase from 2 to 4 weeks) in the posterior pituitary and not the anterior pituitary was observed after prolonged stimulation of the hypothalamus– neurohypophysis axis by salt loading (Gagnon et al., 1978b). On the other hand, there was a progressive and earlier decrease of methyl-acceptor proteins, with the greatest fall occurring between 1 and 2 days after salt loading. Analysis of the methyl-acceptor proteins by gel electrophoresis (two different systems were used) showed a single major methylated peak of $M_r \approx 11,000$, accounting for up to 80% of the total radioactivity. The disappearance of this peak after salt loading suggests that the *in vitro*-methylated protein is neurophysin.

B. Speculations on the Role of Protein-Carboxyl Methylase in Exportable Product Processing

The concept that vasopressin and its associated neurophysin are synthesized through a common precursor protein by neurons with their cell bodies located in the supraoptic nucleus of the hypothalamus was first proposed by Sacks and Takabatake (1964). Subsequently, the identification of separate precursors for vasopressin–neurophysin and oxytocin–neurophysin was reported (Gainer et al., 1977a,b; Brownstein et al., 1977). Additional experiments have indicated that the site of posttranslational processing of the common precursor into smaller peptide products including the hormone and carrier protein is the secretory granules. This posttranslational processing is initiated in the cell body and continues during axonal transport. The final peptide products are stored in the secretory granules in the nerve terminals in the posterior pituitary (Brownstein et al., 1980; Russell et al., 1980).

The proposed structure of the precursor for vasopressin–neurophysin shows vasopressin in the center of the molecule, with a glycopeptide on the amino terminal end and the corresponding neurophysin on the carboxyl terminal end. The three segments of the molecule are separated by basic amino acid residues (Brownstein *et al.*, 1980). Limited proteolysis of this precursor generates peptides with very different chromatographic properties than those of authentic vasopressin (Russell *et al.*, 1980). Thus, it would seem that the tertiary structure of the precursor molecule may be extremely important in order for the processing enzymes to precisely hydrolyze the protein to generate the biologically active peptides.

It is tempting to speculate, therefore, that protein-carboxyl methylation may function as a preprocessing posttranslational modifier of the precursor molecule. This enzyme has the capacity to cause reversible conformational changes in proteins. A temporary change in the tertiary structure of the precursor molecule may be the key to product generation by the proteolytic processing enzymes. The consequences of methylation of the precursor might be inhibition of processing, acceleration of processing, and/or regulation of the types of peptides cleaved by the processing proteolytic enzymes. This hypothesis is supported by several recent findings. Gagnon *et al.* (1978b) showed that, although most of the methylase is in the cytosol fraction, there is a significant portion in the secretory granule fraction that appears to be in part located within these particles. Furthermore, prolonged stimulation of the hypothalamo–neurohypophyseal system caused a significant increase in methylase activity in the pituitary; no change in enzyme activity was observed in supraoptic nuclei of the hypothalamus. Unfortunately, the subcellular localization of protein-carboxyl methylase in the pituitary after salt loading was not determined. If the increase in enzyme activity was indicative of a change in particulate enzyme, it may have suggested a role for this enzyme in precursor processing.

Protein-carboxyl methylation of nascent peptide chains has been demonstrated in an *in vitro* protein translation system that contained wheat germ ribosomes and hen oviduct mRNA. Puromycin-sensitive methylation of the peptides was observed at the stage of nascent chains attached to ribosomes (Chen and Liss, 1978). Thus, posttranslational modification of protein might occur before completion of synthesis of the protein and, therefore, might impose greater control over the tertiary structure of the protein.

Obviously, a suggestion that protein-carboxyl methylase participates in exportable product processing can be only highly speculative at this point. Nonetheless, the data presented here is consistent with such a hypothesis. Appropriate experiments designed to specifically address this question are needed to evaluate whether regulation of secretion by this enzyme operates through this mechanism.

V. FUNCTION OF PROTEIN-CARBOXYL METHYLATION IN PROKARYOTIC AND EUKARYOTIC CHEMOTAXIS

A. Introduction

A behavioral response that causes the directional migration of a cell as a result of an environmental stimuli is called chemotaxis. Bacterial chemotaxis is mediated by a sensory transduction system that comprises the chemoreceptors (which function to detect attractant or repellent concentrations), a signal transduction system (which translates and integrates the chemical message from the receptor), and a response apparatus (which receives the transduced signal and effects an appropriate motor response). In response to a chemical–receptor interaction, information flows from the sensory system through a transduction system to the motor system of the flagella. In bacteria, the direction of the flagella's rotation controls whether the cell will tumble (clockwise rotation) or run (counterclockwise rotation). In response to a stimulus, the frequency of tumbling and the length of a run determine the direction and velocity that the cell moves in a given direction. Thus, when the cell is moving up-gradient in an attractant, tumbling is suppressed and the run is lengthened (Adler, 1975).

B. Bacterial Chemotaxis and Carboxyl Methylation

Although protein-carboxyl methylase was first discovered in mammalian tissues, the identity of specific methyl-acceptor proteins involved in cellular functions remains unknown (see Section II). On the other hand, a well-defined role for this enzyme and specific methyl-acceptor proteins in bacterial chemotaxis is emerging. Early studies by Adler and Dahl (1967) showed that L-methionine is required for chemotaxis but not for motility. Armstrong (1972) discovered that the requirement of L-methionine was actually a requirement for S-adenosyl-L-methionine. These results implied that a transmethylation reaction might be involved in chemotaxis. The participation of methylation of specific cytoplasmic membrane proteins of $M_r = 62,000$ in this behavioral response was soon identified (Kort et al., 1975). Exposure of the mobile bacterium to a chemoattractant results in an increase in methylation of glutamyl residues on this specific group of membrane proteins (Kleene et al., 1977; Van Der Werf and Koshland, 1977). Through the use of bacterial mutants, these investigators have shown that protein-carboxyl methylase is essential for chemotaxis and that in nonchemotactic mutants the methylase or its methyl-accepting chemotaxis proteins are lacking (Springer and Koshland, 1977; Goy *et al.*, 1977). Motile bacteria also contain a methylesterase that catalyzes the deesterification of the methylated proteins, thus influencing their steady-state levels (Stock and Koshland, 1978; Toews and Adler, 1979). In response to attractants, there is an increase in the methylation of the methyl-accepting chemotaxis proteins, whereas dilution of the attractant causes a decrease in the level of methylated chemotaxis proteins. Repellents produce the opposite effect (Goy *et al.*, 1977). These changes in carboxyl methylation are rapid and result in a new steady-state level of methylated chemotaxis proteins. Excitation occurs during the change in level of methylated proteins and is responsible for the behavioral response, i.e., an altered frequency of tumbling, whereas when the new steady-state level is attained the bacteria return to the unstimulated frequency of tumbling. This latter phenomenon is called adaptation (Springer *et al.*, 1979). The precise mechanism involved in the transduction of chemoreception to motor activity is not presently known. It appears, however, that the methyl-accepting chemotaxis proteins are involved in the transduction of the excitation to response, whereas methylation of these proteins is in some way responsible for adaptation. This switching mechanism implicates protein-carboxyl methylase as an important biological regulator in this stimulus–response cycle.

C. Involvement of Methylation in Eukaryotic Chemotaxis

It is apparent that carboxyl methylation plays a crucial role in bacterial chemotaxis. In fact, mutations in this system generally result in nonchemotactic cells. Thus, it would be expected that evolution might conserve this efficient biochemical regulator for eukaryotic chemotaxis. Leukocytes have been shown to respond chemotactically to a variety of peptides of various origins as well as to well-defined synthetic formylated peptides (Showell *et al.*, 1976). In 1978 O'Dea *et al.* (1978b) examined the role of protein-carboxyl methylase in stimulated rabbit neutrophils. The simultaneous addition of the leukoattractant fMet-Leu-Phe (10 nM) and of L-[*methyl*-^{3}H]methionine caused a rapid and transient increase in carboxyl methylation with a peak at 30 seconds. This increase did not result from changes in the uptake of L-[*methyl*-^{3}H]methionine or from an increase in protein synthesis, i.e., inhibition of protein synthesis by cycloheximide did not alter the peptide-induced increase in methylation. Both the behavioral response and the increase in carboxyl methylation could be prevented by the prior addition of an attractant antagonist fPhe-Met (O'Dea et al., 1978b; Diliberto et al., 1979). Subsequently, Pike et al. (1978) and Chiang et al. (1979) showed that inhibitors of protein-carboxyl methylation simultaneously suppressed methylation and the chemotactic response in leukocytes.

These increases in carboxyl-methylated protein(s), however, have not been observed upon exposure of guinea pig macrophages to chemoattractant peptides (Pike et al., 1979). This latter result may not be unexpected in view of the fact that protein-carboxyl methylation involves esterification and deesterification (see Section III,B,4). Venkatasubramanian et al. (1980) determined whether a protein methylesterase was present in neutrophil and, if so, whether this enzyme activity would account for the variability in the changes in methyl ester content with chemotactic stimulation. In these cells, the presence of a chemoattractant evoked a rapid stimulation of methylesterase activity with half-maximal stimulation induced by a 3 nM concentration of fMet-Leu-Phe, a concentration of peptide quite similar to that (1 nM) which produced a half-maximal chemotactic response. The time course for this increase in methylesterase activity is, however, much longer (a plateau is reached by 5 minutes) than the previous increase in protein-carboxyl methylase activity reported by O'Dea et al. (1978b). The short-term stimulation in methyl ester formation was reinvestigated and confirmed (Venkatasubramanian et al., 1980). Thus, in response to a chemotactic stimulus, the earliest event may be an increase in protein-carboxyl methylase activity, which is followed rapidly by an increase in methylesterase activity. The rapid, transient nature of these phenomena are temporally related to the earliest events in the leukotactic response, suggesting that the turnover of protein-carboxyl methyl esters functions in the transduction of the chemotactic signal with directed migration of the mammalian cell.

Another example of eukaryotic chemotaxis is the movement of sperm toward the ovum. The specific activity of protein-carboxyl methylase in the testes was the highest of any peripheral tissue examined (Diliberto and Axelrod, 1976). Dissociation and fractionation of the various cell types of this tissue revealed that spermatids have the highest carboxyl methylase specific activity as well as the highest concentration of methyl-acceptor proteins. This localization was confirmed by the fact that testicular tissue that is reduced in germ cell elements has a correspondingly reduced methylase specific activity (Gagnon et al., 1979a,b; Bouchard et al., 1980a). The enzyme specific activity and methyl-acceptor protein content were also examined in motile spermatozoa. In spermatozoa, the enzymatic activity was lower than either whole testis or spermatids, whereas the methyl-acceptor

protein capacity was increased by 2-fold (Bouchard *et al.*, 1980a). Semen from normal volunteers was examined to determine the localization of enzyme activity in the spermatazoal pellet and the seminal
plasma. The specific activity in the sperm was 60-fold greater than in
the plasma (Gagnon *et al.*, 1980). In the same study, semen from necrospermic patients was analyzed and shown to have reduced methylase
activity in their spermatozoal pellets. Thus, immotile spermatozoa
from necrospermic patients are deficient in methylase activity, suggesting that this enzyme may play a role in sperm motility (Gagnon *et
al.*, 1980). Fractionation of heads and tails of rat spermatozoa on
sucrose gradients and analysis of carboxyl methylase activity revealed
the exclusive localization of this enzyme in the tail fraction, whereas
methyl-acceptor proteins were detected in both fractions (Bouchard *et
al.*, 1980b). The involvement of protein-carboxyl methylase was examined further by testing the effects of *erythro*-9-[3-(2-hydroxynonyl)]-
adenine in the presence or absence of adenosine and homocysteine
thiolactone (see Section III,B,4). Unexpectedly, in rat spermatozoa,
erythro-9-[3-(2-hydroxynonyl)]adenine alone completely inhibited
motility instantaneously, whereas protein methylation was inhibited
only 20% over the first 15 minutes. Furthermore, cycloleucine, an inhibitor of methionine adenosyltransferase, inhibited protein-carboxyl
methylation (approximately 80% by 90 minutes) but did not have a
marked effect on sperm motility. In addition, *erythro*-9-[3-(2-hy-
droxynonyl)]adenine was found to inhibit sperm flagella dynein
ATPase activity; this observation led to the conclusion that inhibition
of the dynein ATPase rather than carboxyl methylation was responsible for the effect of *erythro*-9-[3-(2-hydroxynonyl)]adenine on sperm
motility (Bouchard *et al.*, 1981). Although these data do not exclude
the possibility that protein-carboxyl methylase participates in sperm
motility, the data might be more consistent with a role in chemotaxis.
As in bacterial chemotaxis, where this enzyme is part of the transduction system in the stimulus–response coupling, protein-carboxyl methylase may function in the directional movement of these germ cells to
their target. If this methylase was indeed involved in sperm chemotaxis, then these cells would be an interesting model to study eukaryotic
chemotaxis because the entire apparatus would probably be located in
the tail.

VI. CONCLUDING REMARKS

The purpose for the in-depth analysis of the protein-carboxyl methylase system in this chapter was not only to present current progress

but also to encourage investigators from a variety of disciplines to probe the biological function(s) of this system. In this regard, I hope the extended presentation of data supporting a role for this enzyme in exocytosis will not mislead the reader into assuming that this is the only mode of participation of protein-carboxyl methylase in the process of secretion. In fact, when considering the putative role for this enzyme in secretion and chemotaxis, it is tempting to correlate these cellular responses as occurring through a common biochemical pathway.

In general, the present studies pose a convincing but not conclusive argument that protein-carboxyl methylase has a role in neurotransmission and secretion in general. Whether it functions as an integral part of the exocytotic process or in its regulation has yet to be determined. In a regulatory capacity, protein-carboxyl methylase could act either in controlling the amount of secretory materials released by a given stimulus or in altering exportable product processing of polypeptides. It is hoped that with recent technological advances in protein isolation specific studies will be designed to uncover the precise role(s) for this enzyme system.

The participation of protein-carboxyl methylase in bacterial chemotaxis appears definitive, although a mechanism describing transduction of a signal to the motor response is lacking. Also, the mode of action of methylation of the methyl-accepting chemotaxis proteins in adaptation is not clear at this time. It is perhaps because of the efficiency of such a system that one might expect a similar role for this enzyme in eukaryotic chemotaxis.

ACKNOWLEDGMENTS

The author is grateful for the invaluable assistance provided by Thomasine M. Cozart and Sylvia E. Short in the preparation of this chapter.

REFERENCES

Adler, J. (1975). Chemotaxis in bacteria. *Annu. Rev. Biochem.* **44,** 341–356.
Adler, J., and Dahl, M. M. (1967). A method for measuring the motility of bacteria and for comparing random and non-random motility. *J. Gen. Microbiol.* **46,** 161–173.
Ahkong, Q. F., Fisher, D., Tampion, W., and Lucy, J. A. (1975). Mechanisms of cell fusion. *Nature (London)* **253,** 194–195.
Armstrong, J. B. (1972). An S-adenosylmethionine requirement for chemotaxis in *Escherichia coli. Can. J. Microbiol.* **18,** 1695–1701.
Atassi, M. Z., and Nakhlen, E. T. (1975). Conformational studies on modified proteins and peptides. IX. Conformation and immunochemistry of hemoglobin reduced at some carboxyl groups by diborane. *Biochim. Biophys. Acta* **379,** 1–12.

Atassi, M. Z., and Singhal, R. P. (1972). Conformational studies on modified proteins and peptides. V. Conformation of myoglobin derivatives modified at two carboxyl groups. *J. Biol. Chem.* **247,** 5980–5986.

Axelrod, J., and Daly, J. (1965). Pituitary gland: Enzymic formation of methanol from S-adenosyl-methionine. *Science* **150,** 892–893.

Axelrod, J., and Diliberto, E. J., Jr. (1975). Methylation of pituitary peptide hormones by protein carboxymethylase. *Ann. N. Y. Acad. Sci.* **248,** 90–91.

Batzri, S., and Selinger, Z. (1973). Enzyme secretion mediated by the epinephrine β-receptor in rat parotid slices. *J. Biol. Chem.* **248,** 356–360.

Batzri, S., Selinger, Z., and Schramm, M. (1971). Potassium ion release and enzyme secretion: Adrenergic regulation by α- and β-receptors. *Science* **174,** 1029–1031.

Bernhard, S. A., Berger, A., Carter, J. H., Katchalski, E., Sela, M., and Shalitin, Y. (1962). Cooperative effects of functional groups in peptides. I. Aspartyl-serine derivatives. *J. Am. Chem. Soc.* **84,** 2421–2434.

Blaustein, M. P., and Goldring, J. M. (1975). Membrane potentials in pinched-off presynaptic nerve terminals monitored with a fluorescent probe: Evidence that synaptosomes have potassium diffusion potentials. *J. Physiol. (London)* **247,** 589–615.

Borchardt, R. T. (1980). S-adenosyl-L-methionine-dependent macromolecule methyltransferases: Potential targets for the design of chemotherapeutic agents. *J. Med. Chem.* **23,** 347–357.

Borchardt, R. T., Olsen, J., Eiden, L. E., Schowen, R. L., and Rutledge, C. O. (1978). The isolation and characterization of the methyl acceptor protein from adrenal chromaffin granules. *Biochem. Biophys. Res. Commun.* **83,** 970–976.

Bouchard, P., Gagnon, C., and Bardin, C. W. (1980a). Protein carboxyl-methylase in rat testes and spermatozoa. *In* "Testicular Development, Structure, and Function" (A. Steinberger and E. Steinberger, eds.), pp. 441–446. Raven, New York.

Bouchard, P., Gagnon, C., Phillips, D. M., and Bardin, C. W. (1980b). The localization of protein carboxyl-methylase in sperm tails. *J. Cell Biol.* **86,** 417–423.

Bouchard, P., Penningroth, S. M., Cheung, A., Gagnon, C., and Bardin, C. W. (1981). *Erythro*-9-[3-(2-hydroxynonyl)]adenine is an inhibitor of sperm motility that blocks dynein ATPase and protein carboxylmethylase activities. *Proc. Natl. Acad. Sci. U.S.A.* **78,** 1033–1036.

Brownstein, M. J., Robinson, A. G., and Gainer, H. (1977). Immunological identification of rat neurophysin precursors. *Nature (London)* **269,** 259–261.

Brownstein, M. J., Russel, J. T., and Gainer, H. (1980). Synthesis, transport, and release of posterior pituitary hormones. *Science* **207,** 373–378.

Case, R. M. (1978). Synthesis, intracellular transport, and discharge of exportable proteins in the pancreatic acinar cell and other cells. *Biol. Rev. Cambridge Philos. Soc.* **53,** 211–354.

Chen, J.-K., and Liss, M. (1978). Evidence of the carboxymethylation of nascent peptide chains on ribosomes. *Biochem. Biophys. Res. Commun.* **84,** 261–268.

Chiang, P. K., Venkatasubramanian, K., Richards, H. H., Cantoni, G. L., and Schiffmann, E. (1979). Adenosylhomocysteine hydrolase and chemotaxis. *In* "Transmethylation" (E. Usdin, R. T. Borchardt, and C. R. Creveling, eds.), pp. 165–172. Elsevier/North-Holland, Amsterdam.

Clarke, S., Sparrow, K., Panasenko, S., and Koshland, D. E., Jr. (1980). *In vitro* methylation of bacterial chemotaxis proteins: Characterization of protein methyltransferase activity in crude extracts of *Salmonella typhimurium*. *J. Supramol. Struct.* **13,** 315–328.

Cleland, W. W. (1970). Steady state kinetics. *In* "The Enzymes" (P. D. Boyer, ed.), Vol. II, pp. 1–65. Academic Press, New York.

Curtis, D. R., and Johnston, G. A. R. (1974). Amino acid transmitters in the mammalian central nervous system. *Ergeb. Physiol. Biol. Chem. Exp. Pharmakol.* **69**, 97–188.

Dean, P. M. (1975). Exocytosis modelling: An electrostatic function for calcium in stimulus-secretion coupling. *J. Theor. Biol.* **54**, 289–308.

Dedman, J. R., Potter, J. D., Jackson, R. L., Johnson, J. D., and Means, A. R. (1977). Physicochemical properties of rat testis Ca^{2+}-dependent regulator protein of cyclic nucleotide phosphodiesterase. *J. Biol. Chem.* **252**, 8415–8422.

Deguchi, T., and Barchas, J. (1971). Inhibition of transmethylations of biogenic amines by S-adenosylhomocysteine. *J. Biol. Chem.* **246**, 3175–3181.

DeRobertis, E., and Vaz Ferreira, A. (1957). Electron microscope study of the excretion of catechol-containing droplets in the adrenal medulla. *Exp. Cell Res.* **12**, 568–574.

Diliberto, E. J., Jr., and Axelrod, J. (1974). Characterization and substrate specificity of a protein carboxymethylase in the pituitary gland. *Proc. Natl. Acad. Sci. U.S.A.* **71**, 1701–1704.

Diliberto, E. J., Jr., and Axelrod, J. (1976). Regional and subcellular distribution of protein carboxymethylase in brain and other tissues. *J. Neurochem.* **26**, 1159–1165.

Diliberto, E. J., Jr., Axelrod, J., and Chaiken, I. M. (1976a). The effects of ligands on enzymic carboxyl-methylation of neurophysins. *Biochem. Biophys. Res. Comm.* **73**, 1063–1067.

Diliberto, E. J., Jr., Viveros, O. H., and Axelrod, J. (1976b). Subcellular distribution of protein carboxymethylase and its endogenous substrates in the adrenal medulla: Possible role in excitation-secretion coupling. *Proc. Natl. Acad. Sci. U.S.A.* **73**, 4050–4054.

Diliberto, E. J., Jr., Viveros, O. H., and Axelrod, J. (1976c). Localization of protein carboxymethylase and its endogenous substrate(s) in the adrenal medulla-methylation of the chromaffin vesicle membrane. *Fed. Proc., Fed. Am. Soc. Exp. Biol.* **35**, 326.

Diliberto, E. J., Jr., O'Dea, R. F., and Viveros, O. H. (1979). The role of protein carboxymethylase in secretory and chemotactic eukaryotic cells. *In* "Transmethylation" (E. Usdin, R. T. Borchardt, and C. R. Creveling, eds.), pp. 529–538, Elsevier/North-Holland, Amsterdam.

Diner, O. (1967). L'expulsion des granules de la médullo-surrenale chez le hamster. *C. R. Hebd. Seances Acad. Sci., Ser. D.* **265**, 616–619.

Douglas, W. W. (1966). Calcium-dependent links in stimulus-secretion coupling in the adrenal medulla and neurohypophysis. *In* "Mechanisms of Release of Biogenic Amines" (U. S. von Euler, S. Rosell, and B. Uvnäs, eds.), pp. 267–289. Pergamon, Oxford.

Douglas, W. W. (1968). Stimulus-secretion coupling: The concept and clues from chromaffin and other cells. *Br. J. Pharmacol.* **34**, 451–474.

Douglas, W. W., and Poisner, A. M. (1966). Evidence that the secreting adrenal chromaffin cell releases catecholamines directly from ATP-rich granules. *J. Physiol. (London)* **183**, 236–248.

Dudman, N. P. B., and Zerner, B. (1975). Carboxylesterases from pig and ox liver. *Methods Enzymol.* **35**, 190–208.

Edgar, D. H., and Hope, D. B. (1974). Neurophysin methylation in extracts of bovine posterior pituitary gland: Hormone binding ability. *FEBS Lett.* **49**, 145–148.

Edgar, D. H., and Hope, D. B. (1976). Protein-carboxyl methyltransferase of the bovine posterior pituitary gland: Neurophysin as a potential endogenous substrate. *J. Neurochem.* **27**, 949–955.

Eiden, L. E., Borchardt, R. T., and Rutledge, C. O. (1979). Protein carboxymethylation in neurosecretory processes. *In* "Transmethylation" (E. Usdin, R. T. Borchardt, and C. R. Creveling, eds.), pp. 539–546. Elsevier/North-Holland, Amsterdam.

Fairbanks, G., and Avruch, J. (1972). Four gel systems for electrophoretic fractionation of membrane proteins using ionic detergents. *J. Supramol. Struct.* **1**, 66–75.

Freitag, C., and Clarke, S. (1981). Reversible methylation of cytoskeletal and membrane proteins in intact human erythrocytes. *J. Biol. Chem.* **256**, 6102–6108.

Gagnon, C. (1979). Presence of a protein methylesterase in mammalian tissues. *Biochem. Biophys. Res. Commun.* **88**, 847–853.

Gagnon, C., and Axelrod, J. (1979). Subcellular localization of protein carboxyl-methylase and its substrates in rat pituitary lobes. *J. Neurochem.* **32**, 567–572.

Gagnon, C., Viveros, O. H., Diliberto, E. J., Jr., and Axelrod, J. (1978a). Enzymatic methylation of carboxyl groups of chromaffin granule membrane proteins. *J. Biol. Chem.* **253**, 3778–3781.

Gagnon, C., Axelrod, J., and Brownstein, M. J. (1978b). Protein carboxymethylation: Effects of 2% sodium chloride administration on protein carboxymethylase and its endogenous substrates in rat posterior pituitary. *Life Sci.* **22**, 2155–2164.

Gagnon, C., Axelrod, J., Musto, N., Dym, M., and Bardin, C. W. (1979a). Protein carboxyl-methylation in rat testes: A study of inherited and x-ray-induced seminiferous tubule failure. *Endocrinology (Baltimore)* **105**, 1440–1445.

Gagnon, C., Bardin, C. W., Strittmatter, W., and Axelrod, J. (1979b). Protein carboxyl-methylation in the parotid gland and in the male reproductive system. *In* "Transmethylation" (E. Usdin, R. T. Borchardt, and C. R. Creveling, eds.), pp. 521–528. Elsevier/North-Holland, Amsterdam.

Gagnon, C., Sherins, R. J., Mann, T., Bardin, C. W., Amelar, R. D., and Dubin, L. (1980). Deficiency of protein carboxyl-methylase in spermatozoa and necrospermic patients. *In* "Testicular Development, Structure, and Function" (A. Steinberger and E. Steinberger, eds.), pp. 491–495. Raven, New York.

Gagnon, C., Kelly, S., Manganiells, V., Vaughan, M., Odya, C., Strittmatter, W., Hoffman, A., and Hirata, F. (1981). Modification of calmodulin function by enzymatic carboxyl methylation. *Nature (London)* **291**, 515–516.

Gainer, H., Sarne, Y., and Brownstein, M. J. (1977a). Biosynthesis and axonal transport of rat neurohypophysial proteins and peptides. *J. Cell Biol.* **73**, 366–381.

Gainer, H., Sarne, Y., and Brownstein, M. J. (1977b). Neurophysin biosynthesis: Conversion of a putative precursor during axonal transport. *Science* **195**, 1354–1356.

Galletti, P., Paik, W. K., and Kim, S. (1978). Selective methyl esterification of erythrocyte membrane proteins by protein methylase II. *Biochemistry* **17**, 4272–4276.

Galletti, P., Paik, W. K., and Kim, S. (1979). Methyl acceptors for protein methylase II from human-erythrocyte membrane. *Eur. J. Biochem.* **97**, 221–227.

Gilad, G. M., and Kopin, I. J. (1979). Neurochemical aspects of neuronal ontogenesis in the developing rat cerebellum: Changes in neurotransmitter and polyamine synthesizing enzymes. *J. Neurochem.* **33**, 1195–1204.

Gilad, G. M., McCarty, R., Weise, V. K., and Kopin, I. J. (1979). Strain differences in the regulation of the sympatho-adrenal system. *Brain Res.* **176**, 380–384.

Gilad, G. M., Gagnon, C., and Kopin, I. J. (1980). Protein carboxymethylase activity in the rat superior cervical ganglion during development and after axonal injury. *Brain Res.* **183**, 393–402.

Gilliland, E. L., Turner, N., and Steer, M. L. (1981). The effects of ethionine administration and choline deficiency on protein carboxymethylase activity in mouse pancreas. *Biochim. Biophys. Acta* **672**, 280–287.

Goy, M. F., Springer, M. S., and Adler, J. (1977). Sensory transduction in *Escherichia coli:* Role of a protein methylation reaction in sensory adaptation. *Proc. Natl. Acad. Sci. U.S.A.* **74,** 4964–4968.

Inkerman, P. A., Scott, K., Runnegar, M. T. C., Hamilton, S. E., Bennett, E. A., and Zerner, B. (1975). Carboxylesterases (EC 3.1.1). Purification and titration of chicken, sheep, and horse liver carboxylesterases. *Can. J. Biochem.* **53,** 536–546.

Jamaluddin, M., Kim, S., and Paik, W. K. (1975). Studies on the kinetic mechanism of S-adenosylmethionine: protein O-methyltransferase of calf thymus. *Biochemistry* **14,** 694–698.

Jamaluddin, M., Kim, S., and Paik, W. K. (1976). A comparison of kinetic parameters of polypeptide substrates for protein methylase II. *Biochemistry* **15,** 3077–3081.

Janson, C. A., and Clarke, S. (1980). Identification of aspartic acid as a site of methylation in human erythrocyte membrane proteins. *J. Biol. Chem.* **225,** 11640–11643.

Jarabak, R., and Westley, J. (1974). Enzymic memory: A consequence of conformational mobility. *Biochemistry* **13,** 3237–3243.

Katz, M., and Westley, J. (1979). Enzymic memory: Steady state kinetic and physical studies with ascorbate oxidase and aspartate aminotransferase. *J. Biol. Chem.* **254,** 9142–9147.

Kim, S. (1973). Purification and properties of protein methylase II. *Arch. Biochem. Biophys.* **157,** 476–484.

Kim, S. (1974). S-adenosylmethionine: Protein-carboxyl methyltransferase from erythrocyte. *Arch. Biochem. Biophys.* **161,** 652–657.

Kim, S., and Li, C. H. (1979a). Enzymatic methyl esterification of specific glutamyl residue in corticotropin. *Proc. Natl. Acad. Sci. U.S.A.* **76,** 4255–4257.

Kim, S., and Li, C. H. (1979b). Enzymatic methyl esterification of pituitary polypeptides. *Int. J. Pept. Protein Res.* **13,** 282–286.

Kim, S., and Paik, W. K. (1970). Purification and properties of protein methylase II. *J. Biol. Chem.* **245,** 1806–1813.

Kim, S., and Paik, W. K. (1971a). Studies on the structural requirements of substrate protein for protein methylase II. *Biochemistry* **10,** 3141–3145.

Kim, S., and Paik, W. K. (1971b). Natural inhibitor for protein methylase II. *Biochim. Biophys. Acta* **252,** 526–532.

Kim, S., and Paik, W. K. (1976). Labile protein-methyl ester: Comparison between chemically and enzymatically synthesized. *Experientia* **32,** 982–984.

Kim, S., and Paik, W. K. (1978). Purification and assay of protein methylase II (S-adenosyl-methionine: protein-carboxyl methyltransferase; EC 2.1.1.24) *Methods Cell Biol.* **19,** 79–88.

Kim, S., Wasserman, L., Lew, B., and Paik, W. K. (1975a). Studies on the natural substrate for protein methylase II in mammalian brain and blood. *J. Neurochem.* **24,** 625–629.

Kim, S., Wasserman, L., Lew, B., and Paik, W. K. (1975b). Studies on the effect of hypophysectomy on protein methylase II of rat. *FEBS Lett.* **51,** 164–167.

Kim, S., Pearson, D., and Paik, W. K. (1975c). Studies on S-adenosylmethionine: Protein-carboxyl methyltransferase in the hypothalamo-neurohypophysial complex in organ culture. *Biochim. Biophys. Res. Commun.* **67,** 448–454.

Kim, S., Nochumson, S., Chin, W., and Paik, W. K. (1978). A rapid method for the purification of S-adenosylmethionine: Protein-carboxyl O-methyltransferase by affinity chromatography. *Anal. Biochem.* **84,** 415–422.

Kim, S., Galletti, P., and Paik, W. K. (1980). *In vivo* carboxyl methylation of human erythrocyte membrane proteins. *J. Biol. Chem.* **255,** 338–341.

Kirshner, N., and Viveros, O. H. (1972). The secretory cycle in the adrenal medulla. *Pharmacol. Rev.* **24**, 385–398.

Kleene, S. J., Toews, M. L., and Adler, J. (1977). Isolation of glutamic acid methyl ester from an *Escherichia coli* membrane protein involved in chemotaxis. *J. Biol. Chem.* **252**, 3214–3218.

Kort, E. N., Goy, M. F., Larsen, S. H., and Adler, J. (1975). Methylation of a membrane protein involved in bacterial chemotaxis. *Proc. Natl. Acad. Sci. U.S.A.* **72**, 3939–3943.

Levy, W. B., Haycock, J. W., and Cotman, C. W. (1974). Effects of polyvalent cations on stimulus-coupled secretion of [^{14}C]-γ-aminobutyric acid from isolated brain synaptosomes. *Mol. Pharmacol.* **10**, 438–449.

Li, C. H., and Fraenkel-Conrat, H. (1947). Studies on pituitary lactogenic hormone. XII. Effect of esterification with methyl alcohol. *J. Biol. Chem.* **167**, 495–498.

Liss, M., and Edelstein, L. M. (1967). Evidence for the enzymatic methylation of crystalline ovalbumin preparations. *Biochem. Biophys. Res. Commun.* **26**, 497–504.

Liss, M., Maxam, A. M., and Cuprak, L. J. (1969). Methylation of protein by calf spleen methylase: A new protein methylation reaction. *J. Biol. Chem.* **244**, 1617–1622.

Llinas, R. R. (1977). Calcium and transmitter release in squid synapse. *Soc. Neurosci. Symp.* **2**, 139–160.

McCarty, R., Gilad, G. M., Weise, V. K., and Kopin, I. J. (1979). Strain differences in rat adrenal biosynthetic enzymes and stress induced increases in plasma catecholamines. *Life Sci.* **25**, 747–754.

Matthews, E. K., Evans, R. J., and Dean, P. M. (1972). The ionogenic nature of the secretory-granule membrane: Electrokinetic properties of isolated chromaffin granules. *Biochem. J.* **130**, 825–832.

Means, A. R., and Dedman, J. R. (1980). Calmodulin in endocrine cells and its multiple roles in hormone action. *Mol. Cell. Endocrinol.* **19**, 215–227.

Meves, H. (1966). Experiments on internally perfused squid giant axons. *Ann. N. Y. Acad. Sci.* **137**, 807–817.

Miledi, R. (1973). Transmitter release induced by injection of calcium ions into nerve terminals. *Proc. R. Soc. London, Ser. B* **183**, 421–425.

Morin, A. M., and Liss, M. (1973). Evidence for a methylated protein intermediate in pituitary methanol formation. *Biochem. Biophys. Res. Commun.* **52**, 373–378.

Neet, K. E., and Ainslie, G. R., Jr. (1980). Hysteretic enzymes. *Methods Enzymol.* **64**, 192–226.

O'Dea, R. F., Viveros, O. H., Acheson, A., Gorman, C., and Axelrod, J. (1978a). Protein carboxymethylase and methyl-acceptor proteins in human platelets and erythrocytes. *Biochem. Pharmacol.* **27**, 679– 684.

O'Dea, R. F., Viveros, O. H., Axelrod, J., Aswanikumar, S., Schiffmann, E., and Corcoran, B. A. (1978b). Rapid stimulation of protein carboxymethylation in leukocytes by a chemotactic peptide. *Nature (London)* **272**, 462–464.

O'Dea, R. F., Viveros, O. H., Aswanikumar, S., Schiffmann, E., Chiang, P. K., Cantoni, G. L., and Axelrod, J. (1978c). A protein carboxymethylation stimulated by chemotactic peptides in leucocytes. *Fed. Proc., Fed. Am. Soc. Exp. Biol.* **37**, 1656.

O'Dea, R. F., Viveros, O. H., and Diliberto, E. J., Jr. (1981). Protein carboxymethylation: Role in the regulation of cell functions. *Biochem. Pharmacol.* **30**, 1163–1168.

Paik, W. K., and Kim, S. (1973). Protein methylases during the development of rat brain. *Biochim. Biophys. Acta* **313**, 181–189.

Paik, W. K., and Kim, S. (1975). Protein methylation: Chemical, enzymological, and biological significance. *Adv. Enzymol.* **42**, 227–286.

Paik, W. K., Kim, S., and Lee, H. W. (1972). Protein methylation during the development of rat brain. *Biochem. Biophys. Res. Commun.* **46**, 933–941.

Panasenko, S. M., and Koshland, D. E., Jr. (1979). Methylation and demethylation in the bacterial chemotactic system. *In* "ICN-UCLA Symposium on Covalent and Noncovalent Modulation of Protein Function" (D. E. Atkinson and C. F. Fox, eds.), Vol. 13, pp. 273–284. Academic Press, New York.

Pearson, D., Shainberg, A., Malamed, S., and Sachs, H. (1975). The hypothalamo-neurohypophysial complex in organ culture: Effects of metabolic inhibitors, biologic and pharmacologic agents. *Endocrinology (Baltimore)* **96**, 994–1003.

Peikin, S. R., Costenbader, C. L., and Gardner, J. D. (1979). Actions of derivatives of cyclic nucleotides on dispersed acini from guinea pig pancreas: Discovery of a competitive antagonist of the action of cholecystokinin. *J. Biol. Chem.* **254**, 5321–5327.

Pershadsingh, H. A., McDaniel, M. L., Landt, M., Bry, C. G., Lacy, P. E., and McDonald, J. M. (1980). Ca^{2+}-activated ATPase and ATP-dependent calmodulin-stimulated Ca^{2+} transport in islet cell plasma membrane. *Nature (London)* **288**, 492–495.

Pike, M. C., Kredick, N. M., and Snyderman, R. (1978). Requirement of S-adenosyl-L-methionine-mediated methylation for human monocyte chemotaxis. *Proc. Natl. Acad. Sci. U.S.A.* **75**, 3928–3932.

Pike, M. C., Kredich, N. M., and Snyderman, R. (1979). Phospholipid methylation in macrophages is inhibited by chemotactic factors. *Proc. Natl. Acad. Sci. U.S.A.* **76**, 2922–2926.

Polastro, E. T., Deconinck, M. M., Devogel, M. R., Mailier, E. L., Looza, Y. B., Schnek, A. G., and Léonis, J. (1978). Purification and some molecular properties of protein methylase II from equine erythrocytes. *Biochem. Biophys. Res. Commun.* **81**, 920–927.

Povilaitis, V., Gagnon, C., and Heisler, S. (1981). Stimulus-secretion coupling in exocrine pancreas: Role of protein carboxyl methylation. *Am. J. Physiol.* **240**, G199–G205.

Quick, D. P., Orchard, P. J., and Duerre, J. A. (1981). Carboxyl methylation of nonhistone chromosomal proteins. *Biochemistry* **20**, 4724–4729.

Rabe, C. S., Williams, T. P., and McGee, R., Jr. (1980). Enhancement of depolarization-dependent release of norepinephrine by an inhibitor of S-adenosylmethionine-dependent transmethylations. *Life Sci.* **27**, 1753–1759.

Rubin, R. P. (1970). The role of calcium in the release of neurotransmitter substances and hormones. *Pharmacol. Rev.* **22**, 389–428.

Russell, J. T., Brownstein, M. J., and Gainer, H. (1980). Biosynthesis of vasopressin, oxytocin, and neurophysins: Isolation and characterization of two common precursors (propressophysin and prooxyphysin). *Endocrinology (Baltimore)* **107**, 1880–1891.

Sachs, H., and Takabatake, Y. (1964). Evidence for a precursor in vasopressin biosynthesis. *Endocrinology (Baltimore)* **75**, 943–948.

Satir, B., Schooley, C., and Satir, P. (1973). Membrane fusion in a model system: Mucocyst secretion in *Tetrahymena. J. Cell Biol.* **56**, 153–176.

Schober, R., Nitsch, C., Rinne, U., and Morris, S. J. (1977). Calcium-induced displacement of membrane-associated particles upon aggregation of chromaffin granules. *Science* **195**, 495–497.

Scott, K., and Zerner, B. (1975). Carboxylesterases from chicken, sheep, and horse liver. *Methods Enzymol.* **35**, 208–221.

Showell, H. J., Freer, R. J., Zigmond, S. H., Schiffmann, E., Aswanikumar, S., Corcoran, B. A., and Becker, E. L. (1976). The structure-activity relations of synthetic peptides as chemotactic factors and inducers of lysosomal enzyme secretion for neutrophils. *J. Exp. Med.* **143**, 1154–1169.

Springer, W. R., and Koshland, D. E., Jr. (1977). Identification of a protein methyltransferase as the *cheR* gene product in the bacterial sensing system. *Proc. Natl. Acad. Sci. U.S.A.* **74**, 533–537.

Springer, M. S., Goy, M. F., and Adler, J. (1979). Protein methylation in behavioural control mechanisms and in signal transduction. *Nature (London)* **280**, 279–284.

Stock, J. B., and Koshland, D. E., Jr. (1978). A protein methylesterase involved in bacterial sensing. *Proc. Natl. Acad. Sci. U.S.A.* **75**, 3659–3663.

Stock, J. B., and Koshland, D. E., Jr. (1979). Identification of a methyltransferase and a methylesterase as essential genes in bacterial chemotaxis. *Dev. Neurosci. (Amsterdam)* **5**, 511–520.

Strittmatter, W. J., Gagnon, C., and Axelrod, J. (1978). Beta adrenergic stimulation of protein carboxymethylation and amylase secretion in rat parotid gland. *J. Pharmacol. Exp. Ther.* **207**, 419–424.

Tanford, C. (1962). Contribution of hydrophobic interactions to the stability of the globular conformation of proteins. *J. Am. Chem. Soc.* **84**, 4240–4247.

Terwilliger, T. C., and Clarke, S. (1981). Methylation of membrane proteins in human erythrocytes. *J. Biol. Chem.* **256**, 3067–3076.

Toews, M. L., and Adler, J. (1979). Methanol formation *in vivo* from methylated chemotaxis proteins in *Escherichia coli. J. Biol. Chem.* **254**, 1761–1764.

Ullah, A. H., and Ordal, G. W. (1981). *In vivo* and *in vitro* chemotactic methylation in *Bacillus subtilis. J. Bacteriol.* **145**, 958–965.

Van Der Kloot, W., and Kita, H. (1973). The possible role of fixed membrane surface charges in acetylcholine release at the frog neuromuscular junction. *J. Membr. Biol.* **14**, 365–382.

Van Der Werf, P., and Koshland, D. E., Jr. (1977). Identification of a γ-glutamyl methyl ester in bacterial membrane protein involved in chemotaxis. *J. Biol. Chem.* **252**, 2793–2795.

Venkatasubramanian, K., Hirata, F., Gagnon, C., Corcoran, B. A., O'Dea, R. F., Axelrod, J., and Schiffmann, E. (1980). Protein methylesterase and leukocyte chemotaxis. *Mol. Immunol.* **17**, 201–207.

Viveros, O. H. (1975). Mechanism of secretion of catecholamines from adrenal medulla. *Handb. Physiol. Sect. 7: Endocrinol. 1972–1976* **6**, 389–426.

Viveros, O. H., and Diliberto, E. J., Jr. (1979). Excitation-secretion coupling: Increased protein carboxymethylation during neurogenic stimulation of the adrenal medulla. *In* "Catecholamines: Basic and Clinical Frontiers" (E. Usdin, I. J. Kopin, and J. Barchas, eds.), Vol. I, pp. 283–285. Pergamon, New York.

Viveros, O. H., Diliberto, E. J., Jr., and Axelrod, J. (1977). Protein carboxymethylase and excitation-secretion coupling. *In* "Synapses" (G. A. Cottrell and P. N. A. Usherwood, eds.), pp. 368–369. Blackie, Glasgow and London.

Walter, R., and Hoffman, P. L. (1973). Tentative identification of a binding site of arginine vasopressin to neurophysin. *Fed. Proc., Fed. Am. Soc. Exp. Biol.* **32**, 567.

Weiss, B., Prozialeck, W., Cimino, M., Barnette, M. S., and Wallace, T. L. (1980). Pharmacological regulation of calmodulin. *Ann. N. Y. Acad. Sci.* **356**, 319–345.

Zappia, V., Zydek-Cwick, C. R., and Schlenk, F. (1969). The specificity of S-adenosylmethionine derivatives in methyl transfer reactions. *J. Biol. Chem.* **244**, 4499–4509.

PART III
SUBCELLULAR ARCHITECTURE: ITS ROLE IN SECRETION

6

The Role of the Cytoskeleton in Endocrine Function

PETER F. HALL

I. INTRODUCTION*

Investigation of the functions of the cytoskeleton provides an interesting contrast to earlier studies of muscular contraction, where the phenomenon of shortening was well understood long before the mo-

---

*Throughout this chapter, recent references and reviews will be cited as points of entry to the literature. This is intended to facilitate further exploration by readers who have limited acquaintance with the vast literature on the cytoskeleton. It is not intended to establish priorities in the relevant discoveries, still less to ignore much of the excellent experimental work upon which current thinking in this field is based.

CELLULAR REGULATION OF SECRETION AND RELEASE

lecular basis of contraction could be approached experimentally. On the other hand, the components of the cytoskeleton have been purified, many important molecular properties of these components have been reported, and yet we cannot describe the functions of the cytoskeleton with any certainty. The cytoskeleton consists of microtubules (diameter 25 nm), intermediate filaments (diameter 10 nm) and microfilaments (diameter 6 nm). The basic component of microtubules is tubulin; intermediate filaments contain a number of substances including keratin, desmin, and vimentin (Lazarides, 1980); microfilaments are composed of actin. However, the functions of each of these organelles are greatly influenced by a number of other associated molecules, which are in some cases components of the cytoskeleton. A review of intermediate filaments had little to say about the functions of these structures (Lazarides, 1980). This is a good example of molecular information outstripping our knowledge of function, and, as a result, there are no studies at this time of the role of intermediate filaments in the responses of cells to hormones. The following discussion is therefore limited to microtubules and microfilaments.

II.   THE FUNCTIONS OF MICROTUBULES AND MICROFILAMENTS

A.   Tubulin and Microtubules

Tubulin is capable of rapid polymerization into long hollow tubules and of equally rapid depolymerization to soluble monomer units (Olmsted and Borisy, 1973a,b). The process of polymerization requires GTP (Weisenberg, Borisy, 1973a,b; Frankel, 1976) and is regulated by proteins associated with microtubules (Slobod *et al.*, 1975; Olmsted and Lyon, 1981). As a result of rapid polymerization of tubulin, the cell can construct new organelles at short notice, no doubt to meet changing functional requirements. As a result of rapid depolymerization, which also may require energy (Bershadsky and Gelfand, 1981), the cell can cancel existing organelles. Although at present it is not possible to describe all the consequences of such changes, we can imagine that thrusting out and retracting rigid tubular structures will change the shape of a cell, could be important in movement (formation and function of cellular processes, e.g., pseudopodia, cilia, and flagella) and in internal shortening, in aligning internal structures, and in producing localized changes in the surface of the cell.

B. Actin and Microfilaments

Actin is a highly conserved protein capable of polymerizing from monomer (G form) to filamentous (F) actin (Korn, 1978). As in the case of tubulin, this polymerization (at least *in vitro*) is regulated in part by a number of protein and other molecules (Korn, 1978). In addition, actin (especially G actin) binds a variety of biologically important molecules (Lindberg *et al.*, 1979); and in the presence of myosin and ATP, it can trigger shortening and generate force (Korn, 1978). The widespread occurrence of myosin in tissues other than muscle suggests that shortening may be an important function of extramuscular actin (Pollard and Weihing, 1974). Possible functions of shortening are not difficult to imagine—movement of cells, movement within the cell (e.g., of organelles), changes in cell shape, and local changes in surface configuration. Moreover, these events would be subject to regulation by mechanisms that are integrated into the metabolism of the cell (because ATP is cleaved) and are capable of taking place in predetermined but not necessarily unchanging directions (unlike contraction of muscle). One of the mysteries of the cytoskeleton is the question of whether or not the binding function of G actin is of any physiological importance (Lindberg *et al.*, 1979).

C. Inhibitors of Tubules and Filaments

The study of the cytoskeleton is a relatively recent development in cell biology, and new methods must be devised to extend the current understanding of the functions of these organelles. Inhibitors have proved valuable in exploring the involvement of the cytoskeleton in various cellular functions. For the investigation of microtubules, colchicine and related compounds have been widely used. Colchicine inhibits the polymerization of tubules by combining with dimers of tubulin (Borisy and Taylor, 1967). The colchicine dimers cannot polymerize, and because microtubules turn over (i.e., continuous addition and removal of subunits occurs), existing microtubules eventually disappear in the presence of colchicine; any cellular function that requires microtubules cannot now take place. A note of caution is warranted, however, because colchicine may exert other effects than those directly attributable to inhibition of microtubules. An important control is available in the form of lumicolchicine, which does not inhibit polymerization of tubulin, but which resembles colchicine in chemical structure. Studies reporting positive results with colchicine require the use of this control if they are to be convincing.

For microfilaments, the preferred inhibitors are members of the cytochalasin family (e.g., B, D, E). These agents inhibit polymerization of actin (Lin *et al.*, 1980; MacLean-Fletcher and Pollard, 1980), and as the result of turnover, existing microfilaments are lost. In addition, cytochalasin cleaves (Hartwig and Stossel, 1979) and rearranges (Miranda *et al.*, 1974) microfilaments. Vinblastine, vincristine, and other inhibitors of tubules and filaments have proved less specific. It goes without saying that the use of such inhibitors in cellular and subcellular systems requires scrupulous attention to possible nonspecific effects that will, in the end, limit the usefulness of these inhibitors with such systems. A rather different use of the two inhibitors (colchicine and cytochalasin) is seen in the study of molecular and supramolecular properties of pure tubulin and actin. Here problems of nonspecificity are less serious, and the inhibitors are correspondingly more valuable.

In addition to the preceding generalizations concerning tubulin and actin, there are two more specific features of the cytoskeleton that must be considered at this point: (1) the cytoskeleton influences the movement of molecules in the plasma cell membrane and (2) the cytoskeleton can become attached to a variety of intracellular structures.

The clearest evidence for the first statement comes from recent studies by Wu *et al.* (1981), who showed that the diffusion coefficient (D) for proteins in the plasma membrane is several orders of magnitude greater in the membrane of blebs raised on the surface of lymphocytes than in the normally attached membrane of the cell. This observation convincingly demonstrated what had previously been inferred from numerous ultrastructural and other studies (Ash and Singer, 1976; Lilly *et al.*, 1977; Koch and Smith, 1978), namely, that cytoskeletal attachments to the plasma membrane serve to restrain the movements of surface proteins. When such attachments are severed (as in blebs), the proteins move much as they do in an isolated lipid phase *in vitro*. The implications of such observations are indeed extensive. The first implication would be that the cytoskeleton plays a major role in the gathering of surface molecules in patches and caps and perhaps in the subsequent internalization of surface molecules (Flanagan and Koch, 1978; Condeelis, 1979). The evidence for a reciprocal relationship (i.e., modification of the cytoskeleton by surface events) has been less clearly demonstrated, but the idea that such a relationship exists is rapidly growing. In any case, such reciprocity is at least partly self-evident. If the cytoskeleton is involved in patching, patching in turn results from or requires the combination of an external molecule (ligand) with a surface receptor. Presumably, the combination of the external ligand with the surface receptor influences the structure and function of the cytoskeleton. There is, in addition, evidence that internalization of lipoprotein involves cytoskeletal structures (Ostlund et al., 1979). This would suggest that the cytoskeleton responds to the binding of lipoprotein to a surface receptor.

A second implication arising from the relationship between the cytoskeleton and components of the surface membrane is that changes taking place within the cell may influence the distribution of surface components. Because these surface components are responsible for interactions between the cell and its environment, it is possible to imagine ways in which the cell can modify such environmental interactions in response to internal changes. For example, a unicellular organism could respond to an internal metabolic change by altering the composition of that part of the surface membrane that is directed toward an external source of cell nutrients. Again, the surface of the cell fulfills a number of distinct functions—adhesion to a basement membrane, intercellular junctions, surface exchange of metabolites, etc. The composition of the surface membrane must differ from one part of the cell to another in order to provide the most appropriate membrane composition for each region of the cell surface. The establishment, maintenance, and modification of these arrangements of surface components is likely to involve the cytoskeleton (Stossel, 1978). Presumably, cell division calls for a major reorganization of the distribution of molecules in the surface membrane in order to provide identical daughter cells. Here again, the cytoskeleton must play an important role. It is too early for more than conjecture concerning the functional possibilities for such relationships between the surface and interior of cells, but there is much evidence that they exist (Ash and Singer, 1976; Lilly et al., 1977; Koch and Smith, 1978). It is likely that the cytoskeleton constitutes an important component in such phenomena.

Evidence for the second generalization, i.e., attachment of intracellular structures to the cytoskeleton, is less convincing because of methodological problems. When cytoskeletal organelles are isolated biochemically, it is difficult to determine whether associated molecules and structures were similarly attached to the cytoskeleton in situ within the cell—the brutal confusion of homogenization provides opportunities for structures that are isolated from each other in the cell to encounter and possibly to bind each other. In spite of these limitations, there is good evidence that microfilaments are important in the functional interactions between cell membranes and nuclei (Franke, 1971), and microtubules appear to be associated with mitochondria (Heggeness *et al.*, 1978). In addition, a number of excellent studies have revealed associations between microtubules and granules (Robbins and Gonatas, 1964) and between microtubules and polyribosomes (Lenk *et al.*, 1977).

These considerations suggest the following generalizations about the cytoskeleton: (1) The cytoskeleton may be important in transmitting signals from the surface to the interior of cells and vice versa. (2) The cytoskeleton provides a means of influencing the surface organization of the cell. (3) Microtubules provide support (stiffening, rigidity) and direction—they are vectorial. (4) Microfilaments are potentially contractile and hence capable of local, directed, and regulated internal shortening; microtubules may also cause shortening by a sliding mechanism. Shortening in turn produces force and movement. (5) The cytoskeleton integrates the organelles of the cell; it provides a matrix for cellular activities by enhancing productive encounters and by establishing compartments within the cell. This idea has been well developed by Wolosewick and Porter (1979), who proposed that cells contain a microtrabecular system essential for the coordinated activities of different parts of the cell. In this role the cytoskeleton is a major factor in providing the inhomogeneity that distinguishes a cell from an aqueous solution. In performing these functions, an important attribute of the cytoskeleton lies in the ability of tubulin and actin to polymerize and depolymerize, which permits rapid and extensive reorganization of microtubules and microfilaments.

In the next section, we will consider how these properties are employed in the synthesis and secretion of hormones by endocrine cells.

III.   THE ROLE OF MICROFILAMENTS AND MICROTUBULES IN ENDOCRINE ACTIVITIES

A.   The Secretion of Thyroid Hormone

The thyroid cell has provided the first and in some ways still the best example of the role of the cytoskeleton in endocrine function. The reason for this preeminence is not hard to find—the thyroid cell is equipped to synthesize, store, and secrete its hormones triiodothyronine and thyroxine (T_3 and T_4) in a clearly vectorial process:

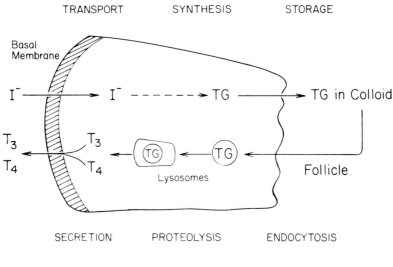

TG: Thyroglobulin
◯ Colloid droplet

Such a process could well require the directing influence of the cytoskeleton—the cell must distinguish its basal from its follicular membrane. Williams and Wolff (1970) studied the secretion of ^{131}I-labeled hormones by isolated thyroid glands *in vitro*. Colchicine was used to test the hypothesis that stimulation of the secretion of thyroid hormones by TSH involves the activity of microtubules (Williams and Wolff, 1970). Thyroglobulin was labeled *in vivo* by administration of ^{131}I. When labeled thyroid glands are incubated *in vitro*, they release or secrete small amounts of labeled hormones (T_3 and T_4) into the surrounding medium; addition of TSH to the medium *in vitro* greatly accelerates this process of secretion. It was observed by Williams and Wolff that the effect of TSH is inhibited by addition to the medium of colchicine, which is a relatively specific inhibitor of microtubules (Wilson and Meza, 1973). Light microscopy of the thyroid glands showed accumulation of colloid droplets in thyroid cells treated with TSH but not those treated with TSH and colchicine. To the extent that release of thyroid hormones *in vitro* represents the process of secretion *in vivo* and to the extent that colchicine is a specific inhibitor of tubule function, these studies strongly support the hypothesis that the action of

TSH in stimulating secretion of thyroid hormones requires microtubules—a finding that is consistent with the proposed roles of microtubules in integration of organelles and in providing direction to cellular events.

Electron microscopy confirmed these findings and clearly showed
that the uptake of colloid droplets from the interior of the follicle into
the cells, which is stimulated by TSH, is greatly inhibited by colchicine
under conditions in which the inhibitor destroys existing microtubules
and prevents polymerization and hence formation of new microtubules
(Nève *et al.*, 1972). The same workers employed cytochalasin B to
inhibit the formation of microfilaments; this inhibitor also prevented
the uptake and transport of colloid droplets, implying that these processes also require microfilaments (Nève *et al.*, 1972). It appears that
the process of engulfing stored colloid involves the development of
elaborate villous processes in the follicular membrane (Wetzel *et al.*,
1965). It is tempting to think of microtubules as thrusting out processes of follicular membrane into the colloid material stored within
the thyroid follicle. Certainly administration of colchicine is associated
with three things: loss of microtubules, absence of well-developed villous processes (Nève *et al.*, 1972), and inhibition of the secretion of
thyroid hormones in response to TSH (Williams and Wolff, 1970). The
uptake or engulfing of colloid might be facilitated by contraction of
microfilaments with internal shortening. However, the molecular
basis of these changes cannot be described at present. Clearly such
morphological studies call for morphometric confirmation. How else
can we be sure that the changes reported in electron micrographs are
reliably associated with hormonal stimulation and are inhibited by
colchicine?

A further development in this field came from Dickson *et al.* (1979),
who showed that TSH promotes an association between lysosomes and
actin. It is known that the intracellular droplets of colloid, produced by
TSH, are subjected to lysosomal proteolysis to release T_3 and T_4 from
the primary structure of thyroglobulin. These workers took considerable care to demonstrate that the association observed was real and
not fortuitous. For example, the association between lysosomes and
actin was increased by addition of TSH. These findings suggest that
the process by which the colloid droplets reach the lysosome may involve actin and hence microfilaments. This would be in keeping with
the role of actin in intracellular transport (in this case, of droplets to
lysosymes) and could come about as the result of actin binding to
various structures (e.g., colloid droplets and lysosomes) or from its
ability to trigger shortening. These studies approach the question of

how TSH promotes secretion of thyroid hormones. Presumably the basal or unstimulated secretion of these hormones takes place by the same mechanism but at a slower rate. In general, the unstimulated process is too slow to be studied by these methods. These findings raise but do not answer the question of how TSH alters the cytoskeleton in such a way as to promote secretion.

We must leave consideration of the thyroid cell with the observation that available evidence strongly suggests involvement of the cytoskeleton in the response of the thyroid gland to TSH and that in part this involvement results in the coordinated activity of organelles (follicular membrane, lysosomes, possibly mitochondria to provide energy, and basal membrane). It is reasonable to suggest that the cytoskeleton provides direction to processes that would not be effective as a series of uncoordinated or random events. It is perhaps too early to give free reign to the imagination in attempting to visualize these events in greater detail. However, the vectorial nature of the processes just described should be emphasized by pointing out that the two limiting membranes in the thyroid cell—the basal membrane facing the interstitial tissue and the follicular membrane facing the interior of the colloid—are different in structure, as Fig. 1 attempts to illustrate (Klinck *et al.*, 1970). The two lateral (intercellular) membranes are probably not directly involved in secretion of the hormones. Clearly the cell must organize the secretory process in a specific direction. It is hard to visualize this as the result of random movement.

B.   Secretion of Insulin

Although the β cells of the pancreas do not provide the striking morphological and functional asymmetry seen in thyroid cells, the role of the cytoskeleton in the secretion of insulin has been studied with important results (also see Chapter 7). Some of the advantages of this system include considerable experience with a sensitive radioimmunoassay for insulin, the development of versatile biochemical systems to study this process *in vitro* (including isolated islets), the fact that insulin is packaged in conspicuous lipid vesicles that can be followed during passage through the cell by electron microscopy much as Palade and co-workers followed amylase granules in the exocrine pancreas (Jamieson and Palade, 1977), and finally the availability of much important background information concerning the regulation of insulin secretion (Hedeskov, 1980). The most popular stimulus used to study secretion of insulin *in vitro* has been glucose. The first studies followed the same general lines as those employed with the thyroid cell, i.e., colchicine was shown to inhibit the secretion of insulin by islets in response to glucose added *in vitro* (Lacy *et al.*, 1972). Pipeleers *et al.* (1976) then showed that this response to glucose is accompanied by polymerization of tubulin. These studies were based upon carefully controlled methods of measuring the degree of polymerization of tubulin (Pipeleers *et al.*, 1977a,b).

A number of difficulties are encountered in attempting to measure the state of polymerization of tubulin in cells. Chief among these is the readiness with which microtubules undergo depolymerization during isolation. To overcome this, it is necessary to use a stabilizing buffer to prevent the polymerized tubulin from undergoing depolymerization. It is then essential to show that this buffer does not alter the proportion of unpolymerized to polymerized tubulin. The details of the various control experiments are not important here and they have been well described elsewhere (Pipeleers *et al.*, 1977a,b).

One publication presented a remarkable electron micrograph of a β cell showing secretory granules aligned in contact with a microtubule (Lacy *et al.*, 1968). Secretory granules in the β cell form by incorporation of insulin into lipid vesicles in preparation for secretion. The inevitable fate of such vesicles therefore involves movement to the surface membrane. The obvious inference from the micrograph in question is that the vesicles were being directed toward the surface membrane of the cell by the microtubule. A detective would describe the evidence as incriminating, a photographer would be anxious to exclude trompe l'oeuil, and a morphologist would regard the association as fortuitous until statistical morphometry proved otherwise. In any case, this micrograph served to give substance to vague ideas of how tubules could function in the secretory process—the tubule showed the vectorial qualities of an arrow (Lacy *et al.*, 1968). Certainly such direction would be a great step forward from a random process in which the secretory vesicles would be left to move through the cytoplasm until chance brought them to the surface membrane.

One interesting approach to the mechanism of secretion of insulin was reported by Aleyassine and Gardiner, who subjected pancreatic tissue to high pressure *in vitro* (Aleyassine and Gardiner, 1976). High pressure resulted in increased secretion of insulin, with a striking quantitative relationship between pressure and rate of secretion (Aleyassine and Gardiner, 1976). The pressures used (up to 45 mm Hg above atmospheric) were well below those required to disrupt microtubules, which would in any case have inhibited secretion of insulin, if we accept the evidence that microtubules are essential for that process. These findings warrant further exploration, but as they stand the results cannot be interpreted. They do, however, serve to remind us that cytochalasin causes decrease in the volume of β cells and increase in secretion of insulin (Orci *et al.*, 1972). It is not clear how inhibition of the polymerization of actin or reorganization of microfilaments could promote secretion of a protein except by some nonspecific mechanism, e.g., withdrawing cytoskeletal support of cell structure may permit those secretory vesicles near the surface of the cell to come in contact with the surface membrane. High external pressure could perhaps produce the same result. Another important possibility is that intact microfilaments are necessary for the transfer of some surface signal to the interior of the cell—without the signal, the vesicles cannot be released to the surface membrane. Although these studies are inconclusive, they emphasize a point that had already emerged from biochemical experiments, namely, that the secretion of insulin is a complex and multistep process. It is entirely conceivable that different elements of the cytoskeleton act at different stages of this process. However, these same experiments should remind us that cytochalasin can be deceptively nonspecific, especially in its effects on cell membranes (Estensen *et al.*, 1971).

One further finding with the β cell system deserves mention, namely, that the secretion of insulin in response to glucose is inhibited by trifluoperazine (Krausz *et al.*, 1980). This could mean that calmodulin is involved in the secretory process, although this evidence is not sufficient to establish proof. Involvement of calmodulin would point to a specific role for Ca^{2+} and that, in turn, would be consistent with involvement of the cytoskeleton, because calmodulin has been implicated in the functions of both tubules (Welsh *et al.*, 1978; Burke and DeLorenzo, 1981) and filaments (Dedman *et al.*, 1978).

We can conclude, then, that the secretion of insulin may involve both tubules and filaments. Tubules would provide direction, and filaments would cause shortening and internal transport. The evidence in both cases is tantalizing but not conclusive.

C. Stimulation of Steroid Synthesis by the Trophic Hormones ACTH and LH

Within a few minutes of exposure to ACTH, adrenal cells convert cholesterol to secreted steroid hormones at an accelerated rate. The cholesterol used in this response must first be transported from cytoplasmic stores to the inner mitochondrial membrane, where steroidogenesis begins with the side chain cleavage of cholesterol to pregnenolone (Hall, 1970). Pregnenolone then leaves the mitochondrion to undergo enzymatic transformation by microsomal enzymes. The steroid must return to the mitochondrion for the last step in the synthetic pathway, namely 11β-hydroxylation (Hall, 1970). The completed hormone is now ready for export by secretion:

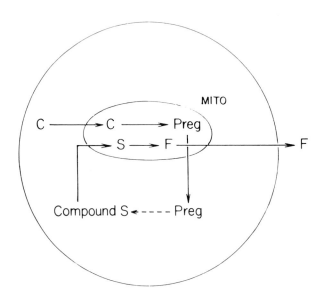

C : Cholesterol
Preg : Pregnenolone
(Compound) S : ll-deoxycortisol
F : Cortisol
MITO : Mitochondrion

Much biochemical evidence suggests that ACTH stimulates the transport of cholesterol to mitochondria. This process appears to limit the rate of steroid synthesis under basal conditions. Stimulation of cholesterol transport is therefore at least partly responsible for the increased synthesis of steroids produced by ACTH in the adrenal (Nakamura *et al.*, 1980) and by LH in the gonads (Hall *et al.*, 1979a, 1980). As a result of these considerations, systems were developed in several laboratories to measure transport of cholesterol from the cytoplasm to mitochondria (Mahaffee *et al.*, 1974) or more specifically, to the inner mitochondrial membrane (Hall *et al.*, 1979a; Nakamura *et al.*, 1980). The basic strategy consists of inhibiting the side chain cleavage of cholesterol by means of the inhibitor aminoglutethimide. In the presence of this inhibitor, cholesterol transported to mitochondria accumulates in the inner membrane because it cannot enter the steroidogenic pathway; side chain cleavage of cholesterol is essential for steroid synthesis. The amount of cholesterol accumulating above the basal level (determined at zero time) provides a measure of the intracellular transport of cholesterol.

Some years ago we discovered that cytochalasin B, added to adrenal cells, inhibits the stimulation of steroid synthesis normally produced by ACTH (Mrotek and Hall, 1975). Because cytochalasin B is known to inhibit microfilaments by preventing polymerization of actin (Lin *et al.*, 1980; MacLean-Fletcher and Pollard, 1980) and by disrupting established filaments (Miranda *et al.*, 1974), this observation rasied the possibility that microfilaments are required for the action of ACTH on steroid synthesis. Unfortunately, this inhibitor shows a variety of nonspecific effects, so that a number of important controls are necessary in using the drug with cells: (1) Because our observations with cytochalasin were made in a simple buffered medium, a major nonspecific effect of cytochalasin, i.e., inhibition of transport of glucose (Estensen and Plagemann, 1972) and amino acids, was excluded. (2) Other cell functions (protein synthesis, energy production, etc.) were not affected by cytochalasin (Mrotek and Hall, 1977). (3) The effect of cytochalasin was rapid and freely reversible (Mrotek and Hall, 1977), like the effect of the drug on actin (Estensen *et al.*, 1971). (4) The effects of four cytochalasins (B, D, E, and reduced B) on the responses of adrenal cells to ACTH and cAMP were examined (Hall *et al.*, 1981a). It was found that for each of these drugs, ED_{50} for inhibition of the steroidogenic responses and ED_{50} for binding to adrenal actin (measured by inhibition of the polymerization of actin) were the same, within the limits of experimental error, for each cytochalasin but very different from one cytochalasin to another (Hall *et al.*, 1981a). Moreover, inhibition by the cytochalasins of the steroidogenic response to ACTH was confined to a single step in the steroidogenic pathway, namely, the action of ACTH (and cAMP) in accelerating the transport of cholesterol to mitochondria (Mrotek and Hall, 1977; Hall *et al.*, 1981a). Because the cytochalasins inhibited the responses of adrenal cells to both ACTH and cAMP, this effect could not be dismissed as a nonspecific action of the inhibitor on the cell plasma membrane, because the second messenger is generally believed to discharge the intracellular responses to ACTH.

In spite of these consistent findings and careful controls, the hypothesis that microfilaments are involved in the response to ACTH rested on indirect evidence with an inhibitor. When Gabbiani and co-workers reported the isolation and characterization of anti-actin antibodies prepared from human serum of patients suffering from hepatitis (Gabbiani *et al.*, 1973; Charponnier *et al.*, 1977), the opportunity was taken to test this hypothesis by means of a much more specific agent. For this purpose, anti-actin was entrapped in liposomes, which were then fused with adrenal cells at 37°C for 1 hour before a second incubation, during which the responses of the cells to ACTH were examined. Anti-actin inhibited the responses to ACTH and cAMP (Hall *et al.*, 1979b). This inhibition was exerted specifically at the step in which cholesterol is transported to mitochondria (Hall *et al.*, 1979b).

These results strongly support the proposal that ACTH stimulates the transport of cholesterol to mitochondria and that this effect is at least partly responsible for increased steroid synthesis produced by that hormone and its second messenger cAMP. Moreover, this action of these stimulating agents (ACTH and cAMP) involves microfilaments. These observations provide excellent evidence for the role of microfilaments in a process of specific vectorial intracellular transport. Studies by Crivello and Jefcoate (1980) presented direct measurements of the rate of transport of cholesterol to mitochondria in adrenal cells and confirmed the increase of this transport by ACTH and the involvement of the cytoskeleton in the response to ACTH.

The significance of these results was emphasized by analogous experiments with steroid synthesis by rat Leydig cells. In these cells the responses to LH and cAMP were also inhibited by anti-actin (Hall *et al.*, 1979a,b, 1980). Evidently these findings apply to the regulation of steroid synthesis by a second trophic hormone. In addition, calmodulin is apparently involved in the intracellular transport of cholesterol in both adrenal and Leydig cells. Not only does trifluoperazine inhibit the steroidogenic actions of ACTH (Osawa *et al.*, 1981) and LH (Hall *et al.*, 1981b), but calmodulin introduced into adrenal and Leydig cells stimulates transport of cholesterol to mitochondria and accelerates the synthesis of steroids (Osawa *et al.*, 1981; Hall *et al.*, 1981b). To the extent that calmodulin and Ca^{2+} are involved in regulating microfilaments (Means and Dedman, 1980), these observations lend further support to the idea that microfilaments are involved in the intracellular transport of cholesterol.

D. Other Hormones

1. *Antidiuretic Hormone*

The response of the epithelial cells of the toad bladder to antidiuretic hormone (ADH) is associated with a remarkable rearrangement of particles in the luminal membranes of these cells. ADH causes a clustering or aggregation of the particles seen on the cytoplasmic surface (P face) of the luminal membrane with complementary depressions on the E face (Bourquet *et al.*, 1976). The particles appear to originate from membranes within the cell, and they take up positions in the luminal membrane as the result of a process of intracellular transport to that membrane, followed by fusion of the internal membrane bearing the aggregated particles with the luminal membrane. These steps (transport and fusion) are inhibited by colchicine and by cytochalasin B; they may, therefore, depend upon microtubules and microfilaments (Katchadorian *et al.*, 1979; Muller *et al.*, 1980). Although more direct evidence is necessary before this idea is accepted, involvement of the cytoskeleton in such a process would be logical. In this case, the transport process resembles the movement of secretory vesicles to the surface membrane, with the important and interesting difference that with ADH the transported particles are inserted in the membrane but not discharged to the exterior as in secretion. In addition, the response to ADH is inhibited by trifluoperazine (Levine *et al.*, 1981). It is perhaps premature to speculate on the possibility that ADH promotes intracellular transport of particles destined for the luminal membrane by a mechanism involving shortening of microfilaments via an ATPase reaction triggered by Ca^{2+}–calmodulin together with the intervention of tubules in some as yet undefined mechanism (possibly providing direction). However, the findings just reviewed would encourage an experimental approach to test such an idea. For example, it will be important to use the sulfoxide derivative of trifluoperazine in order to eliminate nonspecific effects of the molecule; the sulfoxide derivative is much less potent than the parent molecule in inhibiting calmodulin (Hall *et al.*, 1981b). A second approach to investigating the involvement of calmodulin in various cell functions is the use of liposomes to promote entry of calmodulin into cells (Hall *et al.*, 1981b; Osawa *et al.*, 1981).

2. Parathyroid Hormone

The parathyroid gland provides an interesting example of the role of the cytoskeleton in endocrine activity. Morphological evidence shows that destruction of microtubules by colchicine inhibits the secretory response of the parathyroid to phosphate (Reavan and Reaven, 1975). More interesting is the observation of Kemper *et al.* (1975) that colchicine inhibits the conversion of proparathyroid hormone to parathyroid hormone. Cytochalasin B is without effect. Because the conversion of prohormone to the secreted hormone is thought to require intracellular transport of the newly formed prohormone (made on rough ER) to the site of proteolytic cleavage (probably the Golgi complex), the implication is that microtubules are required for this transport (rough ER to Golgi). This transport process was estimated to take some 10 to 20 minutes. It appears that further study of this system might prove rewarding, because the events can be timed with some accuracy. What is now required is the demonstration of a quantitative relationship between the rate of production of the completed hormone and some parameter related to the functions of microtubules in response to a physiological stimulus.

3. Miscellaneous Hormones

Secretion of growth hormone and prolactin by pituitary cells is inhibited by colchicine (Gautwik and Tashjian, 1973; Labrie *et al.*, 1973). Similar studies have been performed with adrenal medulla with a similar result (Poisner and Cooke, 1975; Unsicker *et al.*, 1979).

IV. THE REGULATION OF CYTOSKELETAL FUNCTION

The preceding sections may go some way toward implicating the cytoskeleton in certain functions of endocrine cells. That the cytoskeleton is required for such cellular activities is hardly surprising. How the cell recruits the cytoskeleton and how the cytoskeleton acts in response to hormones is, at present, far from clear. When an investigator of 10 years' experience with microtubules is confronted with the question, "What do microtubules do for the cell?" he is sure to be disarmed. The opening sentence of this chapter attempted to present this problem by asserting that microtubules (and microfilaments) are organelles in search of a function. If we are ignorant of what these organelles do, how can we describe their roles in complex cellular activities? This unsatisfactory state of affairs can only be partly alleviated by studying some of the better-documented examples of cytoskeletal function, and for this purpose we must look outside the endocrine system at cells that are better suited for the first studies in this new area of investigation. We can only hope that these examples are sufficiently typical to provide endocrinologists with some guidelines with which to design experiments aimed at understanding the contributions of these organelles to endocrinology and with the insight to recognize the consequences of tubule and filament activities when they come across them. The following properties of tubules and filaments appear sufficiently documented to warrant discussion in the hope of providing some clues concerning the mechanisms by which the organelles might act in endocrine (and other) cells.

A. Microtubules

1. Sliding Function

The best-understood function of microtubules is to be seen in the workings of the sperm flagellum, in which clear evidence is available to show that microtubules interact with each other and slide past one another. Force is generated with the aid of a protein called dynein, which is a special form of ATPase (Gibbons, 1963). The evidence for sliding is less compelling in the case of the mitotic apparatus, but a similar process may be involved (McIntosh, 1979). Sliding can lead to shortening, to the approximation of two attached ends of microtubules, or to bending. The idea has been expressed that sliding may occur between cytoplasmic microtubules, as in the flagellum, but no clear application of this concept to a specific cellular function has been proposed.

2. Direction

One important feature of microtubules is that they possess two distinct ends, i.e., they can establish direction (Kirschner, 1980). This property has been most successfully established in the filamentous processes of nerve cells, in which direction is of paramount importance to function. The directional properties of microtubules in neurons may be employed in the intracellular transport of substances between cell body and synapse, and perhaps in the reverse direction (Burton and Paige, 1981). When we consider secretion of thyroid hormone (see earlier), it is clear that microtubules could contribute to this process by providing the specific direction required for successful secretory function (i.e., from follicular membrane toward basal membrane). Furthermore, polymerization and depolymerization enable the cell to rearrange the cytoskeleton and hence to provide new directions within the cytoplasm for various cellular activities.

3. Movement

Detailed analysis of the mitotic spindle suggests that depolymerization of tubules causes movement in the spindle, which draws the chromosomes toward the two poles of the spindle (McIntosh, 1979). This was demonstrated by Nicklas (1971), who separated chromosomes from the associated fibers (which contain microtubules). The chromosomes remained motionless until they became associated with new fibers, when they again began to move. It appears that tubules are responsible for the ability of the fibers to move the chromosomes (McIntosh, 1979). Although no other biological system has provided such clear evidence of intracellular movement in response to changes in microtubules, it is reasonable to consider that this mechanism may apply to other examples of cell movement. Movement and direction may, at least partly, account for the role of microtubules in processing proparathyroid hormone (see earlier).

4. Generation of Force

Clearly related to movement is the generation of the forces that cause movement. The theory of Margolis and Wilson (1978) proposes that force can be generated by treadmilling of microtubules. Subunits are added at one end and removed from the other, thus pushing the polymerizing end, and anything attached to it, in the direction of the opposite end, where depolymerization occurs. This process of treadmilling can reach a steady state in which the length of the tubule remains constant—it has been described as giving the illusion of movement. In addition to treadmilling, it has been proposed that dynein may serve to generate force by acting as an ATPase with cytoplasmic microtubules (Dentler et al., 1980).

5. Saltatory Movement

The remarkable experiments of Freed and Lebowitz (1970) showed that the pathways of saltatory movement of particles within the cell are clearly related to the organization of microtubules. It is almost as though the cell possesses a framework on which it organizes intracellular traffic, much as the osseous skeleton dictates the spatial consequences of muscular contraction, with the important difference that microtubules, unlike bone, are capable of extensive and rapid reorganization.

6. Molecular Properties

Although present understanding of the functions of microtubules is incomplete, the molecules of which the tubules are composed have been investigated with striking success. Most studies have been concerned with the regulation of polymerization. It is known that microtubules contain proteins other than tubulin—these are referred to collectively as microtubule associated proteins, for which the acronym MAPs has become the accepted designation. MAPs play an important role in regulating the polymerization of tubulin (Vallee, 1980), and we have seen that one MAP called dynein is a specialized ATPase. This process of polymerization proceeds in a fixed direction by a head-to-tail mechanism in the phenomenon of treadmilling. It is surely relevant to this process of polymerization that MAPs have been shown to be subject to phosphorylation (Vallee, 1980); this would provide one mechanism for controlling the process and would link polymerization with the ubiquitous cAMP. The entry of this cyclic nucleotide into such regulation reminds us that its equally ubiquitous rival Ca^{2+} has also been implicated in regulation of the state of polymerization of tubulin. Increase in the concentration of Ca^{2+} within the physiological (μM) range causes depolymerization of tubules *in vivo* (Kiehart, 1981). These two agents (cAMP and Ca^{2+}) have the important potential of regulating tubular function locally within the cell. In the case of Ca^{2+}, this brings to mind the role of calmodulin in focusing the influence of Ca^{2+} to specific regions or components of the cell (Means and Dedman, 1980). For cAMP, local regulation would involve the specificities and distributions of a variety of protein kinase enzymes. In this connection, it is worth mentioning that as much as one-third of brain cAMP-dependent protein kinase is tightly associated with MAPs (Vallee *et al.*, 1981).

B. Microfilaments

1. Shortening

An increasing number of reports show that many nonmuscle cells contain myosin in addition to actin (Korn, 1978). Moreover, nonmuscle actin *in vitro* interacts with myosin in the same way as muscle actin in that it triggers myosin ATPase activity (Korn, 1978). It is difficult to avoid the conclusion that in nonmuscle cells actin and myosin produce shortening by a sliding mechanism, as in muscle. This could in turn conceivably produce regulated intracellular movement. The equatorial constriction seen during cytokinesis involves shortening produced by a ring of microfilaments known to contain actin (Fujiwara *et al.*, 1978) and myosin (Schroeder, 1973). Based upon these observations, it is possible to develop plausible models to explain cytokinesis by means of a sliding filament mechanism like that generally accepted for the contraction of skeletal muscle (Schroeder, 1973; Fujiwara *et al.*, 1978). Several examples of such a function for actin in endocrine cells were presented earlier, although it is not yet possible to study these cells in sufficient detail to develop the hypothesis completely.

2. Polarity

In addition to providing direction, microfilaments show polarity—both structural polarity and polarity of polymerization. Structural polarity can be demonstrated by decorating cellular microfilaments with heavy meromyosin (Ishikawa *et al.*, 1969). The decorated microfilaments show the classic barbs or arrowheads seen when the thin filaments of muscle are decorated by the same method (Huxley, 1963). The importance of structural polarity lies in the fact that it determines the direction of filament sliding and hence the direction of the forces resulting from the sliding of those filaments that are anchored at both ends; it is known that some microfilaments are anchored to cell membranes. For example, in the microfilament xy,

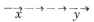

x may be attached to a membrane. A movable organelle attached to the filament at y will, as the result of sliding, be brought closer to x with its attached membrane. It will be realized that the length of the filament xy does not change, because shortening results from sliding. This directional restriction of shortening occurs because the structures of actin and myosin dictate that the cross-bridges that mediate sliding can form only in such a way as to permit shortening in one direction (Huxley, 1963). The importance of direction is obvious in the examples of endocrine cellular functions discussed earlier. For example, intracellular transport of thyroid hormone occurs not merely between two membranes but in a fixed direction (follicular → basal). This polarity is believed to result from the structural polarity of the underlying microfilaments and microtubules.

The structural polarity that determines the direction of shortening should not be confused with the polarity of polymerization. Some microfilaments are attached to the inside of the plasma membrane of the cell and polymerization occurs most rapidly at the end of the microfilament attached to the plasma membrane whereas polymerization away from the point of attachment is much less rapid (Woodrum *et al.*, 1975):

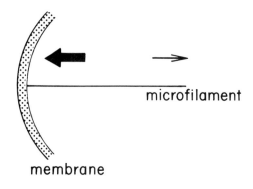

In order to polymerize toward the point of attachment (Fig. 3, heavy arrow), the process of polymerization must displace the attachment of the filament to the membrane (Mooseker *et al.*, 1981). It can be seen that such polymerization at the point of attachment could result in the formation of processes protruding at the cell surface and hence in changes in the surface configuration of the cell.

The ability to form new microfilaments endows the cell with a certain functional versatility because it can create microfilaments where and when they are required. New microfilaments, because of their polarity, give new vectors within the cell. In addition, the cell can dispense with established microfilaments.

3. Rigidity

Microfilaments are to some extent rigid, so that this property may be important in providing local support within cells, much as the stays in a collar serve to maintain shape. The intestinal microvillus offers an excellent example of this, because the many microvilli on the epithelial cells of the intestine are each supported by means of a central core made up of microfilament bundles (Glenney *et al.*, 1981). However, such rigidity should not be considered permanent, because villi can form and collapse in rapid succession so that the shape of the free surface of the intestinal cell is ever-changing. It is interesting to notice that adrenal cells show extensive formation of villous processes when stimulated by ACTH (Kawaoi *et al.*, 1977). Presumably these processes require the support of appropriately directed tubules and filaments. Like the intestinal villus, these adrenal surface villi come and go with great rapidity.

4. Gelation

During amoeboid movement, cytoplasm undergoes a striking change in state as the pseudopodium advances. The cytoplasm exists in two distinct physical states: a fluid state, or sol; and a solid state, or gel. During the formation of the pseudopodium, the fluid cytoplasm flows into the developing process as a sol and at a certain point it undergoes an abrupt transition to the solid or gel form (Taylor and Condeelis, 1979); this process is called gelation. It should be added that gelation occurs in many cells, including certain mammalian cells, e.g., HeLa cells (Weihing, 1977). To make use of variations in the physical state of the cytoplasm, the cytoskeleton must possess the rigidity necessary for the development of tension and the plasticity necessary to permit movement in response to tension. Gelation results from cross-linking of actin filaments under the influence of accompanying proteins; solation results from breakdown of microfilaments and interfilamentous connections. As a result, the microfilaments of amoeba must serve as both muscle and bone, in contrast to the musculoskeletal system of the vertebrate organism, in which these two components are each confined to one role or the other. The gel is sufficiently rigid to permit tension to develop and to be appropriately directed (the function of bone) whereas the sol is sufficiently flexible to allow shortening and movement (the functions of muscle). Local regulation of the physical state of the cytoplasm is provided by a series of proteins capable in some cases of cross-linking microfilaments with the formation of a gel and in other cases of disrupting established filaments to produce a sol. These transitions are closely regulated in extent and location in order to produce the appropriate consistency of cytoplasm where and when changes are required. The most obvious examples of such changes are to be found in movement—both external movement of a cell across a substratum and internal movement of particles within the cell (Taylor and Condeelis, 1979). Internal movement has been most successfully studied in large cells with injected particles or by studying movement of organelles. Such studies are inevitably difficult in mammalian cells, which are for the most part small. Moreover, we are in many cases chiefly interested in the movement of submicroscopic particles. New methods must be developed to meet these challenges.

5. Filament-Associated Proteins

Although the acronym FAP does not appear to have been used, actin is associated with a number of proteins that influence the behavior of microfilaments. G actin is present in cells above the critical concentration that in a solution of actin would result in polymerization to F actin (Korn, 1978). This suggests that polymerization must be prevented in the cell. G actin binds to DNase I and to a protein called profilin (MW 16,000). The interaction with DNase is of no known functional importance, whereas that with profilin prevents polymerization (Carlsson *et al.*, 1976). The protein called filamin (MW 250,000) (which may be the same as actin-binding protein) combines with F actin and promotes polymerization (Korn, 1978). α-Actinin releases G actin from the inhibitory effect of profilin, thereby promoting polymerization (Blikstad *et al.*, 1980). A number of gelation factors combine with F actin to cross-link the actin and cause gelation (Maruta and Korn, 1977). A variety of proteins capable of disrupting microfilaments, to ensure that the process is reversible (solation), have also been isolated (Korn, 1978). Breakdown of filaments is not only important in regulating the directions and positions of the filaments but also in preventing undesirable accumulation of actin in regions of intracellular shortening.

Without removal of the actin filaments from the path of contraction, an inert mass of contracted actomyosin would result from the shortening process. This is most clearly understood by considering skeletal muscle, in which the structural elements of the tissue are attached to each other and in which the two ends of the muscle are permanently fixed. Contraction results from longitudinal sliding. In the cytoskeleton, both ends of a microfilament are not permanently anchored, so that the filaments could be caught up in the contracting processes and become squeezed into bundles between the sliding filaments. One important result of breakdown of microfilaments is that redundant actin escapes from the region of contraction (Taylor and Condeelis, 1979).

In view of analogies between microfilaments and muscle, it is not surprising that Ca^{2+} is involved in the regulation of filament function and that phosphorylation of filament proteins under the influence of cAMP may be important in the functions of microfilaments (Korn, 1978).

ACKNOWLEDGMENTS

The author is extremely grateful to Dr. R. R. Weihing and to Dr. R. B. Vallee (The Worcester Foundation for Experimental Biology, Shrewsbury, Massachusetts, 01545) for helpful discussions during the preparation of this chapter.

REFERENCES

Aleyassine, H., and Gardiner, R. J. (1976). Stimulation of insulin release by elevated pressure gradient. *Endocrinology (Baltimore)* **99**, 1542–1546.

Ash, J. F., and Singer, S. J. (1976). Concanavalin-A-induced transmembrane linkage of con A surface receptors to intracellular myosin-containing filaments. *Proc. Natl. Acad. Sci. U.S.A.* **73**, 4575–4579.

Bershadsky, A. D., and Gelfand, V. I. (1981). ATP-dependent regulation of cytoplasmic microtubule disassembly. *Proc. Natl. Acad. Sci. U.S.A.* **78**, 3610–3613.

Blikstad, I., Eriksson, S., and Carlsson, L. (1980). α-actinin promotes polymerization of actin from profilactin. *Eur. J. Biochem.* **109**, 317–323.

Borisy, G. G., and Taylor, E. W. (1967). The mechanism of action of cholchicine. *J. Cell Biol.* **34**, 535–548.

Bourquet, J., Chevalier, J., and Hugon, J. S. (1976). Alterations in membrane-associated particle distribution during antidiuretic challenge in frog urinary bladder epithelium. *Biophys. J.* **16**, 627–639.

Burke, B. E., and DeLorenzo, R. J. (1981). Ca^{2+} and calmodulin-stimulated phosphorylation of neurotubulin. *Proc. Natl. Acad. Sci. U.S.A.* **78**, 991–995.

Burton, P. R., and Paige, J. L. (1981). Polarity of axoplasmic microtubules in the olfactory nerve. *Proc. Natl. Acad. Sci. U.S.A.* **78**, 3269–3273.

Carlsson, L., Mystrom, L.-E., Lindberg, U., Kannan, K. K., Cid-Dresdner, H., Lovgren,

S., and Jornvall, H. (1976). Crystallization of a non-muscle actin. *J. Mol. Biol.* **105**, 353–366.

Charponnier, C., Kohler, L., and Gabbiani, G. (1977). Fixation of human anti-actin autoantibodies on skeletal muscle fibres. *Clin. Exp. Immunol.* **27**, 278–284.

Condeelis, J. S. (1979). Isolation of Con A caps and their association with actin and myosin. *J. Cell. Biol.* **80**, 751–758.

Crivello, J. F., and Jefcoate, C. R. (1980). Intracellular movement of cholesterol in rat adrenals. *J. Biol. Chem.* **255**, 8144–8151.

Dedman, J. R., Welsh, M. J., and Means, A. R. (1978). Calcium-dependent regulator production and characterization of a monospecific antibody. *J. Biol. Chem.* **253**, 7515–7521.

Dentler, W. L., Pratt, M. M., and Stephens, R. E. (1980). Microtubule-membrane interactions in cilia. II. Identification of a membrane-associated dyneine-like ATPase. *J. Cell Biol.* **84**, 381–403.

Dickson, J. G., Malan, P. G., and Ekins, R. P. (1979). The association of actin with a thyroid lysosomal fraction. *Eur. J. Biochem.* **97**, 471–479.

Estensen, R. D., Rosenberg, M., and Sheridan, I. D. (1971). Cytochalasin B: Microfilaments and contractile processes. *Science* **173**, 356–359.

Estensen, R. O., and Plagemann, P. G. W. (1972). Cytochalasin B inhibition of glucose and glucosamine transport. *Proc. Natl. Acad. Sci. U.S.A.* **69**, 1430–1434.

Flanagan, J., and Koch, G. L. E. (1978). Cross-linked surface Ig attaches to actin. *Nature (London)* **273**, 278–281.

Franke, W. W. (1971). Relationship of nuclear membranes with filaments and microtubules. *Protoplasma* **73**, 263–292.

Frankel, F. R. (1976). Organization and energy-dependent growth of microtubules in cells. *Proc. Natl. Acad. Sci. U.S.A.* **73**, 2798–2801.

Freed, J. J., and Lebowitz, M. M. (1970). The association of a class of saltatory movements with microtubules in cultured cells. *J. Cell Biol.* **45**, 334–354.

Fujiwara, K., Porter, M. E., and Pollard, T. D. (1978). Alpha-actinin localization in the cleavage furrow during cytokinesis. *J. Cell Biol.* **79**, 268–275.

Gabbiani, G., Ryan, G. B., Lamelin, J. P., Vassalli, P., Majno, G., Bouvier, C., Rimchaud, A., and Luscher, E. F. (1973). Human smooth muscle autoantibody. *Am. J. Pathol.* **72**, 473–488.

Gautwik, K. M., and Tashjian, A. H. (1973). Effects of colchicine on release of prolactin and growth hormone by pituitary tumor cells *in vitro. Endocrinology (Baltimore)* **93**, 793–799.

Gibbons, I. R. (1963). Studies on the protein components of cilia from *Tetrahymena pyriformis. Proc. Natl. Acad. Sci. U.S.A.* **50**, 1002–1010.

Glenny, J. R., Kaulfus, P., and Weber, K. (1981). F actin assembly modulated by villin: Ca^{2+}-dependent nucleation and capping of the barbed end. *Cell* **24**, 471–480.

Hall, P. F. (1970). Gonadotrophic regulation of testicular function. *In* "Androgens of the Testis" (K. B. Eik-Nes, ed.), pp. 73–115. Dekker, New York.

Hall, P. F., Charponnier, C., Nakamura, M., and Gabbiani, G. (1979a). The role of microfilaments in the response of Leydig cells to LH. *J. Steroid Biochem.* **11**, 1361–1366.

Hall, P. F., Charponnier, C., Nakamura, M., and Gabbiani, G. (1979b). The role of microfilaments in the response of adrenal tumor cells to ACTH. *J. Biol. Chem.* **254**, 9080–9084.

Hall, P. F., Charponnier, C., and Gabbiani, G. (1980). Role of actin in the response of

Leydig cells to LH. *In* "Testicular Development, Structure and Function" (A. Steinberger and E. Steinberger, eds.), pp. 229–235. Raven, New York.

Hall, P. F., Nakamura, M., and Mrotek, J. J. (1981a). The actions of various cytochalasins on mouse adrenal tumor cells in relation to trophic stimulation of steroidogenesis. *Biochim. Biophys. Acta* **676**, 338–344.

Hall, P. F., Osawa, S., and Mrotek, J. J.(1981b). Influence of Calmodulin on steroid synthesis in Leydig cells from rat testis. *Endocrinology (Baltimore)* **109**, 1677–1682.

Hartwig, J. H., and Stossel, T. P. (1979). Cytochalasin B and the structure of actin gels. *J. Mol. Biol.* **134**, 539–553.

Hedeskov, C. J. (1980). Mechanism of glucose-induced insulin secretion. *Physiol. Rev.* **60**, 447–509.

Heggeness, M. H., Simon, M., and Singer, S. J. (1978). Association of mitochondria with microtubules in cultured cells. *Proc. Natl. Acad. Sci. U.S.A.* **75**, 3863–3866.

Huxley, H. E. (1963). Electron microscope studies on the structure of natural and synthetic protein filaments from striated muscle. *J. Mol. Biol.* **7**, 281–308.

Ishikawa, H., Bischoff, R., and Holtzer, H. (1969). Formation of arrowhead complexes with heavy meromyosin in a variety of cell types. *J. Cell Biol.* **43**, 312–328.

Jamieson, J. D., and Palade, G. E. (1977). Production of secretory proteins in animal cells. *Int. Cell Biol. Pap. Int. Cong., 1st, 1976* pp. 308–317.

Katchadorian, W. A., Ellis, S. J., and Muller, J. (1979). Possible role for microtubules and microfilaments in ADH action. *Am. J. Physiol.* **236**, F14–F20.

Kawaoi, A., Uchida, T., and Okano, T. (1977). Transmission and scanning electron microscope observations of mouse adrenocortical adenoma cells (Y-1) in non-stimulated and stimulated states. *Acta Pathol. Jpn.* **27**, 841–856.

Kemper, B., Habener, J. F., Rich, A., and Potts, J. T. (1975). Microtubules and the intracellular conversion of proparathyroid hormone to parathyroid hormone. *Endocrinology (Baltimore)* **96**, 903–912.

Kiehart, D. P. (1981). Studies on *in vivo* sensitivity of spindle microtubules to Ca^{2+}. *J. Cell Biol.* **88**, 604–617.

Kirschner, M. W. (1980). Implications of treadmilling for the stability and polarity of actin and tubulin polymers *in vivo*. *J. Cell Biol.* **86**, 330–334.

Klinck, G. H., Oertel, J. E., and Winship, T. (1970). Ultrastructure of normal human thyroid. *Lab. Invest.* **22**, 2–22.

Koch, G. L. E., and Smith, M. J. (1978). An association between actin and the major histocompatability antigen H-2. *Nature (London)* **273**, 274–281.

Korn, E. D. (1978). Biochemistry of actomycin-dependent cell motility: A review. *Proc. Natl. Acad. Sci. U.S.A.* **75**, 588–599.

Krausz, Y., Wolheim, C. B., Siegel, W., and Sharp, G. W. G. (1980). Possible role for calmodulin in insulin release. *J. Clin. Invest.* **68**, 603–607.

Labrie, F., Pelletier, G., Gauthier, M., Borgeat, P., Lemay, A., and Gouge, J. J. (1978). Role of microtubules in basal and stimulated release of growth hormone and prolactin in rat adenohypophysis *in vitro*. *Endocrinology (Baltimore)* **93**, 903–914.

Lacy, P. E., Howell, S. L., Young, D. A., and Fink, C. J. (1968). New hypothesis of insulin secretion. *Nature (London)* **219**, 1177–1179.

Lacy, P. E., Walker, M. A., and Fink, C. J. (1972). Participation of the microtubular system in the biphasic release of insulin. *Diabetes* **21**, 987–998.

Lazarides, E. (1980). Intermediate filaments as mechanical integrators of cellular space. *Nature (London)* **283**, 249–256.

Lenk, R., Ransom, L., Kaufmann, Y., and Penman, S. (1977). A cytoskeletal structure with associated polyribosomes obtained from HeLa cells. *Cell* **10,** 67–78.

Levine, S. D., Kachadorian, W. A., Levin, D. N., and Schlondorf, D. (1981). Effects of trifluoperazine on function and structure of toad urinary bladder. *J. Clin. Invest.* **67,** 662–672.

Lilly, Y., Bourgiugnon, W., and Singer, S. J. (1977). Transmembrane interactions and the mechanism of capping of surface receptors. *Proc. Natl. Acad. Sci. U.S.A.* **74,** 5031–5035.

Lin, D. C., Tobin, K. D., Grumet, M., and Lin, S. (1980). Cytochalasins inhibit nuclei-induced actin polymerization by blocking filament elongation. *J. Cell Biol.* **84,** 455–460.

Lindberg, U., Carlsson, L., Markey, F., and Nystrom, L. E. (1979). The unpolymerized form of actin in non-muscle cells. *Methods Achiev. Exp. Pathol.* **8,** 143–170.

McIntosh, J. R. (1979). Cell division. *In* "Microtubules" (K. Roberts and J. S. Hyams, eds.), pp. 381–441. Academic Press, New York.

MacLean-Fletcher, S., and Pollard, T. (1980). Mechanisms of action of cytochalasin B on actin. *Cell* **20,** 329–341.

Mahaffee, D., Reitz, R. C., and Ney, R. L. (1974). The mechanism of action of ACTH. The role of mitochondrial cholesterol accumulation in the regulation of steroidogenesis. *J. Biol. Chem.* **249,** 227–233.

Margolis, R. L., and Wilson, L. (1978). Opposite end assembly and disassembly of microtubules at steady state *in vitro*. *Cell* **13,** 1–8.

Martua, H., and Korn, E. D. (1977). Purification from *Acanthamoeba castellanii* of proteins that induce gelation and synthesis of F-actin. *J. Biol. Chem.* **252,** 399–402.

Means, A. R., and Dedman, J. R. (1980). Calmodulin: An intracellular calcium receptor. *Nature (London)* **285,** 73–77.

Miranda, A. F., Godman, G. G., and Tanenbaum, S. W. (1974). Action of cytochalasin D on cells of established lines. *J. Cell Biol.* **62,** 406–423.

Mooseker, M. S., Bonder, E. D., Grimwade, B. G., Howe, C. L., Keller, T. C. S., Wasserman, R. H., and Weharton, K. A. (1981). Regulation of contractile cytoskeletal structure and filament assembly in the brush boarder of intestinal epithelial cells. *Cold Spring Harbor Symp. Quant. Biol.* **46,** in press.

Mrotek, J. J., and Hall, P. F. (1975). The influence of cytochalasin B on the response of adrenal tumor cells to ACTH and cyclic AMP. *Biochem. Biophys. Res. Commun.* **64,** 891–896.

Mrotek, J. J., and Hall, P. F. (1977). Response of adrenal tumor cells to ACTH: Site of inhibition by cytochalasin B. *Biochemistry* **16,** 3177–3181.

Muller, J., Kachadorian, W. A., and DiScala, V. A. (1980). Evidence that ADH-stimulated intramembrane particle aggregates are transferred from cytoplasmic to luminal membranes in toad bladder epithelial cells. *J. Cell Biol.* **85,** 83–95.

Nakamura, M., Watanuki, M., Tilley, B., and Hall, P. F. (1980). Effect of ACTH on intracellular cholesterol transport. *J. Endocrinol.* **84,** 179–188.

Nève, P., Ketelbant-Balasse, P., Willems, C., and Dumont, J. E. (1972). Effect of inhibitors of microtubules and microfilaments on dog thyroid slices *in vitro*. *Exp. Cell. Res.* **74,** 227–244.

Nicklas, R. B. (1971). Chromosomal movement during cell division. *Adv. Cell Biol.* **2,** 225–297.

Olmsted, J. B., and Borisy, G. G. (1973a). Microtubules. *Annu. Rev. Biochem.* **42,** 507–540.

Olmsted, J. B., and Borisy, G. G. (1973b). Characterization of microtubule assembly in porcine brain extracts by viscometry. *Biochemistry* **12**, 4282–4289.

Olmsted, J. B., and Lyon, H. (1981). A microtubule-associated protein specific to differentiated neuroblastoma cells. *J. Biol. Chem.* **256**, 3507–3511.

Orci, L., Gabbay, K. H., and Malaisse, W. J. (1972). Pancreatic beta cell web: Its possible involvement in insulin secretion. *Science* **175**, 1128–1129.

Osawa, S., Hall, P. F., and Thomasson, C. L. (1981). A role for calmodulin in the regulation of steroidogenesis. *J. Cell Biol.* **90**, 402–407.

Ostlund, R. E., Pfleger, B., and Schonfeld, G. (1979). Role of microtubules in LDL processing in cultured cells. *J. Clin. Invest.* **63**, 75–84.

Pipeleers, D. G., Pipeleers-Marichal, M. A., and Kipnis, D. M. (1976). Microtubule assembly and intracellular transport of secretory granules in pancreatic islets. *Science* **191**, 88–89.

Pipeleers, D. G., Pipeleers-Marichal, M. A., Sherline, P., and Kipnis, D. M. (1977a). A sensitive method for measuring polymerized and depolymerized tubulin in tissues. *J. Cell Biol.* **74**, 341–350.

Pipeleers, D. G., Pipeleers-Marichal, M. A., and Kipnis, D. M. (1977b). Physiological regulation of total tubulin and polymerized tubulin in tissues. *J. Cell Biol.* **77**, 351–357.

Poisner, A. M., and Cooke, P. (1975). Microtubules and the adrenal medulla. *Ann. N. Y. Acad. Sci.* **253**, 653–668.

Pollard, T. D., and Weihing, R. R. (1974). Actin and myosin and cell movement. *CRC Crit. Rev. Biochem.* **2**, 1–65.

Reaven, E. P., and Reaven, G. M. (1975). A quantitative ultrastructural study of microtubule content in parathyroid glands. *J. Clin. Invest.* **56**, 49–55.

Robbins, E., and Gonatas, N. K. (1964). Histochemical and ultrastructural studies on HeLa cell cultures. *J. Histochem. Cytochem.* **12**, 704–711.

Schroeder, T. R. (1973). Actin in dividing cells: Contractile ring filaments bind heavy meromyosin. *Proc. Natl. Acad. Sci. U.S.A.* **70**, 1688–1692.

Slobod, R. D., Rudolph, S. A., Rosenbaum, J. L., and Greengard, P. (1975). Cyclic AMP-dependent endogenous phosphorylation of a microtubule-associated protein. *Proc. Natl. Acad. Sci. U.S.A.* **72**, 177–181.

Stossel, T. P. (1978). Contractile proteins in cell structure and function. *Annu. Rev. Med.* **29**, 427–457.

Taylor, D. L., and Condeelis, J. S. (1979). Cytoplasmic structure and contractility in amoeboid cells. *Int. Rev. Cytol.* **56**, 57–144.

Unsicker, K., Limmeroth-Evert, B., Otten, U., Lindmar, R., Loffelholz, K., and Wolff, U. (1979). Effects of vinblastine on rat adrenal medulla. *Cell Tissue Res.* **196**, 271–288.

Vallee, R. B. (1980). Structure and Phosphorylation of MAPs. *Proc. Natl. Acad. Sci. U.S.A.* **77**, 3206–3210.

Vallee, R. B., Bartolomeis, D., and Theurkary, W. E. (1981). A protein kinase bound to the projection protion of MAPs. *J. Cell Biol.* **90**, 568–576.

Weihing, R. R. (1977). Effect of myosin and heavy meromyosin on actin-related gelation of HeLa cell extract. *J. Cell Biol.* **75**, 95–103.

Weisenberg, R. C. (1972). Microtubule formation *in vitro* in solutions containing low calcium concentrations. *Science* **177**, 1104–1105.

Welsh, M. J., Dedman, J. R., Brinkley, B. R., and Means, A. R. (1978). Calcium-dependent regulator protein: Localization in mitotic apparatus of eukaryotic cells. *Proc. Natl. Acad. Sci. U.S.A.* **75**, 1867–1871.

Wetzel, B. K., Spicer, S. S., and Wollman, S. H. (1965). Changes in fine structure in rat thyroid cells following TSH administration. *J. Cell Biol.* **25,** 593–618.

Williams, J. A., and Wolff, J. (1970). Possible role of microtubules in thyroid secretion. *Proc. Natl. Acad. Sci. U.S.A.* **67,** 1901–1908.

Wilson, L., and Meza, I. (1973). The mechanism of action of colchicine. *J. Cell. Biol.* **58,** 709–719.

Wolosewick, J. J., and Porter, K. R. (1979). Microtrabecular lattice of the cytoplasmic ground substance—artifact or reality? *J. Cell Biol.* **82,** 114–139.

Woodrum, D. T., Rich, S. A., and Pollard, T. D. (1975). Evidence for biased bidirectional polymerization of actin filaments using heavy meromysin prepared by an improved method. *J. Cell Biol.* **67,** 231–237.

Wu, E. S., Tank, D., and Webb, W. W. (1981). Lateral diffusion on Con A receptors in normal and bulbous lymphocytes. *Biophys. J.* **33,** 74a.

7

Cytoskeletal Proteins and Insulin Secretion

A. E. BOYD III

I. INTRODUCTION

"Cytoskeleton" is a term best used to describe a large number of molecules that may regulate the transport and release of insulin in the

223

CELLULAR REGULATION OF SECRETION AND RELEASE

TABLE I

Major Structural and Regulatory Cytoskeletal Elements

Structural Elements	Size (nm)	Composition
Microtubules	24	α and β tubulin, MAPs, tau
Microfilaments	6	Actin
Intermediate filaments	10	Vimentin, desmin, keratin, neuro-filaments, glial filaments
Thick filaments	10	Myosin
Microtrabecular lattice	4–10	Unknown
Regulatory Elements		
Calmodulin		
Cyclic nucleotides		
Ions: Ca^{2+}, Mg^{2+}		
Protein kinases		
Protein kinase inhibitors		
Actin-binding proteins		
Calmodulin-binding proteins		
Ca^{2+}-activated proteases		
MAPs		
Tau proteins		
Tropomyosin		

β cells (see Chapter 6). However, this word suggests a type of plastic rigidity that is not present in the living cells. Morphological studies using immunofluorescence and electron microscopy or biochemical investigations of the isolated elements reveal that the cytoskeleton is composed of a dynamic, fluid, rapidly changing array of proteins that are suspended in a lattice network in the cytoplasm. Four major structural cytoskeletal elements have been identified (Table I) that, with the exception of the red cell, appear to be common to all eukaryotic cells: (1) microtubules, (2) microfilaments, (3) intermediate filaments, and (4) the microtrabecular lattice (MTL). The thick filaments that contain myosin are more difficult to identify in cells. The MTL was only recently described and is seen when cells in culture are examined by high-voltage electron microscopy (Porter, 1976; Wolosewick and Porter, 1979). The MTL is composed of slender, interconnecting strands that vary in diameter from 40 to 100 Å and appear to undergo selective alterations in form in response to cellular regulators such as cAMP or Ca^{2+} (Luby and Porter, 1980). Present studies are not sufficiently developed to provide insight into the role of the intermediate filaments or the MTL in insulin secretion.

In addition to the microtubules, microfilaments, intermediate filaments, and the MTL, there is an ever-expanding group of regulatory proteins of which calmodulin is an example. These proteins, often found in association with the structural cytoskeletal elements, regulate diverse cellular functions such as enzymatic activity, phosphorylation of proteins, cyclic nucleotide metabolism, assembly and disassembly of microtubules and microfilaments, and Ca^{2+} flux into or out of the cell. Many of these processes are intimately involved in the regulation of insulin secretion.

II. MICROTUBULES AND INSULIN SECRETION

Electron microscopy of pancreatic β cells reveals numerous microtubules—25-nm, rodlike structures that are part of the structural cytoskeleton. Tubulin is the subunit protein of microtubules and purifies as a 110,000-molecular weight dimer composed of two polypeptides of similar molecular weights, designated α and β tubulin (Bryan and Wilson, 1971; Lu and Elzinga, 1977). In the β cell, there appears to be a dynamic equilibrium between tubulin and the microtubules (Inoue and Ritter, 1975; Pipeleers et al., 1976). The tubulin–microtubule equilibrium has been studied extensively in vitro (Stephens, 1968; Weisenberg, 1972). Although less is known about the factors that control this reaction in vivo, microtubular polymerization occurs at specific sites in cells called microtubule organizing centers (Brinkley et al., 1975). The polymerization reaction is shifted toward microtubules by two classes of proteins that copurify with microtubules. These proteins are called microtubule associated proteins (MAPs) (Kirkpatrick et al., 1970; Murphy and Borisy, 1975; Sloboda et al., 1976; Murphy et al., 1977) or tau proteins (Weingarten et al., 1975; Penningroth et al., 1976; Cleveland et al., 1977). Microtubule polymerization is a Mg^{2+}-dependent process that is inhibited by Ca^{2+}. However, because the free Ca^{2+} level in cells is approximately 10^{-6} to $10^{-7} M$, the concentration of Ca^{2+} that inhibits tubulin polymerization in vitro ($10^{-3} M$) has been considered to be too high to be of physiological significance (Olmsted, 1976; Solomon, 1976).

In collaboration with B. R. Brinkley, we have used indirect immunofluorescence to identify microtubules in β cells in culture (Boyd et al., 1981a). As seen in Fig. 1, there is an extensive microtubular network that radiates from the perinuclear region of the cell to the plasma membrane. In primary cultures of whole pancreas or in monolayer cultures established from pancreatic islets, it is possible (using a double-label immunofluorescence technique) to identify the insulin secre-

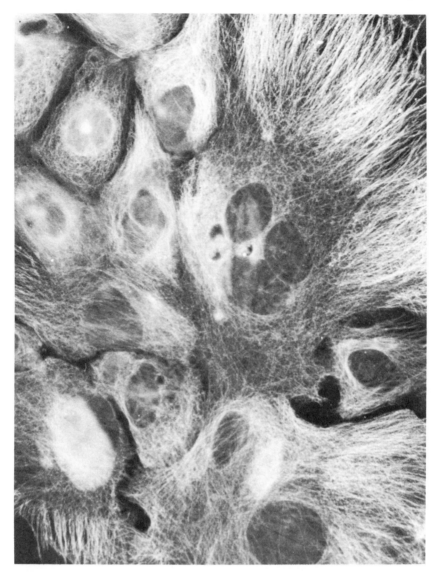

Fig. 1. Monolayer culture of mouse pancreatic epithelial cells stained with a rabbit anti-tubulin antibody and a fluorescein-labeled second antibody to rabbit IgG. Note the extensive microtubular network extending from the perinuclear area of the cell to the plasma membrane. Using double-label immunofluorescence, it is possible to identify many of these cells as β cells × 300. From Boyd et al. (1981a).

tory granules in the same cell. As in cultures of β cells when examined by electron microscopy, the insulin secretory granules often appear to align along the microtubule (Orci, 1974). However, when this relationship has been examined by morphometric analysis of whole islets, the insulin secretory granules and microtubules did not appear to occur together more frequently than would be expected by chance alone (Lacy *et al.*, 1968; Malaisse *et al.*, 1975).

Based on studies showing that colchicine inhibits insulin secretion from pancreatic islets, in 1968 Lacy *et al.* proposed that the microtubules play an important role in the secretory activity of the β cells. These studies have been confirmed and extended (Malaisse *et al.*, 1971; Lacy *et al.*, 1972; Somers *et al.*, 1974; see Malaisse and Orci, 1979, for a review) and show that colchicine retards the movement of insulin from its site of synthesis in the rough endoplasmic reticulum to the plasma membrane (Pipeleers *et al.*, 1976; Malaisse-Lagae *et al.*, 1979). There is a second putative pool of insulin (Grodsky, 1972) that is presumably located in granules near the periphery of the cell and that does not require microtubules for secretion.

Because we developed a method by which we could identify the microtubules in β cells, we quantitated the effect of colchicine on microtubules and insulin secretion more precisely. Although electron microscopy had revealed a decrease in microtubules in β cells treated with colchicine, this technique proved to be too laborious to quantitate the effect of the drug on microtubules (Malaisse and Orci, 1979). In addition, none of the previous colchicine studies of insulin secretion had used inactive lumicolchicine as a control. Following development of techniques for growing adult β cells in primary culture, we studied the role of microtubules in insulin secretion in murine pancreatic monolayer cultures enriched for β cells. To our surprise, glucose-stimulated insulin secretion into the media was usually biphasic. Our studies showed that the initial fall in insulin levels correlated with binding and uptake of insulin into the cells in culture and was not due to degradation of the insulin in the media. In this system, we defined the release of insulin during the first 60 minutes as the first phase of secretion and that from 60 to 180 minutes as the secondary phase of insulin release. Although alterations in the level of Ca^{2+} in the media did not alter the microtubule pattern in the β cell, Ca^{2+} was required for both the initial and secondary release of insulin. Optimum insulin release occurred at a Ca^{2+} concentration of 2.5 mM. We determined the concentration of colchicine required to completely disrupt the microtubules. Colchicine in concentrations of 10^{-10} to 10^{-8} M did not affect the microtubule immunofluorescence pattern. At concentrations of 5×10^{-7} M colchicine, the microtubules decreased in number, and no microtubules could be identified in cultures treated with 10^{-6} M colchicine for 2 hours. After a 2-hour preincubation with 10^{-6} M colchicine, the prolonged release of insulin to either 2.0 or 4.5 mg/ml of glucose was decreased significantly. However, it was obvious that insulin secretion from β cells with no microtubules was continuing at a slower rate. The immediate release of insulin was similar to that in the lumicolchicine controls and occurred in cultures with no identifiable microtubules. Lumicolchicine by itself had no effect on insulin release.

These experiments help to interpret previous studies on the role of microtubules in insulin secretion. Some doubt about their importance had been raised by the fact that the inhibitory concentration of colchicine used (usually 10^{-3} M in perfusion studies) is much higher than that required to alter other microtubule-mediated cell functions. For example, mitosis is blocked in cells grown in culture at 5×10^{-8} M (Taylor, 1965). At the concentrations of colchicine used in most of the insulin secretory studies (10^{-3} M), both the uptake of glucose into fat cells (Cheng and Katsoyannis, 1975) and ATPase activity (Nicklas *et al.*, 1973) are inhibited, and even the Golgi apparatus (Mizel *et al.*, 1972b) is disrupted. Thus, the effects on insulin secretion might not be due to a direct effect on the microtubules. By determining that 10^{-6} M colchicine completely disrupts the microtubules, it is now evident that this dose is three orders of magnitude lower than that which alters glucose uptake, ATPase activity, or disrupts Golgi. In addition, we showed that lumicolchicine at 10^{-6} M had no effect on insulin secretion and that the effect of colchicine on secretion was reversible. Because the secondary release of insulin was not completely inhibited, the microtubules appeared only to facilitate the rate at which the packaged hormone reaches the cell surface. Diffusion of the hormone from β cells with no microtubules can probably keep the hormone moving to the cell surface at a lower rate. There is a pool of insulin that does not require microtubules to be released.

The alignment of the insulin secretory granules along the microtubules of β cells in culture suggests that binding of the secretory granule to a component of the microtubule can occur. Because of the three-dimensional nature of this culture system, it has not been possible to quantitate this relationship. Binding of cytoskeletal proteins to secretory granules may be important in the regulation of secretion. Sherline *et al.* (1977) demonstrated that isolated pituitary secretory granules bind to the microtubules. This binding occurs through the MAPs, which constitute 20–30% of the microtubules (Sloboda *et al.*, 1975).

Several theories attempt to explain the mechanism by which microtubules are involved in insulin secretory granules' movement. In cilia, a sliding filament mechanism with the microtubules moving over each other has been proposed (Satir, 1974). When examined by immunofluorescence or electron microscopy, the microtubules in β cells do not often occur in groups (Lacy *et al.*, 1968; Malaisse *et al.*, 1975). Thus, the sliding filament mechanism appears unlikely as a means of movement of insulin secretory granules. Clues to the role of microtubules in insulin secretion may lie in the assembly–disassembly process. Tubulin monomers bind and hydrolize GTP during polymerization into microtubules. This hydrolysis does not provide energy for assembly, as microtubules assemble readily in the presence of nonhydrolyzable nucleotide triphosphate analogs. Margolis and Wilson (1978), using pulse–chase experiments, have labeled steady-state microtubules with [^{3}H]GTP and quantitated the amount of tubulin polymerizing into the microtubule. They concluded that assembly and disassembly occur at opposite ends of the microtubule. As suggested by Margolis *et al.* for mitosis (1978), this process could function as a treadmill to perform work and translocate the secretory granule down the microtubule. However, this would be an inefficient process and would have to contend with the lack of obvious molecular mechanisms for utilizing subunit flux to do useful work (Kirshner, 1980). The most plausible theory is that the microtubules are not involved in an active way in secretion and merely provide the framework to direct the insulin secretory granules about the cell.

The concentration of microtubules has been quantitated by colchicine binding assays in isolated islets (Montague *et al.*, 1976; Pipeleers *et al.*, 1976; McDaniel *et al.*, 1980). These studies suggested that the polymerization state of the microtubules might be important in the secretion of insulin. In the rat islet, about one-third of the tubulin exists as microtubules. Although there are still technical difficulties to be overcome in separating microtubules and tubulin in cells, the studies on islets indicate that insulin secretagogues, such as glucose and theophylline, increase the polymerization of tubulin and thus would make more microtubules available for interaction with insulin secretory granules.

Although it has been proposed that Ca^{2+} is a regulator of microtubule polymerization, the physiological role of Ca^{2+} on *in vivo* polymerization is unclear. *In vitro*, Ca^{2+} in millimolar concentrations prevents the polymerization of microtubules. In the presence of calmodulin, which has been localized with microtubules to the actin microfilament bundles (Welsh *et al.*, 1978), assembly of microtubules is inhibited in the micromolar range (Brinkley *et al.*, 1978). In our studies we did not observe an effect on the β cell microtubule pattern by increasing concentrations of Ca^{2+} in the media, despite showing that extracellular Ca^{2+} was required for insulin release. This is in agreement with direct measurements of the effect of Ca^{2+} on the amount of microtubule protein in isolated islets (Pipeleers *et al.*, 1976). Thus, the intracellular flow of Ca^{2+} into the β cell does not appear to alter the degree of tubulin polymerization as measured by either colchicine binding or by immunofluorescence.

III. ACTIN IN PANCREATIC ISLETS

Nonmuscle cell extracts prepared in isotonic buffers contain actin in several forms (see Korn, 1978, for a review); G actin is a linear polypeptide of 42,000 daltons, which in the presence of ATP and magnesium polymerizes to filamentous F actin. In addition, a significant amount of unpolymerized actin is complexed with profilin, a low-molecular-weight protein that binds stoichiometrically to G actin and inhibits actin assembly. Actin has been identified in pancreatic islets using either immunofluorescence (Gabbiani *et al.*, 1974) or electron microscopy (Orci *et al.*, 1972) and has been measured directly (Kelly *et al.*, 1980; Swanson-Flatt *et al.*, 1980). An extensive network of actin microfilaments, 4–6 nm in diameter, lies beneath the plasma membrane of the β cell. This area, termed the cell web, varies in thickness from 50 to 300 nm and in unstimulated β cells is usually devoid of insulin secretory granules. The microfilaments are thought to be composed of actin because, like the actin in thin-filament bundles of muscle, the microfilaments bind to a myosin proteolytic fragment, i.e., heavy meromysin (Ishikawa *et al.*, 1969).

Cytochalasin B, a mold metabolite, binds to the barbed ends of polymerizing actin filaments and prevents further F actin elongation (Brenner and Korn, 1979). Treatment of pancreatic islets with cytochalasin B at 10^{-5} M potentiates both phases of insulin secretion (Malaisse *et al.*, 1972b; Lacy *et al.*, 1973; Van Obbergen *et al.*, 1973), although higher concentrations inhibit insulin release (Lacy *et al.*, 1973; Van Obbergen *et al.*, 1973). Following cytochalasin B treatment, the β cell web demonstrates thinning and opposition of insulin secretory granules with the plasma membrane. This observation and the lack of insulin secretory granules in the microfilamentous web led Orci *et al.* (1972) to suggest that the cell web acts as a barrier to insulin secretion.

Further support for an action of cytochalasin B on insulin secretion through effects on the microfilaments comes from several lines of evidence. The drug does not alter the influx of Ca^{2+} into the β cell and also has no effect of insulin biosynthesis (Malaisse *et al.*, 1972b). Furthermore, the viscosity of platelet actin filaments is decreased by cytochalasin (Spudich, 1972), indicating a decrease in F actin. Finally, the effect of cytochalasin B is reversible. Although the drug has other effects on cells, such as inhibition of glucose and glucosamine transport (Mizel and Wilson, 1972a), this does not explain the facilitation of insulin secretion by cytochalasin B because another analog that has no effect on glucose transport (cytochalasin D) also increases insulin secretion (McDaniel *et al.*, 1975).

There appear to be parallels between muscle contraction and force generation in nonmuscle cells. The generation of force is necessary to translocate secreted proteins from the site of synthesis in the rough endoplasmic reticulum to the plasma membrane. Both muscle contraction and secretion require Ca^{2+} (Grodsky, 1966), energy in the form of ATP (Babad *et al.*, 1967; Malaisse *et al.*, 1967; Renold, 1970), and depolarization of the cell membrane (Dean and Matthews, 1968). In nonmuscle cells, immunofluorescent studies indicate that myosin is closely associated with the actin microfilaments (Weber and Groeschel-Stewart, 1974; Fujiwara and Pollard, 1976). Myosin is a large molecule composed of two heavy chains and two pairs of light chains that make up the globular head of the molecule (see Adelstein *et al.*, 1979, for a review). In cells grown in culture, including β cells (Kelly *et al.*, 1980), many of the actin microfilaments are arranged in larger structures up to 1 μm in diameter. These structures are called stress fibers or microfilament bundles and certain epithelial cells also contain myosin, calmodulin (Drenckhahn and Groschel-Stewart, 1980), tropomyosin, and myosin light chain kinase (Yagi *et al.*, 1978). The actin-binding sites and the ATPase activity required to hydrolyze ATP both reside in the globular head of the myosin molecule. In smooth muscle, these activities are Ca^{2+} dependent and require phosphorylation of the myosin light chains by a kinase enzyme, the myosin light chain kinase (MLCK). The Ca^{2+} dependence of this reaction involves calmodulin, which is the regulatory component of the MLCK (Yagi *et al.*, 1978). Phosphorylation of the light chain appears to result in a conformational change in the myosin molecule (Mornet *et al.*, 1981) that enables actin binding, activation of ATPase, hydrolysis of ATP, and generation of energy. In smooth muscle cells, it is possible to correlate phosphorylation of the myosin light chain with the development of tension (Adelstein, 1980). If the analogy with muscle is correct, similar events in the β cell should correlate with insulin secretion (also see Chapter 13).

IV. QUANTITATION OF ACTIN IN ISLETS AND RIN CELLS

Although our initial studies measuring the actin pools in pancreatic islets (Kelly *et al.*, 1980) utilized the DNase I inhibition assay of Blikstad *et al.* (1978), we were interested in developing a faster and more sensitive actin assay. We raised antibodies to rabbit skeletal muscle actin that was cut out of SDS–polyacrylamide gels (SDS–PAGE) and purified these antisera on affinity columns prepared with muscle actin. As previously shown by Lazarides (1975) using indirect immunofluorescence, these antisera revealed wide tissue cross-reactivity. We found, like Morgan *et al.* (1980), that differences in the primary structure of actin from various species or even from different tissues from the same species resulted in marked differences in actin binding and displacement of labeled actin from the actin antibodies. It was therefore difficult to quantitate absolute amounts of nonmuscle actin by radioimmunoassay. However, we knew that actin in various tissues bound to DNase I, and using the enzyme as the ligand, we developed an assay that utilizes the competition between unlabeled rabbit skeletal muscle actin and ^{125}I-labeled actin for DNase I (Snabes *et al.*, 1981a). The actin, labeled by the Bolton-Hunter method (1973), binds to DNase I, inhibits enzymatic activity, and will polymerize. Bound and free actin are separated by a two-step immunoprecipitation of the actin–DNase I complex. Displacement of the tracer by either the rabbit skeletal muscle standards or by actin present in cells and tissue is linear. The sensitivity of the assay can be altered by varying the DNase I concentration. Using 17.5 ng of DNase I and approximately 500 pg of ^{125}I-labeled actin, 50% inhibition of binding is observed with 23 ng of actin. Decreasing the DNase I concentration increases the sensitivity to 200 pg, with a limit of detection of 61 pg per assay tube. The slopes of binding curves from vertebrate and invertebrate actins are all parallel to the rabbit skeletal muscle standard. This observation indicates approximately equal actin–DNase binding affinities and suggests a high degree of conservation of the actin–DNase I binding site. In order to use the assay to measure both G and F actin, it is necessary to separate these forms before assay and to then depolymerize the F actin. The strategy is to rapidly and gently lyse the cells with a nonionic detergent and then to separate a cytoskeletal fraction by centrifugation at 15,000 g for 5 minutes. The supernatant fluid is either diluted directly for assay or is diluted after incubation with guanidine-HCl (Gdn-HCl); the F actin in the cytoskeletal fraction is depolymerized in Gdn-HCl before dilution for assay. This strategy is not unique but does attempt to minimize the potential redistribution of actin during the initial fractionation. During the assay, the concentrations of actin are routinely in the nanogram per milliliter range, i.e., at least 100 times below the critical concentrations for assembly. Therefore, the actin remains in a nonfilamentous form available to DNase I. We have tested the low-speed extracts for the presence of additional F actin by recentrifugation at 100,000 g for 120 minutes. In three cases (β cells, Chinese hamster ovary cells, and sea urchin coelomocytes), we find no further actin sediments at higher gravitational forces and suggest that, under the lysis conditions employed, the bulk of the filamentous actin in these cells is present in a "cytoskeleton" that is sedimentable at relatively low g forces. It should be noted that the criterion for discriminating G and F actin is substantially different from that used by Blikstad *et al.* (1978). The inhibition assay relies upon the substantially higher rate of enzyme binding to G actin to measure soluble actin in the presence of F actin. This assay provides a simple and rapid method for quantitation of filamentous and soluble actin. The sensitivity is increased approximately 1000-fold from the 10 mg/ml reported for the DNase I inhibition method. Using the binding/immunoprecipitation assay, in 2 days it is possible to measure 100 actin samples in duplicate at several dilutions with a coefficient of variation of less than 10%. Because the standard curve is linear after logit transformation, the assay is amenable to the statistics used for radioimmunoassays. Moreover, it is unnecessary to purify individual actins from the tissues or species of interest because all the α, β, and γ actins tested to date displace in parallel. Finally, DNase I is commercially available in an electrophoretically pure form and is highly antigenic. The use of DNase I and anti-DNase I obviates the need for characterization of individual specific actin antibodies.

V. ACTIN LEVELS IN ISLETS AND IN MONOLAYER CULTURES OF BETA CELLS

Our studies measuring actin in islets isolated from fasted and fed hamsters show that actin constitutes 1–2% of the cell protein. Approximately 75–80% of the actin is in the soluble form and 20–25% is found in the sedimentable cytoskeletal pellet (Kelly *et al.*, 1980; Snabes and Boyd, 1982). We have performed a number of experiments to test the hypothesis that the acute secretion of insulin is associated with a change in the polymerization state of actin. During glucose-stimulated insulin secretion, we have seen no change in the total actin concentration or the G/F actin ratio in pancreatic islets or in primary pancreatic monolayer cultures enriched for pancreatic β cells. These studies do not exclude local changes in the polymerization state, which would be difficult to discern using whole cell extracts. Our results differ with those of Swanson-Flatt *et al.* (1980), who reported that incubation of isolated islets increases the amount of F actin.

In prolonged fasting, the polymerization state of the contractile protein is altered. In hamsters fasted for 72 hours, there is a consistent 2- to 3-fold increase in the amount of F actin without a change in the total actin concentration (Kelly *et al.*, 1980; Snabes and Boyd, 1982). If this increase in actin occurs in the cell web, it could alter the access of the secretory granule to the plasma membrane and could decrease insulin secretion during prolonged fasting.

VI. ACTIN-BINDING PROTEINS

A number of actin-associated proteins have been identified and purified from muscle and nonmuscle cells. In nonmuscle cells, proteins that cross-link (Hartwig *et al.*, 1975; Shizuta *et al.*, 1976; Wang *et al.*, 1976; Maruta *et al.*, 1977), bundle (Kane, 1975, 1976; Bryan and Kane, 1978), depolymerize (Yin *et al.*, 1980), and cap (Isenberg *et al.*, 1980) the ends of actin filaments have been identified. Actin filaments have been associated with membrane structures, including binding to red cell membrane protein spectrin (Tilney and Detmers, 1975), intestinal brush border membranes (Mooseker and Tilney, 1975), and membranes of other mammalian cells (Buckley and Porter, 1967). In addition, actin can be shown to bind to adrenal, pituitary, and insulin secretory granules (Burridge and Phillips, 1975; Ostlund *et al.*, 1977; Howell and Tyhurst, 1979). Furthermore, a protein with an M_r similar to actin copurifies with ACTH secretory granules (Gumbiner and Kelly, 1981). Thus, actin could serve to link the secretory granule to the plasma membrane through microfilamentous structures.

VII. ACTIN-BINDING PROTEINS IN RAT INSULINOMA CELLS

Because numerous actin-associated proteins have been identified and purified from nonmuscle cells, we set out to develop a method to identify these proteins in β cells. We used the approach employed to localize calmodulin-binding proteins (Glenney and Weber, 1980) and first worked with platelets because of the enormous amount of actin in those cells. After separation of the proteins on SDS–PAGE, fixation, and elution of the SDS, the proteins are renatured. The gels are incubated with ^{125}I-labeled actin, washed extensively, dried, and processed for autoradiography. The labeled actin binds to several proteins in human platelets. The binding is specific and is displaced by increasing amounts of cold actin. Binding requires the actin to be in the native form because it is abolished by heating the ^{125}I-labeled actin to 90°C for 3 minutes. Binding is not affected by high salt. Prominent actin-binding activities are present at $M_r = 90,000$ and $40,000$. The binding to the 90K protein appears to be Ca^{2+} sensitive, whereas the binding to the 40K protein is not. In addition, we can clearly identify eight minor bands at M_r's of 75,000, 70,000, 65,000, 58,000, 48,000, 33,000, 28,000, and 20,000 (Fig. 2). Because the concentrations of the ^{125}I-labeled G actin is approximately 2 nM, the actin-binding affinity of these proteins must be high (Snabes et al., 1981b).

We have subsequently identified actin-binding proteins in a wide variety of cells and tissues. The proteins have been identified on two-dimensional gels as well as in the first dimension. The major actin-binding activity identified in a homogeneous population of β cells [the rat insulinoma cell line (RIN 5f)] exists at $M_r = 90,000$ with minor components at 70,000, 58,000, 40,000, 37,000, and 18,000. This cloned rat insulinoma was developed by Gazdar, Oie, and Chick (Chick et al., 1977; Gazdar et al., 1980) and was provided to us by Dr. Gazdar. As in the platelets, the binding in β cells is decreased about five-fold in the presence of EGTA. This 90K protein has previously been purified from platelets by Wang and Bryan (1981). On two-dimensional gels, if Ca^{2+} is present, the protein is a doublet with p_I's around 6.2 to 6.4. The 90K protein is partially associated with the membrane fraction but cannot be labeled by surface labeling with lactoperoxidase. Actin-binding proteins of similar M_r have also been identified in smooth, skeletal, and cardiac muscle. In the intestine, an additional actin-binding protein activity is identified at 95,000 and is presumed to be villin (Bretscher and Weber, 1979; Mooseker et al., 1980). The 90K protein in β cells most clearly resembles gelsolin, which is a 90K protein isolated from macrophages (Stossel, 1978; Yin and Stossel, 1979). An analysis of the proposed function of gelsolin may help to predict the possible function of the 90K actin-binding protein in insulinoma cells. Gelsolin binds to Ca^{2+} and the Ca^{2+}–gelsolin complex reduces the viscosity of macrophages by decreasing the length of preformed actin filaments. Local changes in the gel–sol state could facilitate the movement of secreted

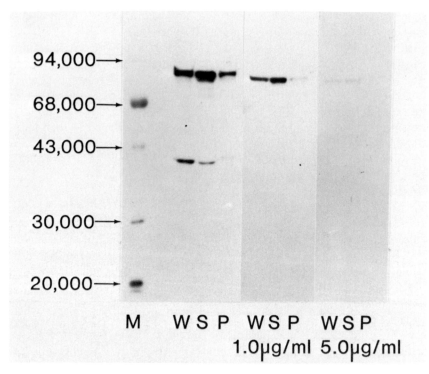

Fig. 2. Displacement of ^{125}I-labeled G actin by increasing concentrations of unlabeled actin. Chloramine-T-iodinated molecular weight standards were applied to lane
M. W refers to the whole platelet lysates; S, a 250,000-g platelet supernatant fraction; P,
the pellet from this centrifugation, which was carried out for 60 minutes. The first three
lanes are platelet fractions incubated only in the presence of ^{125}I-labeled G actin. The
next three lanes, (W, S, P; 1.0 µg/ml) were preincubated with 1.0 µg/ml of unlabeled
rabbit skeletal muscle actin. The last three lanes were preincubated with 5.0 µg/ml
unlabeled actin. Following preincubation for 8 hours, 1.0 µCi/ml ^{125}I-labeled G actin
was added, and after a 12-hour incubation, the gels were washed extensively to remove
unbound ^{125}I-labeled G actin. The washed gels were dried and processed for autoradiography. The major actin-binding proteins in platelets are at M_r = 90,000 and
approximately 40,000. Because the concentration of ^{125}I-labeled G actin is approximately 2 nM, the actin-binding affinities of these proteins must be high. Preincubation
of the gel with a 10-fold (1 µg/ml) excess of unlabeled actin markedly decreases binding,
whereas a 50-fold excess (5 µg/ml) almost completely eliminates the binding. In gels run
in the presence of EGTA, there is a clear decrease in the binding of ^{125}I-labeled G actin
to the 90,000-M_r protein but no effect on binding to the 40,000-M_r protein.

proteins through the cytoplasm; however, the function of the 90K protein in β cells remains to be determined.

VIII. CALCIUM AND INSULIN SECRETION

A rise in the intracellular level of Ca^{2+} is a prerequisite for the release of insulin. Glucose alters the flux of Ca^{2+} across the β cell membrane and increases the free cytoplasmic level of Ca^{2+} (Grodsky and Bennett, 1966; Malaisse et al., 1978), triggering insulin secretion. This effect can be imitated, at least in part, by ouabain, Ca^{2+} ionophores, and depolarization of the β cell by high levels of K^+ (Hales and Milner, 1968; Gomez and Curry, 1973; Wollheim et al., 1975). The requirement for Ca^{2+} in the immediate secretion of insulin is absolute. The secondary release of the hormone can occur, although at a slower rate, in the absence of Ca^{2+} (Henquin, 1978) because prolonged insulin secretion is not abolished by agents like D600, which is an inhibitor of Ca^{2+} influx into the cell.

The free cytoplasmic Ca^{2+} level is altered by three mechanisms: (1) variations in flux across the plasma membrane; (2) shifts of Ca^{2+} from organelles like mitochondria or insulin secretory granules into the cytoplasm; and (3) alterations in binding of Ca^{2+} with Ca^{2+}-binding proteins in the β cell. One proposed mechanism for the facilitation of insulin secretion by cAMP is that this nucleotide stimulates a translocation of the internal Ca^{2+} stores, increasing the free Ca^{2+} level by an alternative mode (Brisson et al., 1972). Conversely, inhibitors of insulin secretion such as epinephrine and diazoxide block glucose-stimulated uptake of Ca^{2+} into the islet (Malaisse et al., 1971). Moreover, when one compares the dose–response for glucose-stimulated Ca^{2+} uptake and insulin release, the curves are both sigmoidal and are quite similar (Malaisse et al., 1971). Thus, the consensus that Ca^{2+} is the major cellular signal for exocytosis is secure.

IX. CALMODULIN: THE INTRACELLULAR CALCIUM RECEPTOR

Calmodulin is the major Ca^{2+}-binding protein in cells and regulates many, if not all, Ca^{2+}-sensitive processes. This protein, which was initially isolated from brain as an activator of phosphodiesterase (Cheung, 1970), has been found in isolated rat islets (Sugden et al., 1979; Valverde et al., 1979; Sharp et al., 1980).

In our laboratory, J. Oberwetter, in collaboration with J. Chafouleas, has measured calmodulin in islets isolated from fasted and fed hamsters using a specific radioimmunoassay for calmodulin (Chafouleas *et al.*, 1979) developed in the laboratory of A. Means. The levels of the intracellular regulator are quite constant (approximately 1 ng/μg protein) and do not change with fasting or when insulin secretion was stimulated *in vitro*. The lack of an effect of glucose on calmodulin levels was then confirmed in the RIN cells. The studies in islets and insulinoma cells are in agreement with other hormone responsive tissues examined with this radioimmunoassay and showed that calmodulin regulates Ca^{2+}-dependent hormonal events by mechanisms that do not require fluctuations in the total intracellular level of this important Ca^{2+} receptor.

X. CALMODULIN REGULATION OF ENZYMES THAT COULD CONTROL INSULIN SECRETION

Calmodulin is involved in the regulation of a wide variety of intracellular enzymes, many of which have been localized to the β cell (see Table II) and could control exocytosis. Because several of these enzymes alter the cellular level of cAMP, an understanding of the role of cAMP in glucose-stimulated insulin release is important (Hedeskov, 1980, has reviewed this subject). The metabolism of glucose to key glycolytic intermediates, phosphoenolpyruvate and pyruvate, results in an accumulation of cAMP in the islet. Other insulin secretagogues as diverse as sulfonyl ureas and glucagon (Morgan, 1976; Schubart *et al.*, 1977) also share this action. The common feature of each of these secretagogues is that the rise in cAMP then increases the free cytosolic Ca^{2+} concentration. It is possible to dissociate a rise in the intracellular level of cAMP from insulin secretion. Some stimuli release insulin without increasing cAMP and others, such as cholera toxin or methylxanthine, increase the level of cAMP dramatically, yet do not stimulate insulin release. These data indicate that an increase in cAMP levels is not a sufficient or necessary condition for insulin secretion. For this reason, Hedeskov (1980) considers cAMP to be a positive modulator rather than a primary trigger of insulin release.

After the identification of both phosphodiesterase and adenylate cyclase as calmodulin-regulated enzymes in brain, a variety of tissues were shown to have calmodulin-responsive, cyclic nucleotide-metabolizing enzymes (Table II). Cyclic nucleotide phosphodiesterase has been identified in islets from three different mammalian species; how-

TABLE II

Calmodulin-Regulated Enzymes That Could Alter Insulin Secretion

Enzyme	Tissue source	Reference
Cyclic nucleotide Phosphodiesterase	Islets/*obob* mice Normal mice	Atkins and Matty (1971) Atkins and Matty (1971) Ashcroft et al. (1972) Bowen and Lazarus (1973) Capito and Hedeskov (1974)
	Guinea pigs	Sams and Montague (1972)
Adenylate cyclase	Normal mouse and rat pancreatic islets	Capito and Hedeskov (1974) Davis and Lazarus (1972) Howell and Montague (1973)
	Normal mouse, rat, and hamster insulinoma cells	Goldfine et al. (1972) Rosen et al. (1971)
	Human insulinoma	Goldfine et al. (1972)
Protein kinase	Hamster insulinoma cells Rat and guinea pig islets	Schubart et al. (1980a,b) Montague and Howell (1972)
Phosphoprotein phosphatase	Islets	Dods and Burdowski (1973) Muller and Sharp (1974) Sharp et al. (1975)
Ca^{2+},Mg^{2+}- ATPase	Rat islets	Pershadsingh et al. (1980)
Phosphorylase	Rat insulinoma cells RIN 5F	G. Slaughter T. Nelson, A. E. Boyd III, and A. R. Means (unpublished observations)
Guanylate cyclase	Guinea pig islets	Howell and Montague (1974)

ever, the studies of the enzyme do not show that it is activated by Ca^{2+}, making it unlikely that calmodulin regulation of phospho-diesterase is an important means of control of insulin secretion. Because of the calmodulin-dependence of this enzyme in at least seven other tissues (see Means and Dedman, 1980, for review), these experiments may require reinvestigation in β cells. Although calmodulin has been shown to activate adenylate cyclase in pancreatic islets (Valverde et al., 1979), the stimulation of adenylate cyclase in these experiments was small, about 10% of that achieved with NaF and was dependent on the Ca^{2+} concentration. In the same study, calmodulin was shown to bind to unidentified substances in the particulate fraction of pancreatic islets.

Cyclic nucleotide-dependent protein kinase has been characterized in islets of guinea pigs and the rat (Table II). In contrast to the calmodulin-dependent kinases, the cAMP-dependent kinases do not require Ca^{2+} for activity. There appear to be only two types of non-Ca^{2+}-dependent protein kinases, which have identical catalytic subunits and differ only in the regulatory subunits. In contrast, there are at least four Ca^{2+}-dependent protein kinases that have been described in various tissues. Schubart et al. (1980a) have demonstrated Ca^{2+} – calmodulin-dependent protein kinase activity within the cytosol of a hamster insulinoma and several proteins in these cells that are phosphorylated in a Ca^{2+}-dependent manner (Schubart et al., 1980a,b). This reaction did not require cyclic nucleotides, was enhanced by the addition of Ca^{2+} or purified calmodulin, and was inhibited by the addition of EGTA or trifluoperazine (TFP). Furthermore, TFP inhibited insulin secretion but did not alter the influx of Ca^{2+} into the cells. Although phosphoprotein phosphatase activity has been demonstrated in pancreatic islets (Muller and Sharp, 1974; Morgan, 1976), no systematic study of these enzymes in β cells or islets has been performed.

Calcium transport is also regulated by calmodulin. The entry of Ca^{2+} into cells occurs readily down a concentration gradient; however, the movement between cellular organelles and removal of Ca^{2+} from the cell is an energy-dependent process. After the demonstration that the stimulation of Ca^{2+}, Mg^{2+}-ATPase activity in red cells required calmodulin, similar activity was demonstrated in pancreatic islets (Pershadsingh et al., 1980). This calmodulin-dependent enzyme might regulate Ca^{2+} levels. As the free level of Ca^{2+} in the β cell rises, the unoccupied binding sites on calmodulin would become filled, converting the calmodulin configuration to an active structure that could bind to the membrane-associated Ca^{2+}, Mg^{2+}-ATPase activating the Ca^{2+} pump. Ca^{2+} would then be pumped out of the cell and calmodulin would again alter its configuration and dissociate from the calmodulin-dependent Ca^{2+} pump.

In collaboration with G. Slaughter and A. Means, we have identified phosphorylase, another calmodulin-dependent enzyme in the rat insulinoma cells (G. Slaughter, T. Nelson, A. E. Boyd III, and A. R. Means, unpublished observation). By indirect immunofluorescence, this enzyme is located in granules that appear to contain glycogen, and it is not seen in the insulin secretory granule. This is not surprising because phosphorylase kinase contains calmodulin as its regulatory subunit and converts the inactive enzyme (phosphorylase B) into an active form (phosphorylase A). Our studies have shown that calmodulin binds more avidly to the inactive form of the enzyme. We identified the phosphorylase enzyme after finding that labeled calmodulin bound to the phosphorylase B enzyme we were using as a molecular weight marker in the calmodulin overlay procedure. Thus, a number of calmodulin-dependent enzymatic activities are present in either islets or β cells and may regulate cyclic nucleotide or glycogen metabolism and control the level of Ca^{2+} in the cell.

XI. PHARMACOLOGICAL STUDIES OF CALMODULIN ANTAGONISTS AND INSULIN SECRETION

The role of calmodulin in insulin secretion has been examined by the use of drugs that were felt to be specific inhibitors of the action of calmodulin. Levin and Weiss (1976) have shown that TFP binds to the Ca^{2+}–calmodulin complex and inhibits the subsequent activation of calmodulin-sensitive enzymes. The specificity of TFP was shown by the lack of Ca^{2+}-dependent binding of TFP to a variety of other proteins; the inhibitory effects were related to the presence of Ca^{2+} at the concentrations required to activate calmodulin-sensitive enzymes and the inhibitory activity correlated with the binding affinity of TFP to calmodulin. Schubart et al. (1980a) showed that 20 µg/ml of TFP inhibited insulin release from transplantable hamster insulinoma cells without affecting the flux of Ca^{2+} into the cells. In contrast, glucagon stimulation of insulin secretion, a hormonal event they had previously demonstrated to be cAMP mediated, was not altered by TFP. These data and the demonstration that TFP also inhibited the phosphorylation of several proteins suggested that cAMP and Ca^{2+} regulated insulin release by different mechanisms and that the Ca^{2+}–calmodulin regulation might occur through a calmodulin-dependent protein kinase. Krausz et al. (1980) showed that 30 to 100 µg/ml of TFP inhibited glucose-stimulated insulin release from rat pancreatic islets in a dose-dependent manner. Because the inhibitory effect was also demonstrated with glyceraldehyde, the site of action of TFP was felt to lie after the metabolism of glucose to the trioses. Finally, the effect of TFP on the synergism between glucose and a phosphodiesterase inhibitor, 3-butyryl-1-methylxanthine (IBMX), on insulin secretion was tested. TFP did not alter this synergy. The conclusions of these two groups were similar: that calmodulin is involved in the Ca^{2+} stimulus–secretion, but that the potentiation of insulin secretion by cAMP and exocytosis itself are not affected by calmodulin.

Anti-calmodulin compounds also inhibit secretion in several other systems, including intestinal ion secretion (Ilundain and Naptalin, 1979), histamine release from mast cells (Sieghart et al., 1978), polymorphonuclear secretion (Elferink, 1979; Naccache et al., 1980), and the release of serotonin by platelets (White and Raynor, 1980). Although initially appealing, there are problems with the interpretation of most of these pharmacological experiments. It is difficult to establish whether the effects of such drugs result from specific interactions with calmodulin or through other effects of these hydrophobic compounds with the plasma membrane. One indication that the latter may be the case is the stimulation of insulin secretion by low concentrations of glucose and 30 μM TFP. In addition, reversal of the drug effects has not been demonstrated in most studies. Although the original studies of Schubart et al. (1980a) indicated that 20 μM TFP did not alter the uptake of Ca^{2+} into insulinoma cells, more complete dose–response studies in the same system show that TFP inhibits Ca^{2+} uptake at doses similar to those that inhibit insulin secretion (N. Fleischer, personal communication). Phenothiazines also bind in a specific fashion to surface receptors to dopamine and α-adrenergic agonists and could alter the uptake of other substances into the cell (Hanbauer et al., 1979; Gnegy and Lau, 1980).

XII. STUDIES OF EFFECTS OF THE W COMPOUNDS ON INSULIN RELEASE

We have taken advantage of another class of calmodulin antagonists—the naphthalenesulfonamides, or W compounds—to study the regulation of exocytosis by calmodulin. These drugs were developed by Hidaka et al. (1978) and have been used by our group in collaboration with J. Chafouleas and A. Means to study the regulation of calmodulin in the cell cycle (Means et al., 1981; Chafouleas et al., 1982). The W compounds are considerably less hydrophobic than the phenothiazines and enter cells more readily, yet have binding affinities to calmodulin (10^{-6}–10^{-7} M) that are similar to the most potent phenothiazines. By deletion of a single Cl from the benzene ring of the active compound W13, it is possible to produce an analog that is 5-fold less active in binding to calmodulin. The biological activity follows the binding affinity and W12 is also 5-fold less active in inhibition of bovine brain cyclic nucleotide phosphodiesterase and myosin light chain kinase activity (Chafouleas et al., 1982).

J. Oberwetter and J. Chafouleas have studied the effects of W12 and

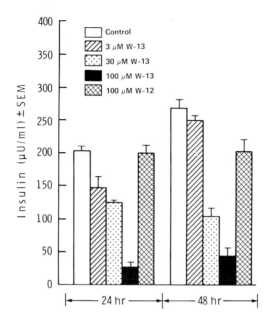

Fig. 3. Effect of three concentrations of the calmodulin antagonist W13 and the inactive analog W12 on insulin secretion. One hundred thousand cells were plated, and insulin was measured at 24 and 48 hours. Note the progressive decrease of insulin in the media at 24 and 48 hours with increasing concentrations of W13. W12 had no effect on insulin release. Each bar is the mean ± SEM of three plates.

W13 on the release of insulin from the RIN 5F cells. As seen in Fig. 3, W13 inhibits insulin release in a dose-dependent manner, whereas W12 has no effect. In the concentrations used, cell survival was not affected, and after removal of the drug, insulin secretion recovers to control levels. In addition, in contrast to the phenothiazines, the W compounds do not appear to alter Ca^{2+} flux (Naccache et al., 1980). Thus, although any drug may have unsuspected actions on cells, these studies add to the evidence that insulin secretion is calmodulin dependent.

XIII. CALMODULIN-BINDING PROTEINS IN RIN 5F CELLS

The binding of Ca^{2+} to calmodulin results in a conformational change in the intramolecular structure of this protein; the conformational change is necessary for the subsequent binding of calmodulin with other enzymes or proteins that it regulates (Dedman et al., 1977).

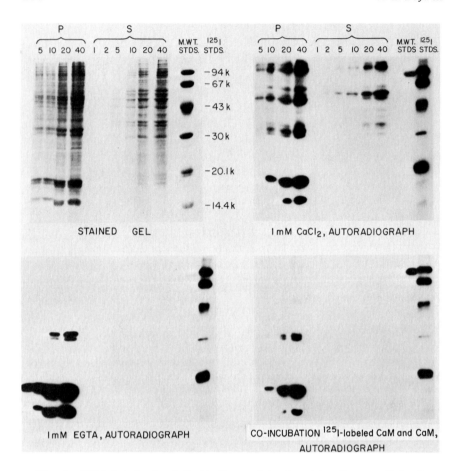

Fig. 4. ^{125}I-Labeled calmodulin-binding proteins in rat insulinoma cell fractions. Increasing amounts of a 1500-*g* pellet (P; 5–40 μg protein) and a supernatant fraction (S; 1–40 μg protein) from RIN 5F cells were electrophoresed on four 12.5% poly-acrylamide gels using the Laemmli buffer system (*Nature* **227**, 680–685, 1970). Calmodulin-binding proteins were identified using the gel overlay technique of Glenney and Weber (1980). The molecular weight standards were iodinated using a chloramine-T method and applied to the right lane. This lane is not visible in the stained gel because of the small amount of protein present but is visible on all of the autoradiographs. The M_r of these markers is depicted on the stained gel. The overlay solutions contained 0.6 μCi ^{125}I-labeled calmodulin/ml and either 1 mM CaCl$_2$, 1 mM EGTA, or 1 mM CaCl$_2$ and 126 nM of unlabeled calmodulin. The autoradiograph in the upper right shows that the ^{125}I labeled calmodulin-binding activity increases with increasing amounts of protein. The binding affinity of the proteins for calmodulin must be high because the concentration of ^{125}I-labeled calmodulin in the overlay solution is low (1.26 nM), and the major bands of binding activity are quite obvious even when the protein bands are barely discernible. Phosphorylase B, used as a molecular weight marker in the stained gel, binds ^{125}I-labeled calmodulin in the CaCl$_2$ autoradiograph. There is no binding activity in the

In order to identify proteins to which calmodulin interacts in a specific fashion in β cells, T. Nelson has applied a gel overlay procedure (Glenney and Weber, 1980) to whole cell extracts and cellular fractions of the cloned rat insulinoma cells (Nelson *et al.*, 1981). The proteins are separated by SDS–PAGE, fixed in the gel matrix, renatured, and incubated with ^{125}I-labeled calmodulin. The iodinated calmodulin retains biological activity. The gels are then washed extensively to remove nonspecifically bound radioactivity and the bound ^{125}I-labeled calmodulin identified by autoradiography. Using this technique, we have identified a number of calmodulin-binding proteins that interact in a Ca^{2+}-dependent and specific fashion. Binding to the label is inhibited by the addition of a 100-fold excess cold calmodulin.

Of particular interest are the two high-molecular-weight calmodulin-binding proteins with apparent M_r of approximately 125,000 and 110,000 and the 56K and 52K proteins (Fig. 4). The higher M_r proteins of 125,000 could be the myosin light chain kinase, which has been purified from smooth muscle, cardiac muscle, and brain and reported to range in M_r from 80,000 to 130,000 (Dabrowska *et al.*, 1977; Guerriero *et al.*, 1981; Pires and Perry, 1977; Walsh *et al.*, 1980; Wolf and Hofman, 1980). It is suggested either that there are mutliple forms of the enzyme or that the proteins with smaller M_r are proteolytic fragments cleaved during purification. We are now performing direct experiments to determine whether the 125 K calmodulin-binding protein in β cells is MLCK. We also have investigated the possibility that the 56K and 52K proteins are the two subunits of tubulin. When highly purified tubulin is run in the gel overlay procedure, the calmodulin probe binds to the leading edge of the tubulin. These gels do not completely resolve α and β tubulin. In less pure preparations of tubulin isolated by three cycles of temperature-dependent polymerization–depolymerization, other calmodulin-binding proteins can be shown to copurify with the tubulin. The nuclear pellet also contains strong calmodulin-binding activities that have molecular weights at

supernatant fraction in the presence of 1 mM EGTA (bottom left). Thus, binding of the ^{125}I-labeled calmodulin to the RIN supernatant fraction proteins and to phosphorylase B is Ca^{2+} dependent. The calmodulin-binding proteins in the 1500-*g* pellet have M_r's similar to histones. This same pattern of binding is observed when histone standards are used. A 100-fold excess of unlabeled calmodulin (bottom right) displaces all binding in the supernatant fraction. Residual binding to the putative histones and phosphorylase B is due to an excess of binding sites and can be decreased further by either increasing the concentration of unlabeled calmodulin or by electrophoresing smaller amounts of protein.

33,000 and 31,000 and at 17,000 and 14,000. These correspond with the histones, and the binding to these proteins is not Ca^{2+} dependent.

We have investigated the effect of the W compounds on the binding of calmodulin to β cell proteins. W13 blocks the binding to calmodulin-binding proteins and inhibits insulin release, whereas the inactive analog had no effect on binding or secretion. Thus, the same compound that alters insulin secretion interferes with the specific interaction of calmodulin with calmodulin-binding proteins in the β cell.

XIV. CA^{2+}-CALMODULIN PHOSPHORYLATION OF BETA CELL PROTEINS

The importance of phosphorylation as a regulatory mechanism in many physiological systems has been a topic of several recent reviews (Greengard, 1978; Krebs and Beavo, 1979; Adelstein, 1980). To date, the only studies on protein phosphorylation and insulin secretion have been performed in a transplantable hamster islet cell tumor (Schubart *et al.*, 1977, 1980a,b). This tissue consists of a relatively homogeneous population of cells. Although the cells do not secrete insulin in response to glucose, two discrete release mechanisms have been defined. The tumors possess glucagon receptors on the plasma membranes (Goldfine *et al.*, 1972) and contain glucagon-responsive adenylate cyclase activity (Rosen *et al.*, 1971). Manipulations that increase the intracellular level of cAMP either by inhibition of the phosphodiesterase or using cAMP analogs trigger insulin secretion. The second stimulus to insulin release is the influx of Ca^{2+} into the cell and is blocked by the calmodulin antagonist TFP.

In stimulated cells, numerous ^{32}P-labeled bands were apparent upon analysis of cells that were incubated with ^{32}P, lysed, and subjected to SDS–PAGE and autoradiography. However, in the presence of agents that raise the intracellular level of cAMP, a significant increase in ^{32}P incorporation occurred in only one band. Characterization of this phosphoprotein revealed a ribosomal protein with a molecular weight of 23,000. The functional significance of ribosomal phosphorylation is unknown. The Ca^{2+}-mediated release of insulin from these cells also involves a Ca^{2+}-activated kinase and phosphorylation of two other proteins with molecular weights of 98,000 and 60,000. Phosphorylation of both proteins can be blocked with TFP and the half-maximal inhibition of K^+-induced insulin release and phosphorylation of the 60,000 protein occur at similar concentrations of TFP.

XV. INSULIN SECRETION IN TYPE II, NON-INSULIN-
DEPENDENT DIABETES

Glucose-stimulated insulin secretion is biphasic (see Pfeifer *et al.*, 1981, for a recent review). One to two minutes after the administration of glucose, insulin levels rise in blood and then decline rapidly. This first phase of insulin release is completed within 10 minutes. The secondary release of insulin begins at about 10 minutes and subsides 60 to 120 minutes after an intravenous bolus of glucose. If the stimulus is more prolonged, the secondary phase of secretion is also more sustained. The first phase of secretion is dependent upon immediate releasable pools of insulin, whereas the secondary release of insulin is dependent on the prestimulus glucose level (Pfeifer *et al.*, 1979).

The earliest defect in type II diabetes is an abnormality in the immediate release of insulin following a glucose stimulation (Cerasi and Luft, 1967; Seltzer *et al.*, 1967; Simpson *et al.*, 1968; Lerner and Porte, 1972). When hyperglycemia is present (fasting glucose levels over 115 mg%), the first-phase insulin release in response to glucose is markedly impaired (Brunzell *et al.*, 1976). There may even be a paradoxical decrease in insulin levels immediately after the glucose stimulus (Metz *et al.*, 1979). Pfeifer *et al.* (1981) reviewed the studies that have shown that the other nonglucose stimuli of secretion result in normal insulin release in such patients. They suggest that the initial delay in insulin secretion results in the hyperglycemia in these patients. The higher levels of glucose then would potentiate the other nonglucose stimuli and result in a normal secondary release of insulin. In 1973, Robertson and Porte proposed that the glucoreceptor may be abnormal in type II diabetes. Although their studies excluded an abnormality in the β receptor in diabetes by showing that the mean insulin responses to the β receptor agonist isoproterenol were normal in type II diabeties, the protocol did not actually test the glucoreceptor. An abnormality in the glucoreceptor is hard to reconcile with the normal secondary release of insulin. Another explanation for these data is that there is an abnormality in the mechanisms by which the cytoskeletal protein triggers the immediate release of insulin. However, direct experiments to test this hypothesis will require a more detailed understanding of the molecular events regulating exocytosis and direct examination of β cells from patients with type II diabetes.

In 1960, Fajans and Cohn first described a group of patients ranging in age from 11 to 35 with impaired carbohydrate tolerance. In contrast to juvenile onset or type I diabetics, these patients had a milder form of the disease without ketonuria. The patients respond to sulfonylurea treatment with striking improvement in glucose disposal and there has been little or no progression in the disease for periods of followup exceeding 20 years. The over-50% frequency of diabetes in the family members of these patients suggests that this disease, now called maturity onset diabetes of the young of MODY, is transmitted by a Mendelian dominant pattern (Tattersall and Fajans, 1975). Although not well characterized, these patients appear to have a secretory defect that results in hyperglycemia and that can be corrected by tolbutamide.

XVI. SECRETORY ABNORMALITIES IN DIABETIC RABBITS

In collaboration with Drs. Conoway and Roth at the University of Arkansas, we have been investigating a colony of diabetic rabbits that appear to develop the disease on the basis of a severe defect in insulin secretion (Roth *et al.*, 1980; Boyd *et al.*, 1981b; Conaway *et al.*, 1981). Between 1 to 3 years of age, 25% of the animals in this inbred colony develop marked hyperglycemia and serum insulin levels that are inappropriately low for the degree of glucose intolerance. The striking morphological feature in the diabetic animals is the marked hypergranularity of the β cells (Fig. 5). Pathological examination of the pancreas reveals no apparent difference in the number of pancreatic islets, although this has not been precisely quantitated.

In vivo, the animals have a global defect in insulin secretion and do not respond to intravenous glucose, β receptor agonists, or amino acids. The defect in insulin release is also found when isolated pancreatic islets from the diabetic rabbits are studied *in vitro*. The islets in diabetic rabbits are slightly smaller, which is reflected in a 50% decrease in the protein content. However, the insulin content is only slightly decreased when expressed per islet and is similar to the content of normal rabbits when expressed per microgram of protein. Thus, these animals appear to have a severe defect in the release of insulin, resulting in diabetes.

Because the only other hypergranulated animal model of diabetes, the Spiny mouse, is felt to have an abnormality of the microtubule (Malaisse-Lagae *et al.*, 1975), we have attempted to measure the amount of tubulin and microtubules in the diabetic rabbits. We encountered problems in the development of a tubulin radioimmunoassay. The antisera we raised to bovine brain tubulin did not cross-react well with tubulin in pancreatic islets and could not be used

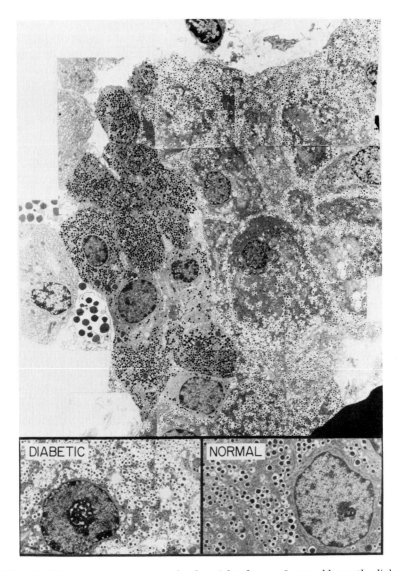

Fig. 5. This composite micrograph of an islet from a 2-year-old overtly diabetic rabbit shows that the outer rim of the islet (top, to the left) is composed primarily of α cells. These glucagon-containing cells can be recognized by the dense secretory granule with little perinuclear space. Note the marked hypergranularity of the β cells that contain characteristic large perinuclear halos around the insulin secretory granules. × 2000. The two panels at the bottom of the figure compare the secretory granules in a diabetic and normal rabbit islet and demonstrate the striking hypergranularity in the diabetic rabbit. These micrographs were prepared by D. Hodges.

to quantitate tubulin in β cells. However, the antisera could be used to identify the pattern of microtubule immunofluorescence in monolayer cultures established from islets isolated from diabetic and normal rabbits. The microtubule pattern was similar to the diabetic and normal rabbits. It should be stressed that the immunofluorescence pattern is only a qualitative method of examining the microtubules. Using this technique we have not seen changes in microtubules with high glucose stimulation of insulin secretion, whereas direct measurements of the amount of microtubules by a colchicine binding assay reveal that glucose increases the amount of microtubules in isolated islets. In future studies, this model should be helpful in dissecting the molecular mechanisms of the secretory defect that leads to diabetes.

XVII. DIABETES IN THE SPINY MOUSE

The Spiny mouse (*Acomys cahirinus*) develops a diabetes-like syndrome with hyperglycemia, obesity, and low serum insulin responses *in vivo*, despite evidence of hyperplasia of the islets (Gonet *et al.*, 1965; Stauffacher *et al.*, 1970; Cameron *et al.*, 1972b). The islet insulin content is similar to the nondiabetic animals (Gonet *et al.*, 1965). *In vivo*, the immediate release of insulin is blunted (Cameron *et al.*, 1972a; Gutzeit *et al.*, 1974), and in perfusion studies there is no clear-cut first phase of insulin release in islets isolated from either young or old animals (Stauffacher *et al.*, 1970; Rabinovitch *et al.*, 1975). With prolonged glucose stimulation (15 to 30 minutes), the rate of insulin release approaches that of other rodents. Tolbutamide, arginine, cAMP, cytochalasin B, and theophylline are also ineffective in releasing insulin from the islets in the presence of substimulatory levels of glucose. In contrast, when theophylline, arginine, and cytochalasin B were perfused in the presence of high concentrations of glucose, there was an increase in glucose-stimulated insulin release similar to that seen in islets isolated from normal rats.

Two theories propose to explain the abnormality in the *Acomys*. Rabinovitch *et al.* (1975) suggest that the failure of all secretagogues tested to stimulate an early release in insulin may reflect a selective impairment in the recognition of glucose as a signal. The other hypothesis (Malaisse-Lagae *et al.*, 1975) is based on observations that the number of paracrystals formed when vincristine binds irreversibly to tubulin is decreased. Because the microtubules and tubulin are in a dynamic equilibrium, this assay should reflect a decrease in microtubule protein. It is difficult to rationalize these data with the observed secretory abnormalities in these animals for several reasons. First, microtubules do not appear to be necessary for the immediate release of insulin, and a defect in the immediate release of the hormone is the primary abnormality in these diabetic mice. Furthermore, as pointed out by Rabinovitch *et al.* (1975), the normal late release of insulin to glucose, as well as the intact potentiating action of other insulin secretagogues demonstrated in *Acomys,* is also difficult to explain on the basis of the decreased microtubules content.

XVIII.   CYTOSKELETAL PROTEINS IN DIABETIC MICE

The C57BLKsJ *db/db* mouse develops a diabetes that evolves through two distinct phases. The first phase is characterized by obesity, hyperphagia, hyperglycemia, degranulation of the β cells, and high serum insulin levels. This lasts until about 8 to 12 weeks of age, after which time the weight gain ceases and the animals show a relative deficiency in insulin. The islets of Langerhans then become atrophic, the animals lose weight, and death usually occurs (Coleman and Hummel, 1967; Like and Chick, 1970; Hummel *et al.,* 1972). Studies on the islets isolated from these animals have revealed a defect in the immediate release of insulin (Siegel *et al.,* 1980). Because the major protein in the microfilamentous cell web is actin, it becomes a candidate protein that could be involved in the secretory defect.

In order to study the possible involvement of actin in the acute release of insulin in these animals, we developed a monolayer culture system to grow pancreatic cells from diabetic and normal mice. Animals were studied at the transition point from the first phase into the second phase of the disease. Insulin secretion into the media of cultures from the normal and diabetic animals was compared with the content of actin, calmodulin, and insulin. As seen in Fig. 6, in diabetic mice there is delay in release of insulin into the media when the glucose concentration is increased. Except for the initial release, the accumulation of insulin occurs at the same rate in normal and diabetic animals and hormone levels ultimately reach the same point. β Cell mass appears to be similar in the two cultures because cell numbers, cell protein, and the amount of extractable insulin is the same in the diabetic and normal animals. The concentration of total actin has been consistently decreased in the diabetic mice, as analyzed with either the enzymatic assay or the actin-binding immunoprecipitation assay. In contrast, the levels of calmodulin and the microtubules identified by indirect immunofluorescence are similar in diabetic and normal cul-

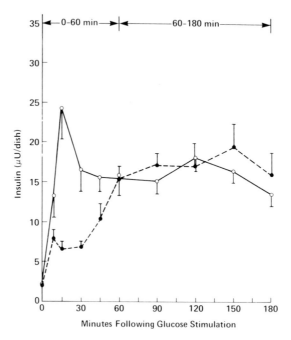

Fig. 6. Equal numbers (approximately 10^5) of pancreatic epithelial cells were plated after homogenizing whole pancreases of diabetic C57KsJ *db/db* mice 14 weeks of age and normal animals from the same strain. Glucose in the media was increased from 50 to 300 mg/ml and insulin measured at frequent time points. Note the delay in the immediate release of insulin (●) from the diabetic cultures. Insulin release from the normal mice (○) occurs promptly. Insulin levels in the diabetic cultures reach the same level by 60 minutes. Each point is the mean ± SEM from six plates.

tures. Thus, the diabetic state in these mice is associated with a defect in the immediate release in insulin and a decrease in the total amount of actin. It is tempting to speculate that the decrease in microfilaments in the β cells accounts for the insulin secretory abnormalities; however, immunofluorescence of the cells in culture shows a generalized decrease in actin microfilaments in all of the cells.

These observations could also provide a clue as to the possible mechanism for the diabetic state. When cells in culture are transformed by tumor viruses, there is a decrease in the actin immunofluorescent pattern that reflects a decrease in the actin bundles (McNutt *et al.*, 1973; Pollack and Rifkin, 1975; Wang and Goldberg, 1976). Several studies have shown that the actin associated with the plasma membrane is decreased in the transformed cell (Wickus *et al.*, 1975; Boxer *et al.*, 1978). Evidently this does not reflect a generalized decrease in actin content because the amount of extractable actin is, if anything, increased (Fine and Taylor, 1976), and the electron microscopic examination of such cells shows more microfilaments in the interior of the cells (McNutt *et al.,* 1973). Because diabetes may be initiated by a virus infection (for a review, see Cahill, 1981), the decrease in actin content in the diabetic cultures might be another clue to the possible viral involvement in this disease.

ACKNOWLEDGMENTS

This research was supported by a grant from the NIH AM 23033 and the Juvenile Diabetes Foundation #79R042. I would like to acknowledge my colleagues B. R. Brinkley, W. E. Bolton, J. Bryan, J. G. Chafouleas, J. Kelly, A. R. Means, T. Nelson, J. G. Oberwetter, M. C. Snabes, and S. Terrell, who were instrumental in performing many of the studies reported in this chapter. Linda Miner was invaluable in the preparation of this manuscript.

REFERENCES

Adelstein, R. S. (1980). Phosphorylation of muscle contraction proteins. *Fed. Proc., Fed. Am. Soc. Exp. Biol.* **39,** 1554–1573.

Adelstein, R. S., Scordilis, S. P., and Trotter, J. A. (1979). The cytoskeleton and cell movement: General considerations. *Methods Archiev. Exp. Pathol.* **8,** 1–41.

Ashcroft, S. J., Randle, P. J., and Taljedal, I. B. (1972). Cyclic nucleotide phosphodiesterase activity in normal mouse pancreatic islets. *FEBS Lett.* **20,** 263–266.

Atkins, T., and Matty, J. (1971). Adenyl cyclase and phosphodiesterase activity in the isolated islets of Langerhans of obese mice and their lean litter mates: The effects of glucose, adrenalin, and drugs on adenyl cyclase activity. *J. Endocrinol.* **51,** 67–78.

Babad, H., Ben-Zvi, R., Bdolah, A., and Schramm, M. (1967). The mechanism of enzyme secretion by the cell. *Eur. J. Biochem.* **1,** 96–101.

Blikstad, I., Markey, F., Carlsson, L., Persson, T., and Lindberg, U. (1978). Selective assay of monomeric and filamentous actin in cell extracts using inhibition of deoxyribonuclease I. *Cell* **15,** 935–943.

Bolton, A. E., and Hunter, W. M. (1973). The labeling of proteins to high specific radioactivities by conjugation to a ^{125}I-containing acylating agent. *Biochem. J.* **133,** 529–538.

Bowen, V., and Lazarus, N. R. (1973). Glucose-mediated insulin release: 3′,5′-cAMP phosphodiesterase. *Diabetes* **22,** 738–743.

Boyd, A. E., III, Bolton, W. E., and Brinkley, B. R. (1981a). Microtubules and beta cell function: Effect of colchicine on microtubules and insulin secretion *in vitro* by mouse beta cells. *J. Cell Biol.,* **92,** 425–434.

Boyd, A. E., III, Bolton, W. E., Conaway, H. H., and Brinkley, B. R. (1981b). Identification of microtubules in normal and diabetic rabbit islets grown in monolayer culture. *Metabolism,* **31,** 154–157.

Boxer, L. A., Richardson, S., and Floyd, A. (1978). Identification of actin-binding protein in membrane of polymorphonuclear leukocytes. *Nature (London)* **263,** 259–261.

Brenner, S. L., and Korn, E. D. (1979). Substoichiometric concentrations of cytochalasin D inhibit actin polymerization. *J. Biol. Chem.* **254,** 9982–9985.

Bretscher, A., and Weber, K. (1979). The major microfilament-associated protein of the intestinal microvillus. *Proc. Natl. Acad. Sci. U.S.A.* **76,** 2321–2325.

Brisson, C. R., Malaisse-Lagae, F., and Malaisse, W. J. (1972). The stimulus-secretion coupling of glucose-induced release. VII. A proposed site of action for adenosine-3′,5′-cyclic monophosphate. *J. Clin. Invest.* **51,** 232–241.

Brunzell, J. D., Robertson, R. P., Lerner, R. L., and Hazzard, W. R., Ensinck, J., Bierman, E. L., and Porte, D. (1976). Relationships between fasting plasma glucose levels and insulin secretion during intravenous glucose tolerance tests. *J. Clin. Endocrinol. Metab.* **42,** 222–229.

Bryan, J., and Kane, R. E. (1978). Separation and interaction of the major components of sea urchin actin gel. *J. Mol. Biol.* **125,** 207–224.

Bryan, J., and Wilson, L. (1971). Are cytoplasmic microtubules heteropolymers? *Proc. Natl. Acad. Sci. U.S.A.* **68,** 1762–1766.

Brinkley, B. R., Fuller, G. M., and Highfield, D. P. (1975). Cytoplasmic microtubules in normal and transformed cells in culture: Analysis by tubulin antibody immunofluorescence. *Proc. Natl. Acad. Sci. U.S.A.* **72,** 4981–4985.

Brinkley, B. R., Marcum, J. M., Welsch, M. J., Dedman, J. R., and Means, A. R. (1978). Regulation of spindle microtubule assembly-disassembly: Localization and possible functional role of calcium-dependent regulator protein. *In* "Cell Reproduction" (E. R. Dirksen, D. M. Prescott, and E. F. Fox, eds.), pp. 229–314. Academic Press, New York.

Buckley, I. K., and Porter, K. R. (1967). Cytoplasmic fibrils in living cultured cells: A light and electron microscope study. *Protoplasma* **64,** 349–380.

Burridge, K., and Phillips, J. H. (1975). Association of actin and myosin with secretory granule membranes. *Nature (London)* **254,** 526–529.

Cahill, G. F. Jr. and McDevitt, H. O. (1981). Insulin-dependent diabetes mellitus: The initial lesion. *New Engl. J. Med.* **24,** 1454–1465.

Cameron, D. P., Stauffacher, W., Orci, L., Amherdt, M., and Renold, Á. E. (1972a). Defective immunoreactive insulin secretion in the *acomys cahirinus. Diabetes* **21,** 1060–1071.

Cameron, D., Stauffacher, W., and Renold, A. E. (1972b). Spontaneous hyperglycemia and obesity in laboratory rodents. *Handb. Physiol., Sect. 7: Endocrinol. 1972–1976* pp. 611–625.

Capito, K., and Hedeskov, C. J. (1974). The effect of starvation on phosphodiesterase activity and the content of adenosine 3′,5′-cyclic monophosphate in isolated mouse pancreatic islets. *Biochem. J.* **142,** 653–658.

Cerasi, E., and Luft, R. (1967). The plasma insulin response to glucose infusion in healthy subjects and in diabetes mellitus. *Acta Endocrinol. (Kbh)* **55,** 278–304.

Chafouleas, J. G., Dedman, J. R., Munjaal, R. P., and Means, A. R. (1979). Calmodulin development and application of a sensitive radioimmunoassay. *J. Biol. Chem.* **254,** 10262–10267.

Chafouleas, J. G., Bolton, W. E., Hidaka, H., Boyd, A. E., III, and Means, A. R. (1982). Calmodulin and the cell cycle: Involvement in regulation of cell cycle progression. *Cell,* **28,** 41–50.

Cheng, K., and Katsoyannis, P. G. (1975). The inhibition of sugar transport and oxidation in fat cell ghosts by colchicine. *Biochem. Biophys. Res. Commun.* **64,** 1069–1075.

Cheung, W. Y. (1970). Cyclic 3′,5′-nucleotide phosphodiesterase. *Biochem. Biophys. Res. Commun.* **38,** 533–538.

Chick, W. L., Warren, S., Chute, R. N., Like, A. A., Lauris, V., and Kitchen, K. C. (1977). A transplantable insulinoma in the rat. *Proc. Natl. Acad. Sci. U.S.A.* **74,** 628–632.

Cleveland, D. W., Hwo, S.-Y., and Kirshner, M. W. (1977). Physical and chemical properties of purified tau factor and the role of tau in microtubule assembly. *J. Mol. Biol.* **116,** 227–247.

Coleman, D. L., and Hummel, K. P. (1967). Studies with the mutation, diabetes in the mouse. *Diabetologia* **3,** 238–240.

Conaway, H. H., Faas, F. H., Smith, S. D., and Sanders, L. L. (1981). Spontaneous diabetes mellitus in the New Zealand white rabbit: Physiologic characteristics. *Metabolism* **30,** 50–56.

Dabrowska, R., Aromatorio, D. K., Sherry, J., and Hartshorne, D. (1977). Composition of the myosin light chain kinase from chicken gizzard. *Biochem. Biophys. Res. Commun.* **78,** 1263–1272.

Davis, B., and Lazarus, N. R. (1972). Insulin release from mouse islets. Effect of glucose and hormones on adenylate cyclase. *Biochem. J.* **129,** 373–379.

Dean, P. M., and Matthews, E. K. (1968). Electrical activity in pancreatic islet cells. *Nature (London)* **219,** 389–390.

Dedman, J. R., Potter, J. D., Jackson, R. L., Johnson, J. D., and Means, A. R. (1977). Physiochemical properties of rat testis Ca^{2+}-dependent regulator protein of cyclic nucleotide phosphodiesterase: Relationship of Ca^{2+}-binding, conformational changes and phosphodiesterase activity. *J. Biol. Chem.* **252,** 8415–8422.

Dods, R. F., and Burdowski, A. (1973). Cyclic adenosine 3′,5′-monophosphate dependent protein kinase and phosphoprotein phosphatase activities in rat islets of Langerhans. *Biochem. Biophys. Res. Commun.* **51,** 421–427.

Drenckhahn, D., and Groschel-Stewart, V. (1980). Localization of myosin, actin, and tropomyosin in rat intestinal epithelium: Immunohistochemical studies at the light and electron microscope levels. *J. Cell Biol.* **86,** 475–483.

Elferink, J. G. R. (1979). Chlorpromazine inhibits phagocytosis and exocytosis in rabbit polymorphonuclear leukocytes. *Biochem. Pharm.* **28,** 965–968.

Fajans, S. S., and Cohn, J. (1960). Tolbutamide-induced improvement in carbohydrate tolerance in young people with diabetes. *Diabetes* **9,** 83–88.

Fine, R. E., and Taylor, L. (1976). Decreased actin and tubulin synthesis in 3T3 cells after transformation by SV-40 virus. *Exp. Cell Res.* **102,** 126–168.

Fujiwara, K., and Pollard, T. D. (1976). Fluorescent antibody localization of myosin in the cytoplasm, cleavage furrow, and the mitotic spindle of human cells. *J. Cell Biol.* **71,** 848–875.

Gabbiani, G., Malaisse-Lagae, F., Blondel, B., and Orci, L. (1974). Actin in pancreatic islet cells. *Endocrinology (Baltimore)* **95,** 1630–1635.

Gazdar, A. F., Chick, W. L., Oie, H. K., Sinis, H. L., King, D. L., Weir, G. C., and Lauris, V. (1980). Continuous, clonal, insulin and somatostatin-secreting cell lines established from a transplantable rat islet cell tumor. *Proc. Natl. Acad. Sci. U.S.A.* **77,** 3519–3523.

Glenney, J. R., Jr., and Weber, K. (1980). Calmodulin-binding proteins of the microfilaments present in isolated brush borders and microvilli of internal epithelial cells. *J. Biol. Chem.* **255,** 10551–10554.

Gnegy, M. E., and Lau, Y. S. (1980). Effects of chronic and acute treatment of antipsychotic drugs on calmodulin release from rat striatal membranes. *Neuropharmacology* **19**, 319–323.

Goldfine, I. D., Roth, J., and Birnbaumer, L. (1972). Glucagon receptors in β-cells. Binding of [125] and activation of adenylate cyclase. *J. Biol. Chem.* **247**, 1211–1218.

Gomez, M., and Curry, D. (1973). Potassium stimulation of insulin release in the perfused rat pancreas. *Endocrinology (Baltimore)* **92**, 1126–1134.

Gonet, A. E., Stauffacher, W., Pietet, R., Mougin, J., and Renold, A. E. (1965). Obesity and diabetes mellitus with striking congenital hyperplasia of the islets of Langerhans in spiny mice (*Acomys cahirinus*). *Diabetologia* **1**, 162–171.

Greengard, P. (1978). Phosphorylated proteins as physiologic effectors. *Science* **199**, 146–152.

Grodsky, G. M. (1972). A threshold distribution hypothesis for packet storage of insulin. II. Effect of calcium. *Diabetes Suppl. 2*, **21**, 584–593.

Grodsky, G. M., and Bennett, L. L. (1966). Cation requirements for insulin secretion in the isolated perfused pancreas. *Diabetes* **15**, 910–918.

Guerriero, V. Jr., Rowley, D. R. and Means, A. R. (1981). Production and characterization of an antibody to myosin light chain kinase and intracellular localization of the enzyme. *Cell* **27**, 449–458.

Gumbiner, B., and Kelly, R. B. (1981). Secretory granules of an anterior pituitary cell line, AtT-20, contain only mature forms of corticotropin and β-lipotropin. *Proc. Natl. Acad. Sci. U.S.A.* **78**, 318–322.

Gutzeit, A., Rabinovitch, A., Studer, P. O., Trueheart, P., Cerasi, E., and Renold, A. E. (1974). Decreased glucose tolerance and low plasma insulin responses in *Acomys cahirinus*. *Diabetologia* **10**, 667–670.

Hales, C. N., and Milner, R. D. G. (1968). The role of sodium and potassium in insulin secretion from rabbit pancreas. *J. Physiol. (London)* **194**, 725–743.

Hanbauer, I., Gimple, J., Sankaran, K., and Sherrard, R. (1979). Modulation of striatal cyclic nucleotide phosphodiesterase by calmodulin: Regulation by opiate and dopamine receptor activation. *Neuropharmacology* **18**, 859–864.

Hartwig, J. H., and Stossel, T. P. (1975). Isolation and properties of actin, myosin, and a new actin-binding protein of rabbit alveolar macrophages. *J. Biol. Chem.* **250**, 5696–5705.

Hedeskov, C. J. (1980). Mechanism of glucose-induced insulin secretion. *Phys. Rev.* **60**, 442–508.

Henquin, J. C. (1978). Relative importance of extracellular and intracellular calcium for the two phases of glucose-stimulated insulin release: Studies with theophylline. *Endocrinology (Baltimore)* **102**, 723–730.

Hidaka, H., Naka, M., and Yamaki, T. (1978). Effect of novel specific myosin light chain kinase inhibitors on Ca^{2+}-activated-Mg^{2+}-ATPase of chicken gizzard actomyosin. *Biochem. Biophys. Res. Commun.* **90**, 694–699.

Howell, S. L., and Montague, W. (1973). Adenylate cyclase activity in isolated rat islets of Langerhans. Effects of agents which alter rates of insulin secretion. *Biochim. Biophys. Acta* **320**, 44–52.

Howell, S. L., and Montague, W. (1974). Regulation of guanylate cyclase in guinea pig islets of Langerhans. *Biochem. J.* **142**, 379–384.

Howell, S. L., and Tyhurst, M. (1979). Interaction between insulin-storage granules and F-actin *in vitro*. *Biochem. J.* **178**, 367–371.

Hummel, K. D., Coleman, D. L., and Lane, P. W. (1972). The influence of the genetic background on the expression of mutations at the diabetes locus in the mouse. *Biochem. Genet.* **7**, 1–13.

Ilundain, A., and Naptalin, R. J. (1979). Role of Ca^{2+}-dependent regulator protein in intestinal secretion. *Nature (London)* **279**, 446–448.

Inoue, S., and Ritter, H., Jr. (1975). Dynamics of mitotic spindle organization and function. *In* "Molecules and Cell Movement" (S. Inoue and R. E. Stephens, eds.), pp. 3–29. Raven, New York.

Isenberg, G., Aebi, U., and Pollard, T. D. (1980). An actin binding protein from *Acanthamoeba* regulates actin filament polymerization and interactions. *Nature (London)* **288**, 455–459.

Ishikawa, H., Bischoff, R., and Holtzer, H. (1969). Formation of arrowhead complexes with heavy meromyosin in a variety of cell types. *J. Cell Biol.* **43**, 312–328.

Kane, R. E. (1975). Preparation and purification of polymerized actin from sea urchin eggs. *J. Cell Biol.* **66**, 305–316.

Kane, R. E. (1976). Actin polymerization and interaction with other proteins in temperature-induced gelation of sea urchin egg extracts. *J. Cell Biol.* **71**, 704–714.

Kelly, J., Boyd, A. E., III, Bryan, J., Bolton, W. E., and Brinkley, B. R. (1980). Actin and insulin secretion. *J. Cell Biol.* **87**, 306A.

Kirkpatrick, J. B., Hyams, L., Thomas, V., and Howley, P. M. (1970). Purification of intact microtubules from brain. *J. Cell Biol.* **47**, 384–394.

Kirschner, M. W. (1980). Implications of treadmilling for the stability and polarity of actin and tubulin polymers *in vivo*. *J. Cell Biol.* **86**, 330–334.

Korn, E. D. (1978). Biochemistry of actomyosin-dependent cell motility: A review. *Proc. Natl. Acad. Sci. U.S.A.* **75**, 588–599.

Krausz, Y., Wollheim, C. B., Siegel, B., and Sharp, G. W. G. (1980). Possible role for calmodulin in insulin release: Studies with trifluoperazine in rat pancreatic islets. *J. Clin. Invest.* **66**, 603–607.

Krebs, E. G., and Beavo, J. A. (1979). Phosphorylation-dephosphorylation of enzymes. *Annu. Rev. Biochem.* **48**, 923–960.

Lacy, P. E., Howell, S. L., Young, D. A., and Fink, C. J. (1968). New hypothesis of insulin secretion. *Nature (London)* **219**, 1177–1179.

Lacy, P. E., Walker, M. M.,and Fink, C. J. (1972). Perifusion of isolated rat islets *in vitro*. Participation of the microtubular system in the biphasic release of insulin. *Diabetes* **21**, 987–998.

Lacy, P. E., Klein, N. J., and Fink, C. J. (1973). Effect of cytochalasin B on the biphasic release of insulin in perifused rat islets. *Endocrinology (Baltimore)* **92**, 1458–1468.

Lazarides, E. (1975). Immunofluorescence studies on the structure of actin filaments in tissue culture cells. *J. Histochem. Cytochem.* **23**, 507–528.

Lerner, R. L., and Porte, D., Jr. (1972). Acute and steady-state insulin responses to glucose in nonobese diabetic subjects. *J. Clin. Invest.* **51**, 1624–1631.

Levin, R. M., and Weiss, B. (1976). Binding of trifluoperazine to the calcium-dependent activator of cyclic nucleotide phosphodiesterase. *Mol. Pharmacology* **4**, 374–388.

Like, A. A., and Chick, W. L. (1970). Studies in the diabetic mutant mouse. Electron microscopy of pancreatic islets. *Diabetologia* **6**, 216–242.

Lu, R. C., and Elzinga, M. (1977). Chromatographic resolution of the subunits of calf brain tubulin. *Anal. Biochem.* **77**, 243–250.

Luby, K. H., and Porter, K. R. (1980). The control of pigment migration in isolated erythropores of *Holocentrus ascensionis* (Osbeck). I. Energy requirements. *Cell* **21**, 13–24.

McDaniel, M., Roth, C., Fink, J., Fyfe, G., and Lacy, P. (1975). Effect of cytochalasins B and D on alloxan inhibition of insulin release. *Biochem. Biophys. Res. Commun.* **66**, 1089–1096.

McDaniel, M. L., Bry, C. G., Homer, R. W., Fink, C. J., Ban, D., and Lacy, P. E. (1980). Temporal changes in islet polymerized and depolymerized tubulin during biphasic insulin release. *Metabolism* **29,** 762–766.

McNutt, N. S., Culp, I. A., and Black, P. H. (1973). Contact inhibited revertant cell lines isolated from SV-40 transformed cells. IV. Microfilament distribution and cell shape in untransformed, transformed, and revertant Balb C 3T3 cells. *J. Cell Biol.* **56,** 412–428.

Malaisse, W. J., and Orci, L. (1979). The role of the cytoskeleton in pancreatic β-cell function. *Methods Achiev. Exp. Pathol.* **9,** 112–136.

Malaisse, W. J., Malaisse-Lagae, F., and Wright, P. H. (1967). A new method for the measurement *in vitro* of pancreatic insulin secretion. *Endocrinology (Baltimore)* **80,** 99–108.

Malaisse, W. J., Malaisse-Lagae, F., Walker, M. O., and Lacy, P. E. (1971). The stimulus secretion coupling of glucose-induced insulin release. V. The participation of a microtubular-microfilamentous system. *Diabetes* **20,** 257–265.

Malaisse, W. J., Mahy, M., Brisson, G. R., and Malaisse-Lagae, F. (1972a). The stimulus-secretion coupling of glucose-induced insulin release. VIII. Combined effects of glucose and sulfonylureas. *Eur. J. Clin. Invest.* **2,** 85–90.

Malaisse, W. J., Hager, D. L., and Orci, L. (1972b). The stimulus-secretion coupling of glucose-induced insulin release. IX. The participation of the beta cell web. *Diabetes Suppl. 2,* **21,** 594–604.

Malaisse, W. J., Malaisse-Lagae, F., Van Obberghen, E., Somers, G., Devis, G., Ravazolla, M., and Orci. L. (1975). Role of microtubules in phasic pattern of insulin release. *Ann. N. Y. Acad. Sci.* **253,** 630–652.

Malaisse, W. J., Herchuelz, A., Devis, G., Somers, G., Boschero, A. C., Hutton, J. C., Kawazu, S., Serner, A., Atwater, I. J., Duncan, G., Ribalet, B., and Rojas, E. (1978). Regulation of calcium fluxes and their regulatory roles in pancreatic islets. *Ann. N. Y. Acad. Sci.* **307,** 562–581.

Malaisse-Lagae, F., and Malaisse, W. J. (1971). The stimulus-secretion coupling of glucose-induced insulin release. III. Uptake of 45 calcium by isolated islets of Langerhans. *Endocrinology (Baltimore)* **88,** 72–80.

Malaisse-Lagae, F., Ravazzola, M., Amherdt, M., Gutzeit, A., Malaisse, W. J., and Orci, L. (1975). An apparent abnormality of the β-cell microtubular system in spiny mice (*Acomys cahirinus*). *Diabetologia* **10,** 71–76.

Malaisse-Lagae, F., Amherdt, M., Ravazzola, M., Sener, A., Hutton, J. C., Orci, L., and Malaisse, W. J. (1979). Role of microtubules in the synthesis, conversion and release of (pro)insulin. A biochemical and radioautographic study in rat islets. *J. Clin. Invest.* **63,** 1284–1291.

Margolis, R. L., and Wilson, L. (1978). Opposite end assembly and disassembly of microtubules at steady-state *in vitro*. *Cell* **13,** 1–8.

Margolis, R. L., Wilson, L., and Kiefer, B. I. (1978). Mitotic mechanisms based on intrinsic microtubule behavior. *Nature (London)* **272,** 450–452.

Maruta, H., and Korn, E. D. (1977). Purification from *Acanthamoeba castellanii* of proteins that induce gelation and syneresis of F-actin. *J. Biol. Chem.* **252,** 399–402.

Means, A. R., and Dedman, J. R. (1980). Calmodulin: An intracellular calcium receptor. *Nature (London)* **285,** 73–77.

Means, A. R., Chafouleas, J. G., Bolton, W. E., Hidaka, H., and Boyd, A. E., III (1981). Calmodulin regulation during the cell cycle of mammalian cells. *Proc. West. Pharmacol. Soc.* **24,** 209–219.

Metz, S. A., Halter, J. B., and Robertson, R. P. (1979). Paradoxical inhibition of insulin secretion by glucose in human diabetes mellitus. *J. Clin. Endocrinol. Metab.* **48**, 827–835.

Mizel, S. B., and Wilson, L. (1972a). Inhibition of the transport of hexoses in mammalian cells by cytochalasin B. *J. Biol. Chem.* **247**, 4102–4105.

Mizel, S. B., and Wilson, L. (1972b). Nucleoside transport in mammalian cells. Inhibition by colchicine. *Biochemistry* **11**, 2573–2578.

Montague, W., and Howell, S. L. (1972). The mode of action of adenosine 3′,5′-cyclic monophosphate in mammalian islets of Langerhans. Preparation and properties of islet-cell protein phosphokinase. *Biochem. J.* **129**, 551–560.

Montague, W., Howell, S. L., and Green, I. C. (1976). Insulin release and the microtubular system of the islets of Langerhans. Effect of insulin secretagogues on microtubule subunit pool size. *Horm. Metab. Res.* **8**, 166–169.

Morgan, J. L. (1976). Myosin light chain phosphatase. *Biochem. J.* **157**, 687–697.

Morgan, J. L., Holladay, C. R., and Spooner, B. S. (1980). Immunologic differences between actins from cardiac muscle, skeletal muscle, and brain. *Proc. Natl. Acad. Sci. U.S.A.* **77**, 2069–2073.

Mornet, D., Bertrand, R., Panntel, P., Audemard, E., and Kassab, R. (1981). Structure of the actin-myosin interface. *Nature (London)* **292**, 301–306.

Mooseker, M. S., and Tilney, L. G. (1975). Organization of an actin filament-membrane complex. Filament polarity and membrane attachment in the microvilli of intestinal epithelial cells. *J. Cell Biol.* **67**, 725–743.

Mooseker, M. S., Graves, T. A., Wharton, K. A., Falco, N., and Howe, C. L. (1980). Regulation of microvillus structure: Calcium-dependent solution and cross-linking of actin filaments in microvilli of intestinal epithelial cells. *J. Biol. Chem.* **87**, 809–822.

Muller, W. A., and Sharp, W. G. (1974). Cyclic-AMP-dependent protein kinase and phosphoprotein phosphatase in rat islets. *Diabetologia* **10**, 380–381.

Murphy, D. B., and Borisy, G. G. (1975). Association of high-molecular weight proteins with microtubules and their role in microtubule assembly *in vitro*. *Proc. Natl. Acad. Sci. U.S.A.* **72**, 2696–2700.

Murphy, D. B., Vallee, R. B., and Borisy, G. G. (1977). Identity and polymerization-stimulatory activity of the nontubulin protein associated with microtubules. *Biochemistry* **16**, 2598–2605.

Naccache, P. H., Molski, T. F. P., Alopaidi, T., Pecker, E. L., Showell, H. J., and Sha'afi, R. I. (1980). Calmodulin inhibitors block neutrophil degranulation at a step distal from the mobilization of calcium. *Biochem. Biophys. Res. Commun.* **97**, 62–68.

Nelson, T. Y., Oberwetter, J. M., Chafouleas, J. G., Oie, H., Gazdar, A., and Boyd, A. E., III (1981). Chalmodulin-binding proteins in beta cells. *J. Cell Biol.* **91**, 405a.

Nicklas, W. J., Puszkin, S., and Berl, S. (1973). Effect of vinblastine and colchicine on uptake and release of putative transmitters by synaptosomes and on brain actomysin-like protein. *J. Neurochem.* **20**, 109–121.

Olmsted, J. B. (1976). The role of divalent cations and nucleotides in microtubule assembly *in vitro*. *Cold Spring Harbor Conf. Cell Proliferation* **3**, 1081–1092.

Orci, L. (1974). A portrait of the pancreatic β-cell. *Diabetes* **10**, 163–187.

Orci, L., Gabbay, K. H., and Malaisse, W. J. (1972). Pancreatic β-cell web: Its possible role in insulin secretion. *Science* **175**, 1128–1130.

Ostlund, R. E., Leung, J. T., and Kipnis, D. M. (1977). Muscle actin filaments bind pituitary secretory granules *in vitro*. *J. Cell Biol.* **73**, 78–87.

Penningroth, S. M., Cleveland, D. W., and Kirschner, M. W. (1976). Microtubules and related proteins. *In* "Cell Motility," (R. Goldman, T. Pollard, and J. Rosenbaum, eds.), pp. 1233–1257. Cold Spring Harbor Lab., Cold Spring Harbor, New York.

Pershadsingh, H. A., McDaniel, M. L., Landt, M., Bry, C. G., Lacy, P. E., and McDonald, J. M. (1980). Ca^{2+}-activated ATPase and ATP-dependent calmodulin-stimulated Ca^{2+} transport in islet cell plasma membrane. *Nature (London)* **288**, 492–495.

Pfeifer, M. A., Halter, J. B., Graf, R., and Porte, D. (1979). Is it necessary to postulate an extrapancreatic action of tolbutamine? *Clin. Res.* **27A**, 48.

Pfeifer, M. A., Halter, J. B., and Porte, D. (1981). Insulin secretion in diabetes mellitus. *Am. J. Med.* **70**, 579–588.

Pipeleers, D. G., Pipeleers-Marichal, M. A., and Kipnis, D. M. (1976). Microtubule assembly and the intracellular transport of secretory granules in pancreatic islets. *Science* **191**, 88–89.

Pires, E. M. V., and Perry, S. V. (1977). Purification and properties of myosin light chain kinase from fast skeletal muscle. *Biochem. J.* **167**, 137–146.

Pollack, R., and Rifkin, D. (1975). Actin-containing cables within anchorage-dependent rat embryo cells are dissociated by plasmin and trypsin. *Cell* **6**, 495–505.

Porter, K. R. (1976). Introduction: Motility in cells. *Cold Spring Harbor Conf. Cell Proliferation* **3**, 1–28.

Rabinovitch, A., Gutzeit, A., Kikuchi, M., Cerasi, E., and Renold, A. E. (1975). Defective early phase insulin release in perifused isolated pancreatic islets of spiny mice (*Acromys cahirinus*). *Diabetologia* **11**, 457–465.

Renold, A. E. (1970). Insulin biosynthesis and secretion: A still unsettled topic. *N. Engl. J. Med.* **282**, 173–182.

Robertson, R. P., and Porte, D., Jr. (1973). The glucose receptor: A defective mechanism in diabetes mellitus distinct from the β-adrenergic receptor. *J. Clin. Invest.* **52**, 870–876.

Rosen, O. M., Hirsch, A. H., and Goren, W. N. (1971). Factors which influence cyclic AMP formation and degradation in an islet cell tumor of the Syrian hamster. *Arch. Biochem. Biophys.* **146**, 660–663.

Roth, S. I., Conaway, H. H., Sanders, L. L., Casali, R. E., and Boyd, A. E., III (1980). Spontaneous diabetes mellitus in the New Zealand white rabbit: Preliminary morphological characteristics. *Lab. Invest.* **42**, 571–579.

Sams, D. J., and Montague, V. (1972). The role of adenosine 3′,5′-cyclic monophosphate in the regulation of insulin release. Properties of islet-cell adenosine 3′,5′-cyclic monophosphate phosphodiesterase. *Biochem. J.* **129**, 945–952.

Satir, P. (1974). How cilia move. *Sci. Am.* **231**, 44–52.

Schubart, U. K., Shapiro, S., Fleischer, N., and Rosen, O. M. (1977). Cyclic adenosine 3′,5′-monophosphate-mediated insulin secretion and ribosomal protein phosphorylation in a hamster islet cell tumor. *J. Biol. Chem.* **252**, 92–101.

Schubart, U. K., Fleischer, N., and Erlichman, J. (1980a). Ca^{2+}-dependent protein phosphorylation and insulin release in intact hamster insulinoma cells. *J. Biol. Chem.* **255**, 11063–11066.

Schubart, U. K., Erlichman, J., and Fleisher, N. (1980b). The role of calmodulin in the regulation of protein phosphorylation and insulin release in hamster insulinoma cells. *J. Biol. Chem.* **255**, 4120–4124.

Seltzer, H. S., Allen, E. W., Herron, A. L., Jr., and Brennan, M. T. (1967). Insulin secretion in response to glycemic stimulus: Relation of delayed initial release to carbohydrate intolerance in mild diabetes. *J. Clin. Invest.* **46**, 323–335.

Sharp, G. W. G., Wollheim, C., Muller, W. A., Gutzeit, A., Trueheart, P. A., Blondel, B.,

Orci, L., and Renold, E. (1975). Studies on the mechanism of insulin release. *Fed. Proc., Fed. Am. Soc. Exp. Biol.* **34**, 1537–1548.

Sharp, G. W. G., Wiedenkeller, D. E., Karlin, D., Siegel, E. G., and Wollheim, C. B. (1980). Stimulation of adenylate cyclase by Ca^{2+} and calmodulin in rat islets of Langerhans. *Diabetes* **29**, 76–76.

Sherline, P., Lee, Y.-D., and Jacobs, L. (1977). Binding of microtubules to pituitary secretory granules and secretory granule membranes. *J. Cell Biol.* **72**, 380–389.

Shizuta, Y., Shizuta, H., Gallo, M., Davies, P., Pastan, I., and Lewis, M. (1976). Purification and properties of filamin, an actin-binding protein from chicken gizzard. *J. Biol. Cehm.* **251**, 6562–6567.

Siegel, E. G., Wollheim, C. B., Sharp, G. W. G., Herberg, L., and Renold, A. E. (1980). Role of Ca^{2+} in impaired insulin release from islets of diabetic (C57BL/KsJ-db/db) mice. *Am. J. Physiol.* **239**, E132–E138.

Sieghart, W., Theoharides, T. C., Alper, S. L., Douglas, W. W., and Greengard, P. (1978). Calcium-dependent protein phosphorylation during secretion by exocytosis in the mast cell. *Nature (London)* **275**, 329–331.

Simpson, R. G., Benedetti, A., Grodsky, G. M., Koram, J. H., and Forsham, P. H. (1968). Early phase of insulin release. *Diabetes* **17**, 684–691.

Sloboda, R. D., Rudolph, S. A., Rosenbaum, J. L., and Greengard, P. (1975). Cyclic AMP-dependent endogenous phosphorylation of a microtubule-associated protein. *Proc. Natl. Acad. Sci. U.S.A.* **72**, 177–181.

Sloboda, R. D., Dentler, W. L., Bloodgood, R. A., Telzer, B. R., Granett, S., and Rosenbaum, J. L. (1976). Microtubule-associated proteins (MAPs) and the assembly of microtubules *in vitro. Cold Spring Harbor Conf. Cell Proliferation* **3**, 1171–1212.

Snabes, M. C., and Boyd, A. E., III (1982). Increased filamentous actin in islets of Langerhans from fasted Hamsters. *Biochem. Biophys. Res. Commun.,* **104**, 207–211.

Snabes, M. C., Boyd, A. E., III, Pardue, R. L., and Bryan, J. (1981a). DNase I Binding/Immunoprecipitation assay for actin. *J. Biol. Chem.* **256**, 6291–6295.

Snabes, M. C., Boyd, A. E., III, and Bryan, J. (1981b). Detection of actin-binding proteins in human platelets by ^{125}I-actin overlay of polyacrylamide gels. *J. Cell Biol.* **90**, 809–812.

Solomon, F. (1976). Characterization of the calcium-binding activity of tubulin. *Cold Spring Harbor Conf. Cell Proliferation* **3**, 1139–1148.

Somers, G., Van Obberghen, E., Devis, G., Ravazzola, M., Malaisse-Lagae, F., and Malaisse, W. J. (1974). Dynamics of insulin release and microtubular-microfilamentous system. III. Effect of colchicine upon glucose-induced insulin secretion. *Eur. J. Clin. Invest.* **4**, 299–305.

Spudich, J. A. (1972). Effect of cytochalasin B on actin filaments. *Cold Spring Harbor Symp. Quant. Biol.* **37**, 535–593.

Stauffacher, W., Orci, L., Amherdt, M., Burr, I. M., Balant, L., Froesch, E. R., and Renold, A. E. (1970). Metabolic state, pancreatic insulin content, and β-cell morphology of normoglycemic spiny mice (*Acomys cahirinus*): Indications for an impairment of insulin secretion. *Diabetologia* **6**, 330–342.

Stephens, R. E. (1968). Reassociation of microtubule protein. *J. Mol. Biol.* **33**, 517–519.

Stossel, T. P. (1978). Contractile proteins in cell structure and function. *Annu. Rev. Med.* **29**, 427–456.

Sugden, M. C., Christie, M. R., and Ashcroft, S. J. H. (1979). Presence and possible role of calcium-dependent regulator (calmodulin) in rat islets of Langerhans. *FEBS Lett.* **105**, 95–100.

Swanson-Flatt, S. K., Carlsson, L., and Gylife, E. (1980). Actin filament formation in pancreatic beta cells during glucose stimulation of insulin secretion. *FEBS Lett.* **117,** 299–302.

Tattersall, R. B., and Fajans, S. S. (1975). A difference between the inheritance and classical juvenile-onset and maturely-onset diabetes. *Diabetes* **24,** 44–53.

Taylor, E. W. (1965). The mechanism of colchicine inhibition of mitosis. I. Kinetics of inhibition and the binding of ^{3}H-colchicine. *J. Cell Biol.* **25,** 145–160.

Tilney, L. G., and Detmers, P. (1975). Actin in erythrocyte ghosts and its association with spectrin: Evidence for a nonfilamentous form of these two molecules *in situ. J. Cell Biol.* **66,** 508–520.

Valverde, I., Vandermeers, A., Anjaneyula, R., and Malaisse, W. J. (1979). Calmodulin activation of adenylate cyclase in pancreatic islets. *Science* **206,** 225–227.

Van Obberghen, E., Somers, G., Devis, G., Vaughan, D., Malaisse-Lagae, F., Orci, L., and Malaisse, W. J. (1973). Dynamics of insulin release and microtubular-microfilamentous system. I. Effect of cytochalasin B. *J. Clin. Invest.* **52,** 1041–1050.

Walsh, M. P., Cavadore, J. C., Vallet, B., and Demaille, J. G. (1980). Calmodulin-dependent myosin light chain kinases from cardiac and smooth muscle: A comparative study. *Can. J. Biochem.* **58,** 299–308.

Wang, E., and Goldberg, A. R. (1976). Changes in microfilament organization and surface topography upon transformation of chick embryo fibroblasts with Rous sarcoma virus. *Proc. Natl. Acad. Sci. U.S.A.* **73,** 4065–4069.

Wang, L. L., and Bryan, J. (1981). Isolation of calcium-dependent platelet proteins that interact with actin. *Cell* **25,** 637–649.

Weber, K., and Groeschel-Stewart, U. (1974). Myosin antibody: The specific visualization of myosin-containing filaments in non-muscle cells. *Proc. Natl. Acad. Sci. U.S.A.* **71,** 4561–4564.

Weingarten, M. D., Lockwood, A. H., Hwo, S.-Y., and Kirschner, M. W. (1975). A protein factor essential for microtubule assembly. *Proc. Natl. Acad. Sci. U.S.A.* **72,** 1858–1862.

Weisenberg, R. C. (1972). Microtubule formation *in vitro* in solutions containing low calcium concentrations. *Science* **177,** 1104–1105.

Welsh, M. J., Dedman, J. R., Brinkley, B. R., and Means, A. R. (1978). Calcium-dependent regulator protein: Localization in mitotic apparatus of eucaryotic cells. *Proc. Natl. Acad. Sci. U.S.A.* **75,** 1867–1871.

White, G. C., II, and Raynor, S. T. (1980). The effects of trifluoperazine, an inhibitor of calmodulin on platelet function. *Thromb. Res.* **18,** 279–284.

Wickus, G., Gruenstein, E., Robbins, P. W., and Rich, A. (1975). Decrease in membrane-associated actin of fibroblasts after transformation by Rous sarcoma virus. *Proc. Natl. Acad. Sci. U.S.A.* **72,** 746–749.

Wolf, H., and Hofmann, F. (1980). Purification of myosin light chain kinase from bovine cardiac muscle. *Proc. Natl. Acad. Sci. U.S.A.* **77,** 5852–5855.

Wollheim, C. B., Blondel, B., Trueheart, P. A., Renold, A. E., and Sharp, G. W. G. (1975). Calcium-induced insulin release in monolayer culture of the endocrine pancreas: Studies with ionophore A23187. *J. Biol. Chem.* **250,** 1354–1360.

Wolosewick, J. J., and Porter, K. R. (1979). Microtubular lattice of the cytoplasm ground substance: Artifact or reality. *J. Cell Biol.* **82,** 114–139.

Yagi, K., Yazawa, M., Kakiuchi, S., Ohshima, M., and Uenishi, K. (1978). Identification of an activator protein for myosin light chain kinase as a Ca^{2+}-dependent modulator protein. *J. Biol. Chem.* **253,** 1338–1340.

Yin, H. L., and Stossel, T. P. (1979). Control of cytoplasmic actin gelsol transformation by gelsolin, a calcium-dependent regulatory protein. *Nature (London)* **281,** 583–586.

Yin, H. L., Zaner, K. S., and Stossel, T. P. (1980). Ca^{2+} control of actin gelation: Interaction of gelsolin with actin filaments and regulation of actin gelation. *J. Biol. Chem.* **255,** 9494–9500.

PART IV
SYNTHESIS, PROCESSING, AND STORAGE OF SECRETORY PRODUCTS

8

Regulation of Prolactin Gene Expression

RICHARD A. MAURER

I. INTRODUCTION

The actual secretion of a protein is only one step in the expression of the gene for that protein. The multiple steps that precede secretion of the protein include transcription of the gene, processing of a precursor messenger RNA, translation of the messenger RNA, modification of the primary translation product, and sequestration of the protein in a secretory granule. Each of these steps provides a possible site for regulation of the production of the protein. Clearly, it would be useful to

267

CELLULAR REGULATION OF SECRETION AND RELEASE

understand how the regulation of these steps is integrated with the regulation of secretion. In this chapter recent studies of the regulation of prolactin gene expression will be reviewed.

The production of prolactin by the pituitary has provided a particularly favorable system for analysis of the regulation of gene expression. Prolactin is a major gene product of the pituitary. Thus, the molecular machinery involved in prolactin gene expression is relatively abundant. This has facilitated both analysis and isolation of some of the relevant molecular species, such as prolactin mRNA. Also, a large number of experiments have identified hormones that regulate prolactin secretion. These hormones have been useful for manipulation of prolactin gene expression. Finally, cell culture systems that synthesize prolactin are available. All of these factors have greatly facilitated the study of prolactin gene expression.

II. BIOSYNTHESIS OF PROLACTIN

A. Synthesis and Intracellular Transport of Prolactin

Prolactin is synthesized in specialized cells in the anterior pituitary. Although there are at least six different hormone-secreting cell types in the anterior pituitary, in female rats prolactin cells are a predominant cell type. Hymer *et al.* (1974) found that in female rat pituitaries 33% of the cells were prolactin-secreting cells (mammotrophs). The prolactin-secreting cells are highly specialized and secrete large amounts of prolactin. Studies of *de novo* synthesis of prolactin have demonstrated that prolactin is synthesized in very large amounts by pituitaries of female rats (Catt and Moffat, 1967; MacLeod and Abad, 1968; Maurer and Gorski, 1977). These studies utilized incubation of pituitary fragments with radiolabeled amino acids to demonstrate that prolactin is the major protein synthesized by the pituitary.

The intracellular movement of newly synthesized prolactin has been examined by autoradiography and electron microscopy (Farquhar, 1961). The synthesis and intracellular transit of prolactin is similar to that of the well-studied secretory proteins of the exocrine pancreas (Palade, 1975). Prolactin is synthesized on ribosomes bound to the rough endoplasmic reticulum. Newly synthesized prolactin moves into the cisternae of the endoplasmic reticulum and then to the Golgi apparatus, where mature secretory granules are formed. Secretion occurs by exocytosis of the secretory granules.

There is some evidence for heterogeneity in the movement of prolactin through the cell. Pulse–chase experiments have suggested that newly synthesized prolactin may be released preferentially (Swearingen, 1971; Walker and Farquhar, 1980; Maurer, 1980a). Autoradiographic analysis of prolactin synthesis per cell indicated that the preferential release of newly synthesized prolactin may be due to functional heterogeneity of mammotrophs (Walker and Farquhar, 1980).

B. Preprolactin

A number of studies have shown that prolactin is synthesized as a precursor—preprolactin. The initial studies that demonstrated the synthesis of preprolactin utilized translation of prolactin mRNA in a cell-free system (Maurer *et al.*, 1976; Evans and Rosenfeld, 1976; Dannies and Tashjian, 1976a). These studies were made possible by the fact that wheat germ extracts contain little endogenous mRNA activity but will readily translate added mRNA. Analysis of translation products by immunoprecipitation and electrophoresis demonstrated that a product larger than prolactin, but containing the antigenic determinants of prolactin, was synthesized in a wheat germ translation system (Fig. 1A). Comparison of the tryptic peptides from preprolactin and prolactin demonstrated that preprolactin does contain the amino acid sequence of prolactin (Maurer *et al.*, 1976). Thus, it seems likely that preprolactin is, in fact, a precursor for prolactin.

If preprolactin is a precursor for prolactin, then it should be possible to demonstrate the conversion of preprolactin to prolactin. Several studies have suggested that it is possible to convert preprolactin to prolactin in cell-free translation systems (Lingappa *et al.*, 1977; Shields and Blobel, 1978; Maurer and McKean, 1978). These studies have shown that addition of microsomal membranes to cell-free translation systems results in the apparent conversion of preprolactin to prolactin (Fig. 1B). Sequence analysis of prolactin produced by membrane-mediated cleavage of preprolactin has shown that the cleavage is accurate, as the known amino-terminal sequence of prolactin was produced (Lingappa *et al.*, 1977; Maurer and McKean, 1978).

Several lines of evidence suggest that cleavage of preprolactin to prolactin occurs before the nascent peptide is completed. This includes the finding that addition of membranes to cell-free translation systems results in cleavage of preprolactin to prolactin only when the membranes are present during translation and not when membranes are added after translation (Lingappa *et al.*, 1977). Studies utilizing polysomes have also suggested that cleavage occurs before the nascent peptide is complete (Blobel and Dobberstein, 1975; Szczesna and

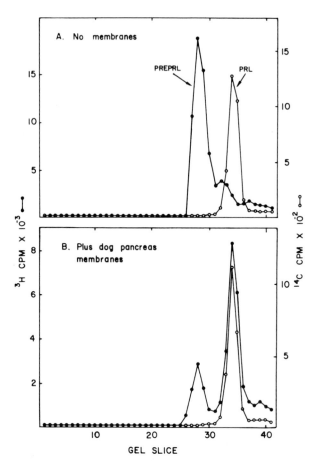

Fig. 1. Electrophoretic analysis of the synthesis of preprolactin and conversion to prolactin in a cell-free system. (A) Pituitary RNA was translated in a wheat germ cell-free reaction. The products synthesized in the cell-free reaction (●) were then immunoprecipitated by the addition of carrier ^{14}C-labeled prolactin (○) and anti-prolactin. The immunoprecipitate was dissolved in a sodium dodecyl sulfate-containing buffer and analyzed on a 12% polyacrylamide gel. The ^{14}C-labeled prolactin carrier serves as a marker for prolactin. (B) Pituitary RNA was translated in a wheat germ assay containing membranes prepared from dog pancreas. The reaction was immunoprecipitated with anti-prolactin and electrophoresed on a 12% polyacrylamide gel. The addition of the membranes resulted in the synthesis of a substantial amount of product (●), which comigrates with the prolactin standard (○). Reprinted from Maurer and McKean (1978) with permission.

Boime, 1976; Spielman and Bancroft, 1977). If preprolactin is always cleaved before completion of the peptide chain, then it would be impossible to detect complete, intact preprolactin in intact cells. However, the use of very brief pulse-labeling of monolayer cultures of pituitary cells has permitted the detection of newly synthesized proprolactin in intact cells (Maurer and McKean, 1978). Even when using very brief pulse-labeling conditions, the amount of preprolactin was relatively small compared to the amount of mature prolactin in the cells (Fig. 2). This finding demonstrates that some complete preprolactin is synthesized in cells, but it is not clear if this is the usual pathway for prolactin synthesis. Cleavage of the precursor segment could occur at ran-

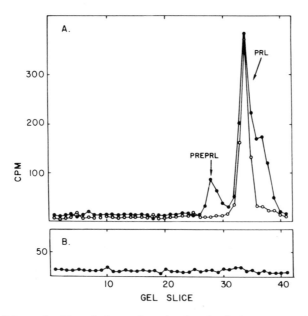

Fig. 2. Polyacrylamide gel electrophoresis of prolactin immunoreactive material synthesized when pituitary cells were incubated with [^{3}H]leucine for 3 minutes. (A) The 10,000-g supernatant fraction from the homogenized cells was incubated with antiprolactin overnight, and the immunoprecipitate was isolated by adsorption to fixed *Staphylococcus aureus*. The immunoprecipitate was dissolved in a sodium dodecyl sulfate-containing buffer, combined with a ^{14}C-labeled prolactin standard and electrophoresed on a 10% polyacrylamide gel. The peaks with a mobility of preprolactin (PREPRL) and prolactin (PRL) are indicated. (B) A cell extract was incubated with antiprolactin plus 100 μg of unlabeled rat prolactin and then processed as above. (●), ^{3}H-labeled immunoprecipitate; (○), ^{14}C-labeled prolactin standard. Reprinted from Maurer and McKean (1978) with permission.

dom times during the synthesis of preprolactin. Some prolactin could be synthesized as complete preprolactin and then cleaved, whereas other precursor segments could be removed before the completion of the protein. Alternatively, the small amount of preprolactin detected in the cells may represent aberrant protein synthesis that does not actually lead to prolactin production. At the present time it is not possible to distinguish between these possibilities. Thus, although considerable evidence suggests that cleavage of preprolactin is a co-translational event, it remains possible that at least some preprolactin is cleaved after the completion of translation.

It is likely that preprolactin is involved in the movement of newly synthesized prolactin into the cisternae of the endoplasmic reticulum. Sequence analysis of rat preprolactin has shown that it differs from prolactin by the presence of a 29-amino acid, amino-terminal extension (Maurer et al., 1977). The amino-terminal precursor segment has been completely sequenced (McKean and Maurer, 1978), and the sequence is   Met-Asn-Ser-Gln-Val-Ser-Ala-Arg-Lys-Ala-Gly-Thr-Leu-Leu-Leu-Leu-Met-Met-Ser-Asn-Leu-Leu-Phe-Cys-Gln-Asn-Val-Gln-Thr-.   This sequence contains a large number of hydrophobic amino acid residues. These hydrophobic amino acids are likely important in interacting with the membranes of endoplasmic reticulum and facilitating the movement of preprolactin across the membrane of the endoplasmic reticulum. The role of precursor segments in possible mechanisms for the movement of secretory proteins across membranes is discussed in detail in Chapter 9.

III.   REGULATION OF PROLACTIN SYNTHESIS AND PROLACTIN mRNA LEVELS

A.   Effects of Estradiol

17β-Estradiol is well established as a physiological regulator of prolactin production. Perhaps the most direct demonstration that estradiol is involved in physiological regulation of prolactin was provided by the passive immunization experiments of Neill et al. (1971). They demonstrated that antibodies against estradiol blocked the proestrous peak of prolactin secretion. Thus, neutralization of endogenous estradiol prevented the normal proestrous secretion of prolactin. This clearly demonstrates that physiological concentrations of estradiol are involved in regulating prolactin production. Furthermore, ovariectomy results in a marked decline in prolactin production, and treatment of ovariectomized rats with estradiol results in a dramatic stimulation of prolactin production (Amenomori et al., 1970). Studies examining incorporation of radiolabeled amino acids have demonstrated that estradiol increases the de novo synthesis of prolactin. MacLeod et al. (1969) found that de novo prolactin synthesis was increased 8 days after a single injection of polyestradiol phosphate. Yamamoto et al. (1975) observed that prolactin synthesis was increased after either a single injection or eight daily injections of estradiol.

Administration of daily estradiol injections to ovariectomized female or intact male rats results in a gradual stimulation of prolactin synthesis (Maurer and Gorski, 1977). In females, prolactin synthesis appeared to be maximally stimulated after 2 or 3 days of estradiol treatment. In males, prolactin synthesis was still increasing after a week of estradiol injections. This relatively slow time course of estradiol effects suggests that the molecular events mediating the estradiol response likely have a slow turnover, so that a new steady state is reached only slowly. The specificity of estradiol effects on prolactin is illustrated by the fact that growth hormone synthesis did not increase, but tended to slightly decrease, after estradiol treatment in both males and females. Interestingly, estradiol treatment did not significantly alter the protein or DNA content of the pituitary, but it did increase DNA synthesis by the pituitary. Several studies have shown that estradiol can stimulate DNA synthesis by the pituitary (Baker and Everett, 1944; Mastro and Hymer, 1973; Davies et al., 1974). As only a very small percentage of pituitary cells are dividing in the basal state (Crane and Loomes, 1967; Mastro et al., 1969), it seems likely that even though estradiol may cause a considerable increase in the number of dividing cells, the number of dividing cells is too small to affect total DNA content of the pituitary. However, estradiol effects on proliferation of prolactin-secreting cells could be very physiologically important. For instance, long-term treatment of rats with estradiol leads to the development of pituitary tumors in a large percentage of rats (Clifton and Meyer, 1956).

The ability of estradiol to stimulate prolactin synthesis is likely due to a direct effect of estradiol on pituitary cells. Early studies using organ culture systems demonstrated that high doses of estradiol could stimulate prolactin accumulation in the system (Nicoll and Meites, 1962; Lu et al., 1971). More recent studies utilizing monolayer cultures of dispersed pituitary cells have shown that physiological concentrations of estradiol will directly stimulate prolactin synthesis (Lieberman et al., 1978). It was found that treatment of cultured pituitary cells with 10 nM estradiol specifically stimulated prolactin synthesis, but not synthesis of the bulk of other pituitary proteins. A concentration of 10 nM was maximal, and approximately 0.5 nM estradiol produced half-maximal effects. As estradiol concentrations during the estrous cycle of the rat range from approximately 0.1 nM to greater than 2 nM (Butcher et al., 1974), the concentrations of estradiol that alter prolactin synthesis by the cultured pituitary cells are clearly in the physiological range. The effects were specific for estrogens, as estradiol, estriol, and diethylstilbestrol stimulated prolactin synthesis whereas testosterone, dihydrotestosterone, progesterone, and corticosterone had little or no effect. Other studies utilizing monolayer cultures of dispersed bovine pituitary cells (Vician et al., 1979), pituitary tumor cells (Haug and Gautvik, 1976), or a clonal cell line derived from Rathke's pouch (Herbert et al., 1978) have also shown specific, direct effects of estradiol on the stimulation of prolactin production.

The studies demonstrating estradiol effects on prolactin synthesis prompted further studies concerning the mechanisms involved in this response. Changes in the synthesis of prolactin could be due either to changes in the amount of prolactin mRNA in pituitary cells or to changes in the efficiency of translation of prolactin mRNA. A number of studies have examined effects of estradiol on prolactin mRNA levels. The initial studies made use of cell-free translation systems to assay prolactin mRNA levels (Stone et al., 1977; Shupnik et al., 1979; Vician et al., 1979; Seo et al., 1979a). For these studies RNA was isolated from control and estradiol-injected rats and the isolated RNA translated in a cell-free system. The translation of prolactin mRNA was quantitated by immunoprecipitation of preprolactin synthesized in the cell-free reaction. The results of such studies demonstrated that in male rats there was a maximum 3-fold increase in prolactin synthesis after treatment with estradiol for 7 days (Stone et al., 1977). Similar increases in prolactin mRNA levels have been detected in the other studies. This increase in prolactin mRNA is very similar in magnitude to the increase in prolactin synthesis observed by Maurer and Gorski (1977). Therefore, it seems likely that the estradiol-induced increases in prolactin synthesis are mediated by increases in prolactin mRNA. However, the possibility remained that a factor that copurified with the RNA may have altered the translation of the mRNA in the cell-free system. For further analysis of the estrogenic regulation of prolactin mRNA levels, it would be desirable to have a specific hybridization probe that would measure prolactin mRNA sequences independently of the biological activity of the sequences.

Specific hybridization probes can be prepared from a purified mRNA through the use of the enzyme reverse transcriptase from avian my-

eloblastosis virus. Under the appropriate conditions, reverse transcriptase will use an mRNA as a template to synthesize a copy DNA
(cDNA). If the mRNA is highly purified, then the cDNA will be a
specific hybridization probe for that mRNA. Therefore, to obtain a
specific hybridization probe for prolactin mRNA, it was necessary to
first purify prolactin mRNA. Highly purified prolactin mRNA was
prepared by immunoprecipitation of polysomes (Maurer, 1980b). This
technique makes use of the fact that antibodies can specifically bind to
the nascent chains of polysomes. Polysomes were incubated with anti-
prolactin and then with a second antibody directed against the first

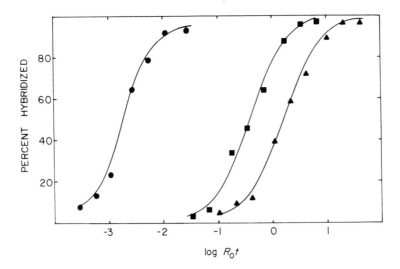

Fig. 3. Analysis of prolactin mRNA content of pituitary RNA from control and
estradiol-treated rats. Female rats, 60 days old, were ovariectomized 2 weeks prior to the
start of injections. Estrogen-treated rats received for 2 weeks daily injections of 10 μg
estradiol dissolved in oil. Controls received only the oil. After the treatments, total RNA
was prepared from the pituitaries. Purified prolactin mRNA (●), RNA from control rats
(▲), and RNA from estradiol-treated rats (■) was hybridized to prolactin ^{3}H-labeled
cDNA for various periods of time and the percentage of cDNA hybridized was determined by S1 nuclease digestion. Percentage of hybridization is plotted against log R_ot,
where R_ot is the product of the initial concentration of RNA in moles of nucleotides per
liter and time in seconds. The $R_ot_{1/2}$ is the R_ot (mol•sec/liter) at which the hybridization
of the cDNA is half completed, and this value should be inversely related to proportion of
the RNA that is complementary to the cDNA. As $R_ot_{1/2}$ for purified prolactin mRNA was
0.0018 mol•sec/liter, for RNA from controls was 1.6 mol•sec/liter, and for RNA from
estradiol-treated rats was 0.39 mol•sec/liter, the results suggest that 0.11 and 0.46% of
RNA are prolactin mRNA in pituitaries from control and estradiol-treated rats, respectively. Reprinted from Maurer (1980b) with permission.

antibody. RNA was isolated from the immunoprecipitated polysomes and then prolactin mRNA was separated from ribosomal RNA by chromatography on oligo(dT)-cellulose. Finally, the mRNA was further purified by sedimentation through a 5–20% sucrose gradient. The purification and yield of prolactin mRNA during each step was determined by cell-free translation of the RNA. The final RNA obtained from the sucrose gradient was purified 320-fold with a 14% yield. Analysis of the translation products directed by this RNA demonstrated that the isolated RNA was greater than 95% pure in terms of prolactin mRNA activity. This mRNA was used to synthesize a radiolabeled cDNA and the cDNA used as a hybridization probe to investigate the effects of estradiol on the concentration of prolactin mRNA sequences in the pituitary (Fig. 3). Comparison of the kinetics of hybridization of the cDNA probe to purified prolactin mRNA and total cellular RNA from control or estradiol-treated rats suggested that estradiol resulted in a considerable increase in the concentration of prolactin mRNA. In control rats 0.11% of total cellular RNA was prolactin mRNA, whereas in estradiol-treated rats 0.46% of total cellular RNA was prolactin mRNA. This 4-fold increase in prolactin mRNA is similar to that seen using the translation assay and would account for the effects of estradiol on prolactin synthesis. Ryan *et al.* (1979) and Seo *et al.* (1979b,c) have also demonstrated similar estrogenic effects on prolactin mRNA sequences. Thus, it seems clear that estradiol stimulates the accumulation of increased prolactin mRNA levels in the pituitary and that this increase in prolactin mRNA leads to increased synthesis of prolactin.

B. Effects of Dopamine

The control of prolactin appears to be relatively unique among the hormones secreted by the mammalian pituitary in that the major regulatory mechanism involves inhibition of prolactin production. This can be demonstrated by removal of the pituitary from the influence of the hypothalamus, which results in a high rate of prolactin secretion (Chen *et al.*, 1970; Bishop *et al.*, 1971). Hypothalamic extracts inhibit the *in vitro* release of prolactin (Talwalker *et al.*, 1963) and decrease prolactin secretion when infused into a pituitary portal vessel (Kamberi *et al.*, 1971). These findings clearly suggest that the hypothalamus has a net inhibitory effect on prolactin production by the pituitary.

A large body of evidence suggests that dopamine is the hypothalamic hormone that is responsible for the inhibition of prolactin production. Several laboratories have shown that dopamine and dopamine agonists are able to inhibit the ability of pituitary explants to secrete prolactin *in vitro* (MacLeod *et al.*, 1970; Birge *et al.*, 1970; Smalstig *et al.*, 1974). Also, the concentration of dopamine in hypophyseal portal blood is sufficient to inhibit prolactin secretion and varies inversely with prolactin secretion (Ben-Jonathan *et al.*, 1977; Plotsky *et al.*, 1978; Ben-Jonathan *et al.*, 1980). Furthermore, dopamine receptors are located on the plasma membrane of pituitary cells, and there is a good

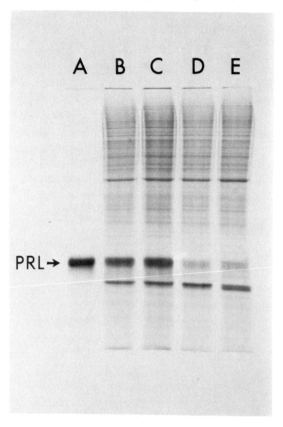

Fig. 4. Electrophoretic analysis of proteins synthesized by control pituitary cell cultures and cultures treated with 10 nM ergocryptine for 4 days. Monolayer cultures of pituitary cells were maintained in serum-free medium for 6 days. During the last 4 days in culture, one-half of the cultures were treated with 10 nM ergocryptine. The cells were then incubated with [^{35}S]methionine for 1 hour and a soluble cell extract was prepared. An aliquot from control cells was immunoprecipitated (A) and aliquots of total soluble proteins from duplicate control cultures (B and C) and ergocryptine-treated cultures (D and E) were subjected to electrophoresis on a 12% polyacrylamide sodium dodecyl sulfate-containing slab gel. The gel was stained, destained, dried, and exposed to X-ray film. An unlabeled prolactin (PRL) standard was also electrophoresed on the gel; the migration of this standard is indicated by the arrow. Reprinted from Maurer (1980c) with permission.

correlation between the ability of various dopamine agonists to bind to this receptor and their ability to inhibit prolactin secretion (Brown *et al.*, 1976; Calabro and MacLeod, 1978; Caron *et al.*, 1978; Creese *et al.*, 1977; Cronin *et al.*, 1978).

Dopamine and dopamine agonists have also been shown to inhibit *de novo* synthesis of prolactin (Maurer, 1980c). These studies utilized cul-

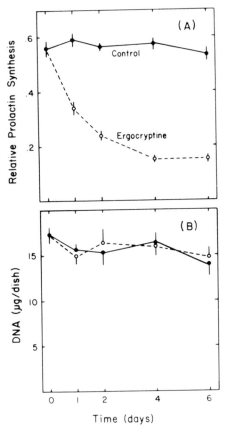

Fig. 5. Time course of ergocryptine effects on prolactin synthesis. Pituitary cell cultures were maintained in control medium (●) or in medium containing 10 nM ergocryptine (○). At the start of the ergocryptine treatment (time 0) and 1, 2, 4, and 6 days thereafter, cultures were incubated with [³H]leucine for 1 hour. Prolactin synthesis (A) was determined by immunoprecipitation. Relative prolactin synthesis is the ratio of radioactivity incorporated into prolactin to radioactivity incorporated in nonprolactin proteins. An aliquot of each cell homogenate was also assayed to determine the DNA content of cultures (B). All values are means ± SE for three determinations per group. Reprinted from Maurer (1980c) with permission.

tures of dispersed rat pituitary cells maintained in serum-free medium. In the initial experiment, pituitary cells were pulse labeled with radiolabeled methionine and the soluble proteins electrophoresed on a sodium dodecyl sulfate-containing polyacrylamide slab gel (Fig. 4). The results demonstrate that even after several days in serum-free medium, control cells synthesize large amounts of prolactin. Cultures treated with the potent dopaminergic agonist ergocryptine synthesized much less prolactin than control cultures. The results also demonstrate the specific inhibition of prolactin synthesis by ergocryptine. Analysis of the time course of ergocryptine effects demonstrated that prolactin synthesis decreased rather slowly (Fig. 5A). Maximal inhibition of prolactin synthesis occurred after 4 to 6 days of ergocryptine treatment. The time course of the dopaminergic inhibition of prolactin synthesis seen in this study is similar to the time course of the estrogenic stimulation of prolactin synthesis seen previously (Maurer and Gorski, 1977). Thus, for both regulatory systems it seems likely

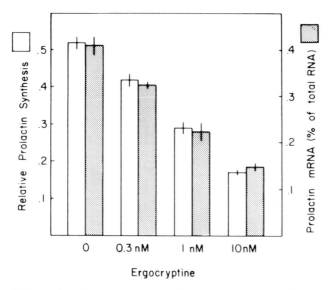

Fig. 6.   Effects of various concentrations of ergocryptine on prolactin synthesis and prolactin mRNA levels. Pituitary cell cultures were treated with the indicated concentration of ergocryptine for 4 days; and then one-half of the cultures were incubated with [3H]leucine for analysis of prolactin synthesis by immunoprecipitation and one-half of the cultures were used to prepare total RNA for analysis of prolactin mRNA levels. Prolactin mRNA levels were determined by hybridization of RNA to prolactin 3H-labeled cDNA. All values are means ± SE for three determinations per groups. Reprinted from Maurer (1980c) with permission.

that there is some rate-limiting step that involves a molecule with a long half-life. Ergocryptine did not affect the DNA content of the cultures, suggesting that the treatment did not cause major changes in cell populations (Fig. 5B). The inhibition of prolactin synthesis was reversed by removal of the ergocryptine from the culture medium. The reversibility of the inhibitory effects of ergocryptine argues that the inhibition is not likely due to a toxic effect of the drug. To determine whether changes in prolactin mRNA were involved in mediating the dopaminergic inhibition of prolactin synthesis, cultured cells were treated with varying doses of ergocryptine, and prolactin synthesis and prolactin mRNA levels were determined (Fig. 6). The results indicate that there was a very good correspondence between the inhibition of prolactin synthesis and prolactin mRNA levels. Brocas *et al.* (1981) have also shown that ergocryptine inhibits prolactin synthesis and prolactin mRNA levels. Thus, these studies demonstrate the ability of dopaminergic treatment to specifically inhibit prolactin synthesis and decrease prolactin mRNA levels.

The rate of production of a protein is dependent on both the rate of synthesis and the rate of degradation of a protein. The studies discussed earlier indicate that dopaminergic stimuli inhibit the synthesis of prolactin. Interestingly, dopamine agonists have also been shown to alter the degradation of prolactin (Dannies and Rudnick, 1980; Maurer, 1980a). The dopamine agonist bromoergocryptine was found to induce maximal prolactin degradation after 1 day of treatment, whereas maximal inhibition of prolactin synthesis required several days of treatment (Fig. 7). Thus, this degradatory mechanism is probably necessary because dopamine agonists act rather slowly to inhibit prolactin synthesis, leading to accumulation of excess prolactin. It seems likely that this mechanism allows for removal of excess prolactin, which accumulates in the pituitary when prolactin secretion is blocked. The studies of prolactin degradation are described in more detail in Chapter 16.

As dopamine receptors are located on the plasma membrane of pituitary cells (Caron *et al.*, 1978), it seems likely that the dopaminergic regulation of prolactin mRNA levels will involve a second messenger such as a cyclic nucleotide. Several studies have shown that dopamine agonists inhibit pituitary adenylate cyclase (De Camilli *et al.*, 1979; Giannattasio *et al.*, 1981) and decrease pituitary cAMP levels (Barnes *et al.*, 1978; Adams *et al.*, 1979). This offers some evidence that pituitary dopamine receptors are coupled to adenylate cyclase. As dopamine has been shown to inhibit pituitary adenylate cyclase, it is expected that cAMP analogs should stimulate prolactin secretion if cAMP is really involved in the regulation of prolactin. Although there is some

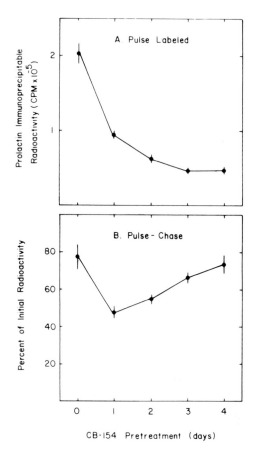

Fig. 7. Effect of various periods of bromoergocryptine (CB-154) pretreatment on prolactin synthesis and degradation. Monolayer cultures of pituitary cells were pretreated for 1, 2, 3, or 4 days with 10 n*M* CB-154; control cultures (0 pretreatment) received no CB-154. The cells were labeled for 30 minutes with [³H]leucine and one-half were incubated in a chase medium containing a 400-fold excess of unlabeled leucine for 4 hours. Treatments were arranged so that all cells were labeled at the same time. Prolactin synthesis (A) was estimated by determination of the amount of radioactivity incorporated in prolactin during the 30-minute pulse. Prolactin degradation (B) was estimated by determining the percentage of labeled prolactin that remained after the 4-hour chase incubation. Values are means ± SE for three determinations per point. Reprinted from Maurer (1980a) with permission. Copyright (1980) American Chemical Society.

evidence that cAMP analogs can stimulate prolactin secretion, the results have been inconclusive (Hill *et al.*, 1976; Dannies *et al.*, 1976; Naor *et al.*, 1980; Dannies and Tashjian, 1980; Tam and Dannies, 1981). Also, most of these studies examined prolactin secretion. It is possible that cAMP could be involved in regulation of prolactin synthesis but not in the regulation of prolactin secretion. Certainly further studies are required to examine the possible role of cAMP in mediating the dopaminergic regulation of prolactin gene expression.

C. Effects of Thyrotropin-Releasing Hormone

The hypothalamic peptide thyrotropin-releasing hormone (TRH) has been shown to increase prolactin secretion in female and estrogen–progesterone-treated or propylthiouracil-treated male rats (Vale *et al.*, 1973; Rivier and Vale, 1974). TRH stimulates *de novo* prolactin synthesis in GH3 cells, a clonal pituitary tumor cell line (Dannies and Tashjian, 1973). GH3 cells have high-affinity receptors for TRH (Hinkle and Tashjian, 1973), and the biological activity of various TRH analogs correlates with their affinity for the receptor (Hinkle *et al.*, 1974). Analysis of the effects of different analogs of TRH has suggested that release and synthesis of prolactin are regulated independently by TRH (Dannies and Tashjian, 1976b; Dannies and Markell, 1980). Immunocytochemical studies have shown that TRH acts on GH3 cells by increasing the prolactin content of individual cells rather than by altering the proportion of GH3 cells that synthesize prolactin (Hoyt and Tashjian, 1980). TRH-induced increases in prolactin synthesis are mediated by increases in prolactin mRNA (Evans and Rosenfeld, 1976; Dannies and Tashjian, 1976b; Evans *et al.*, 1978; Brennessel and Biswas, 1980).

D. Effects of Other Hormones

A number of hormones may have some role in the regulation of prolactin. For instance, pituitary tumor cells have been found to contain receptors for epidermal growth factor and this hormone stimulates prolactin synthesis and inhibits cellular proliferation in GH3 cells (Schonbrunn *et al.*, 1980; Johnson *et al.*, 1980). Vasoactive intestinal peptide has been reported to alter the *in vitro* production of prolactin (Ruberg *et al.*, 1978; Shaar *et al.*, 1979; Nicosia *et al.*, 1980; Samson *et al.*, 1980). Somatostatin receptors have been identified on pituitary tumor cells and somatostatin inhibits prolactin release (Schonbrunn and Tashjian, 1978). It is possible that 1,25-dihydroxyvitamin D_3 also has effects on prolactin production, as receptors have been found in the pituitary (Stumpf *et al.*, 1980; Haussler *et al.*, 1980) and prolactin stimulates 1,25-dihydroxyvitamin D_3 production by chicken kidney (Bikle *et al.*, 1980). Also, thyroid hormone may be involved in the regulation of prolactin synthesis (Tsai and Samuels, 1974; Perrone and Hinkle, 1978). For most of these hormones, the physiological role of the hormone in the regulation of prolactin synthesis has not been defined.

E. Effects of Hormonal Interactions

With a large number of regulators, the potential interactions of these regulators could be very complicated. Although this area has not been extensively investigated, the available data reveal several interesting hormonal interactions. Estradiol greatly decreases the ability of dopamine to inhibit prolactin secretion (Raymond *et al.*, 1978; West and Dannies, 1980; de Quijada *et al.*, 1980). Probably at least a portion of the *in vivo* ability of estradiol to stimulate prolactin production is due to this antidopaminergic effect. The ability of estradiol to block dopamine effects is not due to effects of estradiol on dopamine receptors (DiPaolo *et al.*, 1979). Estradiol has been shown to increase the number of TRH receptors on pituitary cells (De Lean *et al.*, 1977; Gershengorn *et al.*, 1979) and to increase the biological response to TRH (De Lean *et al.*, 1977). Thyroid hormone also has been found to alter the number of TRH receptors and the biological response to TRH (De Lean *et al.*, 1977; Perrone and Hinkle, 1978; Hinkle *et al.*, 1981). Furthermore, glucocorticoids have been found to alter the number of TRH receptors and the effects of thyroid hormone on TRH receptors (Tashjian *et al.*, 1977; Perrone *et al.*, 1980).

IV. ANALYSIS OF THE PROLACTIN GENE

A. Cloning of a DNA Containing the Prolactin Coding Sequence

The studies described in the preceding section demonstrate that several hormones regulate the concentration of prolactin mRNA in pituitary cells. Altered levels of prolactin mRNA could be due to changes in either the synthesis or the degradation of prolactin mRNA. For further studies of the metabolism of prolactin mRNA, it is essential to have large quantities of a homogeneous hybridization probe. Although prolactin cDNA could be prepared from highly purified prolactin mRNA, this cDNA is available in only small quantities (Maurer, 1980b). Recombinant DNA techniques can provide an essentially unlimited supply of a homogeneous hybridization probe for analysis of specific gene sequences. Therefore, recombinant DNA containing the prolactin gene was prepared and cloned in bacteria (Gubbins *et al.,* 1979).

As a starting point for cloning the prolactin structural gene, RNA enriched in prolactin mRNA sequences was prepared. Fischer 344 rats received diethylstilbestrol implants and their pituitaries were removed 1 month later. This treatment results in a considerable increase in pituitary weight and high levels of prolactin mRNA. Poly(A)-containing RNA was prepared from pituitary RNA by oligo(dT)-cellulose chromatography. The mRNA fraction was then size fractionated by sedimentation through a 5–20% sucrose gradient. Translation of RNA from the sucrose gradient fractions revealed a 12S RNA peak that was highly enriched in prolactin mRNA activity. Prolactin mRNA activity accounted for about 70% of the total mRNA activity in this peak fraction. This enriched prolactin mRNA was then used as a starting point for the preparation of recombinant DNA containing prolactin sequences (Fig. 8). The RNA was used to direct the synthesis of cDNA using reverse transcriptase. The mRNA was removed from the single-stranded cDNA by alkaline hydrolysis. The single-stranded cDNA was converted to duplex DNA in a second reaction using viral reverse transcriptase. After digestion with the single strand-specific nuclease S1 to remove the hairpin loop at one end, dCMP residues were added to the 3'-termini using terminal transferase. This tailed cDNA was annealed to plasmid pBR322, which had been digested with restriction endonuclease *Pst*I and to which dGMP residues were added by terminal transferase. The annealed mixture was used to transform *E. coli* strain X1776. After transformation, bacterial colonies were allowed to grow, and colonies containing plasmids were selected on the basis of growth on tetracycline-containing plates. To identify colonies containing prolactin sequences, the colonies were screened using the *in situ* colony hybridization technique (Grunstein and Hogness, 1975). Several colonies that hybridized strongly to the prolactin probe were selected for further analysis. Digestion of plasmids from these colonies with restriction endonuclease *Pst*I followed by gel electrophoresis demonstrated the presence of DNA inserts. Two plasmids containing the largest inserts were then analyzed by restriction enzyme mapping and finally sequenced using the Maxam and Gilbert technique (1977). Plasmid pPRL-1 contains most of the coding sequence of prolactin plus a large segment of 3' untranslated sequence, and pPRL-2 contains the complete coding sequence of prolactin. Analysis of the DNA sequence of both of these plasmids has yielded the complete 681-nucleotide cod-

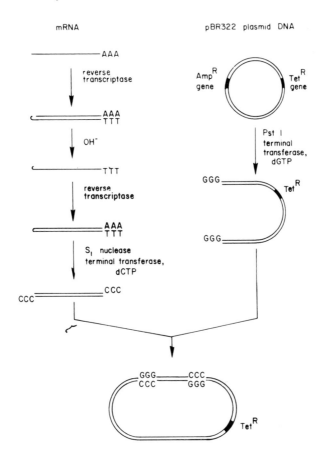

Fig. 8. Outline of the procedure for the synthesis of a double-stranded DNA containing the coding sequence of prolactin and insertion of that DNA into a bacterial plasmid.

ing sequence of preprolactin as well as 17 nucleotides preceding the initiation codon and 90 nucleotides following the termination codon (Fig. 9). The amino acid sequence predicted from the cloned DNA sequence agrees quite well with the known sequence of preprolactin (Parlow and Shome, 1976; McKean and Maurer, 1978). This offers unambiguous evidence that prolactin cDNA sequences have been cloned in the bacterial plasmid. Thus, these plasmids can be used as hybridization probes for prolactin mRNA sequences. Cooke *et al.* (1980) have also cloned the rat prolactin structural gene. A portion of the bovine preprolactin gene has also been cloned (Nilson *et al.*, 1980; Miller *et al.*, 1980).

The possible expression of the cloned prolactin gene in bacteria has

```
                  -29                                    -20
                  Met Asn Ser Gln Val Ser Ala Arg Lys Ala Gly Thr Leu Leu Leu
     UCCCAGUGGUCAUCACC AUG AAC AGC CAA GUG UCA GCC CGG AAA GCA GGG ACA CUC CUC CUG

              -10                                   -1  1
     Leu Met Met Ser Asn Leu Leu Phe Cys Gln Asn Val Gln Thr Leu Pro Val Cys Ser Gly
     CUG AUG AUG UCA AAC CUU CUG UUC UGC CAA AAU GUG CAG ACC CUG CCA GUC UGU UCU GGU

              10                                  20
     Gly Asp Cys Gln Thr Pro Leu Pro Glu Leu Phe Asp Arg Val Val Met Leu Ser His Tyr
     GGC GAC UGC CAG ACA CCU CUC CCG GAG CUG UUU GAC CGU GUG GUC AUG CUU UCU CAC UAC

              30                                  40
     Ile His Thr Leu Tyr Thr Asp Met Phe Ile Glu Phe Asp Lys Gln Tyr Val Gln Asp Arg
     AUC CAU ACC CUG UAU ACA GAU AUG UUU AUU GAA UUU GAU AAA CAG UAU GUC CAA GAU CGU

              50                                  60
     Glu Phe Ile Ala Lys Ala Ile Asn Asp Cys Pro Thr Ser Ser Leu Ala Thr Pro Glu Asp
     GAG UUU AUU GCC AAG GCC AUC AAU GAC UGC CCC ACU UCU UCC CUA GCU ACU CCU GAA GAC

              70                                  80
     Lys Glu Gln Ala Gln Lys Val Pro Pro Glu Val Leu Leu Asn Leu Ile Leu Ser Leu Val
     AAG GAA CAA GCC CAG AAA GUC CCU CCG GAA GUU CUU UUG AAC CUG AUC CUC AGU UUG GUG

              90                                  100
     His Ser Trp Asn Asp Pro Leu Phe Gln Leu Ile Thr Gly Leu Gly Gly Ile His Glu Ala
     CAC UCC UGG AAU GAC CCU CUG UUU CAA CUA AUA ACU GGA CUA GGU GGA AUC CAU GAA GCU

              110                                 120
     Pro Asp Ala Ile Ile Ser Arg Ala Lys Glu Ile Glu Glu Gln Asn Lys Arg Leu Leu Glu
     CCU GAU GCU AUC AUA UCA AGA GCC AAA GAG AUU GAG GAA CAA AAC AAG CGG CUU CUU GAA

              130                                 140
     Gly Ile Glu Lys Ile Ile Ser Gln Ala Tyr Pro Glu Ala Lys Gly Asn Glu Ile Tyr Leu
     GGG AUU GAA AAG AUA AUU AGC CAG GCC UAU CCU GAA GCC AAA GGA AAU GAG AUC UAC UUG

              150                                 160
     Val Trp Ser Gln Leu Pro Ser Leu Gln Gly Val Asp Glu Glu Ser Lys Asp Leu Ala Phe
     GUU UGG UCA CAA CUC CCA UCC CUG CAA GGA GUU GAU GAA GAA UCC AAA GAC UUG GCU UUU

              170                                 180
     Tyr Asn Asn Ile Arg Cys Leu Arg Arg Asp Ser His Lys Val Asp Asn Tyr Leu Lys Phe
     UAU AAC AAC AUU CGG UGC CUG CGC AGG GAU UCC CAC AAG GUU GAC AAU UAU CUC AAG UUC

              190                              197
     Leu Arg Cys Gln Ile Val His Lys Asn Asn Cys
     CUG AGA UGC CAA AUU GUC CAU AAA AAC AAC UGC UAAGCCUACAUUCAUUCCAUGUACAUCUGAGAUGU
```

UCUUAAAAGUCUAUUUCUUCAAAGGUUCUAUUUGCAUUACAACUUUCAGCACAUGCUU

Fig. 9. The nucleotide sequence of prolactin mRNA determined from the sequence of the cDNA inserts in plasmids pPRL-1 and pPRL-2. The predicted amino acid sequence is also indicated. The numbers indicate the position of the amino acid in prolactin. Negative numbers are used for amino acids in the precursor segment. Data taken from Gubbins *et al.* (1980).

been explored (Erwin *et al.*, 1980). Restriction enzyme mapping was used to identify three plasmids in which the prolactin sequence was in the same orientation as the ampicillin-resistance gene of pBR322. These plasmids were used to transform the minicell-producing strain X1411. Minicells do not usually contain chromosomal DNA, but they do contain plasmid DNA. Thus, gene products directed by the plasmid will be synthesized in relatively large amounts. Minicells were prepared from the bacteria by three successive sucrose gradient centrifugations. The minicells were then pulse labeled with radiolabeled methionine, and lysates of the minicells were prepared. Immunoprecipitation of these lysates with anti-prolactin demonstrated that minicells containing one of the plasmids synthesized considerable amounts of a protein with the antigenic determinants of prolactin. Analysis of the immunoprecipitated protein on a polyacrylamide gel demonstrated that the protein recognized by anti-prolactin was much larger than rat prolactin. This protein is probably a read-through fusion product containing a bacterial protein sequence fused to the rat prolactin protein sequence. Thus, by inserting prolactin DNA sequences into a bacterial gene, a protein containing prolactin sequences and the bacterial gene sequences was produced. This demonstrates how eukaryotic protein sequences can be synthesized by bacteria and illustrates that minicell-producing bacteria can be used for analysis of the expression of cloned genes. Other plasmid vectors allowing highly efficient expression of inserted genes are available for facilitating the expression of eukaryotic genes in bacteria (Guarente *et al.*, 1980).

B.   Cloning of the Chromosomal Prolactin Gene

Analysis of the prolactin chromosomal gene might provide some insight into structures involved in the regulation of gene expression. For instance, symmetrical, self-complementary DNA sequences might form loop-out structures that would be recognized by regulatory proteins. Furthermore, prolactin is part of a gene family that includes growth hormone and chorionic somatomammotropin. Analysis of the amino acid sequence (Sherwood, 1967; Catt *et al.*, 1967; Li *et al.*, 1970; Niall *et al.*, 1971) as well as the nucleotide sequence of cloned structural genes (Seeburg *et al.*, 1977; Shine *et al.*, 1977; Martial *et al.*, 1979; Gubbins *et al.*, 1980; Cooke *et al.*, 1980) has shown considerable homology among the sequences of these three hormones. This had led to the hypothesis that the three different hormones arose from a common precursor gene via gene duplication (Niall *et al.*, 1971). When the chromosomal genes for all three of these hormones have been isolated, comparison of the gene structures may yield some insight into the mechanisms that allow the differential expression and regulation of these genes.

Genomic DNA containing prolactin DNA sequences has been isolated (Chien and Thompson, 1980; Gubbins *et al.*, 1980; Maurer *et al.*, 1981). The prolactin clones were isolated from a library of rat chromosomal DNA fragments cloned in bacteriophage lambda (Sargent *et al.*, 1979). The library was screened for prolactin sequences using the plaque hybridization technique (Benton and Davis, 1977) with labeled prolactin cDNA as the hybridization probe. To date no single clone has been isolated that contains the complete prolactin gene. Chien and Thompson (1980) have obtained several overlapping clones that together contain the complete gene. Gubbins *et al.* (1980) have obtained a clone containing the 3′ end of the gene, and Maurer *et al.* (1981) have obtained a clone containing the 5′ end of the gene. The coding sequence of the prolactin gene, like most eukaryotic genes (Abelson, 1979; Breathnach and Chambon, 1981), is split by intervening sequences. Analysis of the cloned prolactin gene has shown that the gene consists of five exons, or regions that are represented in the mature mRNA, and four introns, or intervening sequences (Fig. 10). The five exons and four intervening sequences comprise approximately 10 kilobases of DNA. Thus, although prolactin mRNA is only approximately 1 kilobase long (Maurer, 1980b), the chromosomal gene is 10 times longer as a result of the presence of large introns.

The putative transcription initiation site of the prolactin gene has been mapped using the S1 nuclease sensitivity procedure (Maurer *et*

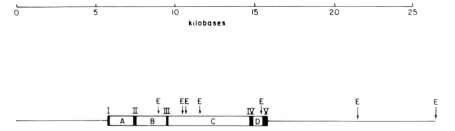

Fig. 10.   Physical map of the rat prolactin chromosomal gene. The five exons of the prolactin gene are labeled I through V and are indicated by the dark boxes. The four introns are lettered A through D and are indicated by the open boxes. Cleavage sites for the restriction endonuclease *Eco*R1 (E) are also indicated. This map was constructed using data from Chien and Thompson (1980), Gubbins *et al.* (1980), and Maurer *et al.* (1981).

al., 1981). Sequence analysis of the 5' flanking sequence has revealed several interesting features. The sequence TATAAA was found at positions −27 to −22 from the transcription initiation site. This sequence is similar to the TATA box that has been found approximately 30 nucleotides from the transcription initiation site of a number of eukaryotic genes (Breathnach and Chambon, 1981). This TATA sequence probably serves as a promoter site involved in facilitating the initiation of transcription. Also, at positions −62 to −45, a large palindrome—TGATTATATATATATTCA—was found. This symmetrical sequence may be involved in binding regulatory proteins. However, this is clearly speculative at the present time. Perhaps further studies utilizing purified hormone receptors will yield some insight into this possibility.

C. Potential Nuclear Precursors for Prolactin mRNA

The finding that the prolactin gene is considerably larger than prolactin mRNA suggests that prolactin mRNA may be synthesized as a large precursor, which is then processed to produce the final mature mRNA. Studies of other genes have demonstrated that eukaryotic genes are transcribed as a unit and then intervening sequences are accurately removed from the RNA (Tilghman *et al.*, 1978). To examine this possibility, cytoplasmic and nuclear RNA were prepared from rat pituitaries and then electrophoresed on agarose gels in the presence of the potent RNA denaturant methylmercury hydroxide (Maurer *et al.*, 1980). The RNA was then transferred to diazobenzyloxymethyl paper. This derivatized paper has been shown to covalently bind RNA (Alwine *et al.*, 1977). The paper was then hybridized to a prolactin recombinant DNA probe, which had been radiolabeled *in vitro*. The prolactin probe hybridized to several large RNA species from pituitary nuclear RNA but to only a single RNA species from cytoplasmic RNA (Fig. 11). The results were specific for pituitary nuclear RNA as no prolactin sequences were detected in liver nuclear RNA and no large species of prolactin mRNA were detected when liver nuclear RNA was mixed with pituitary cytoplasmic RNA. The large species of prolactin mRNA detected in pituitary nuclear RNA are likely precursors of prolactin mRNA. The largest prolactin mRNA species had a size of approximately 7.0 kilobases. This is considerably smaller than the estimated 10-kilobase size of the chromosomal gene. It is likely that the 7.0-kilobase species is not the primary transcript of the gene. Hoffman *et al.* (1981) have detected larger potential precursors for prolactin mRNA. However, the largest of these potential precursors had a size of

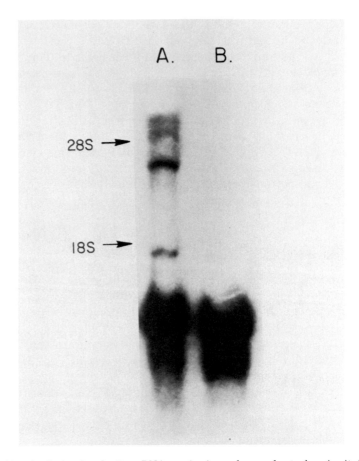

Fig. 11. Analysis of prolactin mRNA species in nuclear and cytoplasmic pituitary RNA. Nuclear (lane A, 30 μg) and cytoplasmic (lane B, 5 μg) pituitary RNA was electrophoresed on a 1.5% agarose gel containing 10 mM methylmercury hydroxide, transferred to diazobenzyloxymethyl paper, and hybridized to pPRL-1 DNA labeled with ^{32}P by nick translation to a specific activity of 200 cpm/pg. The paper was washed, dried, and exposed to X-ray film. The position of ribosomal RNA markers and purified prolactin mRNA was determined by staining of parallel gel tracks with ethidium bromide. The slowest migrating band prolactin RNA species in nuclear RNA has a size of about 7.0 kilobases. The broad band at the bottom of the autoradiogram in both the nuclear and cytoplasmic samples was greatly overexposed. Shorter exposures indicate the presence of a much sharper band with the appropriate mobility for the 1.0-kilobase mature prolactin mRNA. Reprinted from Maurer et al. (1980) with permission.

about 14 kilobases, which is considerably larger than the estimated 10-kilobase size of the gene. This discrepancy may be due to the difficulty in sizing these large nucleic acids. Thus, one or both of the size estimates may be inaccurate. Alternatively, large prolactin mRNA precursors may be transcripts of prolactin genes that have not yet been isolated.

V. SUMMARY AND FUTURE PROSPECTS

A number of studies have shown that several hormones, including estradiol, dopamine, and thyrotropin-releasing hormone, regulate the biosynthesis of prolactin. The hormonal regulation of prolactin synthesis is likely mediated by changes in prolactin mRNA levels. The finding that the levels of prolactin mRNA correlate very well with prolactin synthesis suggests that the regulation of prolactin mRNA levels is the principal regulatory mechanism for controlling the biosynthesis of prolactin. Thus, a considerable amount of information has accumulated concerning one aspect of prolactin gene expression. However, there are a great many important areas requiring further study.

One important question concerns the relationship of prolactin synthesis and secretion. Clearly, it would seem desirable to coordinate regulation of prolactin synthesis and secretion. In fact, the data indicate that hormones such as estradiol and thyrotropin, which stimulate prolactin synthesis, also stimulate prolactin secretion. Furthermore, dopamine, which inhibits prolactin synthesis, also inhibits prolactin secretion. Thus, there is coordinate regulation of synthesis and secretion. The fact that dopamine and TRH are able to affect prolactin secretion much more rapidly than they affect prolactin synthesis suggests that changes in synthesis are probably not the mechanism responsible for changes in secretion. It remains possible that secretion-induced changes in intracellular prolactin content regulate prolactin synthesis. Thus, the total number of secretory granules in a prolactin-producing cell might regulate prolactin synthesis. However, the finding that analogs of TRH have different effects on prolactin synthesis and secretion (Dannies and Tashjian, 1976b; Dannies and Markell, 1980) argues against such a model. It may be that there are parallel regulatory mechanisms that independently regulate prolactin synthesis and secretion. I hope that further studies on the mechanisms regulating the processes will yield insight into the relationship between synthesis and secretion.

Another important question concerns the intracellular mediators of the hormonal regulation of prolactin production. For estradiol, it seems likely that intracellular steroid receptors mediate the estrogenic regulation of prolactin (Leavitt *et al.*, 1969; Notides, 1970; Keefer *et al.*, 1976; Keefer, 1981). However, TRH and dopamine have plasma membrane receptors, and it seems likely that their effects are mediated by second messengers. Although a number of studies implicate cAMP or calcium as possible intracellular regulators of prolactin release and/or synthesis, the role of these agents as second messengers remains unclear.

The mechanism involved in regulating prolactin mRNA levels is another important topic that remains to be explored. Changes in prolactin mRNA could be due to changes in the transcription of the prolactin gene or to changes in the stability of prolactin mRNA sequences. The availability of cloned prolactin DNA sequences should facilitate analysis of these possibilities. In fact, studies have suggested that dopaminergic regulation of prolactin involves changes in the transcription of the prolactin gene (Maurer, 1981). Further studies will be required to confirm this finding and to determine whether the effects of estradiol and TRH are also mediated by changes in transcription.

ACKNOWLEDGMENTS

Research in the author's laboratory was supported by NIH grant AM 21803. I thank B. Maurer for aid in preparing this manuscript.

REFERENCES

Abelson, J. (1979). RNA processing and the intervening sequence problem. *Annu. Rev. Biochem.* **48**, 1035–1069.

Adams, T. E., Wagner, T. O. F., Sawyer, H. R., and Nett, T. M. (1979). GnRH interaction with anterior pituitary. II. Cyclic AMP as an intracellular mediator in the GnRH activated gonadotroph. *Biol. Reprod.* **21**, 735–747.

Alwine, J. C., Kemp, D. J., and Stark, G. R. (1977). Method for detection of specific RNAs in agarose gels by transfer to diazobenzyloxymethyl-paper and hybridization with DNA probes. *Proc. Natl. Acad. Sci. U.S.A.* **74**, 5350–5354.

Amenomori, Y., Chen, C. L., and Meites, J. (1970). Serum prolactin levels in rats during different reproductive states. *Endocrinology (Baltimore)* **86**, 506–510.

Baker, B. L., and Everett, N. B. (1944). The effect of small doses of diethylstilbestrol on the anterior hypophysis of the immature rat. *Endocrinology (Baltimore)* **34**, 254–264.

Barnes, G. D., Brown, B. L., Gard, T. G., Atkinson, D., and Ekins, R. P. (1978). Effect of TRH and dopamine on cyclic AMP levels in enriched mammotroph and thyrotroph cells. *Mol. Cell. Endocrinol.* **12**, 273–284.

Ben-Jonathan, N., Oliver, C., Weiner, H. J., Mical, R. S., and Porter, J. C. (1977). Dopamine in hypophysial portal plasma of the rat during the estrous cycle and throughout pregnancy. *Endocrinology (Baltimore)* **100**, 452–458.

Ben-Jonathan, N., Neill, M. A., Arbogast, L. A., Peters, L. L., and Hoefer, M. T. (1980). Dopamine in hypophysial portal blood: Relationship to circulating prolactin in pregnant and lactating rats. *Endocrinology (Baltimore)* **106**, 690–696.

Benton, W. D., and Davis, R. (1977). Screening λgt recombinant clones by hybridization to single plaques *in situ*. *Science* **196**, 180–182.

Bikle, D. D., Spencer, E. M., Burke, W. H., and Rost, C. R. (1980). Prolactin but not growth hormone stimulates 1,25-dihydroxyvitamin D_3 production by chick renal preparations *in vitro*. *Endocrinology (Baltimore)* **107**, 81–84.

Birge, C. A., Jacobs, L. S., Hammer, C. T., and Daughaday, W. H. (1970). Catecholamine inhibition of prolactin secretion by isolated rat adenohypophyses. *Endocrinology (Baltimore)* **86**, 120–130.

Bishop, W., Krulich, L., Fawcett, C. P., and McCann, S. M. (1971). The effect of median eminence (ME) lesions on plasma levels of FSH, LH, and prolactin in the rat. *Proc. Soc. Exp. Biol. Med.* **136**, 925–927.

Blobel, G., and Dobberstein, B. (1975). Transfer of proteins across membranes. I. Presence of proteolytically processed and unprocessed nascent immunoglobulin light chains on membrane-bound ribosomes of *murine myeloma*. *J. Cell Biol.* **67**, 835–851.

Breathnach, R., and Chambon, P. (1981). Organization and expression of eukaryotic split genes coding for proteins. *Annu. Rev. Biochem.* **50**, 349–383.

Brennessel, B. A., and Biswas, D. K. (1980). Regulated expression of the prolactin gene in rat pituitary tumor cells. *J. Cell Biol.* **87**, 6–13.

Brocas, H., Coevorden, A. V., Seo, H., Refetoff, S., and Vassart, G. (1981). Dopaminergic control of prolactin mRNA accumulation in the pituitary of the male rat. *Mol. Cell. Endocrinol.* **22**, 25–30.

Brown, G. M., Seeman, P., and Lee, T. (1976). Dopamine/neuroleptic receptors in basal hypothalamus and pituitary. *Endocrinology (Baltimore)* **99**, 1407–1410.

Butcher, R. L., Collins, W. E., and Fugo, N. W. (1974). Plasma concentration of LH, FSH, prolactin, progesterone and estradiol-17B throughout the 4-day estrous cycle of the rat. *Endocrinology (Baltimore)* **94**, 1704–1708.

Calabro, M. A., and MacLeod, R. M. (1978). Binding of dopamine to bovine anterior pituitary gland membranes. *Neuroendocrinology* **25**, 32–46.

Caron, M. G., Beaulieu, M., Raymond, V., Gagne, B., Drouin, J., Lefkowitz, R. J., and Labrie, F. (1978). Dopaminergic receptors in the anterior pituitary gland. Correlation of [^{3}H]dihydroergocryptine binding with the dopaminergic control of prolactin release. *J. Biol. Chem.* **253**, 2244–2253.

Catt, K., and Moffat, B. (1967). Isolation of internally labeled rat prolactin by preparative disc electrophoresis. *Endocrinology (Baltimore)* **80**, 324–328.

Catt, K. J., Moffat, B., and Niall, H. D. (1967). Human growth hormone and placental lactogen: Structural similarity. *Science* **157**, 321.

Chen, C. L., Amenomori, Y., Lu, K. H., Voogt, J. L., and Meites, J. (1970). Serum prolactin levels in rats with pituitary transplants or hypothalamic lesions. *Neuroendocrinology* **6**, 220–227.

Chien, Y.-H., and Thompson, E. B. (1980). Genomic organization of rat prolactin and growth hormone genes. *Proc. Natl. Acad. Sci. U.S.A.* **77**, 4583–4587.

Clifton, K. H., and Meyer, R. K. (1956). Mechanism of anterior pituitary tumor induction by estrogen. *Anat. Rec.* **125**, 65–81.

Cooke, N. E., Coit, D., Weiner, R. I., Baxter, J. D., and Martial, J. A. (1980). Structure of cloned DNA complementary to rat prolactin messenger RNA. *J. Biol. Chem.* **255,** 6502–6510.

Crane, W. A., and Loomes, R. S. (1967). Effect of age, sex, and hormonal state on tritiated thymidine uptake by rat pituitary. *Br. J. Cancer* **21,** 787–792.

Creese, I., Schneider, R., and Snyder, S. H. (1977). ^{3}H-spiroperidol labels dopamine receptors in pituitary and brain. *Eur. J. Pharmacol.* **46,** 377–381.

Cronin, M. J., Roberts, J. M., and Weiner, R. I. (1978). Dopamine and dihydroergocryptine binding to the anterior pituitary and other brain areas of the rat and sheep. *Endocrinology (Baltimore)* **103,** 302–309.

Dannies, P. S., and Markell, M. S. (1980). Differential ability of thyrotropin-releasing hormone and N^{3im}-methyl-thyrotropin-releasing hormone to affect prolactin and thyrotropin production in primary rat pituitary cell cultures. *Endocrinology (Baltimore)* **106,** 107–112.

Dannies, P. S., and Rudnick, M. S. (1980). 2-Bromo-α-ergocryptine causes degradation of prolactin in primary cultures of rat pituitary cells after chronic treatment. *J. Biol. Chem.* **255,** 2776–2781.

Dannies, P. S., and Tashjian, A. H., Jr. (1973). Effects of thyrotropin-releasing hormone and hydrocortisone on synthesis and degradation of prolactin in a rat pituitary cell strain. *J. Biol. Chem.* **248,** 6174–6179.

Dannies, P. S., and Tashjian, A. H., Jr. (1976a). Thyrotropin-releasing hormone increases prolactin mRNA activity in the cytoplasm of GH-cells as measured by translation in a wheat germ cell-free system. *Biochem. Biophys. Res. Commun.* **70,** 1180–1189.

Dannies, P. S., and Tashjian, A. H., Jr. (1976b). Release and synthesis of prolactin by rat pituitary cell strains are regulated independently by thyrotropin releasing hormone. *Nature (London)* **261,** 707–710.

Dannies, P. S., and Tashjian, A. H., Jr. (1980). Action of cholera toxin on hormone synthesis and release in GH cells: Evidence that adenosine 3′,5′-monophosphate does not mediate the decrease in growth hormone synthesis caused by thyrotropin-releasing hormone. *Endocrinology (Baltimore)* **106,** 1532–1536.

Dannies, P. S., Gautvik, K. M., and Tashjian, A. H., Jr. (1976). A possible role of cyclic AMP in mediating the effects of thyrotropin-releasing hormone on prolactin release and on prolactin and growth hormone synthesis in pituitary cells in culture. *Endocrinology (Baltimore)* **98,** 1147–1159.

Davies, C., Jacobi, J., Lloyd, H. M., and Meares, J. D. (1974). DNA synthesis and the secretion of prolactin and growth hormone by the pituitary gland of the male rat: Effects of diethylstilboestrol and 2-bromo-α-ergocryptine methanesulphonate. *J. Endocrinol.* **61,** 411–417.

De Camilli, P., Macconi, D., and Spada, A. (1979). Dopamine inhibits adenylate cyclase in human prolactin-secreting pituitary adenomas. *Nature (London)* **278,** 252–254.

De Lean, A., Garon, M., Kelly, P. A., and Labrie, F. (1977). Changes in pituitary thyrotropin releasing hormone (TRH) receptor level and prolactin response to TRH during the rat estrous cycle. *Endocrinology (Baltimore)* **100,** 1505–1510.

de Quijada, M., Timmermans, H. A. T., Lamberts, S. W. J., and MacLeod, R. M. (1980). Tamoxifen enhances the sensitivity of dispersed prolactin-secreting pituitary tumor cells to dopamine and bromocriptine. *Endocrinology (Baltimore)* **106,** 702–706.

Di Paolo, T., Carmichael, R., Labrie, F., and Raynaud, J.-P. (1979). Effects of estrogens on the characteristics of [^{3}H]spiroperidol and [^{3}H]RU24213 binding in rat anterior pituitary gland and brain. *Mol. Cell. Endocrinol.* **16,** 99–112.

Erwin, C. R., Maurer, R. A., and Donelson, J. E. (1980). A bacterial cell that synthesizes a protein containing the antigenic determinants of rat prolactin. *Nucleic Acids Res.* **8,** 2537–2546.

Evans, G. A., and Rosenfeld, M. G. (1976). Cell-free synthesis of a prolactin precursor directed by mRNA from cultured rat pituitary cells. *J. Biol. Chem.* **251,** 2842–2847.

Evans, G. A., David, D. N., and Rosenfeld, M. G. (1978). Regulation of prolactin and somatotropin mRNAs by thyroliberin. *Proc. Natl. Acad. Sci. U.S.A.* **75,** 1294–1298.

Farquhar, M. G. (1961). Origin and fate of secretory granules in cells of the anterior pituitary gland. *Trans. N. Y. Acad. Sci.* **23,** 346–351.

Gershengorn, M. C., Marcus-Samuels, B. E., and Geras, E. (1979). Estrogens increase the number of thyrotropin-releasing hormone receptors on mammotropic cells in culture. *Endocrinology (Baltimore)* **105,** 171–176.

Giannattasio, G., De Ferrari, M. E., and Spada, A. (1981). Dopamine-inhibited adenylate cyclase in female rat adenohypophysis. *Life Sci.* **28,** 1605–1612.

Grunstein, M., and Hogness, D. S. (1975). Colony hybridization: A method for the isolation of cloned DNAs that contain a specific gene. *Proc. Natl. Acad. Sci. U.S.A.* **72,** 3961–3965.

Guarente, L., Roberts, T. M., and Ptashne, M. (1980). A technique for expressing eukaryotic genes in bacteria. *Science* **209,** 1428–1430.

Gubbins, E. J., Maurer, R. A., Hartley, J. L., and Donelson, J. E. (1979). Construction and analysis of recombinant DNAs containing a structural gene for rat prolactin. *Nucleic Acids Res.* **6,** 915–930.

Gubbins, E. J., Maurer, R. A., Lagrimini, M., Erwin, C. R., and Donelson, J. E. (1980). Structure of the rat prolactin gene. *J. Biol. Chem.* **255,** 8655–8662.

Haug, E., and Gautvik, K. M. (1976). Effects of sex steroids on prolactin secreting rat pituitary cells in culture. *Endocrinology (Baltimore)* **99,** 1482–1489.

Haussler, M. R., Manolagas, S. C., and Deftos, L. J. (1980). Evidence for a 1,25-dihydroxyvitamin D_3 receptor-like macromolecule in rat pituitary. *J. Biol. Chem.* **255,** 5007–5010.

Herbert, D. C., Ishikawa, H., Shiino, H., and Rennels, E. G. (1978). Prolactin secretion from clonal pituitary cells following incubation with estradiol, progesterone, thyrotropin releasing hormone, and dopamine. *Proc. Soc. Exp. Biol. Med.* **157,** 605–609.

Hill, M. K., MacLeod, R. M., and Orcutt, P. (1976). Dibutyryl cyclic AMP, adenosine and guanosine blockage of the dopamine, ergocryptine and apomorphine inhibition of prolactin release *in vitro. Endocrinology (Baltimore)* **99,** 1612–1617.

Hinkle, P. M., and Tashjian, A. H., Jr. (1973). Receptors for thyrotropin-releasing hormone in prolactin-producing rat pituitary cells in culture. *J. Biol. Chem.* **248,** 6180–6186.

Hinkle, P. M., Woroch, E. L., and Tashjian, A. H., Jr. (1974). Receptor-binding affinities and biological activities of analogs of thyrotropin-releasing hormone in prolactin-producing pituitary cells in culture. *J. Biol. Chem.* **249,** 3085–3090.

Hinkle, P. M., Perrone, M. H., and Schonbrunn, A. (1981). Mechanism of thyroid hormone inhibition of thyrotropin-releasing hormone action. *Endocrinology (Baltimore)* **108,** 199–205.

Hoffman, L. M., Fritsch, M. K., and Gorski, J. (1981). Probable nuclear precursors of preprolactin mRNA in rat pituitary cells. *J. Biol. Chem.* **256,** 2597–2600.

Hoyt, R. F., Jr., and Tashjian, A. H., Jr. (1980). Immunocytochemical analysis of prolactin production by monolayer cultures of GH3 rat anterior pituitary tumor cells. I. Long-term effects of stimulation with thyrotropin-releasing hormone (TRH). *Anat. Rec.* **197,** 153–162.

Hymer, W. C., Snyder, J., Wilfinger, W., Swanson, N., and Davis, J. A. (1974). Separation of pituitary mammotrophs from the female rat by velocity sedimentation at unit gravity. *Endocrinology (Baltimore)* **95**, 107–122.

Johnson, L. K., Baxter, J. D., Vlodavsky, I., and Gospodarowicz, D. (1980). Epidermal growth factor and expresion of specific genes: Effects on cultured rat pituitary cells are dissociable from the mitogenic response. *Proc. Natl. Acad. Sci. U.S.A.* **77**, 394–398.

Kamberi, I. A., Mical, R. S., and Porter, J. C. (1971). Pituitary portal vessel infusion of hypothalamic extract and release of LH, FSH, and prolactin. *Endocrinology (Baltimore)* **88**, 1294–1299.

Keefer, D. A. (1981). Quantification of *in vivo* ^{3}H-estrogen uptake by individual anterior pituitary cell types of male rats: A combined autoradiographic-immunocytochemical technique. *J. Histochem. Cytochem.* **29**, 167–174.

Keefer, D. A., Stumpf, W. E., and Petrusz, P. (1976). Quantitative autoradiographic assessment of ^{3}H-estradiol uptake in immunocytochemically characterized pituitary cells. *Cell. Tissue Res.* **166**, 25–35.

Leavitt, W. W., Friend, J. P., and Robinson, J. A. (1969). Estradiol: Specific binding by pituitary nuclear fraction *in vitro*. *Science* **165**, 496–498.

Li, C. H., Dixon, J. S., Lo, T.-B., Schmidt, K. D., and Pankov, Y. A. (1970). Studies on pituitary lactogenic hormone. XXX. The primary structure of the sheep hormone. *Arch. Biochem. Biophys.* **141**, 705–737.

Lieberman, M. E., Maurer, R. A., and Gorski, J. (1978). Estrogen control of prolactin synthesis *in vitro*. *Proc. Natl. Acad. Sci. U.S.A.* **75**, 5946–5949.

Lingappa, V. R., Devillers-Thiery, A., and Blobel, G. (1977). Nascent prehormones are intermediates in the biosynthesis of authentic bovine pituitary growth hormone and prolactin. *Proc. Natl. Acad. Sci. U.S.A.* **74**, 2432–2436.

Lu, K.-H., Koch, Y., and Meites, J. (1971). Direct inhibition by ergocornine of pituitary prolactin release. *Endocrinology (Baltimore)* **89**, 229–233.

McKean, D. J., and Maurer, R. A. (1978). Complete amino acid sequence of the precursor region of rat prolactin. *Biochemistry* **17**, 5215–5219.

MacLeod, R. M., and Abad, A. (1968). On the control of prolactin and growth hormone synthesis in rat pituitary glands. *Endocrinology (Baltimore)* **83**, 799–806.

MacLeod, R. M., Abad, A., and Eidson, L. L. (1969). *In vivo* effect of sex hormones on the *in vitro* synthesis of prolactin and growth hormone in normal and pituitary tumor-bearing rats. *Endocrinology (Baltimore)* **84**, 1475–1483.

MacLeod, R. M., Fontham, E. H., and Lehmeyer, J. E. (1970). Prolactin and growth hormone production as influenced by catecholamines and agents that affect brain catecholamines. *Neuroendocrinology* **6**, 283–294.

Martial, J. A., Hallewell, R. A., Baxter, J. D., and Goodman, H. M. (1979). Human growth hormone: Complementary DNA cloning and expression in bacteria. *Science* **205**, 602–607.

Mastro, A., and Hymer, W. C. (1973). The effects of age and oestrone treatment on DNA polymerase activity in anterior pituitary glands of male rats. *J. Endocrinol.* **59**, 107–119.

Mastro, A., Hymer, W. C., and Therrian, C. D. (1969). DNA synthesis in adult rat anterior pituitary glands in organ culture. *Exp. Cell Res.* **54**, 407–414.

Maurer, R. A. (1980a). Bromoergocryptine-induced prolactin degradation in cultured pituitary cells. *Biochemistry* **19**, 3573–3578.

Maurer, R. A. (1980b). Immunochemical isolation of prolactin messenger RNA. *J. Biol. Chem.* **255**, 854–859.

Maurer, R. A. (1980c). Dopaminergic inhibition of prolactin synthesis and prolactin messenger RNA accumulation in cultured pituitary cells. *J. Biol. Chem.* **255,** 8092–8097.

Maurer, R. A. (1981). Transcriptional regulation of the prolactin gene by ergocryptine and cyclic AMP. *Nature (London)* **294,** 94–97.

Maurer, R. A., and Gorski, J. (1977). Effects of estradiol-17B and pimozide on prolactin synthesis in male and female rats. *Endocrinology (Baltimore)* **101,** 76–84.

Maurer, R. A., and McKean, D. J. (1978). Synthesis of preprolactin and conversion to prolactin in intact cells and a cell-free system. *J. Biol. Chem.* **253,** 6315–6318.

Maurer, R. A., Stone, R., and Gorski, J. (1976). Cell-free synthesis of a large translation product of prolactin messenger RNA. *J. Biol. Chem.* **251,** 2801–2807.

Maurer, R. A., Gorski, J., and McKean, D. J. (1977). Partial amino acid sequence of rat pre-prolactin. *Biochem. J.* **161,** 189–192.

Maurer, R. A., Gubbins, E. J., Erwin, C. R., and Donelson, J. E. (1980). Comparison of potential nuclear precursors for prolactin and growth hormone messenger RNA. *J. Biol. Chem.* **255,** 2243–2246.

Maurer, R. A., Erwin, C. R., and Donelson, J. E. (1981). Analysis of 5' flanking sequences and intron-exon boundaries of the rat prolactin gene. *J. Biol. Chem.* **256,** 10524–10528.

Maxam, A. M., and Gilbert, W. (1977). A new method for sequencing DNA. *Proc. Natl. Acad. Sci. U.S.A.* **74,** 560–564.

Miller, W. L., Thirion, J.-P., and Martial, J. A. (1980). Cloning of DNA complementary to bovine prolactin mRNA. *Endocrinology (Baltimore)* **107,** 851–854.

Naor, Z., Snyder, G., Fawcett, C. P., and McCann, S. M. (1980). Pituitary cyclic nucleotides and thyrotropin-releasing hormone action: The relationship of adenosine 3',5'-monophosphate and guanosine 3',5'-monophosphate to the release of thyrotropin and prolactin. *Endocrinology (Baltimore)* **106,** 1304–1310.

Neill, J. D., Freeman, M. E., and Tillson, S. A. (1971). Control of the proestrus surge of prolactin and luteinizing hormone secretion by estrogens in the rat. *Endocrinology (Baltimore)* **89,** 1448–1453.

Niall, H. D., Hogan, M. L., Sauer, R., Rosenblum, I. Y., and Greenwood, F. C. (1971). Sequences of pituitary and placental lactogenic and growth hormones: Evolution from a primoridal peptide by gene reduplication. *Proc. Natl. Acad. Sci. U.S.A.* **68,** 866–869.

Nicoll, C. S., and Meites, J. M. (1962). Estrogen stimulation of prolactin production by rat adenohypophysis *in vitro. Endocrinology (Baltimore)* **70,** 272–277.

Nicosia, S., Spada, A., Borghi, C., Cortelazzi, L., and Giannattasio, G. (1980). Effects of vasoactive intestinal polypeptide (VIP) in human prolactin (PRL) secreting pituitary adenomas. *FEBS Lett.* **112,** 159–162.

Nilson, J. H., Thomason, A. R., Horowitz, S., Sasavage, N. L., Blenis, J., Albers, R., Salser, W., and Rottman, F. M. (1980). Construction and characterization of a cDNA clone containing a portion of the bovine prolactin sequence. *Nucleic Acids Res.* **8,** 1561–1573.

Notides, A. C. (1970). Binding affinity and specificity of the estrogen receptor of the rat uterus and anterior pituitary. *Endocrinology (Baltimore)* **87,** 987–992.

Palade, G. (1975). Intracellular aspects of the process of protein synthesis. *Science* **189,** 347–358.

Parlow, A. F., and Shome, B. (1976). Rat prolactin: The entire linear amino acid sequence. *Fed. Prod., Fed. Am. Soc. Exp. Biol.* **35,** 219.

Perrone, M. H., and Hinkle, P. M. (1978). Regulation of pituitary receptors for thyrotropin-releasing hormone by thyroid hormones. *J. Biol. Chem.* **253**, 5168–5173.

Perrone, M. H., Greer, T. L., and Hinkle, P. M. (1980). Relationship between thyroid hormone and glucocorticoid effects in GH3 pituitary cells. *Endocrinology (Baltimore)* **106**, 600–605.

Plotsky, P. M., Gibbs, D. M., and Neill, J. D. (1978). Liquid chromatographic-electrochemical measurement of dopamine in hypophysial stalk blood of rats. *Endocrinology (Baltimore)* **102**, 1887–1894.

Raymond, V., Beaulieu, M., Labrie, F., and Boissier, J. (1978). Potent antidopaminergic activity of estradiol at the pituitary level on prolactin release. *Science* **200**, 1173–1175.

Rivier, C., and Vale, W. (1974). *In vivo* stimulation of prolactin secretion by thyrotropin releasing factor, related peptides, and hypothalamic extracts. *Endocrinology (Baltimore)* **95**, 978–983.

Ruberg, M., Rotsztejn, W. H., Arancibia, S., Besson, J., and Enjalbert, A. (1978). Stimulation of prolactin release by vasoactive intestinal peptide. *Eur. J. Pharmacol.* **51**, 319–320.

Ryan, R., Shupnik, M. A., and Gorski, J. (1979). Effect of estrogen on preprolactin messenger ribonucleic acid sequences. *Biochemistry* **18**, 2044–2048.

Samson, W. K., Said, S. I., Snyder, G., and McCann, S. M. (1980). *In vitro* stimulation of prolactin release by vasoactive intestinal peptide. *Peptides* **1**, 325–332.

Sargent, T. D., Wu, J.-R., Sala-Trepat, J. M., Wallace, R. B., Reyes, A. A., and Bonner, J. (1979). The rat serum albumin gene: Analysis of cloned sequences. *Proc. Natl. Acad. Sci. U.S.A.* **76**, 3256–3260.

Schonbrunn, A., and Tashjian, A. H., Jr. (1978). Characterization of functional receptors for somatostatin in rat pituitary cells in culture. *J. Biol. Chem.* **253**, 6473–6483.

Schonbrunn, A., Krasnoff, M., Westendorf, J. M., and Tashjian, A. H., Jr. (1980). Epidermal growth factor and thyrotropin-releasing hormone act similarly on a clonal pituitary cell strain. *J. Cell Biol.* **85**, 786–797.

Seeburg, P. H., Shine, J., Martial, J. A., Baxter, J. D., and Goodman, H. M. (1977). Nucleotide sequence and amplification in bacteria of structural gene for rat growth hormone. *Nature (London)* **270**, 486–494.

Seo, H., Refetoff, S., Martino, E., Vassart, G., and Brocas, H. (1979a). The differential stimulatory effect of thyroid hormone on growth hormone synthesis and estrogen on prolactin synthesis due to accumulation of specific messenger ribonucleic acids. *Endocrinology (Baltimore)* **104**, 1083–1090.

Seo, H., Refetoff, S., Scherberg, N., Brocas, H., and Vassart, G. (1979b). Isolation of rat prolactin messenger ribonucleic acid and synthesis of the complementary deoxyribonucleic acid. *Endocrinology (Baltimore)* **105**, 1481–1487.

Seo, H., Refetoff, S., Vassart, G., and Brocas, H. (1979c). Comparison of primary and secondary stimulation of male rats by estradiol in terms of prolactin synthesis and mRNA accumulation in the pituitary. *Proc. Natl. Acad. Sci. U.S.A.* **76**, 824–828.

Shaar, C. J., Clemens, J. A., and Dininger, N. B. (1979). Effect of vasoactive intestinal polypeptide on prolactin release *in vitro*. *Life Sci.* **25**, 2071–2074.

Sherwood, L. M. (1967). Similarities in the chemical structures of human placental lactogen and pituitary growth hormone. *Proc. Natl. Acad. Sci. U.S.A.* **58**, 2307–2314.

Shields, D., and Blobel, G. (1978). Efficient cleavage and segregation of nascent presecretory proteins in a reticulocyte lysate supplemented with microsomal membranes. *J. Biol. Chem.* **253**, 3753–3756.

Shine, J., Seeburg, P. H., Martial, J. A., Baxter, J. A., and Goodman, H. M. (1977). Construction and analysis of recombinant DNA for human chorionic somatomammotropin. *Nature (London)* **270**, 494–499.

Shupnik, M. A., Baxter, L. A., French, L. R., and Gorski, J. (1979). *In vivo* effects of estrogen on ovine pituitaries: Prolactin and growth hormone biosynthesis and messenger ribonucleic acid translation. *Endocrinology (Baltimore)* **104**, 729–735.

Smalstig, E. B., Sawyer, B. D., and Clemens, J. A. (1974). Inhibition of rat prolactin release by apomorphine *in vivo* and *in vitro*. *Endocrinology (Baltimore)* **95**, 123–129.

Spielman, L. L., and Bancroft, F. C. (1977). Pregrowth hormone: Evidence for conversion to growth hormone during synthesis on membrane-bound polysomes. *Endocrinology (Baltimore)* **101**, 651–658.

Stone, R. T., Maurer, R. A., and Gorski, J. (1977). Effect of estradiol-17B on preprolactin messenger ribonucleic acid activity in the rat pituitary gland. *Biochemistry* **16**, 4915–4921.

Stumpf, W. E., Sar, M., Reid, F. A., Tanaka, Y., and DeLuca, H. (1980). Target cells for 1,25-dihydroxyvitamin D_3 in intestinal tract, stomach, kidney, skin, pituitary, and parathyroid. *Science* **206**, 1188–1190.

Swearingen, K. C. (1971). Heterogeneous turnover of adenohypophysial prolactin. *Endocrinology (Baltimore)* **89**, 1380–1388.

Szczesna, E., and Boime, I. (1976). mRNA-dependent synthesis of authentic precursor to human placental lactogen: Conversion to its mature hormone form in ascites cell-free extracts. *Proc. Natl. Acad. Sci. U.S.A.* **73**, 1179–1180.

Talwalker, P. K., Ratner, A., and Meites, J. (1963). *In vitro* inhibition of pituitary prolactin synthesis and release by hypothalamic extract. *Am. J. Physiol.* **205**, 213–218.

Tam, S. W., and Dannies, P. S. (1981). The role of adenosine 3′,5′-monophosphate in dopaminergic inhibition of prolactin release in anterior pituitary cells. *Endocrinology (Baltimore)* **109**, 403–408.

Tashjian, A. H., Jr., Osborne, R., Maina, D., and Knaian, A. (1977). Hydrocortisone increases the number of receptors for thyrotropin-releasing hormone on pituitary cells in culture. *Biochem. Biophys. Res. Commun.* **79**, 333–340.

Tilghman, S. M., Curtis, P. J., Tiemeier, D. C., Leder, P., and Weissman, C. (1978). The intervening sequence of a mouse B-globin gene is transcribed within the 15S B-globin mRNA precursor. *Proc. Natl. Acad. Sci. U.S.A.* **75**, 1309–1313.

Tsai, J. S., and Samuels, H. H. (1974). Thyroid hormone action: Stimulation of growth hormone inhibition of prolactin secretion in cultured GH1 cells. *Biochem. Biophys. Res. Commun.* **59**, 420–428.

Vale, W., Blackwell, R., Grant, G., and Guillemin, R. (1973). TRF and thyroid hormones on prolactin secretion by rat anterior pituitary cells *in vitro*. *Endocrinology (Baltimore)* **93**, 26–33.

Vician, L., Shupnik, M. A., and Gorski, J. (1979). Effects of estrogen on primary ovine pituitary cell cultures: Stimulation of prolactin secretion, synthesis and preprolactin messenger ribonucleic acid activity. *Endocrinology (Baltimore)* **104**, 736–743.

Walker, A. M., and Farquhar, M. G. (1980). Preferential release of newly synthesized prolactin granules is the result of functional heterogeneity among mammotrophs. *Endocrinology (Baltimore)* **107**, 1095–1104.

West, B., and Dannies, P. S. (1980). Effects of estradiol on prolactin production and dihydroergocryptine-induced inhibition of prolactin production in primary cultures of rat pituitary cells. *Endocrinology (Baltimore)* **106,** 1108–1113.

Yamamoto, K., Kasai, K., and Ieiri, T. (1975). Control of pituitary functions of synthesis and release of prolactin and growth hormone by gonadal steroids in female and male rats. *Jpn. J. Physiol.* **25,** 645–658.

9

Signal Peptides: Properties and Interactions

LAWRENCE CHAN AND WILLIAM A. BRADLEY

I. INTRODUCTION

Considerable attention has been focused recently on the occurrence of intracellular precursors to various proteins during their biosynthesis (Zimmerman *et al.,* 1980). The initial observation that secretory proteins were synthesized on membrane-bound ribosomes as outlined by Palade (1975), coupled with the findings of Blobel and Sabatini (1971) suggesting that ribosome attachment to the rough endoplasmic reticulum was mediated by the nascent polypeptide chain, eventually

CELLULAR REGULATION OF SECRETION AND RELEASE

led to the concept of the central role of the signal or leader peptide in the transmembrane translocation of proteins. This concept is termed the "signal hypothesis" (Blobel and Dobberstein, 1975a,b) and will be examined in detail later. The "signal" or "leader" peptide, the essential structural component in this model, is an amino-terminal peptide (usually 15–30 residues in length) that is thought to anchor the nascent polypeptide to the rough endoplasmic reticulum, thereby initiating its translocation across the lipid barrier. Although the basic steps of this mechanism are still under active investigation, the concept of a hydrophobic leader domain interacting with the lipid matrix (whatever the mechanism) has had fundamental impact, not only in the study of protein secretion but also in the area of assembly of proteins within the membrane (i.e., integral and transmembrane proteins).

In this chapter some of the major hypotheses concerning the leader peptide will be outlined. Furthermore, we will examine the possible structure–function relationship of the leader peptide, especially in relationship to its interaction with membranes.

II. GENERAL STRUCTURAL CONSIDERATIONS

A. Hydrophobicity

Probably the most distinctive feature of leader peptide sequences is the relatively high frequency of occurrence of hydrophobic residues. That this observation is significant and probably meaningful can be understood when one considers the putative role of the leader. Ostensibly it is the penetration of the apolar phospholipid-rich bilayer membrane of the endoplasmic reticulum. It has been noted by various authors (Austen, 1979; Chan et al., 1980; Inouye and Halegoua, 1980; von Heijne, 1981) that the general feature of the leader peptide is a hydrophobic stretch of amino acids flanked by polar (charged, or hydroxylated) residues on the N and C termini. This linear amphipathic structure might be considered common to transmembrane structure(s) as opposed to the amphipathic helical structures (Morrisett et al., 1975; Jackson et al., 1976) that interact with phospholipid interfacially to form surface monolayers of polar lipid and protein. Using the hydrophobicity scale of Bull and Breeze (1974), we have estimated that the average hydrophobicity of 23 known leader sequences is greater than 1063 kcal (mol•residue) (Chan et al., 1980). Comparing this value to an average hydrophobicity of 900 kcal (mol•residue) for soluble proteins and 1030 kcal (mol•residue) for membrane-bound segments of proteins such as cytochrome b_5, a semiquantitative estimate of the degree of hydrophobicity of these peptide segments can be appreciated.

Von Heijne (1981) analyzed a number of signal peptides, prokaryotic as well as eukaryotic, in terms of their gross amino acid composition and hydrophobicity. Although several assumptions are involved in his calculations concerning charged residues and the secondary structure of the bound leader peptide, the hydrophobic free energy gained is more than necessary to overcome the unfavorable H-bond breaking energies, which suggests that the driving force for leader insertion into the membrane is essentially hydrophobic in nature. The spontaneous insertion of a leader peptide into the membrane has been reiterated by Engelman and Steitz (1981) in their helical hairpin hypothesis, which will be considered later. Their emphasis again is similar to that of von Heijne (1981) and suggests that the interaction is driven by the free energy gained by burying hydrophobic helical surfaces in the apolar lipid membrane.

B. Secondary Structure

Although the hydrophobic character of the leader peptide is obviously important because it is universal among leader peptides from numerous proteins, each of the aforementioned analyses assumes an α-helical structure as the major secondary structural feature of the leader segment. Consideration of the probable secondary structures, using predictive schemes, has been attempted with interesting results. Austen (1979) predicted the secondary structures of 21 known leader sequences using Chou–Fasman (Chou and Fasman, 1978) criteria. His calculations revealed that the central portion of all the leader sequences would contain regular structures, either α-helices or β-sheets. We (Chan et al., 1980) also have analyzed a number of presequences by Chou–Fasman criteria, including β-turn probabilities. The results are similar to those of Austen in that regular structures are predicted in all sequences analyzed. However, our calculations indicate a higher frequency of β-sheet. The actual conformational structure that inserts and/or is found in the membrane in any specific case may still, however, be helical, based on energetic considerations. Remembering that these values are probabilities, a comparison of the values for p_α and p_B of various segments of sequences (Table I) indicates that both structures are probable ($p > 1$). Upon interaction with the lipid bilayer, the helical structure could be preferred.

Evidence for this hypothesis is found in a study by Rosenblatt et al. (1980). Using a 30-residue synthetic peptide representing the amino

TABLE I

Conformational Predictions on Leader Peptides[a]

Protein	Number of residues	Position number	α-Helix $p\alpha$	β-Sheet $p\beta$	β-Turn p_T
Human β-chorio-gonadotropin[b]	25	6–24	1.07	1.21	
Rat growth hormone[c]	25	1–8	1.07	0.88	
		8–25	1.03	1.07	
		6–22	1.00	1.15	
Rat proalbumin[d]	18	1–13	1.12	1.26	
		12–15	0.80	0.96	1.22
Chick ovomucoid[e]	24	1–16	1.08	1.19	
		17–24	1.06	0.95	
		5–18	1.00	1.28	
		18–21	1.05	0.81	1.06
Chick conalbumin[f]	19	1–12	1.04	1.18	
		11–19	1.11	1.15	
Chick lysozyme[g]	18	1–13	1.07	1.19	
		3–14	1.05	1.25	
MOPC 104 E light chain[h]	19	1–16	1.08	1.10	
		3–11	1.07	1.25	
		13–16	0.83	0.89	1.25
		14–17	0.88	0.77	1.27
MOPC 41 light chain[h]	22	5–19	1.04	1.09	
		7–18	1.08	1.18	
		17–20	0.77	0.97	1.17
		19–22	0.77	1.01	1.17
Lipoprotein (*E. coli*)[i]	20	1–15	1.08	1.10	
		4–9	1.01	1.16	
α-Lactalbumin[j]	19	1–19	1.11	1.19	
K-Casein[k]	21	1–17	1.08	1.20	
		4–21	1.09	1.26	
α-S$_2$-Casein[k]	15	1–15	1.23	1.14	
α-S$_1$-Casein[k]	15	1–15	1.18	1.21	
MOPC-315 light chain[l]	18	1–8	1.10	1.20	
		12–18	1.05	1.04	
		3–13	1.08	1.28	
Preproparathyroid hormone[m]	25	1–25	1.14	1.08	
		7–22	1.18	1.25	
		22–25	0.83	0.74	1.35
Leu-specific binding protein[n]	23	1–7	1.15	0.90	
		5–23	1.16	1.07	
Rabbit uteroglobin[o]	21	1–18	1.11	1.12	
		3–17	1.12	1.19	
		17–20	0.88	0.72	1.26

(continued)

TABLE I (*Continued*)

Protein	Number of residues	Position number	α-Helix $p\alpha$	β-Sheet $p\beta$	β-Turn p_T
α-Lactoglobulin[p]	18	1–15	1.11	1.06	
Bovine promelanocortin[q]	26	10–21	1.13	1.06	
		6–9	0.82	0.80	1.31
β-Casein[k]	15	1–15	1.22	1.19	
Rat prolactin[r]	29	12–20	1.11	1.13	
		20–29	0.97	1.20	
		18–21	1.03	1.00	1.25
Chicken apoVLDL-II[s,t]	24	5–21	1.07	1.24	

[a] Calculations were based on criteria set by Chou and Fasman (1978).
[b] Birken *et al.* (1981).
[c] Seeburg *et al.* (1977).
[d] Strauss *et al.* (1977).
[e] Palmiter *et al.* (1977a).
[f] Thibodeau *et al.* (1978).
[g] Palmiter *et al.* (1977).
[h] Burstein and Schechter (1978).
[i] Inouye *et al.* (1977).
[j] Blobel and Dobberstein (1975a,b).
[k] Gaye *et al.* (1977).
[l] Jilka and Pestrka (1979).
[m] Habener *et al.* (1978).
[n] Oxender *et al.* (1980).
[o] Malsky *et al.* (1979).
[p] Mercier *et al.* (1978).
[q] Nakamishi *et al.* (1979).
[r] McKean and Maurer (1978).
[s] Chan *et al.* (1980).
[t] Dugaiczyk *et al.* (1981).

terminal leader sequence of preproparathyroid hormone, these authors studied by circular dichroism the secondary structure in two environments of different polarity. Chou–Fasman analysis of this peptide predicted both high helical potential ($p_\alpha = 1.14$, or approximately 83% α-helix, 0% β-sheet, and 17% random + β-turn). Beta-sheet also had a high potential with $< p_B >$ calculated at 1.18, which would then predict approximately 57% β-sheet with 20% α-helix and 23% random coil + β-turn. In aqueous buffer, the circular dichroism measurements revealed 27% α-helix, 43% β-sheet, and 30% random coil. However, when these measurements were made in 1,1,1,3,3,3-hexafluoro-2-propranol (a solvent selected to mimic the intramembranous nonpolar environment), only 46% α-helix was observed with 54% random coil; no β-sheet was observed in the circular dichroism spectrum.

Although the emphasis has been placed on the α-helical structure in most analyses, the 3_{10} helix is also a possible secondary structure, particularly for short leader sequences of approximately 15 residues. As pointed out by Engelman and Steitz (1981), the rise per amino acid for the 3_{10} helix (Dickerson and Geis, 1969) is 2.0 Å, so that approximately 15 residues are required to span a 30 Å bilayer. This structure would not be distinguishable from the α-helix by circular dichroism measurements.

C. Beta-Turns and the Signal Peptidase

One additional structural feature of leader peptides, which may be involved in cleavage site recognition by the signal peptidase, is the β-turn structure near the carboxy terminus of the leader (Austen, 1979; Rosenblatt et al., 1980; Boecke et al., 1980; von Heinje, 1981). No distinctive primary structural feature emerges upon comparison of leader sequences. However, signal peptidase(s) from different species are able to cleave presequences with fidelity, yielding the correct N terminus of the mature protein. It has been suggested that the peptidase identifies a regular common structural feature, such as the β-turn, to yield its specific cleavage. If one includes the residues of the N terminus of the mature or secreted protein in the structural predictions, many of these sequences will have a β-turn near the site of cleavage of the leader sequence. Table I also indicates the possibility of β-turns in at least eight cases, when just the presequence residues are considered.

D. Tertiary Structure

Although no direct evidence exists, energetic considerations indicate that the tertiary structure may play an important role in the interaction of the leader segment with the membrane. In the helical hairpin model (a tertiary structure) of Engelman and Steitz (1981), two helices are thought to form, the first from the leader peptide and the second from the first 20–25 residues of the mature protein. From both enthalpic and entropic considerations, it can be calculated that a hydrophobic helical hairpin formed in solution (perhaps after some type of initial binding to the membrane surface) would spontaneously insert into the lipid bilayer driven by approximately −60 kcal/mol of hydrophobic free energy gain. Other tertiary structures may also be involved in this interaction, but until appropriate model systems are available and physical measurements made (i.e., NMR, X ray, etc.), we are left with speculative models and mechanisms.

E. Conclusions

In general then, the basic structural features of a leader peptide include the following.

1. The leader peptide must have sufficient length to be able to span the lipid bilayer; therefore, 15 residues would seem to be the lower limit. Leader sequences of as long as 30 residues (or more for some sequences of nonsecreted proteins that are not cleaved) have been reported.
2. The leader peptide must have a sequence with a high potential for helix formation, at least in the central region of the peptide segment that would be in contact with nonpolar lipid bilayer.
3. The leader peptide must have a central core region that has a highly hydrophobic character and consists of residues such as leucine, isoleucine, valine, phenylalanine, tyrosine, and tryptophan.
4. Basic residues, such as arginine and lysine, seem to prefer the amino terminal region of the leader; acidic residues, such as glutamic acid and aspartic acid, are preferred in the carboxy terminus.
5. Finally, residues with sterically small side chains, such as alanine, glycine, serine, threonine, and cysteine, are very often located at, or near, the site of cleavage of the leader peptide from the mature protein. These residues are also preferred in β-turn regions that may be involved in the recognition for cleavage by the signal peptidase.

III. INTERACTION OF THE LEADER PEPTIDE WITH MEMBRANES

This particular aspect of the probable role of leader sequences is especially controversial. There are two main schools of thought concerning the general mechanism by which the leader peptide interacts with the membrane. One school (signal hypothesis) favors a receptor-mediated mechanism, whereas the other postulates a direct insertion of the helix into the lipid matrix. Each of the conceptual models will be discussed in more detail later. In this section we will attempt to analyze data from several different systems in order to detail the kinds of protein–protein and protein–lipid interactions that might participate in the translocation process.

The early proponents of the signal hypothesis suggested that the leader peptide of the nascent protein chain might be recognized by an integral membrane protein on the rough endoplasmic reticulum. This binding would result in the formation of a transient pore (or channel) through which the peptide could be extruded into the cisternal side of the endoplasmic reticulum. Although this has been an attractive hypothesis, the bulk of the data to support this proposal consists of the ability of leader sequences, such as that of preproparathyroid hormone, to inhibit translocation and processing of other preproteins (Rosenblatt *et al.*, 1979; Majzoub *et al.*, 1980). Unfortunately, high concentrations of the synthetic peptide had to be used for such experiments. Few model systems, if any, exist in which the receptor-mediated process has been critically tested. With synthetic leaders, saturation kinetics of the receptor should be demonstrable. If a protein receptor is involved, then use of synthetic leaders should allow measurement of the equilibrium constants for protein–protein interactions. These are all testable interactions, and the fate of the hypothesis lies in the results.

IV. MODEL SYSTEMS OF LEADER-LIKE PEPTIDES INTERACTING WITH MEMBRANES

The lack of sufficient quantities of native signal peptide as just described has indeed hindered the definitive experiments that would be most useful in elucidating its role in protein translocation. However, alternative model systems do exist in which one can test the interaction of leader-like peptides with lipid matrices. In the membrane-trigger hypothesis as espoused by Wickner (1979), the leader is thought to be involved only in the pathway of folding, which in turn directs the peptide to assemble into the membrane without the necessity for a receptor process. Wickner (1975, 1976, 1977) has used as a model system the procoat capsid protein of the filamentous coliphage M13. This protein is a 50-residue peptide consisting of a hydrophobic core with an acidic N terminus and a basic C terminus. Once synthesized, the protein can be shown posttranslationally to interact with *E. coli* membrane vesicles or liposomes (Wickner *et al.*, 1978). In addition, Wickner (1976) described the asymmetric incorporation of M13 capsid proprotein into synthetic lipid vesicles, or dimyristoylphosphatidylcholine vesicles, again suggesting that this leader-like peptide controls the vectorial insertion into the lipid. Asymmetry of orientation of the peptide in the lipid matrix was determined by accessibility to specific proteases. These experiments do indicate that the protein can exert thermodynamic control over its orientation in the lipid matrix, but it has not been demonstrated in a completely defined system that spontaneous, asymmetric insertion occurs. The assembly experiments with the M13 capsid proteins were performed by the Racker cholate dilution technique (Racker *et al.*, 1975). Although the products are thermodynamically stable, the kinetic barrier to their formation may be large, and for practical purposes their rates of formation may be infinitely slow. One argument against this, of course, is the observation that the capsid procoat protein inserts into the liposome of *E. coli* membranes. However, this is not a defined fraction and interpretation is not as straightforward as in the case of well-defined synthetic lipid vesicles such as dimyristoylphosphatidylcholine vesicles (Pownall *et al.*, 1981). If spontaneous insertion of a leader-like peptide, or better still, a synthetic leader (Rosenblatt *et al.*, 1980) can be demonstrated, conformational changes of the leader peptide upon binding could be monitored for change (Mao *et al.*, 1980) by optical methods and asymmetric insertion could be determined by several methods, depending upon the leader sequence of the isolated protein–lipid vesicle.

Another system used to model leader peptide interaction with membrane is the peptide melittin (Knöppel *et al.*, 1979) from bee venom. This 26-residue polypeptide is linearly amphipathic, the N-terminal 20 residues are hydrophobic whereas the C-terminal 6 residues are charged. Although the nascent peptide of melittin does possess an additional leader peptide, several investigators have studied the spontaneous interaction of the mature melittin peptide with natural and synthetic lipid membranes (Dawson *et al.*, 1978; Drake and Hider, 1979). Melittin is predicted to have β-sheet structure (about 70%) based on Chou–Fasman calculations, but the potential for α-helix formation exists ($p_\alpha = 0.96$, $p_B = 1.15$ for residues 1–12; and $p_\alpha = 1.07$, $p_B = 1.06$ for residues 13–26). In micelles of deoxycholate, Brij, and sodium dodecyl sulfate, the major structural feature discernable by circular dichroism is the α-helix. Knöppel *et al.* (1979) suggest that melittin might interact with these various types of detergents by mechanisms similar to those involved in the interaction of secretory preproteins and integral membrane proteins with membranes. Using egg yolk phosphatidylcholine liposomes (at a melittin:phospholipid ratio of 1:13 and at a temperature of 20°C, where melittin did not cause liposome fusion), Drake and Hider (1979) measured the secondary structure of the peptide. The main secondary structural feature was indeed an α-helix. Based on their data, under these conditions melittin consists of approximately 70% α-helix, which would be consistent with residues 2–20 being involved in an α-helical structure within the lipid matrix. Unfortunately, the orientation of the peptide in the liposome was unknown.

The most appropriate model studied to date on the interaction of leader peptide with membranes involves the synthetic leader pre-proparathyroid peptide described earlier. Circular dichroism studies on the peptide again revealed α-helix formation (α = 46%; β = 0%) in the presence of a nonpolar solvent (1,1,1,3,3,3-hexafluoro-2-propanol), whereas substantial β-sheet (43%) was present in an aqueous buffer.

Finally, another mechanism has been proposed to explain the interaction of plasma apolipoproteins with phospholipids (Pownall *et al.*, 1981) and the permeation of small molecules (Kanehisa and Tsong, 1978) with phospholipid surfaces. It involves the interaction at a defect site within the matrix and is known as the cluster-model theory. A similar type of interaction could be important in any of the postulated spontaneous insertion mechanisms (membrane trigger, helical hairpin, or direct transfer mechanism; see Section V). The defect or pore can be the result of local fluctuations in the lipid matrix and/or the presence of perturbants in the matrix, such as cholesterol or membrane proteins, in other words, any local packing mediator in the phospholipid matrix. The model predicts that in pure lipid systems, the rate of permeation is a function of the size of the permeant and the temperature of the system with respect to the lipid transition temperature. The association of a hydrophobic peptide (such as the leader) with the lipid can be viewed as that of a large permeant. According to this model, the rate of association of the peptide with the lipid would be kinetically maximal at the transition temperature of the lipid.

V. HYPOTHESES ON TRANSMEMBRANE TRANSLOCATION OF PROTEINS

It is generally appreciated that membrane-associated proteins assume a conformation such that specific domains with an apolar face are in close proximity with the lipid bilayer and the hydrophilic residues tend to protrude into the aqueous environment. Although this is thermodynamically the favored conformation, it is not known how a nascent peptide chain inserts into the cell organellar membranes, because in many instances (e.g., bacteriorhodopsin) the proteins span the membrane numerous times. A more common situation involves eukaryotic secretory proteins as well as the prokaryotic periplasmic and outer membrane proteins where the nascent chain is vectorially discharged across either the endoplasmic reticulum in the eukaryote or the cytoplasmic membrane in the prokaryote. The mechanism of such transport is again unknown. Some hypotheses have been advanced, and of these, some offer conflicting evidence and conclusions, whereas others are by no means mutually exclusive. We will review the most popular and plausible hypotheses and briefly examine the evidence for each of them.

A.   The Signal Hypothesis

In explaining why secretory proteins were synthesized on bound ribosomes whereas other proteins were synthesized on free ribosomes, Blobel and Sabatini (1971) proposed that mRNA for the former group of proteins encoded for a special sequence that was located at the amino terminus of the polypeptide chain and that might be recognized by a membrane-binding factor. The following year, Milstein *et al.* (1972) independently found that, when mouse myeloma mRNA was used to direct protein synthesis in the rabbit reticulocyte lysate system, the translation product for immunoglobulin light chain took the form of a protein approximately 1500 daltons larger than authentic light chain itself. However, when the myeloma rough endoplasmic reticulum was added instead of the mRNA, the protein was identical in size to mouse immunoglobulin light chain. Peptide mapping showed an altered amino terminus for the mRNA-directed larger protein. Milstein *et al.* (1972) postulated that a short amino acid sequence at the amino terminus of secretory protein precursor might serve as a *signal* for segregating the translation of these proteins on rough endoplasmic reticulum. They further showed that the addition of homologous membrane fragments converted the precursor to the final authentic product (Cowan *et al.*, 1973). Blobel and Dobberstein (1975a,b) extended the observation and showed that heterologous stripped rough endoplasmic reticulum also effected the "processing" of the precursor and that the processed mature protein was sequestered within the rough endoplasmic reticulum and was inaccessible to exogenously added proteases. The results formed the basis for the "signal hypothesis."

The essential feature of the signal hypothesis as it was originally formulated is the occurrence of a unique sequence of codons on mRNAs that upon translation results in a unique sequence of amino acid residues on the amino terminus of the nascent chain. Translation of the mRNA is initiated on free ribosomes. However, emergence of this amino-terminal sequence (the "signal peptide" triggers the attachment of the ribosome to the membrane. This attachment would occur by specific membrane receptor proteins and the attachment process would lead to "tunnel" formation by the receptor(s) and/or other integral membrane protein(s) through which the lengthening nascent chain is translocated across the membrane. A protease on the luminal aspect of the rough endoplasmic reticulum would cleave the signal peptide from the mature protein, usually before the termination of translation. In the original hypothesis, translocation was envisioned as exclusively cotranslational. Subsequently, refinement of the hypothesis extends it to include instances where translocation may be posttranslational (Blobel, 1980), i.e., uncoupled from translation.

Blobel (1980) has extended his initial hypothesis to explain the location and asymmetrical distribution of integral membrane proteins, as well as the unidirectional translocation of proteins across various membranes. He postulated that the information for the location in and translocation of proteins across membranes, a process that he termed protein topogenesis, is encoded in discrete "topogenic" sequences that constitute a permanent or transient part of the polypeptide chain. Four types of topogenic sequences were predicted by Blobel: signal sequences, stop-transfer sequences, sorting sequences, and insertion sequences. Signal sequences initiate translocation of proteins across specific membranes. Stop-transfer sequences interrupt the translocation process and yield asymmetrical integration of proteins into translocation-competent membranes. Sorting sequences would act as determinants for posttranslational traffic of subpopulations of proteins to various organellar membranes. Insertion sequences would initiate unilateral integration of proteins into the lipid bilayer without the mediation of a distinct protein effector. Putative examples of the various sequences were given by Blobel in his review, and various possible exceptions were also discussed.

Blobel's signal hypothesis has stimulated considerable interest and intense research activity in the areas of secretory and integral membrane protein biosynthesis. Confirmation of the hydrophobic signal peptide as a common feature of most secretory proteins has come from numerous laboratories, and signal peptidase activity has been repeatedly demonstrated. The signal hypothesis has been used to explain the cotranslational extrusion of membrane proteins through a protein pore. Proper insertion of a number of nascent peptides into exogenously added stripped rough endoplasmic reticulum *in vitro* has been demonstrated for many integral membrane proteins. An 11 S protein has been isolated from dog pancreas microsomal membranes in Blobel's laboratory (Walter and Blobel, 1980, 1981a,b; Walter *et al.,* 1981). This protein has been termed the signal recognition protein. The protein bound selectively to wheat germ ribosomes engaged in the synthesis of secretory protein (bovine preprolactin) and inhibited the translocation of the latter. It did not bind to the ribosomes involved in cytoplasmic protein (α and β chains of rabbit globin) synthesis. Furthermore, microsomal membrane vesicles were shown to bind selectively to nascent, *in vitro*-assembled polysomes synthesizing secretory protein, but not those synthesizing cytoplasmic protein. This selective polysome binding capacity was abolished when the microsomal vesicles were salt-extracted but was restored by addition of the partially purified signal recognition protein. The description of the latter protein adds support to the Blobel hypothesis, but its exact function remains to be established. Other aspects of the signal hypothesis, e.g., the demonstration of specific receptors on rough endoplasmic reticulum from various tissues and organs and the creation of a protein "pore" through which the nascent chain is translocated remains to be confirmed. His hypothesis on topogenic sequences will likely stimulate intense debate as well as experimental work on the forces behind the asymmetric location of proteins in membranes and those behind the "homing" mechanism for various proteins to particular organelles.

B.   The Membrane-Triggered Folding Hypothesis

Wickner (1979) proposed the membrane-triggered folding hypothesis to explain the translocation of proteins across membranes. In this model, the thermodynamics of protein folding are postulated to be the major, if not the only, force behind translocation. The process of the protein translocation takes place co- or posttranslationally. In the case of proteins with a transient or permanent hydrophobic leader sequence, the sequence is thought to allow the growing peptide chain to fold in a manner compatible with the aqueous environment. The subsequent removal of the leader sequence is thought to render the folding pathway irreversible (Wickner, 1980). Upon entering a membrane, the proteins may be triggered to refold by the availability of the hydrocarbon core of the bilayer. The mechanism for membrane recognition is thought to depend on the physical properties of the membrane, and assembly is independent of any protein pore or specific receptors on the membrane.

Wickner's argument against the requirement for a specific protein receptor in translocation is supported mainly by experiments in his laboratory on the biosynthesis of the major coat protein (gene 8 product) of coliphage M13. As discussed in Section IV, coat protein is initially synthesized as a precursor, termed "procoat," with an extra 23 amino acid-residue on the amino terminus. Procoat has been demonstrated in the soluble cytoplasmic compartment and will posttranslationally assemble into large *E. coli* membrane vesicles or even large protein-free lysosomes. Furthermore, solubilized signal peptidase cleaved procoat into coat protein in the presence of *E. coli* membrane vesicles.

The Wickner model is important because it points out that there are alternatives to specific membrane proteins that might facilitate the translocation of proteins. In neither the signal hypothesis nor the membrane-triggered folding hypothesis were the energetics of the translocation adequately treated. The following model is based on careful consideration of the thermodynamics of the translocation or membrane insertion (in the case of integral proteins) process.

C. The Direct Transfer Hypothesis

Von Heijne and Blomberg (1979) examined the passage of nascent peptide chains through the membrane from a physicochemical point of view. An analysis of the free energies involved in each step of the translocation process was made. From such calculations they have developed the "direct transfer model," which is based on the following assumptions: First, any segment of a polypeptide chain can bind to a membrane if it is sufficiently hydrophobic. Second, all parts of the chain that are embedded in the membrane have an α-helical conformation. Third, the subsequent binding of the ribosome to a binding site on the membrane [possibly a ribophorin (Kreibich *et al.*, 1978a,b)] will force even strongly polar or charged residues into the membrane. Hence, the nascent chain of secretory proteins emerging from the large ribosomal subunit binds to the rough endoplasmic reticulum and the ribosome anchors on the ribophorin. The energetics of partitioning of the amino acid residues between the aqueous (cytoplasmic) phase and lipid (membranous) phase directly "push" the peptide chain across the membrane as the latter assumes an α-helical conformation, in the form of a hairpin loop structure with the amino terminus remaining on the cytoplasmic side of the membrane. When stable domains can be formed by the extruded parts of the chain (i.e., 50–100 residues), the folding of this part of the chain is thought to provide an additional "pull" through the membrane.

The quantitative estimates of the energetics of translocation have been applied to both secreted proteins as well as integral membrane proteins. In the latter instance, the hydrophobic membrane-spanning sequence must be followed by a strongly hydrophilic part in order to detach the ribosome from the binding site on the membrane. Von Heijne (1980) has further examined quantitatively a number of secretory and membrane proteins by his hypothesis. Using a computer model, he correctly predicted that a number of proteins with known sequences would be either secreted or lodged in membranes. There were several instances that were especially interesting. For example, ovalbumin is a very special type of secretory protein. The nascent chain has no hydrophobic leader sequence at its amino terminus, which is blocked and uncharged. If inserted into a membrane as a single helix, the relatively hydrophobic residues at the amino terminus, together with the paucity of charged residues, would provide more than enough hydrophobic free energy to compensate for the helix initiation free energy. Based on such calculations, von Heijne proposed that ovalbumin is the first known representative of a class of proteins that initiate translocation directly, without the need for a cleavable leader sequence. Such a class of proteins is predicted to be "ovalbumin-like" at its amino terminal region, i.e., an abundance of hydrophobic residues (about 10), and a paucity of charged residues up to a distance of perhaps 20–30 residues from the amino terminus. Another prediction from the von Heijne model is that the C-terminal "tail" left on the cytoplasmic side of the membrane upon termination of translation may, in many cases, significantly reduce the rate of detachment of the mature protein from the membrane. This is another testable premise of the model.

D. The Helical Hairpin Hypothesis

Using similar calculations involving specific energetics and structural considerations, Engelman and Steitz (1981) have arrived at the "helical hairpin" hypothesis. The specifics of the hypothesis are not too different from those proposed by von Heijne and Blomberg (1979) and von Heijne (1980). The initial event in the secretion of proteins across membranes and their insertion into membranes is the spontaneous penetration of the hydrophobic portion of the bilayer by a helical hairpin. Only α- and 3_{10} helices are predicted in the hydrophobic interior of membranes. Insertion of a polypeptide is accomplished by a hairpin structure composed of two helices, which will partition into membranes if the free energy arising from burying hydrophobic helical surfaces exceeds the free energy "cost" of burying potentially charged and hydrogen-bonding groups. The hydrophobic leader sequence thus functions by "pulling" polar portions of a protein into the membrane as the second helix of the hairpin. The occurrence of all categories of membrane proteins can be explained by the hydrophobic or hydrophilic character of the two helices of the inserted hairpin and, for some integral membrane proteins, by events in which a single terminal helix is inserted. Hence, according to this hypothesis, secretion and insertion of membrane proteins are spontaneous processes that do not require the participation of additional membrane receptors or transport proteins (or channels).

E. Other Models

A number of other less well developed models for translocation of proteins across membranes have been proposed. For example, the "loop model" of Inouye and Halegoua (1980) is topographically very similar to the direct transfer and helical hairpin hypotheses. They postulated that the first few residues of the leader sequence, which are often basic in nature, bind to the acidic phospholipid surface. As polypeptide chain elongation continues, the growing chain forms a loop that extrudes through the bilayer without the participation of specific membrane proteins. The energetics involved in such interactions were not calculated. Davis and Tai (1980) have postulated an organized membrane structure actively transporting the growing peptide chain across the membrane. This model is thus quite similar to the signal hypothesis. The authors, however, have failed to observe any direct attachment of ribosomes to the membranes in bacteria, though such an event could not be excluded.

Various other studies using genetic manipulations indicated that hybrid molecules of signal peptide attached to other proteins were often secreted. However, additional evidence indicated that a signal sequence was not sufficient to lead β-galactosidase out of the cytoplasm (Moreno *et al.*, 1980). Furthermore, the importance of the C-terminal region of various proteins in the translocation process also seemed to vary with the particular proteins studied. For example, Koshland and Botstein (1980) found that chain-terminated (amber) fragments of the periplasmic protein β-lactamase lacking the C-terminal end of the protein failed to be secreted into the periplasmic space in *Salmonella typhimurium*. On the other hand, in the case of the maltose-binding protein in *E. coli*, Ito and Beckwith (1981) found that an amber fragment lacking up to two-thirds of the residues at the C terminus was secreted at normal levels, suggesting that this part of the sequence was not required for secretion. These different results might indicate that there are different mechanisms of secretion for different proteins. However, another possible explanation is that differences in experimental conditions [e.g., ionic environment and method of cell disruption (Ito *et al.*, 1981)] might affect the apparent localization of unusual proteins.

In summary, the various experiments involving recombinant molecules indicate that signal peptides seem to be necessary, but insufficient, for protein translocation. The contribution of other regions of these proteins seem to vary according to the specific system under investigation. Such experiments involving genetic manipulations have provided significant and interesting information in various model systems. They underscore the complexity of the mechanism of protein translocation. Until additional observations are made and compiled, the contribution of nonleader sequences to this process is still unclear.

VI. CONCLUSIONS

Since the first description of the leader peptide about 10 years ago, many experiments on the properties and interactions of the peptide have been published. A number of hypotheses have been proposed, some of which are contradictory, others of which seem to be complimentary to each other. In addition to the various hypotheses reviewed in the last section, the authors believe that the cluster-model theory discussed at the end of Section IV is an attractive alternative and the concept should be incorporated into hypotheses explaining the mechanism of translocation of proteins across membranes. Further experimentation, especially on the purification and characterization of the putative signal receptor from a variety of tissues, the direct measurement of the interaction of synthetic leader sequences and their analogs with lipid bilayers, and further studies by genetically modifying peptide structures will likely help us understand the significance of signal peptides and their role in translocation of proteins across membranes.

ACKNOWLEDGMENTS

Work by the authors described in this chapter was supported in part by grants SCOR HL27341, HL-23470 and HL-16512 from the National Institute of Health and grant 80-875 from the American Heart Association. The authors thank M. Scheib for typing the manuscript.

REFERENCES

Austen, B. M. (1979). Predicting secondary structure of the amino-terminal extension sequence of secreted proteins. *FEBS Lett.* **103**, 308–313.
Birken, S., Fetherston, J., Canfield, R., and Boime, I. (1981). The amino acid sequences of

the peptides contained in the subunits of human chriogonadotropin. *J. Biol. Chem.* **256,** 1816–1823.

Blobel, G. (1980). Intracellular protein topogenesis. *Proc. Natl. Acad. Sci. U.S.A.* **77,** 1496–1500.

Blobel, G., and Dobberstein, B. (1975a). Transfer of protein across membranes. I. Presence of proteolytically processed and unprocessed nascent immunoglobulin light chains on membrane-bound ribosomes of *murine myeloma. J. Cell Biol.* **67,** 835–851.

Blobel, G., and Dobberstein, B. (1975b). Transfer of proteins across membranes. II. Reconstitution of functional rough microsomes from heterologous components. *J. Cell Biol.* **67,** 852–862.

Blobel, G., and Sabatini, D. D. (1971). Ribosome-membrane interaction in eukaryotic cells. *In* "Biomembranes" (L. A. Manson, ed.), Vol. 2, 193–195. Plenum, New York.

Boecke, J. D., Russel, M., and Model, P. (1980). Processing of filamentous phage pre-coat protein. Effect of sequence variations near the signal peptidase cleavage site. *J. Mol. Biol.* **144,** 103–116.

Bull, H. B., and Breeze, K. (1974). Surface tension of amino acid solutions. A hydrophobicity scale of the amino acid residues. *Arch. Biochem. Biophys.* **161,** 665–670.

Burstein, Y., and Schechter, I. (1978). Primary structures of N-terminal extra peptide segments linked to the variable and constant regions of immunoglobulin light chain precursors: Implication in the organization and controlled expression of immunoglobin genes. *Biochemistry* **17,** 2392–2400.

Chan, L., Bradley, W. A., and Means, A. R. (1980). Amino acid sequence of the signal peptide of apoVLDL-II, a major apoprotein in avian very low density lipoproteins. *J. Biol. Chem.* **255,** 1006–10063.

Chou, P. Y., and Fasman, G. D. (1978). Empirical predictions of protein conformation. *Annu. Rev. Biochem.* **47,** 251–276.

Cowan, N. J., Harrison, T. M., Brownlee, G. G., and Milstein, C. (1973). The cell-free synthesis of immunoglobulin chains. *Biochem. Soc. Trans.* **1,** 1247–1250.

Davis, B. D., and Tai, P.-C. (1980). The mechanism of protein secretion across membranes. *Nature (London)* **283,** 433–438.

Dawson, C. R., Drake, A. F., Helliwell, J., and Hider, R. C. (1978). The interaction of bee melittin with lipid bilayers. *Biochim. Biophys. Acta* **510,** 75–86.

Dickerson, R. E., and Geis, I. (1969). *In* "The Structure and Action of Protein" p. 26. Harper & Row, New York.

Drake, A. F., and Hider, R. C. (1979). The structure of melittin in lipid bilayer membranes. *Biochim. Biophys. Acta* **55,** 371–373.

Dugaiczyk, A., Inglis, A. S., Strike, P. M., Burley, R. W., Beattie, W. G., and Chan, L. (1981). Comparison of the nucleotide sequence of cloned cDNA coding for an apolipoprotein (apoVLDL-II) from avian blood and the amino acid sequence of an egg-yolk protein (apovitellenin I): Equivalence of the two sequences. *Gene* **14,** 175–182.

Engelman, D. M., and Steitz, T. A. (1981). The spontaneous insertion of proteins into and across membranes: The helical hairpin hypothesis. *Cell* **23,** 411–422.

Gaye, P., Gautron, J.-P., Mercier, J.-C., and Haze, G. (1977). Amino terminal sequences of the precursors of ovine caseins. *Biochem. Biophys. Res. Commun.* **79,** 903–911.

Habener, J. F., Rosenblatt, M., Kemper, B., Kronenberg, H. M., Rich, A., and Potts, J. T., Jr. (1978). Preproparathyroid hormone: Amino acid sequence, chemical synthesis, and some biological studies of the precursor region. *Proc. Natl. Acad. Sci. U.S.A.* **73,** 1964–1968.

Inouye, M., and Halegoua, S. (1980). Secretion and membrane localization of proteins in *Escherichia coli. CRC Crit. Rev. Biochem.* **10**, 339–371.

Inouye, S., Wang, S., Sekizawa, J., Halegona, S., and Inouye, M. (1977). Amino acid sequence for the peptide extension in the prolipoprotein of the *E. coli* outer membrane. *Proc. Natl. Acad. Sci. U.S.A.* **74**, 1004–1008.

Ito, K., and Beckwith, J. R. (1981). Role of the mature protein sequence of maltose-binding protein in its secretion across the *E. coli* cytoplasmic membrane. *Cell* **25**, 143–150.

Ito, K., Bassford, J. P., and Beckwith, J. R. (1981). Protein localization in *E. coli:* Is there a common step in the secretion of periplasmic and outer-membrane proteins. *Cell* **24**, 707–717.

Jackson, R. L., Morrisett, J. D., and Gotto, A. M. (1976). Lipoprotein structure and metabolism. *Physiol. Rev.* **56**, 255–316.

Jelka, R. L., and Pestka, S. (1979). Precursor sequence of MOPC-315 mouse immunoglobulin light chains. *J. Biol. Chem.* **254**, 9270–9276.

Kanehisa, M. I., and Tsong, T. Y. (1978). Cluster model of lipid phase transitions with application to passive permeation of molecules and structure relaxations in lipid bilayers. *J. Amer. Chem. Soc.* **100**, 424–432.

Knöppel, E., Eisenberg, D., and Wickner, W. (1979). Interactions of melittin, a preprotein model, with detergents. *Biochemistry* **18**, 4177–4181.

Kosland, D., and Botstein, D. (1980). Secretion of beta-lactamase requires the carboxy end of the protein. *Cell* **20**, 749–760.

Kreibich, G., Freienstein, C. M., Pereyra, B. N., Ulrich, B. L., and Sabatini, D. D. (1978a). Proteins of rough microsomal membrane related to ribosome binding. II. Cross-linking of bound ribosomes to specific membrane proteins exposed at the binding sites. *J. Cell Biol.* **77**, 488–506.

Kreibich, G., Ulrich, B. L., and Sabatini, D. D. (1978b). Proteins of rough microsomal membranes related to ribosome binding. I. Identification of ribophorins I and II, membrane proteins characteristic of rough microsomes. *J. Cell Biol.* **77**, 464–487.

McKean, D. J., and Maurer, R. A. (1978). Amino acid sequence of the precursor region of rat. *Biochemistry* **17**, 5215–5219.

Malsky, M. L., Bullock, D. W., Willard, J. J., and Ward, D. N. (1979). Progesterone-induced secretory protein. NH_2-terminal sequence of the pre-uteroglobin. *J. Biol. Chem.* **254**, 1580–1585.

Majzoub, J. A., Rosenblatt, M., Fennick, S., Maunces, R., Kronenberg, H. M., Potts, J. T., Jr., and Habener, J. F. (1980). Synthetic pre-proparathyroid hormone leader sequence inhibits cell-free processing of placental, parathyroid and pituitary prehormones. *J. Biol. Chem.* **255**, 11478–11483.

Mao, S. J. T., Jackson, R. L., Gotto, A. M., and Sparrow, J. T. (1980). Mechanism of lipid-protein interaction in the plasma lipoproteins: Identification of a lipid-binding site in apolipoprotein A-II. *Biochemistry* **20**, 1676–1680.

Mercier, J.-C., Haze, G., Gaye, P., and Hue, D. (1978). Amino terminal sequence of the precursor of ovine α-lactoglobulin. *Biochem. Biophys. Res. Commun.* **82**, 1236–1245.

Milstein, C., Brownlee, G. G., Harrison, T. M., and Mathews, M. B. (1972). A possible precursor of immunoglobulin light chains. *Nature (London) New Biol.* **239**, 117–120.

Moreno, F., Fowler, A. V., Hall, M., Silhavy, T. J., Zabin, I., and Schwartz, M. (1980). A signal sequence is not sufficient to lead β-galactosidase out of the cytoplasm. *Nature (London)* **286**, 356–359.

Morrisett, J. D., Jackson, R. L., and Gotto, A. M. (1975). Lipoproteins: Structure and function. *Annu. Rev. Biochem.* **44,** 183–207.

Nakamishi, S., Inoue, A., Keta, T., Nakamura, M., Chang, A. C. Y., Cohen, S. N., and Numa, S. (1979). Nucleotide sequence of cloned cDNA for bovine corticotropin-β-lipotropin precursor. *Nature (London)* **278,** 423–427.

Oxender, D. L., Anderson, J. T., Daniels, C. J., Lindick, R., Gunsalus, R. P., Zurawski, G., and Yanofsky, C. (1980). Amino-terminal sequence and processing of the precursor of the leucine-specific binding protein, and evidence for conformational differences between precursor and mature form. *Proc. Natl. Acad. Sci. U.S.A.* **77,** 2005–2009.

Palade, G. E. (1975). Intracellular aspects of the process of protein synthesis. *Science* **189,** 347–358.

Palmiter, R. D., Thibodeau, S. N., Gagnon, J., and Walsh, K. A. (1977a). *FEBS Meet.* **47,** 89–101.

Palmiter, R. D., Gagnon, J., Ericsson, L. H., and Walsh, K. A. (1977b). Precursor of egg white lysozyme. Amino acid sequence of the NH_2-terminal extension. *J. Biol. Chem.* **252,** 6386–6394.

Pownall, J. H., Pao, Q., Hickson, D., Sparrow, J. T., Jusserow, S. K., and Massey, J. B. (1981). Kinetics and mechanism of association of human plasma apolipoproteins with dimyristoylphosphatidylcholine: Effect of protein structure and lipid clusters on reaction rates. *Biochemistry* **20,** 6630–6635.

Racker, E., Chien, T.-F., and Kandrach (1975). A cholate-dilution procedure for the reconstitution of the Ca^{++} pump, $^{32}P_i$-ATP exchange, and oxidative phosphorylation. *FEBS Lett.* **57,** 14–18.

Rosenblatt, M., Majzoub, J. A., Kronenberg, H. M., Habener, J. F., and Potts, J. T. (1979). The precursor-specific region of pre-proparathyroid hormone: Chemical synthesis and preliminary studies in its effect in post-translational modification of hormone. *Pept., Proc. Am. Pept. Symp., 6th,* pp. 535–538.

Rosenblatt, M., Beaudette, N. V., and Fasman, G. D. (1980). Conformational studies of the synthetic precursor-specific region of preproparathyroid hormone. *Proc. Natl. Acad. Sci. U.S.A.* **77,** 3983–3987.

Seeburg, P. H., Shine, J., Martial, J. A., Baxter, J. D., and Goodman, H. M. (1977). Nucleotide sequence and amplification in bacteria of structural gene for rat growth hormone. *Nature (London)* **270,** 486–494.

Strauss, A. W., Bennett, C. D., Donahue, A. M., Rodkey, J. A., and Alberts, A. W. (1977). Conversion of rat pre-proalbumin to proalbumin *in vitro* by ascites membranes. *J. Biol. Chem.* **252,** 6846–6855.

Thibodeau, S. N., Lee, D. C., and Palmiter, R. D.(1978). Identical precursors for serum transferrin and egg white conalbumin. *J. Biol. Chem.* **253,** 3771–3774.

von Heijne, G. (1980). Trans-membrane translocation of proteins. A detailed physico-chemical analysis. *Eur. J. Biochem.* **103,** 431–438.

von Heijne, G. (1981). On the hydrophobic nature of signal sequences. *Eur. J. Biochem.* **116,** 419–422.

von Heijne, G., and Blomberg, C. (1979). Trans-membrane translocation of proteins. The direct transfer model. *Eur. J. Biochem.* **97,** 175–181.

Walter, P., and Blobel, G. (1980). Purification of a membrane-associated protein complex required for protein translocation across the endoplasmic reticulum. *Proc. Natl. Acad. Sci. U.S.A.* **77,** 7112–7116.

Walter, P., and Blobel, G. (1981a). Translocation of proteins across the endoplasmic reticulum. II. Signal recognition protein (SRP) mediates the selective binding to microsomal membranes of *in vitro*-assembled polysomes synthesizing secretory protein. *J. Cell Biol.* **91,** 551–556.

Walter, P., and Blobel, G. (1981b). Translocation of proteins across the endoplasmic reticulum. III. Signal recognition protein (SRP) causes signal sequence-dependent and site-specific arrest of chain elongation that is released by microsomal membranes. *J. Cell Biol.* **91,** 557–561.

Walter, P., Ibrahimi, I., and Blobel, G. (1981). Translocation of proteins across the endoplasmic reticulum. I. Signal recognition protein (SRP) binds to *in vitro*-assembled polysomes synthesizing secretory protein. *J. Cell Biol.* **91,** 545–550.

Wickner, W. (1975). Asymmetric orientation of a phage coat protein in cytoplasmic membrane of *Escherichia coli. Proc. Natl. Acad. Sci. U.S.A.* **72,** 4749–4753.

Wickner, W. (1976). Asymmetric orientation of phage M13 coat protein in *Escherichia coli* cytoplasmic membranes and in synthetic lipid vesicles. *Proc. Natl. Acad. Sci. U.S.A.* **73,** 1159–1163.

Wickner, W. T. (1977). Role of hydrophobic forces in membrane protein asymmetry. *Biochemistry* **16,** 254–258.

Wickner, W. (1979). The assembly of proteins into biological membranes: The membrane trigger hypothesis. *Annu. Rev. Biochem.* **48,** 23–45.

Wickner, W. (1980). Assembly of proteins into membranes. *Science* **210,** 861–868.

Wickner, W., Model, G., Zwizinski, C., Bates, M., and Killick, T. (1978). Synthesis of phage M13 coat protein and its assembly into membranes *in vitro. Proc. Natl. Acad. Sci. U.S.A.* **75,** 1754–1758.

Zimmerman, M., Munford, R. A., and Steiner, D. F., eds. (1980). Precursor processing in the biosynthesis of proteins. *Ann. N. Y. Acad. Sci.* **343.**

10

Diseases of Secretion

MERRILY POTH AND RAYMOND S. GREENBERG

I. INTRODUCTION

There is a considerable fund of basic scientific knowledge regarding the control of secretion and the mechanism of secretory processes but a

323

relative paucity of clinical applications of this knowledge. This interface of richness and poverty is the stage for our discussion.

Most of this book involves regulation of endocrine secretion. Clinical diseases of the endocrine system with abnormal secretion of specific hormones are common and the causes for abnormal secretion are varied. In some cases, such as idiopathic hypopituitarism, the secreting organ may be dysplastic and appear to be nonspecifically dysfunctional. There are a few instances where the gene for a hormone is lacking and the appropriate hormone is, therefore, not synthesized (Phillips *et al.*, 1981).

In addition, there are examples of autoimmune diseases where the gland is attacked by the immune system and the resulting inflammatory process leads to inadequate or inappropriate secretion from the affected gland. However, in no case is a fundamental defect in the secretory process itself known to be responsible for an abnormal level of hormone secreted.

The following mechanisms must be intact for appropriate hormonal secretion to occur: (1) the cellular mechanism to synthesize and perhaps store the hormone in adequate quantities; (2) the mechanism for hormonal release from the glandular cell into the bloodstream (These first two processes also involve many metabolic requirements, such as amino acid uptake, and availability of energy sources. Some of these requirements may be specific to secretory cells.); (3) a system to monitor the requirements for the hormone at any given time (e.g., receptors, neuronal pathways); (4) effective mechanisms to translate the signal in (3) into appropriate changes in synthesis and release of the hormone.

From a clinical perspective, the consequences of an error in any part of the secretory process would be indistinguishable from a lack of the structural gene for the hormone, or even from total glandular aplasia. Each of these defects would result in diminished circulating hormone. To implicate the secretory process as the source of hormonal inadequacy, the following might be anticipated:

1. The gene for the hormone would be present.
2. The gland would contain adequate and active hormone.
3. The defect might involve several glands and therefore result in multiple hormonal deficiencies.

If all of these conditions are satisfied, the secretory process itself would be suspect. In the past, endocrine diseases have not been conceptualized in this fashion.

Therefore, we turn to another type of secretion—the exocrine system. Cystic fibrosis may be considered as a generalized disease of exocrine secretions because available research and clinical data suggest that the actual secretory process may be disordered in this disease. We will devote the remainder of this chapter to the exocrine system, focusing on cystic fibrosis. This discussion will emphasize exocrine pancreatic function.

II.   CYSTIC FIBROSIS

A.   Background

Cystic fibrosis of the pancreas is a generalized disorder of exocrine tissues. With a prevalence of approximately 1 in 2000 white children (di Sant'Agnese and Talamo, 1967), cystic fibrosis is the most common lethal genetic disease in Caucasians. The disorder is much less common in other races. Genetic studies suggest that cystic fibrosis is inherited in an autosomal recessive pattern, with a gene frequency of about 5% in the United States population (Steinberg and Brown, 1960). Heterozygotes do not manifest any clinical symptoms of the disease.

The prognosis in cystic fibrosis has benefited from advances in clinical management. Nevertheless, most patients still do not survive to the fourth decade of life (Wood *et al.*, 1976). As a result, cystic fibrosis remains a major cause of chronic disability and death in childhood.

B.   Clinical Entity

1.   General Description

Anderson (1938) presented the first description of the clinical and pathological findings in cystic fibrosis. Subsequent reports have extended our appreciation of the diverse manifestations of this disease. There are a variety of recognized presenting symptoms and a wide spectrum of clinical severity. A classic triad of chronic obstructive pulmonary disease, pancreatic insufficiency, and abnormal sweat electrolytes are the hallmarks of the disease. Virtually all patients exhibit the pulmonary and sweat abnormalities, whereas only 80 to 90% of homozygotes have pancreatic insufficiency (Wood *et al.*, 1976). Table I presents the primary characteristics and some attendant secondary manifestations of cystic fibrosis.

TABLE I

Primary Defect and Secondary Clinical Manifestations Encountered in Cystic Fibrosis Patients

Primary defect	Secondary manifestation
Increased sweat electrolytes	Excessive salt loss
	Vascular collapse
Pulmonary infection	Obstructive emphysema
	Bronchopneumonia
	Atelectasis
	Hemoptysis
	Pneumothorax
	Cor pulmonale
	Respiratory failure
Pancreatic insufficiency	Intestinal obstruction
	Rectal prolapse
	Failure to thrive
	Delayed maturation
	Fat-soluble vitamin deficiency
	Biliary cirrhosis
	Pancreatitis
	Diabetes mellitus

2. Eccrine Sweat

The altered sweat electrolyte concentrations are present from birth and persist throughout life. It is often observed by a parent, who kisses the affected child and notes a "salty" taste. The first scientific documentation of this defect was made by di Sant'Agnese and co-workers (1953). These investigators found that cystic fibrosis patients had a consistent elevation in their sweat sodium and chloride concentrations, with a smaller rise in potassium. Only a few other conditions with elevated sweat electrolytes have been identified, as depicted in Fig. 1. It is interesting that the other conditions in which elevated sweat chloride concentrations are seen do not show any of the other significant clinical characteristics of cystic fibrosis. Thus, measurement of sweat electrolytes is the accepted method of laboratory diagnosis of cystic fibrosis. The only potentially serious consequence of this sweat electrolyte defect is that excessive salt loss and secondary vascular collapse may occur, especially in hot weather (di Sant'Agnese et al., 1953).

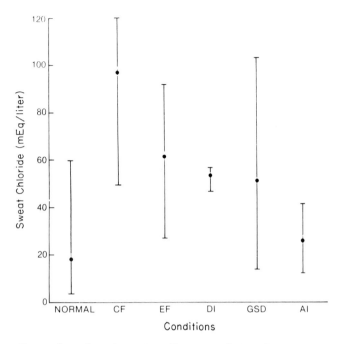

Fig. 1. Sweat electrolytes in various disease conditions. Bar represents range of observed values; mean (●). CF, Cystic fibrosis; ED, ectodermal dysplasia; DI, diabetes insipidus (■); GSD, glycogen storage disease; AI, adrenal insufficiency.

3. Respiratory Compromise

The pulmonary manifestations of cystic fibrosis vary in time of onset; some patients have involvement during infancy, whereas others remain symptom-free for years. However, all homozygotes eventually suffer respiratory disability. Typically, the patient will experience a series of acute respiratory infections, with a progressive decline in pulmonary function. Even between acute episodes, patients usually exhibit a chronic cough. As the disease progresses, a characteristic thick sputum is produced. Culture of this sputum usually reveals bacterial colonization, especially with *Staphylococcus aureus* and mucoid *Pseudomonas aeruginosa* (Mearns *et al.,* 1972). The roentgenographic findings of cystic fibrosis include peribronchial thickening, hyperinflation, patchy atelectasis, and increased anteroposterior diameter (Hodson and France, 1962). Pulmonary function tests show an obstructive pattern, with reduced vital capacity and expiratory flow rates, whereas residual volume and functional residual capacity are increased (West *et al.*, 1954).

The terminal stages of cystic fibrosis are characterized by pulmonary insufficiency. Patients are then subject to a number of serious complications. Hemoptysis is a common finding, which occasionally leads to excessive blood loss. Rupture of emphysematous blebs can produce pneumothoraces, with a range of clinical severity. Progressive hypoxemia and acidosis frequently lead to pulmonary hypertension and cor pulmonale. Even in the absence of acute complications, the pulmonary disability in cystic fibrosis is unremitting and eventually results in death.

4. Pancreatic Insufficiency

The gastrointestinal manifestations of cystic fibrosis are diverse and are often the first sign of the disease. Some newborns present with intestinal obstruction, referred to as meconium ileus. Other infants may exhibit prolapse of the rectum. In older children, pancreatic insufficiency often leads to poor growth, delayed maturation, and fat-soluble vitamin deficiencies. The symptoms of maldigestion include a ravenous appetite, poor growth, and frequent, bulky, greasy stools. Laboratory documentation of pancreatic insufficiency is rarely necessary to make a diagnosis of cystic fibrosis. If an assessment of an infant's pancreatic function is required, measurement of stool trypsin may prove to be useful.

5. Other Manifestations

In addition to the classic triad of increased sweat chloride, respiratory disease, and pancreatic insufficiency, patients with cystic fibrosis may exhibit other findings. Recurrent episodes of pancreatitis have been observed in patients who are spared from pancreatic insufficiency (Shwachman *et al.*, 1975). Glucose intolerance is more common in cystic fibrosis patients than in the general population, but does not correlate with disease severity. A spectrum in extent of hepatic disease may occur, ranging from focal biliary cirrhosis to occasional cases of diffuse cirrhosis and portal hypertension (de Sant'Agnese and Blanc, 1956).

Virtually all males with cystic fibrosis are sterile, with an absence of the epididymis, vas deferens, and seminal vesicles (Taussig *et al.*, 1972). Females with cystic fibrosis have normal reproductive anatomy and function, although delayed menarche is common. The female cervical mucus is abnormal but this has not been correlated with reproduction dysfunction. Other common clinical findings include nasal polyps and chronic purulent sinusitis.

C. Pathology

The pathology of cystic fibrosis parallels its clinical manifestations, with compromise of many exocrine tissues. At necropsy, the debilitating nature of this disease is evident in the spectrum of morphological derangement. Although a general progression of findings can be inferred, considerable individual variation is apparent. In the following sections, common patterns of organ involvement in cystic fibrosis are summarized.

1. Pancreas

The pathological changes seen in the pancreas were the source for the original name: "fibrocystic disease of the pancreas." On gross inspection, the pancreas appears firm and lobulated. On histological examination, the process is characterized by accumulation of hyaline, eosinophilic material in pancreatic ducts. As the ductal lumen occludes, there is secondary cystic dilation with compression and atrophy of the epithelial wall. Fibrosis occurs in periductular elements, eventually leading to replacement of acini by fat and fibrous tissue. It is estimated that maldigestion from pancreatic insufficiency requires destruction of 90% of the exocrine tissue. The islets of Langerhans are not primarily involved, but severe fibrosis may eventually compromise nonexocrine tissue (Oppenheimer and Esterly, 1975b). The postulated sequence of pancreatic disease goes from head to tail of the organ.

Newborns with cystic fibrosis, who die of meconium ileus and other causes, already have demonstrable pancreatic pathology. A recent study showed that the ratio of pancreatic acinar to connective tissue in cystic fibrosis was normal at 32 weeks postconception, but this ratio was reduced to 15% of normal within 4 months (Imrie et al., 1979). The sequence and mechanisms of pancreatic dysfunction is schematized in Fig. 2.

2. Respiratory Tract

The chronic progressive course of cystic fibrosis is typified by the pulmonary pathology. At birth, few lung abnormalities are present, whereas multiple changes occur by late infancy. The earliest microscopic finding is hyperplasia of the bronchial glands, especially the mucus-secreting elements. In addition, squamous metaplasia of the bronchial epithelium and submucosal infiltrations of inflammatory cells are observed (Bedrossian et al., 1976).

The viscid secretory material accumulates in airways, producing mucous plugs. Both airway obstruction and epithelial metaplasia com-

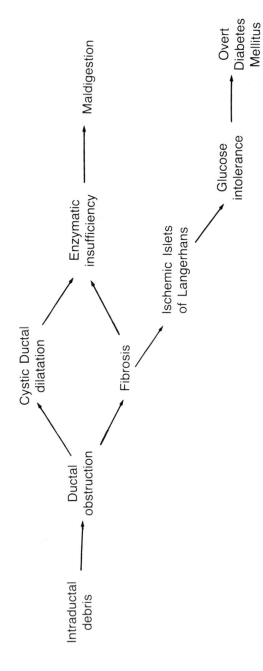

Fig. 2. Speculated pathogenesis of pancreatic disease in cystic fibrosis.

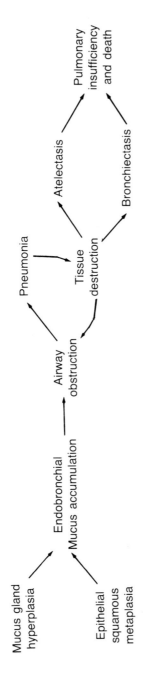

Fig. 3. Speculated pathogenesis of pulmonary disease in cystic fibrosis.

promise the normal pulmonary defense mechanisms and predispose to infection. A recurrent cycle of obstruction, followed by infection and secondary tissue destruction, eventually leads to bronchiectasis. By the age of 2 years, all patients with cystic fibrosis at autopsy manifest bronchiectasis (Stephen *et al.*, 1980).

Abnormalities of the lung parenchyma are less common than airway disease in cystic fibrosis. Nevertheless, most patients experience multiple bouts of pneumonia in the course of their disease. Occasional patients will go on to develop lobar atelectasis and obstructive emphysema (de Sant'Agnese, 1953). This sequence of pulmonary compromise is summarized in Fig. 3.

3. Eccrine Sweat Glands

Despite the clinical importance of abnormal sweat electrolytes in cystic fibrosis, no associated morphological change is apparent in the sweat glands by light or electron microscopic examination. Of particular importance is the absence of intraductal obstructive debris, which is so prominent in the pancreatic and pulmonary disease (Oppenheimer and Esterly, 1975b).

4. Other Pathology Findings

a. Salivary Gland. The mucus-producing salivary glands (submandibular, sublingual, and submucosal glands) all contain intraductal mucous accumulations. This typically progresses to postobstructional ductal dilatation and secondary gland enlargement. Of interest is the lack of corresponding changes in the parotid gland, which produces serous secretions (Barbero and Sibinga, 1962).

b. Gastrointestinal Tract. Other gastrointestinal pathology of cystic fibrosis includes dilatation of Brunner's glands and the crypts of Lieberkuhn in the intestine. The goblet cells of the rectum are increased in number and produce abnormal secretions (Oppenheimer and Esterly, 1975b).

c. Liver. The liver is also a common site of structural change in cystic fibrosis. The most common hepatic lesion is fatty change, which occurs despite seemingly adequate pancreatic enzyme replacement (Craig *et al.*, 1957). Biliary tract disease may also occur in newborns with cystic fibrosis. The microscopic appearance is characterized by inspissated eosinophilic material within the biliary tree. Fibrous tissue proliferation may produce focal biliary cirrhosis, which occasionally is associated with prolonged neonatal jaundice. In older pa-

The exocrine pancreas is responsible for two types of secretion, each with its own regulating stimuli, anatomical sites, and intracellular controls. The functional unit of the exocrine pancreas is depicted in Fig. 4. The electrolyte solution is made in the ductular cells that are referred to as centroacinar and intercalated cells. In contrast, pancreatic enzymes come from the acinar cells (Dixon, 1979). The details of stimulus–secretion coupling of the exocrine pancreas are presented in the next sections.

A. Electrolyte Secretions

The original stimulus for pancreatic electrolyte secretion is dietary intake. The process begins when partially digested, acidic food enters the duodenum, stimulating the release of secretin (a polypeptide hormone) from the intestinal mucosa. Secretin travels to pancreatic ductal cells, where it attaches to a membrane-bound receptor (Fig. 5). This secretin–receptor complex activates adenylate cyclase, which converts adenosine triphosphate to cyclic 3',5'-adenosine monophosphate (cAMP) (Schulz et al., 1974). The cAMP then serves as a second messenger between an extracellular stimulus and its intracellular physiological response. A rise in cytosolic cAMP is followed by electolyte secretion from pancreatic ductular cells. Biochemical analysis of this electrolyte solution reveals detectable levels of cAMP (Domschke et al., 1976). The mode of cAMP action is unclear but probably involves changes in membrane permeability to ions (Case et al., 1969).

Several schemes have been proposed for movement of electrolytes into pancreatic juice. The ultimate solution is rich in both sodium and bicarbonate, with smaller amounts of potassium and chloride (Escour-

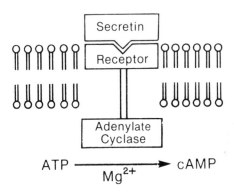

Fig. 5. Mechanism of secretin stimulation of ductalar cell.

tients with cystic fibrosis, chronic and diffuse scarring ʳ
severe hepatobiliary disease (Oppenheimer and Esterly, .

d. Reproductive System. The reproductive system is ɪ
most cases of cystic fibrosis. As previously described, viɪ
males are sterile because of organ dysgenesis. The vas dᵉ
atrophied, the seminal vesicles are absent, and occasionally
didymis is also absent. Females with cystic fibrosis are fertile ł
dilated mucous glands of the uterine cervix (Oppenheimer and ł
1975b).

III. THE NORMAL EXOCRINE PANCREAS

The mechanisms of pancreatic exocrine secretion are not fully
derstood. Nevertheless, vigorous research on this subject has yield
important insights. When considered together, these findings proviᵈ
a useful model of exocrine function. In this section, we will present aɪ
overview of normal pancreatic exocrine secretion. The discussion is
simplified by the omission of experimental details. Admittedly, this
may create an illusion of consensus on issues that remain controversial. Where research findings conflict, we have tried to present the
more internally consistent view.

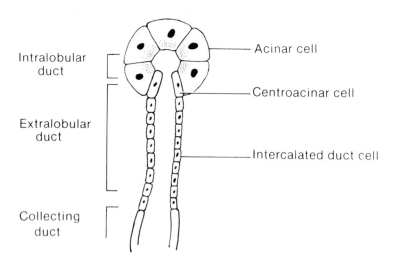

Intralobular
duct

Extralobular
duct

Collecting
duct

Acinar cell

Centroacinar cell

Intercalated duct cell

Fig. 4. Schematic diagram of the anatomy of pancreatic exocrine unit.

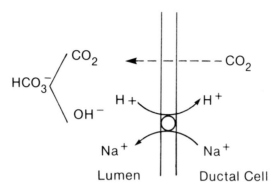

Fig. 6. Mechanism for bicarbonate and sodium ion formation in pancreatic electrolyte secretion.

rou *et al.*, 1978). The bicarbonate is predominantly derived from extracellular sources (Case *et al.*, 1970), with a smaller amount coming from intracellular metabolic carbon dioxide (Pascal *et al.*, 1976). Sodium ions are actively transported into pancreatic juice, in exchange for hydrogen ions (Swanson and Solomon, 1975). Energy to support active ion transport is derived from oxidative metabolism of glucose (Case and Scratcherd, 1974). Intracellular transport of hydrogen ion leaves a free hydroxyl group, which combines with carbon dioxide to produce bicarbonate in the ductal lumen (Fig. 6). This electrolyte secretion flows into the collecting duct and ultimately empties into the duodenum.

B. Enzyme Secretions

Pancreatic digestive enzymes are synthesized and stored in acinar cells. Jamieson and Palade (1967a,b) described an intricate transport mechanism for enzymes (see also Chapter 9). In brief, these secretory proteins are initially synthesized on polysomes. By sequential transfer, the proteins move to cisternae and then to transitional elements of the rough endoplasmic reticulum. Next, the proteins are packaged in smooth transport vesicles, in which they travel to the Golgi complex. Here, the proteins may undergo modification, before discharge in condensing vacuoles. These vacuoles increase in density until mature "zymogen granules" are formed; zymogen granules are predominantly composed of protein and are the principal site of secretory enzyme storage. Figure 7 depicts schematically this secretory process. During quiescence, zymogen granules accumulate at the apical end of acinar cells. In contrast, during secretion, these zymogen granules are pro-

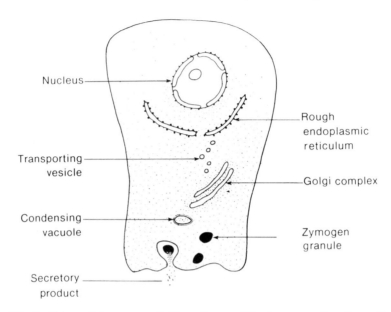

Fig. 7. Intracellular transport of secretory proteins in pancreatic acinar cell.

gressively depleted. The process of secretion occurs by fusion of a granule's membrane with the luminal cell membrane and exocytosis of granular contents (Jamieson and Palade, 1967b). More other studies suggest that granule membranes are recycled, i.e., removed from the cell membrane by endocytosis (Herzog and Reggio, 1980).

The stimuli for pancreatic enzyme secretion, like electolyte production, arise from ingested food. In the case of enzyme secretion, two important mediators are responsible. First, the cephalic and gastric phases of digestion cause the release of acetylcholine from the vagus nerve, which innervates the pancreas. Second, as partially digested proteins and fats enter the duodenum, pancreozymin (a 33-amino acid polypeptide hormone) is released from the intestinal mucosa (Bloom and Polak, 1978) and travels in the bloodstream to the pancreas. Both pancreozymin and acetylcholine interact with specific membrane receptors on the pancreatic cells. These mediator–receptor complexes cause a conformational change in the membrane (Mathews, 1974), with a consequent rise in cytosol calcium ion (Douglass, 1966). For many years, investigators have debated the source of this calcium ion. Some believe that calcium is released from the plasma membrane (Matthews, 1974), whereas others contend that it derives from intracellular stores (Iwatsuki and Peterson, 1977). The only apparent role of extracellular calcium is to replenish calcium supplies in prolonged secretion (Ginsburg and House, 1980). Regardless of the source of calcium, this ion has been proposed as the central mediator of pancreatic enzymatic secretion. In support of this role, intracellular injection of calcium produces a normal secretion of enzymes (Iwatsuki and Peterson, 1978). The precise action of calcium is less clear, but it is thought to bind to zymogen granule membranes, thereby neutralizing surface charges and facilitating fusion with the luminal cell membrane (Dean, 1974). Interestingly enough, calcium is present in the secreted proteinaceous material. Pancreatic digestive enzymes are discharged in an inactive precursor state and flow with electrolyte solution to the intestine, where the enzymes are activated by proteolytic cleavage.

The roles of cyclic adenosine (Bonting and de Pont, 1974) and guanosine (Albano et al., 1979) monophosphates as second messengers in pancreatic enzyme secretion have been proposed. Nevertheless, most experimental work supports calcium as the principal mediator. Discrepant findings may be explained in part by intraspecies differences (Robberecht, 1976).

IV. THE EXOCRINE PANCREAS IN CYSTIC FIBROSIS

Eighty percent of cystic fibrosis patients have symptoms of maldigestion and have no detectable pancreatic enzyme activity. Of the remaining 20%, approximately one-half exhibit a partial loss in pancreatic enzyme activity (de Sant'Agnese, 1955). Although pancreatic insufficiency is not an obligate manifestation of cystic fibrosis, it often leads to the initial clinical presentation. Cystic fibrosis remains a common organic cause of failure to thrive during infancy. This may occur in a child without any specific symptoms or signs of malabsorption. On occasion, the diagnosis may be unnecessarily delayed until the full clinical picture is apparent. The clinician must maintain a high level of suspicion and should consider an early sweat electrolyte test in children with unexplained failure to thrive.

Several research groups have studied pancreatic function in cystic fibrosis. Hadorn and co-workers (1968a) examined a group of cystic fibrosis patients with no clinical evidence of maldigestion. In these patients, the volume of pancreatic juice was decreased to less than one-sixth of normal amounts. The bicarbonate concentration was reported as roughly 20% of that found in controls, whereas pancreatic enzyme concentrations were all above normal. The elevated enzyme concentration is due to the inappropriately low fluid volume, and the absolute amount of secreted enzyme was less than controls. Analysis of specific enzymes revealed variation in relative diminution. The most severely affected enzyme was amylase, which was decreased in the fibrosis patients to 25% of control output. Lipase and trypsin were similarly reduced to 32 and 36% of normal production, respectively. Carboxypeptidase and chymotrypsin were least affected, at 52 and 63% of control values, respectively.

In another study, Zoppi and colleagues (1970a,b) found a comparable reduction in pancreatic juice volume in cystic fibrosis patients. These authors reported an even greater reduction in bicarbonate concentration to 9% of normal. They reported a decrease in sodium concentration to 18% of normal, whereas potassium and calcium were less severely affected at 25 and 33% of normal secretion, respectively.

Analysis of the proteinaceous material in pancreatic secretions of cystic fibrosis patients revealed a predominance of soluble, non-enzymatic proteins. These patients have increased amounts of cellular debris in their pancreatic juice, which is not morphologically different from material found in normal secretions. Electrophoresis of pancreatic proteins revealed elevated concentration of serum proteins in the pancreatic secretion of cystic fibrosis patients, possibly related to the loss of degradative enzyme activity.

The pattern of secretion in cystic fibrosis is distinctly different from that seen as a result of other causes of pancreatic insufficiency. For instance, in pancreatitis, both enzyme and bicarbonate concentrations tend to be reduced below normal (Hadorn et al., 1968b). In children with pancreatic insufficiency of other origin, the pancreatic secretion is normal in volume but exhibits low enzyme and bicarbonate concentrations (Hadorn et al., 1968b). These observations led them to speculate that the pathogenesis of pancreatic insufficiency in cystic fibrosis must primarily involve the fluid and electrolyte secretion. They suggested three possible mechanisms for this dysfunction: (1) absence of secretin stimulation; (2) altered ductal cell function; and (3) loss of normal ductal cell control. The first possibility can be excluded by the documentation of normal secretin levels in cystic fibrosis patients (Gibbs and Gershbein, 1950). Hadorn favored the loss of cellular control hypothesis because ductal cell function seemed relatively intact in some cystic fibrosis patients. Since this hypothesis was advanced, much has been learned about the normal control of pancreatic exocrine secretion. As already noted, the control of enzyme and electrolyte secretion are distinct processes. It is thus clearly feasible for one secretory system to be deranged, with minimal effect on the other secretion process. A subtle disturbance in electrolyte regulation might not alter production of pancreatic enzymes. In contrast, a disease such as pancreatitis causes diffuse parenchymal destruction, with limitation of both electrolyte and enzyme secretion. The caveat to be remembered during speculation about cystic fibrosis pathogenesis is that any explanation must account for all of the exocrine dysfunctions.

V.   OTHER SECRETIONS IN CYSTIC FIBROSIS

In the preceding discussion, we have emphasized the abnormality of pancreatic exocrine secretions in cystic fibrosis. Also, reference was made to associated alterations in eccrine sweat, tracheobronchial, and gastrointestinal secretions. The generalized nature of this disease suggests that the basic defect is shared by each of these gland types. It is important to recognize that not all bodily secretions are affected by cystic fibrosis. Comparison of the altered and unaffected secretions might provide insight into the underlying pathogenesis of cystic fibrosis.

A.   Apocrine Sweat Glands

The apocrine sweat glands discharge a thick fluid product in response to sympathetic stimulation. In contrast to eccrine sweat glands, adrenergic (not cholinegic) mediators are responsible for apocrine stimulation. Located in the groin, axilla, chest, and scalp, the apocrine glands are present from birth, but do not become functional until puberty.

In cystic fibrosis, the apocrine glands have no clinical dysfunction, but microscopic examination often reveals eosinophilic debris in the ductal lumen. As a consequence, the duct dilates progressively, with the passage of time. Histochemical analysis indicates that the luminal material consists of neutral and acid mucopolysaccharides. Although this apocrine ductal obstruction is rare in normal children, it is seen occasionally in normal adults. The etiologic and functional significances of this morphological change in cystic fibrosis is not known.

B.   Breast

We are unaware of any published information on the physiology and biochemistry of lactation in cystic fibrosis. A study of breast pathology in cystic fibrosis was reported, but because it is based upon a single patient, the generalizability of results is unclear. In the reported case, the breast was of normal size, but microscopic examination revealed lobular agenesis with absence of ductule budding. The authors noted a reduction of intraductal secretion, but no mucous inspissation was present (Ward, 1972).

C. Kidney

Robson *et al.* (1971) reported on renal function in a series of patients with cystic fibrosis. A normal glomerular filtration rate was observed in all patients, but they suffered restriction in free water clearance that correlated with disease severity. The patients were able to decrease salt excretion when dietary salt was restricted. However, the authors noted an abnormally high proximal sodium reabsorption associated with diminished sodium delivery to the distal tubule. No pathological specimens were obtained, so it is uncertain whether these functional changes were associated with morphological abnormalities.

D. Endocrine Glands

1. Growth Hormone

Growth hormone is a polypeptide hormone that stimulates protein synthesis, lipolysis, and hyperglycemia. It is released from the anterior pituitary under stimulation from various neurotransmitters: norepinephrine, dopamine, and serotonin. There is also a hypothalamic peptide (somatostatin) that inhibits somatotropin release. One study showed normal growth hormone levels in children with cystic fibrosis, despite manifest growth retardation (Rosenfield *et al.*, 1981).

2. Somatomedin

Somatomedin is produced by the liver (and probably other tissues) in response to growth hormone stimulation. Somatomedin then circulates to the cartilage growth plates, where it stimulates collagen and protein synthesis. A bioassay of somatomedin levels in cystic fibrosis suggested low plasma levels (Lee *et al.*, 1980). These authors speculated that the growth retardation in cystic fibrosis results from suppression of somatomedin generation secondary to protein malnutrition. However, a more reliable radioimmunoassay for somatomedin in growth-retarded cystic fibrosis patients revealed normal levels (Rosenfield *et al.*, 1981). Alternative explanations for the poor growth in cystic fibrosis include a defect in the receptor for somatomedin, diminished responsiveness to somatomedin secondary to tissue hypoxia, or a metabolic derangement. The most likely explanation is that insufficient food stuffs are absorbed for optimal growth and development.

3. Prolactin

Prolactin is a polypeptide hormone that stimulates lactation (see chapters 8 and 16). It is released from the anterior pituitary, under stimulation by thyrotropin-releasing hormone and probably another prolactin-releasing factor. Prolactin secretion is reduced by a specific prolactin-inhibiting factor, mediated by dopaminergic neurotransmission. Serum prolactin levels in children with cystic fibrosis are comparable to levels in normal children (Biswas et al., 1976).

4. Thyroid Hormones

The thyroid hormones participate in the regulation of many processes: body temperature maintenance, body weight control, heart stimulation, protein synthesis, and cholesterol and triglyceride metabolism. In brief, hypothalamic thyroid-releasing hormone stimulates the anterior pituitary to secrete thyrotropin. Thyrotropin (TSH), in turn, stimulates the thyroid to release the thyroid hormones thyroxine and triiodothyronine. By negative feedback control, the thyroid hormones inhibit TSH secretion. One study revealed a normal thyrotropin response to thyroid-releasing hormone in cystic fibrosis patients (Segall-Blank et al., 1981). In addition, circulating thyroxine levels were normal, but triiodothyronine was decreased. The authors attribute the latter finding to a diminished peripheral conversion of thyroxine to triiodothyronine in cystic fibrosis. The reason for the abnormality is unclear, but one explanation is that chronic hypoxia is the cause because children with cyanotic heart disease also have decreased triiodothyronine (Moshag et al., 1980).

5. Parathormone

The release of parathormone by the parathyroids is stimulated by hypocalcemia and inhibited by hypercalcemia. The end organs of parathormone action are bones and the kidney. The renal parathormone-induced calcium reabsorption is mediated by cAMP. Simopoulos and colleagues (1972) reported that patients with cystic fibrosis do not suppress parathormone levels normally in response to calcium infusions. Nevertheless, injection of parathyroid extract into patients resulted in normal end-organ calcium conservation. This suggests that the parathormone-responsive cAMP system in cystic fibrosis must be intact.

6. Gonadotropins and Testosterone

The gonadotropins (follicle-stimulating hormone and luteinizing hormone) are released from the anterior pituitary in response to gonadotropin-releasing hormone from the hypothalamus (see Chapters 14 and 15). Follicle-stimulating hormone stimulates follicle growth in females and spermatogenesis in males. Luteinizing hormone induces ovulation and maintains the corpus luteum in females and stimulates testosterone production by the testes in males. By negative feedback control, estrogens inhibit the release of both follicle-stimulating and luteinizing hormone. In males, testosterone inhibits the release of luteinizing hormone. In males with cystic fibrosis, despite infertility, follicle-stimulating hormone, luteinizing hormone, and testosterone levels are present in normal concentrations (Rosen and Weintraub, 1971). We are not aware of corresponding information on gonadotropins in females with cystic fibrosis.

7. Renin–Angiotensin

Renin is secreted by the juxtaglomerular cells of the kidney in response to decreased glomerular filtration, diminished glomerular pressure, or increased sympathetic stimulation. In the circulation, renin acts on renin substrate to produce a peptide angiotensin II, which causes renal efferent arterioles to constrict. The principal consequence of arteriolar constriction is increased renal tubular reabsorption and fluid conservation. Angiotensin II also stimulates the release of aldosterone from the adrenal cortex. Aldosterone acts to augment renal sodium reabsorption and also to elevate potassium excretion. In patients with cystic fibrosis, basal plasma renin activity is increased over controls but varies normally with body position change (Simopoulos *et al.*, 1971). This results in an elevation in plasma aldosterone. The most logical explanation for these changes are the increased extrarenal sodium losses seen in these patients.

8. Gastrointestinal Hormones

There are a variety of gastrointestinal hormones that control the digestive process. In cystic fibrosis, some of these substances are present in normal amounts and others are secreted in abnormal quantities. For instance, gastrin, which stimulates gastric acid secretion, is found to be normal in these patients (Adrian *et al.*, 1980). Of particular interest is the fact that secretin (the stimulus for pancreatic electrolyte production) is also present in normal levels in cystic fibrosis. Other gastrointestinal hormones are found in abnormal concentrations in cystic fibrosis. Pancreozymin is detected in low basal levels and does not respond to a test meal. Similarly, gastric inhibitory peptide, which is secreted from the upper small intestine and suppresses gastric acid secretion, is basally depressed and responds poorly to food stimulus. Finally, enteroglucagon, which slows intestinal transit, is present at elevated basal levels but does not respond to ingested food (Adrian *et al.*, 1980). There is no good explanation for these defects in gut hormone secretion.

9. Insulin

Handwerger and co-workers (1969) reported that 42% of all patients with cystic fibrosis manifest insulinopenia to some degree. These authors demonstrated a progression from glucose intolerance to fasting hyperglycemia and glycosuria. They speculated that islet cell destruction secondary to diffuse pancreatic fibrosis was the causal mechanism. It has also been demonstrated that patients with cystic fibrosis have an impaired insulin and glucagon response to arginine infusion (Stahl *et al.*, 1974).

VI. CYSTIC FIBROSIS RESEARCH

Cystic fibrosis is a disease of exocrine secretion, with apparently normal secretion of most hormones, immunoglobulins and other white cell products, and even some exocrine products such as parotid saliva. Differences between the basic mechanisms involved in these kinds of secretions must exist, and in these differences lies a clue to the defective gene causing cystic fibrosis.

Although many gifted and creative physicians and scientists have exerted themselves in an effort to find the fundamental error in this disease, there is no real consensus at this time (di Sant'Agnese and Davis, 1976). A discussion of cystic fibrosis research attempting to relate it to exocrine secretion may lead to some insights into the genetic defect.

Research to determine the defect in cystic fibrosis may be divided somewhat arbitrarily into several areas.

A. Cystic Fibrosis "Factors"

The first significant findings in the search for an abnormal gene product in cystic fibrosis was reported by Spock and collaborators in 1967. They reported the presence of a factor in the serum of cystic fibrosis patients that caused disruption of the normal ciliary beating of rabbit tracheal explants. Multiple attempts to expand and quantify these findings have led to a complicated and confusing body of research. There does appear to be a "factor," which is at least quantitatively different from normal serum components, in cystic fibrosis secretions and serum. This substance binds to immunoglobulins, is heat labile, and is destroyed by proteolytic enzymes. Its molecular weight is estimated to be between 4,000 and 10,000. It may also be produced in tissue culture by cells from cystic fibrosis patients.

The major problems in identification of the factor or factors are the lack of a reproducible and quantitative assay system and the seeming instability of the substance. The ciliary dyskinesia assay is subjective, time consuming, and difficult. In addition, bronchial ciliary movement in cystic fibrosis patients appears to be normal, which somewhat confuses the issue. Attempts to develop a better and possibly more relevant assay continue in many laboratories.

Kurlandsky *et al.* (1980) developed an intriguing assay. Their system involves hypersecretion of mucus by a urn cell complex of a marine invertebrate in response to cystic fibrosis factor. The active factor in the assay appears to be similar or identical to the ciliary dyskinesia factor previously reported. This new assay system appears to be somewhat more quantitative, although certainly not simple. Because mucus-containing secretions of cystic fibrosis patients are abnormal, this is an intriguing finding. Confirmation and extension of this work may prove enlightening.

Many of the secretions of cystic fibrosis patients have been noted to have properties of increased tenacity, which is not explained in terms of simple viscosity changes alone. Attempts have been made to quantify and account for this characteristic difference in cystic fibrosis secretions. Litt *et al.* (1976) reported on a factor in parotid saliva from cystic fibrosis patients; this factor is present to a lesser extent in heterozygotes for the cystic fibrosis gene and reduced the zeta potential of tracheal mucus from dogs. (The zeta potential is a measure of the net charge on colloid particles and is related to the structure of the water molecules around the particles. As the zeta potential is reduced, the particles become unstable.) This characteristic change might account for some of the abnormalities in mucous secretions of cystic fibrosis patients. It would, however, not specifically explain the abnormalities in sweat electrolytes of cystic fibrosis patients.

Increased sodium and chloride in sweat of cystic fibrosis patients arises from decreased sodium reabsorption. Cystic fibrosis secretions, saliva, and sweat, when perfused through a rat parotid duct or normal sweat gland, have the capacity to block subsequent reabsorption of sodium by the duck (Mangos and McSherry, 1967). This is a difficult assay and is not in general use, but it appears to be consistent with the clinical defect. Further exploration of the mechanism of this phenomena may be fruitful.

Banchini et al. (1981) found that a "cystic fibrosis factor" that inhibited glucose-dependent sodium transport also appeared to be present in patients with Shwachman's disease. These patients have pancreatic insufficiency but none of the other stigmata and presumably not the gene defect of cystic fibrosis. This would imply that at least this "factor" is a result of nonspecific nutritional defects or other secondary problems rather than a true indication of the primary problem in cystic fibrosis.

B. Membrane Structure and Function in Cystic Fibrosis Tissue

Because ion transport and secretory processes are dependent on intact and functional plasma membranes, there has been extensive research to characterize membranes in cystic fibrosis patients in terms of ultrastructure, enzymes, and membrane structural components. Ward and Bowman (1976) examined cultured cells of cystic fibrosis patients, assaying surface enzymes at different times in the cell cycle. They found no change between cystic fibrosis and normal cells. Baur et al. (1976) reported on studies using scanning electron microscopy in which fibroblasts derived from cystic fibrosis homozygotes and heterozygotes were compared with normal fibroblasts. They could find no difference in the cell surface characteristics of the cell lines. In addition, Baig et al. (1975) characterized membrane components from fibroblasts grown in the presence of radioactive leucine, glucosamine, and fucose and did not find differences between plasma membranes of cystic fibrosis and normal cells.

Mahler and Riordan (1980) characterized plasma membranes from cultured fibroblasts from cystic fibrosis and normal patients. They measured phospholipid per unit of protein, cholesterol content, and the proportions of the individual phospholipid classes and their fatty acid compositions. In addition, they measured the fluidity of the membranes, the carbohydrate composition of the cell surface, and fucose content of the membranes. They found no difference between cystic fibrosis and normal patients in any of these parameters.

C.   Sodium–Potassium ATPase

Because one of the classic triad of disturbances in cystic fibrosis patients is the increased sodium chloride content of sweat, the membrane enzymes involved in sodium and potassium transport have been looked at by many groups. This has been extensively reviewed by di Sant'Agnese and Davis (1976). Breslow *et al.* (1981) looked at radioactive sodium influx in fibroblasts from patients, heterozygotes, and normal controls in the presence of ouabain. They found that fibroblasts from both homozygotes and heterozygotes accumulated less sodium than normal cells. Although they could not separate the heterozygotes from the homozygotes in their assay, there was no overlap between these two groups and normal controls. However, ouabain binding in cystic fibrosis cells has been reported to be normal (Quissell and Pitot, 1974). It will be interesting to see whether other labs can confirm these findings.

D.   Cyclic AMP Systems

Because cAMP has been implicated as the second messenger in pancreatic secretion of electrolyte solution as well as in many other systems in the body, this is a logical area to look for a defect in cystic fibrosis patients. There have been many problems with cAMP research in cystic fibrosis. Most research has been done using human fibroblasts and comparing normal with the cystic fibrosis cells. Because the fibroblast cAMP response to isoproterenol fluctuates during the cell cycle, it was important that Davis *et al.* (1980b) compared cAMP to isoproterenol at various times of the cell cycle. They found that the cellular cAMP content in response to both β-adrenergic stimulation and PGE_1 were comparable in normal and cystic fibrosis-derived fibroblast lines. However, cystic fibrosis fibroblasts appear to be relatively resistant to the toxic effects of isoproterenol, theophylline, and dibutyryl cAMP. This insensitivity might imply a lesion in this pathway distal to the adenylate cyclase (Epstein *et al.*, 1978).

E.   Calcium

Calcium plays an integral part in all secretory mechanisms. Some, but not all, exocrine secretions of cystic fibrosis patients have been reported to have increased calcium concentrations. This excess calcium may complex with glycoproteins in the secretions to increase turbidity. However, this does not take place in the duodenum or bronchus, so that the obstruction seen in these systems is not directly explained by this mechanism.

Christophe *et al.* (1974) contrast endocrine secretion of hormones, which is modulated by calcium uptake from the extracellular milieu, with pancreatic exocrine secretion, where intracellular transport of calcium from some specific pool is mobilized and results in elevation of cytoplasmic free calcium and thereby an increased rate of calcium flux. The difference between these two kinds of calcium actions may hold a clue to the specific exocrine dysfunctions in cystic fibrosis.

F. Glycoproteins

Increased sulfation of mucous glycoproteins in nasal and bronchial secretions in cystic fibrosis as well as increased acidity of these glycoproteins have been reported (Butcher, 1976). It is not clear yet whether this is a primary or secondary defect (Boat and Cheng, 1976).

G. Autonomic Nervous System

Exocrine secretion is in part regulated by the autonomic nervous system. Because of this, multiple attempts have been made to relate possible dysfunction in this system to cystic fibrosis. The most direct research with positive findings was done by Rubin *et al.* (1963), who reported impairment in the rate and magnitude of pupillary dilatation during dark adaptation. More recently, this has been extended by Davis *et al.* (1980a), who looked at the responses of cystic fibrosis patients versus controls to α-adrenergic, β-adrenergic, and cholinergic agents. They confirmed Rubin's work and found that, in addition, the cystic fibrosis patients had reduced cardiovascular sensitivity to β-adrenergic stimulation. Both patients and parents of cystic fibrosis patients were more sensitive to α-adrenergic stimulation than normal subjects. A similar increased sensitivity to cholinergic stimulation was seen in both patients and parents. They suggest that some lesion at or beyond the receptor level accounts for this abnormality. Because heterozygotes also show these abnormal responses, it is difficult to explain them in terms of secondary effects of the cystic fibrosis disease process.

Rats injected with autonomically active drugs have been shown to reproduce some of the pathology seen in cystic fibrosis patients (Mawhinney *et al.*, 1980). These experiments include injections of large doses of isoproterenol, which produces the salivary gland hyperplasia with increased sodium concentration and decreased flow rates in saliva. These isoproterenol-treated rats also exhibit hypertrophy of bronchial submucosal glands and hyperplasia of goblet cells as well. Similar findings have also been reported in rats that have been treated with reserpine (Martinez *et al.*, 1975). However, cystic fibrosis patients do not exhibit gross abnormalities of the autonomic nervous systems in terms of inability to regulate blood pressure, heart rate, or gastric or urinary tract motility.

The defect in autonomic responsivity in patients with cystic fibrosis, combined with the analogy of exocrine dysfunction in rats treated with autonomically active drugs, make this one of the most promising areas of investigation at the present time.

H. Polyamines and Methylation

Polyamine metabolism in cystic fibrosis has been reviewed by Farrell and Lundgren (1976). They note that polyamines may influence glycoprotein metabolism at physiological concentrations and that spermine can inhibit membrane ATPases, including membrane Ca^{2+}-ATPase activity. This enzyme has been reported to be different in cystic fibrosis. Polyamine metabolism is accelerated in isoproterenol-stimulated salivary glands, which are a model for cystic fibrosis. In addition, absolute changes in amounts of polyamines or changes in the ratio of spermidine and spermine may affect protein synthesis. They noted that human blood concentrations of polyamines vary widely and are particularly variable in females under the influence of hormonal changes in the menstrual cycle. However, they did find a significantly elevated spermidine to spermine ratio in whole blood extracts and erythrocytes from male cystic fibrosis homozygotes and heterozygotes.

Methionine deficiency during development in the rat has been shown to cause cystic degeneration and fibrosis of the pancreas (Veghelyi *et al.*, 1955). Although this finding has led several groups to study methylation reactions (particularly RNA methylation) in fibroblasts and lymphocytes, no consistent differences have been seen between cystic fibrosis and normal cells.

I. Enzymes

A defective enzyme has been sought in cystic fibrosis patients to account for the abnormalities. Although many different enzymes have been assayed and reported at one time or another to be abnormal in cystic fibrosis patients and/or persons heterozygous for the cystic fibrosis gene, no consistent and reproducible defect has been shown to be present.

VII. CONCLUSION

It has been said in clinical medicine that when there are many different treatments for a given disease it is because no treatment has been found to be effective. We think that a parallel analogy to clinically relevant research is obvious. At the present time there are many positive findings in cystic fibrosis research. Perhaps tomorrow there will be only one relevant result. Meanwhile, increased understanding of the basic process of secretion may come from scientists looking for the answer to this disease. When the "answer" to cystic fibrosis is found, it will certainly teach us more about the basic mechanisms of secretions. This circle of basic science and clinical medicine is the reason for this chapter, which may stand alone in this volume as containing no new data and certainly no answers.

ACKNOWLEDGMENTS

The authors wish to thank Pat Rattal for expert typing of the manuscript.

REFERENCES

Adrian, T. E., McKiernan, J., Johnstone, D. I., Hiller, E. J., Vyas, H., Sarson, D. L., and Bloom, S. R. (1980). Hormonal abnormalities of the pancreas and gut in cystic fibrosis. *Gastroenterology* **79**, 460–465.

Albano, J., Bhoola, K. D., and Harvey, R. F. (1979). The messenger role of cyclic GMP and calcium in the exocrine pancreas. *J. Physiol. (London)* **293**, 49P–50P.

Anderson, D. H. (1938). Cystic fibrosis of pancreas and its relation to celine disease: Clinical and pathological study. *Am. J. Dis. Child.* **56**, 344–399.

Baig, M. M., Citorelli, J. J., and Roberts, R. M. (1975). Plasma membrane components of skin fibroblasts from normal individuals and patients with cystic fibrosis. *J. Pediatr. (St. Louis)* **86**, 72–76.

Banchini, G., Harries, J. Z., Milla, P. J., Muller, O. P. R., Romm, E., and Tripp, J. H. (1981). Short communication: Cystic fibrosis "factor" present also in sera of Shwachman's pancreatic insufficiency. *Pediatr. Res.* **15**, 1073–1075.

Barbero, G. J., and Sibinga, M. S. (1962). Enlargement of the submaxillary salivary glands in cystic fibrosis. *Pediatrics* **29**, 788–793.

Baur, P. S., Bolton, W. E., and Barranco, S. C. (1976). Electron microscopy and microchemical analysis of cystic fibrosis diploid fibroblasts *in vitro*. *Tex. Rep. Biol. Med.* **34**, 113–134.

Bedrossian, C. W. M., Greenberg, S. D., and Singer, D. B. (1976). The lung in cystic fibrosis. *Hum. Pathol.* **7**, 195–204.

Biswas, S., Norman, A. P., Baffoe, G., and Graves, L. (1976). Prolactin, growth hormone, and alpha-Fetalprotein in children with cystic fibrosis. *Clin. Chim. Acta* **69**, 541–542.

Bloom, S. R., and Polak, J. M. (1978). Gut hormone overview. *In* "Gut Hormones" (S. R. Bloom, ed.), pp. 3–18. Churchill, London.

Boat, T. F., and Cheng, P. W. (1976). Mucus glycoproteins. *In* "Cystic Fibrosis: Projections into the Future" (J. A. Mangos and R. C. Talamo, eds.), pp. 165–178. Symposium Specialist Medical Books, New York.

Bonting, S. L., and de Pont, J. J. H. H. M. (1974). Adenylate cyclase and phosphodiesterase in rat pancreas. *In* "Secretory Mechanisms of Exocrine Pancreas" (N. A. Thorn and O. H. Petersen, eds.), pp. 363–376. Academic Press, New York.

Breslow, J. L., MacPherson, J., and Epstein, J. (1981). Distinguishing homozygous and heterozygous cystic fibrosis fibroblasts from normal cells by differences in sodium transport. *N. Engl. J. Med.* **304**, 1–5.

Butcher, F. R. (1976). Mucus glycoproteins. *In* "Cystic Fibrosis: Projections into the Future" (J. A. Mangos and R. C. Talamo, eds.), pp. 165–178. Symposium Specialists Medical Books, New York.

Case, R. M., and Scratcherd, T. (1974). The secretion of alkali metal ions by the perfused cat pancreas as influenced by the composition and osmolality of the external environment and by inhibitors of metabolism and Na^+, K^+ ATPase activity. *J. Physiol. (London)* **242**, 415–428.

Case, R. M., Harper, A. A., and Scratcherd, T. (1969). Water and electrolyte secretion by the pancreas. *In* "The Exocrine Gland" (S. Y. Bothelo, F. Brooks, and W. B. Shelly, eds.), pp. 39–56. Univ. of Pennsylvania Press, Philadelphia.

Case, R. M., Scratcherd, T., and Wayne, R. A. (1970). The origin and secretion of pancreatic juice bicarbonate. *J. Physiol. (London)* **210**, 1–15.

Christophe, J., Robberecht, P., Deschodt-Lanckman, M., Lambert, M., Van Leemput-Contrez, and Camus, J. (1974). Molecular basis of enzyme secretion by the exocrine pancreas. *Adv. Cytopharmocol.* **2**, 47–61.

Craig, J. M., Haddad, H., and Shawachmon, H. (1957). The pathological changes in the liver in cystic fibrosis of the pancreas. *Am. J. Dis. Child.* **93**, 357–369.

Davis, P. B., Shelhamer, J. R., and Kaliner, M. (1980a). Abnormal adrenergic and cholinergic sensitivity in cystic fibrosis. *N. Engl. J. Med.* **302**, 1453–1456.

Davis, P. B., Hill, S. C., and Ulane, M. M. (1980b). Hormone-stimulated cyclic AMP production by skin fibroblasts cultured from healthy persons and patients with cystic fibrosis. *Pediatr. Res.* **14**, 863–868.

Dean, P. M. (1974). The electokinetic properties of isolated secretory particles. *In* "Secretory Mechanisms of Exocrine Pancreas" (N. A. Thorn and O. H. Peterson, eds.), pp. 152–161. Academic Press, New York.

di Sant'Agnese, P. A. (1953). Bronchial obstruction with lobar atelectasis and emphysema in cystic fibrosis of the pancreas. *Pediatrics* **12**, 178–190.

di Sant'Agnese, P. A. (1955). Fibrocystic disease of pancreas with normal or partial pancreatic function: Current views on pathogenesis and diagnosis. *Pediatrics* **15**, 683–696.

di Sant'Agnese, P. A., and Blanc, W. A. (1956). A distinctive type of biliary cirrhosis of the liver associated with cystic fibrosis of the pancreas. *Pediatrics* **18**, 387–409.

di Sant'Agnese, P. A., and Davis, P. (1976). Research in cystic fibrosis. *N. Engl. J. Med.* **295**, 481–485, 534–541, 597–602.

di Sant'Agnese, P. A., and Talamo, R. C. (1967). Pathogenesis and physiopathology of cystic fibrosis of the pancreas. *N. Engl. J. Med.* **277**, 1287–1294, 1344–1352, 1399–1458.

di Sant'Agnese, P. A., Darling, R. C., Perera, G. A., and Shea, E. (1953). Abnormal electrolyte composition of sweat in cystic fibrosis of the pancreas. *Pediatrics* **12**, 549–563.

Dixon, J. S. (1979). "Histology: Ultrastructure in the Exocrine Pancreas" (H. T. Howat and H. Sarles, eds.), pp. 31–49. Saunders, Philadelphia, Pennsylvania.

Domschke, S., Domshke, W., Rosch, W., Konturek, S. J., Wunsch, E., and Demling, L. (1976). Bicarbonate and cAMP content of pure human pancreatic juice in response to graded doses of secretin. *Gastroenterology* **70**, 533–536.

Douglass, W. W. (1966). Calcium dependent links in stimulus-secretion coupling in the adrenal medulla and neurohypophysis. *Wenner-Gren Cent. Symp. Ser.* pp. 267–290.

Epstein, J., Breslow, J. L., Fitzsimmons, M. J., and Vayo, M. M. (1978). Pleiotropic drug resistance in cystic fibrosis fibroblasts: Increased resistance to cyclic AMP. *Somatic Cell Genet* **4**, 451–460.

Escourrou, J., Frexinus, J., and Ribet, A. (1978). Biochemical studies of pancreatic juice collected by duodenal aspiration and endoscopic cannulation of the main pancreatic duct. *Am. J. Dig. Dis.* **23**, 173–177.

Farrell, P. M., and Lundgren, D. W. (1976). Recent observations concerning RNA methylation and polyamines metabolism in cystic fibrosis. *In* "Cystic Fibrosis: Projections into the Future" (J. A. Mangos and R. C. Talamo, eds.), pp. 223–241. Symposium Specialist Medical Books, New York.

Feigal, R., and Shapiro, B. L. (1979). Altered intracellular calcium in fibroblasts from patients with cystic fibrosis and heterozygotes. *Pediatr. Res.* **13**, 764–768.

Gibbs, G. E., and Gershbein, L. L. (1950). Presence of secretion in cystic fibrosis of the pancreas. *Proc. Soc. Exp. Biol. Med.* **74**, 336–337.

Ginsburg, B. L., and House, C. R. (1980). Stimulus response in coupling in gland cells. *Annu. Rev. Biophys. Bioeng.* **9**, 55–80.

Hadorn, B., Johansen, P. G., and Anderson, C. M. (1968a). Pancreozymin secretin test of exocrine pancreatic function in cystic fibrosis and significance of the result for the pathogenesis of the disease. *Can. Med. Assoc. J.* **98**, 377–385.

Hadorn, B., Zoppi, G., Shmerling, D. H., Prader, A., McIntyre, I., and Anderson, C. M. (1968b). Quantitative assessment of exocrine pancreatic function in infants and children. *J. Pediatr.* **73**, 39–50.

Handwerger, S., Roth, J., Gorden, P., di Sant'Agnese, P. A., Carpenter, D. F., and Peter, G. (1969). Glucose intolerance in cystic fibrosis. *N. Engl. J. Med.* **281**, 451–461.

Herzog, V., and Reggio, H. (1980). Pathways of endocytosis from luminal plasma membrane in rat exocrine pancreas. *Eur. J. Cell Biol.* **21**, 141–150.

Hodson, C. J., and France, N. E. (1962). Pulmonary changes in cystic fibrosis of the pancreas a radio-pathological study. *Clin. Radiol.* **13**, 54–161.

Imrie, J. R., Fagan, D. G., and Sturgess, J. M. (1979). Quantitative evaluation of the development of the exocrine pancreas in cystic and control infants. *Am. J. Pathol.* **95**, 697–707.

Iwatsuki, N., and Petersen, O. H. (1977). Acetylcholine-like effects of intercellular calcium application in pancreatic acinar cells. *Nature (London)* **268**, 147–149.

Iwatsuki, N., and Petersen, O. H. (1978). Electrical coupling and uncoupling of exocrine acinar cells. *J. Cell Biol.* **79**, 533–545.

Jamieson, J. D., and Palade, G. E. (1967a). Intracellular transport of the secretory proteins in the pancreatic exocrine cell. I. Role of the peripheral elements of the golgi complex. *J. Cell Biol.* **34**, 577–596.

Jamieson, J. D., and Palade, G. E. (1967b). Intracellular transport of the secretory proteins in the pancreatic exocrine cell. II. Transport to condensing vacuoles and zymogen granules. *J. Cell Biol.* **34**, 597–615.

Kurlandsky, L. E., Berninger, R. W., and Talamo, R. C. (1980). Mucus-stimulating activity in the sera of patients with cystic fibrosis: Demonstration and preliminary fractionation. *Pediatr. Res.* **14**, 1263–1268.

Lee, J. A., Dickinson, L. S., Kilgore, B. S., Warren, R. H., and Elders, M. J. (1980). Somatomedin activity in cystic fibrosis and reserpinized rats: Possible explanation for growth retardation. *Ann. Clin. Lab. Sci.* **10,** 227–233.

Litt, M., Khan, M. A., Kiwart, H., and Rosenlund, M. L. (1976). Detection of cystic fibrosis heterozygotes using the zeta potential reduction method. *Tex. Rep. Biol. Med.* **34,** 151–154.

Maler, T., and Riordan, J. R. (1980). Isolation and characterization of the plasma membranes of cultured lymphoblasts from patients with cystic fibrosis and normal individuals. *Biochim. Biophys. Acta* **598,** 1–15.

Mangos, J. A., and McSherry, N. R. (1967). Sodium transport: Inhibitory factor in sweat of patients with cystic fibrosis. *Science* **158,** 135–137.

Martinez, J. R., Adelstein, E., Quissell, D. U., and Barbero, G. J. (1975). The chronically reserpinized rat as a possible model for cystic fibrosis. *Pediatr. Res.* **9,** 463–475.

Mathews, E. K. (1974). Bioelectrical properties of secretory cells. *In* "Secretory Mechanisms of Exocrine Pancreas" (N. A. Thorn and O. H. Peterson, eds.), pp. 185–194. Academic Press, New York.

Mawhinney, T. P., Martinez, J. R., Feather, M. S., and Barbero, D. J. (1980). Composition of pulmonary lavage fluid in control and treated rats following isoproterenol and pilocarpine administration. *Pediatr. Res.* **14,** 872–875.

Mearns, M. B., Hart, G. H., and Rushworth, R. (1972). Bacterial flora of respiratory tract in patients with cystic fibrosis. *Arch. Dis. Child.* **47,** 902–907.

Moshag, T., Chance, K. H., Kaplan, M. M., Utiger, R. D., and Takahashi, O. (1980). Effects of hypoxia on thyroid function tests. *J. Pediatr.* **97,** 602–604.

Oppenheimer, E. H., and Esterly, J. R. (1975a). Hepatic changes in young infants with cystic fibrosis: Possible relation to focal biliary cirrhosis. *J. Pediatr.* **86,** 683–689.

Oppenheimer, E. H., and Esterly, J. R. (1975b). Pathology of cystic fibrosis review of the literature and comparison with 146 autopsied cases. *Perspect. Pediatr. Pathol.* **2,** 241–278.

Pascal, J. P., Roux, P., Vaysse, N., Lacroix, A., Martinel, C., and Ribet, A. (1976). Respirator exchanges and acid-base balance during perfusion of *ex vivo* isolated pancreas. *Am. J. Dig. Dis.* **21,** 381–388.

Phillips, J. A., Hjelle, B. L., Seeburg, P. H., and Zachmann, M. (1981). Molecular basis for familial isolated growth hormone deficiency. *Proc. Natl. Acad. Sci. U.S.A.* **78,** 6372–6375.

Quissel, D. O., and Pitot, H. C. (1974). Number of ouabain-binding sites in fibroblasts from normal subjects and patients with cystic fibrosis. *Nature (London)* **247,** 115–116.

Robberecht, P. (1976). The role of cyclic nucleotides in pancreatic enzyme and electrolyte secretion. *In* "Stimulus-Secretion Coupling in Gastrointestinal Tract" (R. M. Case and H. Goebell, eds.), pp. 203–226. MTP Press, Lancaster.

Robson, A. M., Tateishi, S., Ingelfinger, J. R., Strominger, D. B., and Klahr, S. (1971). Renal function in patients with cystic fibrosis. *J. Pediatr.* **79,** 42–50.

Rosen, S. W., and Weintraub, B. D. (1971). Monotropic increase in serum FSH correlated with low sperm count in young men with idiopathic oligospermia and aspermia. *J. Clin. Endocrinol. Metab.* **32,** 410–416.

Rosenfield, R. G., Landon, C., Lewiston, N., Nagashima, R., and Hintz, R. L. (1981). Demonstraion of normal plasma somatomedin concentrations in cystic fibrosis. *J. Pediatr.* **99,** 252–254.

Rubin, L. S., Barbero, G. J., Chernick, W. S., and Sibinga, M. S. (1963). Pupillary reactivity as a measure of antonomic balance in cystic fibrosis. *J. Pediatr* **63,** 1120–1129.

Schulz, I., Pederson, R., Wizemann, V., and Kondo, S. (1974). Stimulatory process of the exocrine pancreas and their inhibition by a non-penetrating SH-reagent. *In* "Secretory Mechanisms of Exocrine Glands" (N. A. Thorn and O. H. Petersen, eds.), pp. 88–95. Academic Press, New York.

Schwachman, H., Lebenthal, E. and Khaw, K. T. (1975). Recurrent acute pancreatitis in patients with cystic fibrosis with normal pancreatic enzymes. *Pediatrics* **55**, 86–95.

Segall-Blank, M., Vagenakis, A. G., Shwachman, H., Ingbar, S. H., and Braverman, L. E. (1981). Thyroid gland function and pituitary TSH reserve in patients with cystic fibrosis. *J. Pediatr.* **98**, 218–222.

Simopoulos, A. P., Lapey, A., Boat, T. F., di Sant'Agnese, P. A., and Bartter, F. C. (1971). The renin-angiotensin-aldosterone system in patients with cystic fibrosis of the pancreas. *Pediatr. Res.* **5**, 626–632.

Simopoulos, A. P., Taussig, L. M., Murad, F., Arnaud, C. D., di Sant'Agnese, P. A., Kattwinkel, J., and Bartter, F. C. (1972). Parathyroid function in patients with cystic fibrosis. *Pediatr. Res.* **6**, 355.

Spock, A., Heich, H. M. C., Cress, H., and Logan, W. S. (1967). Abnormal serum factor in patients with cystic fibrosis of the pancreas. *Pediatr. Res.* **1**, 173–177.

Stahl, M., Girard, J., Rutishauser, M., Nars, P. W., and Zuppinger, K. (1974). Endocrine function of the pancreas in cystic fibrosis evidence for an impaired glucagon and insulin response following arginine infusion. *J. Pediatr.* **84**, 821–824.

Steinberg, A. G., and Brown, D. C. (1960). On the incidence of cystic fibrosis of the pancreas. *Am. J. Hum. Genet.* **12**, 416–424.

Stephen, V., Gotz, M., and Stephen, K. (1980). Cystic fibrosis. *Ergeb. Inn. Med. Kinderheilkd.* **44**, 73–174.

Swanson, C. H., and Solomon, A. K. (1975). Micropuncture analysis of the cellular mechanisms of electrolyte secretion by the *in vitro* rabbit pancreas. *J. Gen. Physiol.* **65**, 22–45.

Taussig, L. M., Lobeck, C. C., di Sant'Agnese, P. A., Ackerman, D. R., and Kattwinkel, J. (1972). Fertility in males with cystic fibrosis. *N. Engl. J. Med.* **278**, 586–589.

Veghelyi, P. V., Sos, J., and Kemeny, T. T. (1955). Prenatal lesions of the pancreas. *Am. J. Dis. Child.* **90**, 28–34.

Ward, A. M. (1972). The structure of the breast in mucoviscidosis. *J. Clin. Pathol.* **25**, 119–122.

Ward, J. B., Jr., and Bowman, B. H. (1976). Surface enzymes in cultured fibroblasts from cystic fibrosis patients. *Tex. Rep. Biol. Med.* **34**, 83–96.

West, J. R., Levin, S. M., and di Sant'Agnese, P. A. (1954). Pulmonary function in cystic fibrosis of the pancreas. *Pediatrics* **13**, 155–164.

Wood, R. E., Boat, T. F., and Doershuk, C. F. (1976). Cystic fibrosis. *Am. Rev. Respir. Dis.* **113**, 833–878.

Zoppi, G., Schmerling, D. H., Gaburro, D., and Prader, A. (1970a). The electrolyte and protein contents and outputs in duodenal juice after pancreatin and secretin stimulation in normal children and in patients with cystic fibrosis. *Acta Paediat. Scand.* **59**, 692–696.

Zoppi, G., Shmerling, D. M., Gaburro, D., and Prader, A. (1970b). Protein content and pancreatic enzyme activities of duodenal juice in normal children and in children with exocrine pancreatic insufficiency. *Meh. Paediat. Acta* **23**, 577–590.

PART V
MECHANISMS AND MODULATION OF SECRETION AND RELEASE

11

Regulation of Steroidogenesis in Leydig Cells

ANITA H. PAYNE, DAVID J. CHASE, AND
PETER J. O'SHAUGHNESSY

I. INTRODUCTION

Leydig cells, which are found in the interstitial tissue between semi-niferous tubules, are the site of testosterone synthesis in the testis. In addition to Leydig cells, interstitial tissue also contains macrophages,

355

fibroblasts, capillaries, and lymph vessels (Christensen, 1975). In the rat, approximately 16% of testicular volume is occupied by interstitial tissue and less than 3% by Leydig cells (Mori and Christensen, 1980). Luteinizing hormone (LH), which is secreted by the anterior pituitary gland, has been shown to be the only hormone essential for maintenance of testicular testosterone production (Zipf et al., 1978a). The effects of LH on steroidogenesis are initiated by its binding to high-affinity receptors on the surface of Leydig cell plasma membranes. The binding of LH to its receptor stimulates adenylate cyclase activity and results in an increase in intracellular accumulation of cAMP, activation of protein kinase (Dufau et al., 1978), and steroid production.

The relationship between changes in LH receptors of Leydig cells and changes in steroid production has been the subject of numerous investigations during the past decade. Hypophysectomy results in a decrease in testicular LH receptors and LH-stimulated testosterone production (responsiveness). The decrease in LH receptors precedes the decrease in responsiveness by at least 2 days (Hauger et al., 1977). It appears, therefore, that the decrease in LH-stimulated testosterone production is not closely coupled to the decrease in LH receptors. Twice daily treatment of hypophysectomized adult rats for 6 days with increasing doses of LH results in a dose-dependent decrease in testicular LH receptor concentration accompanied by a dose-dependent increase in testicular responsiveness (Zipf et al., 1978a). This observation provides additional evidence of the dissociation between changes in LH-stimulated testosterone production and changes in LH receptor concentration.

Pituitary hormones other than LH have been shown to regulate Leydig cell function. Treatment of hypophysectomized adult rats with prolactin partially prevents the decrease in LH receptors but has no influence on LH-stimulated testosterone production. Treatment with ovine growth hormone also partially prevents the loss of LH receptors observed after hypophysectomy (Zipf et al., 1978b). The effects of prolactin and growth hormone on testicular LH receptors are additive. When small amounts of LH are administered together with prolactin and growth hormone to hypophysectomized rats, LH receptors and testosterone production in response to LH are maintained (Zipf et al., 1978b). Studies reported by Huhtaniemi and Catt (1981) suggest that during sexual maturation in the rat normal serum concentrations of prolactin are essential for the increase in testicular LH receptor concentration observed between 25 and 47 days of age but are not necessary for the maintenance of normal serum testosterone concentrations. Thus, LH is responsible for maintenance of steroidogenic responsiveness, whereas prolactin and growth hormone act mainly on maintenance of LH receptors. The effects of prolactin and growth hormone on LH receptor concentration appear to be by different mechanisms. Treatment with prolactin, but not with growth hormone, allows low doses of LH to have a positive effect on homologous receptor concentration and prevents the dose-dependent decrease in LH receptors caused by higher doses of LH (Zipf et al., 1978b; Payne and Zipf, 1978).

Follicle-stimulating hormone (FSH) has no effect on LH receptor concentration or on responsiveness to LH in mature hypophysectomized rats (Hauger et al., 1977), but in immature hypophysectomized rats, FSH treatment increases both testicular LH receptors and responsiveness to LH. This effect of FSH in immature rats will be described in Section VI,D.

Not only do pituitary hormones have diverse effects on LH receptors and on responsiveness to LH, but the mode of administration of LH treatment can also markedly affect responsiveness to subsequent stimulation by LH. Studies from our laboratory have demonstrated that administration of a single dose of LH (100 μg or greater) to mature rats causes a decrease in testosterone production in response to subsequent stimulation by LH, whereas twice daily injection of LH for 6 days or longer is accompanied by a time-related increase in in vivo testicular testosterone secretion in response to a subsequent stimulatory dose of LH (Zipf et al., 1978a; Payne and Zipf, 1978). The LH-induced losses of testicular LH receptors were similar in rats that received a single high dose of LH and in rats that received twice daily injections.

The studies described in this section on regulation of Leydig cell function in immature and mature rats cannot distinguish between effects of pituitary hormones on Leydig cell receptor concentration and responsiveness to LH and effects of the hormones on the number of Leydig cells. To clarify the mechanism by which pituitary hormones regulate Leydig cell function, the number of LH receptors and the intracellular reactions leading to steroid hormone production must be assessed in the same cell.

II. PURIFICATION OF LEYDIG CELLS

To obtain isolated Leydig cells, decapsulated testes have been incubated with various concentrations of collagenase and for various periods of time (Moyle and Ramachandran, 1973; Dufau et al., 1974; Janszen et al., 1976). These treatments with collagenase yield cell suspensions that are enriched with Leydig cells in comparison to intact testes. The percentage of Leydig cells in mixed cell suspensions obtained by collagenase dissociation of testes is usually between 6 and 15% (Janszen *et al.*, 1976; Conn *et al.*, 1977; Browning *et al.*, 1981; Quinn *et al.*, 1981). With the availability of new types of density gradient materials, methods have been developed to separate testicular cells, yielding more highly purified preparations of Leydig cells. Janszen *et al.* (1976) obtained a preparation containing 59% Leydig cells by centrifugation of a rat testicular cell suspension through a 13% Ficoll–albumin solution, followed by centrifugation through a 6% dextran solution. When Leydig cells purified by this method were incubated in the presence of LH, testosterone production increased in proportion to the increase in the percentage of Leydig cells, which indicates that Leydig cells were not damaged during these purification procedures. Conn *et al.* (1977) reported obtaining 94% pure prepara-

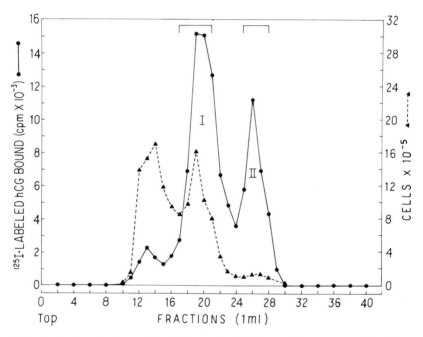

Fig. 1. Sedimentation profile of dispersed cells from whole rat testes after density gradient centrifugation of cells in 0–40% Metrizamide. Cells obtained by treatment of decapsulated testes with 0.3 mg/ml collagenase were layered on a Metrizamide gradient. After centrifugation for 5 minute at 3300 g, 1-ml fractions were collected. Specific binding of ^{125}I-labeled hCG (●) and the total number of cells (▲) were determined in the indicated 1-ml fractions. The bars (⌐) indicate fractions combined from peaks I and II to represent populations I and II Leydig cells, respectively. From Payne *et al.* (1980a).

tions of rat Leydig cells by centrifugation of testicular cell suspensions in continuous gradients consisting of 0 to 80% Metrizamide. Leydig cells obtained in this manner were highly responsive to stimulation by human chorionic gonadotropin (hCG) *in vitro*. Our laboratory has purified rat Leydig cells from collagenase-dispersed cell preparations from whole testes (Fig. 1) and from isolated interstitial tissue (Fig. 2) by centrifugation in continuous gradients of 0 to 40% Metrizamide (Payne *et al.*, 1980a). This method of purifying Leydig cells yields two populations of Leydig cells, the characteristics of which will be described in Section III. In more recent studies from our laboratory (O'Shaughnessy *et al.*, 1981; Payne *et al.*, 1981), dispersed testicular cells have been separated using discontinuous gradients of

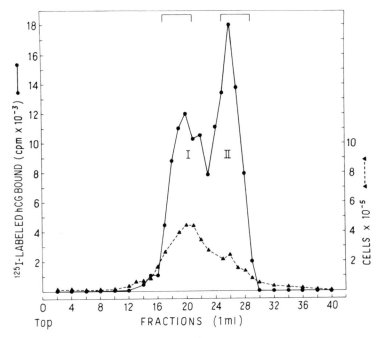

Fig. 2. Sedimentation profile of dispersed cells from isolated interstitial tissue of rat testes after density gradient centrifugation of cells in 0–40% Metrizamide. Cells obtained by collagenase treatment of isolated interstitial tissue were layered on a Metrizamide gradient. After centrifugation for 5 minutes at 3300 *g*, 1-ml fractions were collected. Specific binding of ^{125}I-labeled hCG (●) and the total number of cells (▲) were determined in the indicated 1-ml fraction. The bars (⌐) indicate the fractions combined from peaks I and II to represent populations I and II Leydig cells, respectively. From Payne *et al.* (1980a).

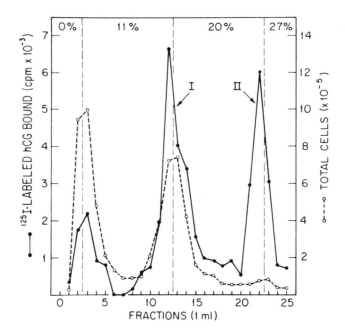

Fig. 3. Sedimentation profile of dispersed testicular cells following centrifugation at 3300 g for 5 minutes in a discontinuous Metrizamide gradient (from bottom to top: 5 ml 27%, 10 ml 20%, 10 ml 11%, and 2 ml 0% Metrizamide). One-milliliter fractions were collected from the top of the gradient. Specific binding of ^{125}I-labeled hCG (●) and total cell number (○) in each fraction were determined as described for Fig. 1.

Metrizamide comprising, from the bottom to the top, 5 ml of 27%, 10 ml of 20%, and 10 ml of 11% Metrizamide. The use of discontinuous Metrizamide gradients results in a better separation of germ cells from other testicular cells. The majority of the germ cells do not enter the gradient. As with continuous gradients, two distinct populations of Leydig cells are observed after centrifugation of testicular cell suspensions in discontinuous Metrizamide gradients (Fig. 3).

Percoll density gradients have been used to obtain purified preparations of mouse and rat Leydig cells. Schumacher *et al.* (1978) described the isolation of 90–95% pure Leydig cells from a crude murine testicular cell suspension (2–4% Leydig cells) prepared by nonenzymatic tissue disintegration and centrifugation in a linear 0 to 90% Percoll gradient. In investigations using Percoll gradient centrifugation for purification of murine and rat testicular cells, at least two peaks of Leydig cells were observed (Cooke *et al.,* 1981a,b; Browning *et al.,* 1981).

Because the methods commonly used to obtain "Leydig cell-enriched" suspensions achieve only partial dissociation of the testis and yield only a small fraction of the total Leydig cells (which may not be a representative sample of all the Leydig cells in the testis), we have devised a method to dissociate testes completely. This method disperses essentially all of the Leydig cells and has thus enabled us to

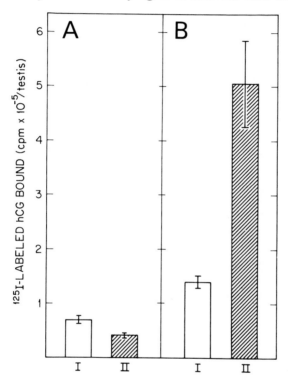

Fig. 4. Relative numbers of populations I and II Leydig cells in testicular cell suspensions after partial dissociation (A) followed by complete dissociation (B) of testes from 55-day-old rats. (A) Partial dissociation. Decapsulated testes were treated for 15 minutes with collagenase (0.3 mg/ml) in Medium 199 and 0.1% BSA. At the end of this treatment, dispersed cells were collected in the supernatant fluid after allowing the undissociated tissue to sediment. The dispersed cells were centrifuged in a discontinuous gradient of Metrizamide as described in Fig. 3. Fractions 11–17 were combined for population I and fractions 20–24 were combined for population II Leydig cells. The relative number of Leydig cells in each population was determined by measuring the amount of specific binding of ^{125}I-labeled hCG. (B) Complete dissociation. The tissue remaining after partial dissociation was completely dissociated by further treatment for 10 minutes with collagenase 1 mg/ml) in Medium 199 and 1.5% BSA. The completely dispersed cells were centrifuged in a discontinuous gradient of Metrizamide. Fractions were combined and numbers of Leydig cells in the two populations were determined as described for A.

evaluate changes in the distribution of Leydig cells between the two populations during sexual maturation. This method uses a higher concentration of collagenase (1 mg/ml) and 15 mg of bovine serum albumin (BSA) per milliliter; this high concentration of BSA is included to protect LH receptors from damage by nonspecific proteolytic activity of the collagenase. Comparisons of the relative numbers of populations I and II Leydig cells in testicular cell suspensions obtained by the commonly used partial dissociation and by our complete dissociation have indicated that the former method does not yield a representative sample of all the Leydig cells in the testis but rather liberates population I Leydig cells preferentially, as illustrated in Fig. 4. Cells were obtained from a partial dissociation and the relative numbers of populations I and II Leydig cells were measured by ^{125}I-labeled hCG binding following Metrizamide gradient centrifugation (Fig. 4A). The tissue remaining after the partial dissociation was then completely dissociated, and the relative numbers of populations I and II Leydig cells were again determined (Fig. 4B). Figure 4 illustrates that approximately 33% of all population I Leydig cells, but only about 7% of all population II Leydig cells, were liberated by the partial dissociation. Thus, about 63% of the Leydig cells obtained by partial dissociation were population I Leydig cells, although, as shown by Fig. 4A and B together, only about 28% of Leydig cells in the whole testis were population I Leydig cells. Preferential liberation of population I Leydig cells by partial dissociation of testes can also be seen by comparing the profiles of ^{125}I-labeled hCG binding after Metrizamide gradient centrifugation of cells from partially dissociated testes (Fig. 3) and from completely dissociated testes (Fig. 16) of 55-day-old rats.

III. LH RECEPTORS AND TESTOSTERONE PRODUCTION IN DIFFERENT POPULATIONS OF LEYDIG CELLS

The first evidence for the existence of two populations of Leydig cells in the mature rat was reported by Janszen et al. (1976). Isopycnic centrifugation of a crude testicular cell preparation in a gradient of Ficoll metrizoate yielded two discrete bands of Leydig cells, distinguished on the basis of 3β-hydroxysteroid dehydrogenase activity and phenylesterase activity, in fractions with densities of 1.049 to 1.055 gm/cm^3 (band I) and 1.068 to 1.088 gm/cm^3 (band II). Leydig cells from each of these bands produced testosterone in vitro in the absence of LH, but only band II responded to LH with increased testosterone production (Janszen et al., 1976). These authors did not investigate LH receptors or other characteristics of these presumably distinct populations of Leydig cells.

In a more recent study, our laboratory demonstrated the existence of two populations of Leydig cells in cell suspensions obtained by collagenase dissociation of whole testes or isolated interstitial tissues of mature rats (Payne et al., 1980a). Centrifugation of either type of cell suspension in 0 to 40% Metrizamide gradients yielded two distinct populations of Leydig cells as identified by specific binding of ^{125}I-labeled hCG. One population (I) was found in fractions with densities of 1.085 to 1.117 gm/cm^3 and the other population (II) was found in fractions with densities of 1.128 to 1.145 gm/cm^3 (Figs. 1 and 2). A major peak of cells with a small amount of ^{125}I-labeled hCG binding was found in fractions with densities of 1.055 to 1.065 gm/cm^3 only in gradients of dispersed cells from whole testes (Fig. 1). The vast majority of cells in this peak are germ cells. The number of LH/hCG receptor sites (as measured by specific binding of ^{125}I-labeled hCG) and the hCG-binding affinities in each Leydig cell population were determined using cells from isolated interstitial tissue following centrifugation of each population in a second continuous Metrizamide gradient. This second centrifugation step was included to eliminate cross-contamination of Leydig cells between the two populations (Payne et al., 1980a). Scatchard analysis of hCG binding indicated that both populations of Leydig cells have a single class of binding sites with essentially the same binding affinity (K_a): 0.64×10^{10} M^{-1} and 0.67×10^{10} M^{-1} for populations I and II Leydig cells, respectively. Binding capacity, when expressed per total cells, was considerably greater for fractions containing population II Leydig cells than for fractions containing population I Leydig cells (Fig. 5) as a result of the large number of non-Leydig interstitial cells found in fractions containing population I Leydig cells. When binding capacity was expressed per equal number of Leydig cells (identified histochemically by the presence of 3β-hydroxysteroid dehydrogenase), no significant difference was observed between the two populations. Binding capacity, expressed as femtomoles per 10^6 Leydig cells (mean ± SE), was 86 ± 20 ($n = 3$) and 91 ± 21 ($n = 3$) for Leydig cell populations I and II, respectively (Payne et al., 1980a). These values are equivalent to approximately 50,000 binding sites per Leydig cell.

Testosterone production in response to hCG was determined for each population of Leydig cells obtained from isolated interstitial tissue (Fig. 6) (Payne et al., 1980a). During a 3-hour incubation, basal testosterone production (expressed as nanograms of testosterone produced per femtomole of LH receptor sites) was similar in the two populations

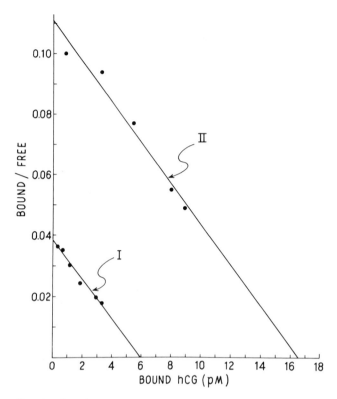

Fig. 5. Scatchard analysis of hCG binding derived from the incubation of interstitial cells from fractions 17–21 of peak I and from fractions 25–29 of peak II obtained after centrifugation in a second continuous gradient of 0–40% Metrizamide. The specific binding of ^{125}I-labeled hCG was determined by incubating aliquots of cells from each peak with increasing concentrations of ^{125}I-labeled hCG. A representative plot of three separate experiments is shown. From Payne *et al.* (1980a).

of Leydig cells. Population I Leydig cells responded to increasing concentrations of hCG with only a small increase in testosterone production. In sharp contrast, testosterone production by population II Leydig cells increased markedly in the presence of hCG, with maximal production observed at 3 pM hCG (Fig. 6). The marked differences in testosterone production between the two populations of Leydig cells were also observed when cells were incubated with various concentrations of dibutyryl cAMP (0.25–2 mM) (Fig. 7). Similar differences in testosterone production in response to various concentrations of hCG were observed during incubations of population I and population II Leydig cells obtained from whole testes. Maximum production of tes-

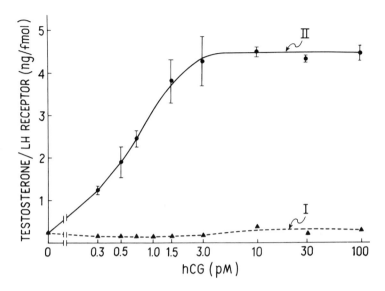

Fig. 6. Testosterone production in response to hCG by two populations of Leydig cells obtained from isolated interstitial tissue. Aliquots of Leydig cells from fractions 17–21 representing population I or fractions 25–29 representing population II obtained after a second centrifugation in a continuous gradient of 0–40%. Metrizamide were incubated for 3 hours at 34°C with increasing concentrations of hCG. Testosterone in cells plus medium was measured by radioimmunoassay. Separate aliquots from each peak were incubated with a saturating concentration of ^{125}I-labeled hCG to measure LH receptor concentration. Testosterone production is expressed as nanograms of testosterone per femtomole LH receptor sites. Each point represents the mean of values obtained in two separate experiments. The range of values is indicated, except where the range is smaller than the dimensions of the symbol. From Payne *et al.* (1980a).

tosterone was observed at similar concentrations of hCG in the two populations of Leydig cells. As seen with Leydig cells obtained from isolated interstitial tissue, the two populations exhibited similar numbers of LH receptor sites per 10^6 Leydig cells (Fig. 8).

Cooke *et al.* (1981b), using Percoll density gradient centrifugation for the separation of adult rat and murine testicular cells, reported three bands of cells that specifically bound ^{125}I-labeled hCG, but only one of these bands contained Leydig cells that exhibited an increase in testosterone production *in vitro* in response to LH. Furthermore, these authors reported that after fractionation of the gradients some fractions containing 100% Leydig cells did not respond to LH with increased testosterone production. Browning *et al.* (1981), using continuous Percoll gradients for the separation of dispersed testicular cells

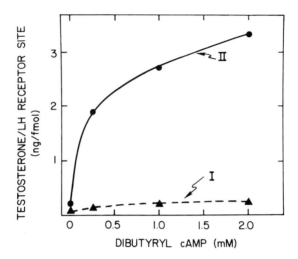

Fig. 7. Testosterone production in response to dibutyryl cAMP by two populations of Leydig cells obtained from isolated interstitial tissue. Leydig cells representing each population (as described for Fig. 6) were incubated for 3 hours at 34°C with increasing concentrations of dibutyryl cAMP. Testosterone in cells plus medium was measured by radioimmunoassay. Separate aliquots from each peak were incubated with a saturating concentration of ^{125}I-labeled hCG to measure LH receptor concentration. Testosterone production is expressed as nanograms of testosterone per femtomole LH receptor sites. Each point represents the mean of duplicate incubations.

from adult rats, described two peaks of cellular ^{125}I-labeled hCG binding, but cells in only one of these peaks exhibited increased testosterone production in response to hCG *in vitro*.

In studies of the aging Leydig cell, Chen *et al.* (1981) observed two populations of Leydig cells in both 60- to 90-day-old and 24-month-old rats. Centrifugation of collagenase-dispersed testicular cells in 0–32% Metrizamide gradients resulted in five bands of cells, of which bands 2 and 3 were used in the reported study. Cells in band 2 from young rats increased testosterone production only 2.5-fold, whereas cells in band 3 increased testosterone production 10- to 16-fold when incubated in the presence of LH. The increases in testosterone production by cells in the two bands from 24-month-old rats were similar (3-fold). Maximum testosterone and cAMP production were markedly lower in band 2 than in band 3. These data are difficult to interpret because the authors did not distinguish between responses per Leydig cell and total cells, and no allowance was made for differences in percentage of Leydig cells present in each band.

It is clear from these studies on purification of testicular cells from

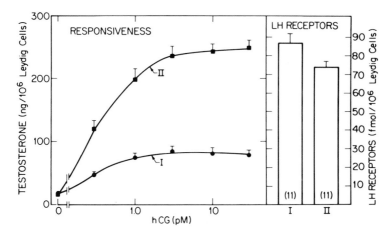

Fig. 8. Number of LH receptor sites and testosterone production in response to hCG in two populations of Leydig cells obtained from whole testes. For testosterone production, duplicate aliquots of Leydig cells from fractions 17–21 (population I) and from fractions 25–28 (population II) obtained after centrifugation in a continuous 0–40% gradient of Metrizamide were incubated for 3 hours at 34°C with increasing concentrations of hCG. Testosterone in cells plus medium was measured by radioimmunoassay. The number of LH receptor sites, expressed as femtomoles per 10^6 Leydig cells, was measured by incubating separate duplicate aliquots of each population with a saturating concentration of ^{125}I-labeled hCG. Results are the mean of 11 separate experiments. From Payne *et al.* (1980b).

adult rats and mice by density gradient centrifugation that more than one population of Leydig cells exist. Leydig cells in these different populations appear to differ in density and in their capacity to produce testosterone when stimulated by LH/hCG. However, because the various reports on the heterogeneity of Leydig cells are based on different techniques of obtaining and purifying testicular cells, as well as on differences in the way of expressing functional responses (i.e., based on numbers of Leydig cells or total cells), it is difficult to make comparisons among these investigations.

IV.   GONADOTROPIN REGULATION OF LH RECEPTORS AND STEROIDOGENESIS IN LEYDIG CELLS

The initial response of Leydig cells to a single *in vivo* injection of LH or the analogous placental hormone (hCG) is an increase in production of LH receptors (Huhtaniemi *et al.*, 1981) and an increase in testosterone production (Catt *et al.*, 1980). The initial increase in LH receptor

concentration is followed by a decrease, the degree of which is dependent on the type of gonadotropin (i.e., LH or hCG) (Payne *et al.*, 1980b),
the dose (Tsuruhara *et al.*, 1977; Payne *et al.*, 1980b), and the mode of
administration of the gonadotropin (Sharpe and McNeilly, 1978;
Cigorraga *et al.*, 1978; Payne *et al.*, 1980b). Maximum loss of testicular
LH receptors is observed between 2 and 3 days after administration of
LH (Zipf *et al.*, 1978a) or hCG (Catt *et al.*, 1980). Replenishment of
testicular LH receptors is a slow process, and even 5 days after a
subcutaneous administration of 200 μg of LH, testicular LH receptor
concentrations have not been restored to normal (Zipf *et al.*, 1978a).
The apparent decrease in LH receptor concentration 24 hours after the
administration of hCG is largely due to occupancy of the receptors by
the administered hormone (Hsueh *et al.*, 1977; Sharpe and McNeilly,
1978). The decrease in receptor concentration 2 days after administration of LH or hCG, however, is due to actual loss of receptors (Hsueh *et
al.*, 1977; Zipf *et al.*, 1978a). Studies using murine Leydig tumor cells
indicate that the loss of receptors is most likely due to internalization
and lysosomal degradation of the hormone–receptor complex (Ascoli
and Puett, 1978a). It should be noted, however, that internalization of
the gonadotropin–receptor complex has been demonstrated only with
the placental analog (hCG) but never with the natural hormone (LH).
Although the two gonadotropins appear to bind to the same receptor,
the affinity of LH is only about one-tenth that of hCG (Ascoli and
Puett, 1978b). Whether loss of gonadotropin binding to Leydig cell LH
receptors is a result of internalization of the hormone–receptor complex normally or occurs only with the analog (hCG) remains to be
demonstrated experimentally.

Although LH and hCG cause a loss of Leydig cell LH receptors regardless of their mode of administration, LH- and hCG-induced
changes in hCG-stimulated testosterone production *in vitro* depend on
the mode of administration of the gonadotropin and do not appear to be
related to the loss of LH receptors (Payne *et al.*, 1980b). It has been
suggested that the decrease in hCG-stimulated testosterone production *in vitro* observed after *in vivo* administration of a single high dose

Fig. 9.   Testosterone production and LH receptor sites in populations I and II Leydig
cells after 6 days of treatment with LH. Rats were injected subcutaneously twice daily
for 6 days with either saline (●), 6 μg (■), or 12.5 μg (▲) of ovine LH. Animals were
killed on day 7 and Leydig cells from fractions 17 to 21, population I (A), and from
fractions 25–28, population II (B), were incubated in duplicate as described in the legend
to Fig. 8. Each point represents the mean ± SE of data from two separate experiments.
The number in parentheses represents the percentage of LH receptor sites per 10^6
Leydig cells relative to control. From Payne *et al.* (1980b).

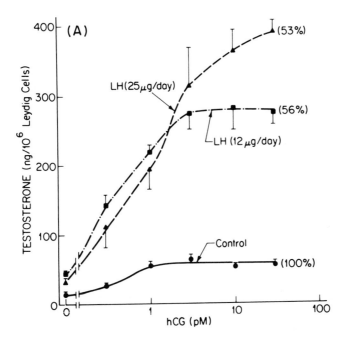

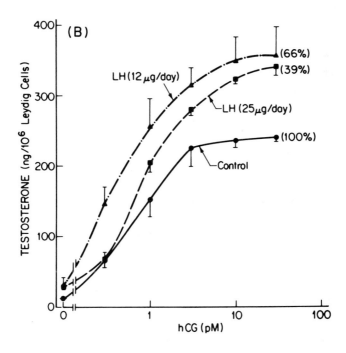

of hCG is a result of decreased C_{17}–C_{20} lyase and 17α-hydroxylase activities (Cigorraga *et al.*, 1978; Chasalow *et al.*, 1979).

Our laboratory has investigated the effect of different modes of *in vivo* administration of LH and hCG on LH receptor concentration and on *in vitro* testosterone production in response to hCG in each of the two populations of Leydig cells. Twice daily treatment of adult rats with 6 or 12.5 μg of LH for 6 days caused a marked increase in *in vitro* responsiveness of population I Leydig cells to hCG (Fig. 9A) but only a small increase in testosterone production in population II Leydig cells (Fig. 9B). After 6 days of treatment, Leydig cells of the two populations produced similar amounts of testosterone *in vitro* in response to hCG. The change in responsiveness of population I Leydig cells after chronic LH treatment was not accompanied by a change in their sedimentation when subjected to centrifugation in a Metrizamide gradient. The concentration of LH receptors was decreased in both populations of Leydig cells following the *in vivo* treatment with LH. Preliminary studies from our laboratory indicate that the increase in Leydig cell responsiveness observed after chronic treatment with LH or hCG may be due to increases in certain enzyme activities associated with the smooth endoplasmic reticulum (P. J. O'Shaughnessy and A. H. Payne, 1982).

A single subcutaneous injection of 150 μg LH (a dose equivalent to the total amount of LH that was administered in the twice daily regimen of 12.5 μg for 6 days) resulted in decreases in LH receptor concentration of 57 and 79% in Leydig cell populations I and II, respectively, after 72 hours. This treatment had no effect on *in vitro* responsiveness of population I Leydig cells to hCG (Fig. 10A) but markedly decreased maximum testosterone production in response to hCG in population II Leydig cells (Fig. 10B). Testosterone production in these Leydig cells could not be stimulated to maximum values of Leydig cells from saline-injected control rats, even when the *in vitro* concentration of hCG was increased to 1000 pM.

A single subcutaneous injection of 100 IU of hCG caused a complete loss of responsiveness to *in vitro* hCG stimulation and greater than 90% loss of LH receptors in both populations of Leydig cells after 72 hours (Payne *et al.*, 1980b).

These data demonstrate that the effects of LH and hCG on Leydig cell steroidogenesis depend on the mode of administration of the hormone and do not appear to relate to loss of LH receptor sites. Reports that gonadotropin-induced loss of testicular LH receptors (down-regulation) is accompanied by a decrease in *in vitro* LH/hCG-stimulated testosterone production (steroidogenic desensitization) were based on studies using a single injection of hCG or LH (Hsueh *et al.*, 1977;

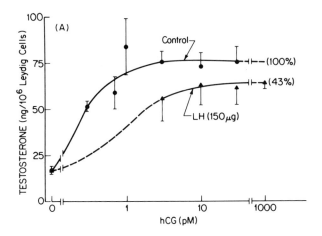

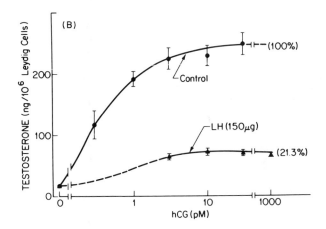

Fig. 10. Testosterone production and LH receptor sites in populations I and II Leydig cells after a single administration of LH. Rats were injected once subcutaneously with either saline (●) or 150 μg of LH (▲) and killed 72 hours later. Aliquots of Leydig cells from fractions 17–21, population I (A), and fractions 25–28, population II (B), were incubated in duplicate as described in the legend to Fig. 8. Each point represents the mean ± SE of data from two separate experiments. Note the difference in the scales of the ordinates in A and B. The number in parentheses represents the percentage of LH receptor sites per 10^6 Leydig cells relative to control. From Payne *et al.* (1980b).

Tsuruhara *et al.*, 1977; Zipf *et al.*, 1978a; Saez *et al.*, 1978). Studies in our laboratory using mature male rats indicated that, although all variations of treatment with LH caused a loss of testicular LH receptors, only a single dose (100 μg or greater) was accompanied by a decrease in *in vivo* testicular responsiveness to a subsequent stimulatory dose of LH. Injection of 15 μg of LH twice daily for up to 10 days caused a loss of testicular LH receptors similar to that caused by a single high dose of LH but caused a time-related increase in *in vivo* testicular responsiveness (Zipf *et al.*, 1978a). Our studies clearly demonstrate that Leydig cell steroidogenic desensitization does not occur except after administration of a single high, nonphysiological dose of LH or hCG. Because the testis is normally exposed to only small pulsatile LH discharges and not massive LH surges, LH-induced steroidogenic desensitization as described by several authors (Hsueh *et al.*, 1977; Tsuruhara *et al.*, 1977; Zipf *et al.*, 1978a; Saez *et al.*, 1978) is not likely to occur under physiological or even under most pathological conditions but only in situations that result in hyperstimulation of Leydig cells, i.e., administration of high doses of hCG. The demonstration that LH has different effects on the two populations of Leydig cells must be considered in future studies on hormonal regulation of Leydig cell function.

Data from our laboratory may provide an explanation for the cause of steroidogenic desensitization that follows the administration of a single high dose of hCG (Quinn *et al.*, 1981). Three days after the administration of 50 IU of hCG to mature rats, serum testosterone concentrations were elevated 3-fold and basal testosterone production by Leydig cells *in vitro* was elevated 2-fold compared to values for saline-injected control rats. These findings indicate that Leydig cells from rats that had been injected with a single high dose of hCG were hyperstimulated, for at least as long as 3 days after the administration of the hormone. However, these hyperstimulated Leydig cells produced markedly less testosterone *in vitro* than those from control rats in response to hCG. Addition of high-density lipoprotein particles (HDL) to the incubation medium completely restored maximal hCG-stimulated testosterone production of the desensitized Leydig cells to that found in normal Leydig cells (Fig. 11) but had no effect on testosterone production by normal Leydig cells. Addition of low-density lipoprotein particles (LDL) also stimulated *in vitro* testosterone production of desensitized Leydig cells, but not to the same extent as was observed with HDL. These data suggest that steroidogenic desensitization caused by high doses of hCG may be due to increased utilization of endogenous Leydig cell cholesterol and thus depletion of the precursor

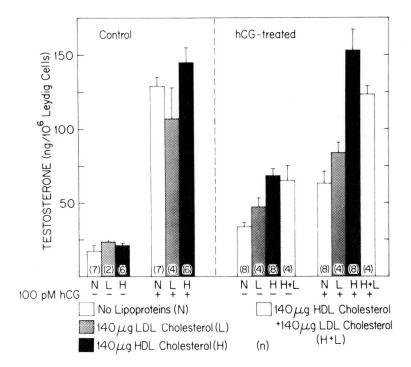

Fig. 11. The effect of high-density (HDL) and low-density (LDL) lipoproteins and/or hCG on testosterone production by Leydig cells from control and from hCG-desensitized rats. Rats 55–60 days of age were injected subcutaneously with either 50 IU of hCG (hCG-treated) or isotonic saline (control) 72 hours prior to the experiment. Leydig cell-enriched suspensions were prepared and $\sim 3 \times 10^6$ cells were incubated for 6 hours at 34°C with or without hCG and the indicated amount of HDL and/or LDL. Testosterone in cells plus medium was measured by radioimmunoassay. Values are the mean ± SE; n represents the number of determinations. From Quinn *et al.* (1981).

for testosterone synthesis. Furthermore, the data indicate that under these conditions serum lipoproteins can provide the precursor cholesterol in the form of high- or low-density lipoprotein particles.

V. STEROIDOGENIC ENZYMES

As discussed in Section III, differences in testosterone production between population I and population II Leydig cells were evident when cells were incubated with either hCG or dibutyryl cAMP. This observation suggested that the difference in responsiveness between the two populations is due to biochemical events distal to LH/hCG binding and

Cholesterol
$\downarrow$
Pregnenolone
$\quad \downarrow \;\; \leftarrow \; \Delta^5\text{-}3\beta\text{-hydroxysteroid dehydrogenase-isomerase}$
$\qquad\qquad (3\beta\text{HSD})$
Progesterone
$\quad \downarrow \; \leftarrow \; 17\text{-hydroxylase}$
17-Hydroxyprogesterone
$\quad \downarrow \; \leftarrow \; C_{17}\text{-}C_{20} \; \text{lyase}$
Androstenedione
$\quad \downarrow \; \leftarrow \; 17\text{-ketosteroid reductase}$
Testosterone

Fig. 12. Biosynthetic pathway from pregnenolone to testosterone.

stimulation of cAMP production. Therefore, we measured the activities of several of the key steroidogenic enzymes responsible for the production of testosterone in the different populations of Leydig cells. The enzymes studied are those responsible for the conversion of pregnenolone to testosterone in the rat Leydig cell: Δ^5-3β-hydroxysteroid dehydrogenase–isomerase, 17α-hydroxylase, C_{17}–C_{20} lyase, and 17-ketosteroid reductase (Fig. 12). All of these enzymes are associated with the smooth endoplasmic reticulum (SER) of the rat Leydig cell, and it has been shown that species differences in testosterone production are correlated with SER volume and density (Zirkin *et al.*, 1980). Metabolism of testosterone by 5α-reductase and aromatase in the different Leydig cell populations was also measured.

For these studies, Leydig cells were separated by centrifugation in discontinuous Metrizamide gradients, as described in Section II. In preliminary experiments, it was found that hCG-stimulated testosterone production per 10^6 Leydig cells in individual 1-ml fractions representing population I (fractions 10–15; Fig. 3) was markedly higher in fractions 13–15 than in fractions 10–12. This finding suggested that fractions 10–12 and 13–15 may represent different subpopulations of Leydig cells. These subpopulations have been termed IA (fractions 10–12) and IB (fractions 13–15). No differences were observed among individual 1-ml fractions representing population II Leydig cells (fractions 20–24). In view of these findings, enzyme studies were carried out using subpopulations IA and IB as well as population II Leydig cells.

Testosterone production by Leydig cells from each population, in response to increasing concentrations of hCG, is shown in Fig. 13. Testosterone production, per 10^6 Leydig cells, was stimulated 12-fold to 250 ng in population II, 10-fold to 180 ng in population IB, and 4- to

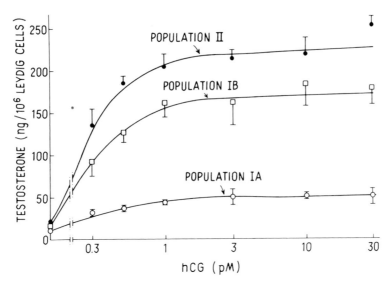

Fig. 13. Testosterone production, in response to hCG, by three populations of Leydig cells *in vitro.* Cells from populations IA (○), IB (□), and II (●) were collected from a discontinuous Metrizamide gradient and incubated for 3 hours at 34°C in the presence of increasing concentrations of hCG. Testosterone concentration in cells and medium was measured by radioimmunoassay. The mean ± SE of duplicate determination is shown. Analysis of variance (not including basal testosterone production) showed that there was a significant ($p < .001$) difference between hCG-stimulated levels of testosterone protion in populations IB and II. From O'Shaughnessy *et al.* (1981).

5-fold to 50 ng in population IA. The concentrations of LH receptor sites, expressed as femtomoles of ^{125}I-labeled hCG bound per 10^6 Leydig cells, were similar in all three populations: 102 ± 6 (mean ± SE, $n = 5$), 108 ± 15 ($n = 5$) and 99 ± 9 ($n = 5$) in Leydig cell populations IA, IB, and II, respectively (O'Shaughnessy *et al.,* 1981).

A. Δ^5-3β-Hydroxysteroid Dehydrogenase–Isomerase

In the rat testis, pregnenolone is converted to progesterone by the action of 3β-hydroxysteroid dehydrogenase and 3-oxosteroid-Δ^5-Δ^4-isomerase. Pregn-5-ene-3,20-dione has been shown to be an intermediate in this conversion in the human placenta (Edwards *et al.,* 1976). 3β-Hydroxysteroid dehydrogenase requires NAD^+ as a hydrogen acceptor, and it has been suggested that NAD^+ may stimulate bovine adrenal 3-oxosteroid-Δ^5-Δ^4-isomerase by accelerating the breakdown of the enzyme–substrate complex (Neville and Engel, 1968). In general, 3β-

hydroxysteroid dehydrogenase and 3-oxosteroid-Δ^5–Δ^4-isomerase have been studied using adrenal tissue, and little information is available on the characteristics of these enzymes in the testis.

The enzymes are located primarily in the SER. A certain amount of activity has been reported to exist in the mitochondria (Basch and Finegold, 1971), although this may be an artifact (Cowan et al., 1974). Although it has been suggested that both oxidation and isomerization are catalyzed by one enzyme (Ford and Engel, 1976), more recent work by Gallay et al. (1978) has shown physical separation of 3β-hydroxy-steroid dehydrogenase and 3-oxosteroid-Δ^5–Δ^4-isomerase solubilized from adrenal microsomes. The existence of single or multiple forms of both 3β-hydroxysteroid dehydrogenase and 3-oxosteroid-Δ^5–Δ^4-iso-merase in steroid-producing cells is, however, still in dispute (Ewald et al., 1964; Neville et al., 1969; Gibb and Hagerman, 1976; Geynet, 1977; Gallay et al., 1978). It is possible that the 3-oxosteroid-Δ^5–Δ^4-isomerase gives the Δ^5-3β-hydroxysteroid dehydrogenase–isomerase complex substrate specificity. The specificity of this enzyme complex and of 17α-hydroxylase and/or C_{17}–C_{20} lyase may determine the preferred path-way of testosterone synthesis from pregnenolone in different species.

The activity of Δ^5-3β-hydroxysteroid dehydrogenase–isomerase was determined in the three Leydig cell populations by measuring the conversion of a saturating (5 μM) concentration of [^{3}H]pregnenolone to [^{3}H]progesterone by cell-free homogenates in the presence of 0.5 mM NAD^+ (Murono and Payne, 1976; O'Shaughnessy et al., 1981). Because ^{125}I-labeled hCG binding per 10^6 Leydig cells was found to be essen-tially identical in all populations of Leydig cells, Δ^5-3β-hydroxysteroid dehydrogenase–isomerase activity was expressed as picomoles of pro-gesterone produced per femtomole of ^{125}I-labeled hCG bound. As shown in Table I, no difference in the activity of this enzyme was observed

TABLE I

Δ^5-3β-**Hydroxysteroid Dehydrogenase–Isomerase Activity in Different Populations of Leydig Cells**

Cell population	Progesterone formed (pmol/fmol ^{125}I-labeled hCG bound·10 min)[a]
IA	27.09 ± 0.19
IB	25.59 ± 2.91
II	12.95 ± 0.61

[a] Mean ± SE of duplicate incubations.

between populations IA and IB, but both of these subpopulations showed markedly higher activity than population II. Results shown here would suggest that this enzyme is not rate-limiting for androgen synthesis in the mature rat testis (at least in populations IA and IB) because testosterone production is highest in population II.

B.   17α-Hydroxylase and C$_{17}$–C$_{20}$ Lyase

17α-Hydroxylase and C$_{17}$–C$_{20}$ lyase are responsible for the conversion of the C$_{21}$ steroids pregnenolone and progesterone to the corresponding C$_{19}$ steroids dehydroepiandrosterone and androstenedione, respectively. These enzymes are being considered together here because it has been shown that in the neonatal pig testis both enzyme activities are associated with a single protein (Nakajin and Hall, 1981; Nakajin et al., 1981b) and probably a single active site (Nakajin et al., 1981a). This will be discussed further later.

17α-Hydroxylase is a microsomal mixed-function oxidase that requires cytochrome P-450 reductase for the transfer of electrons from NADPH to cytochrome P-450 (McMurty and Hagerman, 1972; Betz et al., 1975, 1976). In the presence of molecular oxygen, this enzyme catalyzes the hydroxylation of the C$_{21}$ steroids pregnenolone and progesterone at the C-17 position to form 17α-hydroxypregnenolone and 17α-hydroxyprogesterone. C$_{17}$–C$_{20}$ lyase is also a microsomal cytochrome P-450 requiring molecular oxygen, NADPH, and reductase (McMurty and Hagerman, 1972; Betz and Michels, 1973; Betz et al., 1976). This enzyme catalyzes the cleavage of the bond between C-17 and C-20 of 17α-hydroxylated pregnenolone and progesterone to form the C$_{19}$ steroids dehydroepiandrosterone and androstenedione.

Results obtained in studies by Hochberg et al. (1975, 1976), using steroid substrate analogs and rat testicular microsomes, led them to propose that both hydroxylation and cleavage reactions occur as a single concerted process. This mechanism is consistent with a single cytochrome that mediates the conversion of C$_{21}$ to C$_{19}$ steroids. As mentioned earlier, Nakajin and co-workers have isolated from neonatal pig testes a single heme protein (cytochrome P-450) with activity for both 17α-hydroxylase and C$_{17}$–C$_{20}$ lyase. Both activities require NADPH and a flavoprotein P-450 reductase. The enzyme is a glycoprotein possessing a single subunit of molecular weight equivalent to 59,000 (Nakajin and Hall, 1981). Spectral studies indicated that there may be a single active site for the substrates of both reactions (Nakajin et al., 1981a).

Kinetic studies showed that the affinity of the enzyme for Δ^5 substrates was markedly higher than for Δ^4 substrates, which may explain the preferential use of the Δ^5 pathway by the pig testis (Nakajin et al., 1981a). Thus, as suggested earlier, species differences in the use of the Δ^5 or Δ^4 pathway may be due to relative affinities of Δ^5-3β-hydroxysteroid dehydrogenase–isomerase and 17α-hydroxylase/C_{17}–C_{20} lyase for pregnenolone and progesterone. Alternatively, it is possible that the organization of the enzymes within the membrane of the SER may determine the preferred pathway.

It is not known whether both C_{17}–C_{20} lyase and 17α-hydroxylase activities are present in a single enzyme in other species. Results from Purvis et al. (1973), who used microsomes from rat testes, are compatible with the idea that hydroxylase and lyase act as a single enzyme. It was shown that there is a parallel response of both enzymes to in vivo gonadotropic hormone manipulations. Using rat testicular microsomes, Betz et al. (1976) concluded that 17α-hydroxylation and C_{17}–C_{20} cleavage reactions were catalyzed by two different enzymes. The results, however, could not differentiate conclusively between two different enzymes and a single enzyme with two active sites. In addition, complexities in the partition of lipophilic compounds when using microsomal enzymes may confuse interpretation of results (Matsumoto and Samuels, 1969). Betz et al. (1980) purified a cytochrome P-450 that possessed C_{17}–C_{20} lyase activity when reconstituted with reductase and phospholipid. They were, however, unable to determine whether this protein also contained 17α-hydroxylase activity because of detergent interference with chromatographic separation of the reactants.

Results of double-label experiments using rat and mouse microsomes (Matsumoto and Samuels, 1969; Chasalow, 1979) have provided evidence that 17α-hydroxyprogesterone may not be a free intermediate in the conversion of progesterone to androstenedione. Although there may be problems in the partition of steroids, as mentioned earlier, these data would be consistent with a single enzyme with one active site.

It has been known for some time that substrates for the 17α-hydroxylation reaction can inhibit C_{17}–C_{20} lyase activity in microsomal preparations from mouse and rat testes (Neher and Kahnt, 1965; Matsumoto et al., 1974). Using the purified enzyme preparation, Nakajin et al. (1981a) confirmed this forward inhibition and showed that it was competitive. In addition, it was shown that estradiol can inhibit both 17α-hydroxylase and C_{17}–C_{20} lyase activities for progesterone and pregnenolone metabolism (Onoda and Hall, 1981). Inhibition was shown to be noncompetitive for both enzymes using Δ^5 substrates, whereas inhibition of C_{17}–C_{20} lyase was competitive and of 17α-hydroxylase noncompetitive, using Δ^4 substrates. Using microsomes prepared from human testes, Hosaka *et al.* (1980) showed that estradiol was a competitive inhibitor of C_{17}–C_{20} lyase when 17α-hydroxyprogesterone was the substrate but did not act as an inhibitor when 17α-hydroxypregnenolone was the substrate. Testosterone was shown to inhibit 17α-hydroxyprogesterone metabolism competitively and 17α-hydroxypregnenolone metabolism uncompetitively. From these data, the authors concluded that there are two different active sites on the enzyme for the two substrates. In addition to the enzyme inhibitions mentioned earlier, 17α-hydroxylated pregnenolone and progesterone will inhibit 17α-hydroxylase activity in rat and marmoset testicular microsomes (Kremers, 1976; Preslock and Steinberger, 1979). Inhibition of 17α-hydroxylase and C_{17}–C_{20} lyase by the various steroids described earlier may have some importance *in vivo* under certain conditions. Results from this laboratory and from others (reviewed later in Section V,E) have shown that Leydig cells from mature rats produce estradiol, and it is possible that androgen production in the testis may be modulated by estradiol if the concentration in the SER reaches sufficiently high levels. As discussed in Section IV, injection of a single very high dose of hCG *in vivo* causes a decrease in *in vitro* hCG-stimulated testosterone production. This change in testosterone production is associated with an increase in progesterone and 17α-hydroxyprogesterone accumulation (Dufau *et al.,* 1979), which may be at least partly due to an increase in the production of estradiol (Cigorraga *et al.,* 1980). An increase in estradiol concentrations would be expected to inhibit C_{17}–C_{20} lyase activity, with corresponding inhibition of 17α-hydroxylase by 17α-hydroxyprogesterone and further inhibition of C_{17}–C_{20} lyase by progesterone.

We have investigated 17α-hydroxylase and C_{17}–C_{20} lyase activities in the three populations of Leydig cells using intact cell preparations. Cells were incubated for 1 hour at 34°C with a saturating concentration of the appropriate ^{3}H-labeled substrate, and steroid products were separated by thin-layer chromatography (O'Shaughnessy *et al.,* 1981).

The 17α-hydroxylase activity was determined by measuring the conversion of 10 μM progesterone to 17α-hydroxyprogesterone, androstenedione, and testosterone. As shown in Table II, the 17α-hydroxylase activity was twice as high in populations IB and II as in population IA; there was no difference in activity between populations IB and II.

C_{17}–C_{20} lyase activity was determined by measuring the conversion of 2 μM 17α-hydroxyprogesterone to androstenedione and testosterone. As shown in Table III, the activity of this enzyme was different in all three populations of Leydig cells. Both populations IB and II showed higher activity than population IA; activity in population IB was 2.45-

TABLE II

17α-Hydroxylase Activity in Different Populations of Leydig Cells[a]

Cell population	Products formed (nmol/10^6 Leydig cells)[b]			Total 17α-hydroxylase activity (nmol/10^6 Leydig cells·hr)[c]
	17α-Hydroxy-progesterone	Androstenedione	Testosterone	
IA	3.28 ± 0.01	0.83 ± 0.14	0.13 ± 0.01	4.24 ± 0.15
IB	8.45 ± 0.40	1.30 ± 0.02	0.23 ± 0.04	9.98 ± 0.50
II	8.12 ± 0.51	1.1 ± 0.01	0.27 ± 0.05	9.46 ± 0.53

[a] From O'Shaughnessy et al., 1981.
[b] Mean ± SE of duplicate independent incubations.
[c] 17α-Hydroxylase activity was determined as the sum of 17α-hydroxyprogesterone, androstenedione, and testosterone formed.

fold higher and activity in population II 3.6-fold higher than in population IA.

Differences in the activity of $C_{17}-C_{20}$ lyase among the three populations closely paralleled the differences in hCG-stimulated testosterone production shown in Fig. 13. As discussed previously (Section IV), a decrease in the activities of 17α-hydroxylase and $C_{17}-C_{20}$ lyase is associated with a marked decrease in testosterone production by testes from rats that have received a single very high dose of hCG (Chasalow et al., 1979). In addition, because hCG desensitization leads to an accumulation of 17α-hydroxylated precursors of the C_{19} steroids, it is

TABLE III

$C_{17}-C_{20}$ Lyase Activity in Different Populations of Leydig Cells[a]

Cell population	Products formed (nmol/10^6 Leydig cells)[b]		Total $C_{17}-C_{20}$ lyase activity (nmol/10^6 Leydig cells·hr)[c]
	Androstenedione	Testosterone	
IA	0.96 ± 0.01	0.08 ± 0.01	1.04 ± 0.01
IB	2.12 ± 0.01	0.43 ± 0.03	2.55 ± 0.02
II	2.71 ± 0.01	1.05 ± 0.05	3.76 ± 0.02

[a] From O'Shaughnessy et al., 1981.
[b] Mean ± SE of duplicate independent incubations.
[c] $C_{17}-C_{20}$ lyase activity was determined as the sum of androstenedione and testosterone formed.

possible that differences in the activity of C_{17}–C_{20} lyase may be reflected in differences in testosterone production. These observations suggest that the lower testosterone production seen in populations IA and IB may be, at least partly, a consequence of decreased C_{19} steroid production from 17α-hydroxyprogesterone.

C.   17-Ketosteroid Reductase and 17β-Hydroxysteroid Dehydrogenase

The final step in the synthesis of testosterone by the testis is reduction of androstenedione to testosterone, a reaction catalyzed by the microsomal enzyme 17-ketosteroid reductase. The reverse reaction (testosterone to androstenedione) is catalyzed by 17β-hydroxysteroid dehydrogenase. This enzyme is present in many non-steroid-producing cells. $NADP^+$ is the preferred cofactor for the oxidation reaction whereas NADPH is the preferred cofactor for the reduction reaction. The pH optima for 17-ketosteroid reductase and 17β-hydroxysteroid dehydrogenase in the rat have been shown to be 5 and 9, respectively (Bogovich and Payne, 1980). Similar pH optima were found using cell-free homogenates from human testes (Oshima and Ochiai, 1973; Oshima et al., 1977; P. J. O'Shaughnessy and A. H. Payne, unpublished results).

Several reports from Oshima and co-workers have indicated that in rat and human testicular microsomes both 17-ketosteroid reductase and 17β-hydroxysteroid dehydrogenase are activated by the product of the reaction (Oshima and Ochiai, 1973; Oshima et al., 1977, 1980). They concluded that results from their kinetic data are consistent with two sites on one enzyme: one specific for androstenedione and one for testosterone, each site being both an active site for the substrate and an activation site for the reverse reaction (Oshima et al., 1980). Other workers, however, have failed to show product activation with partially purified 17-ketosteroid reductase from porcine testes (Inano and Tamaoki, 1974) and with homogenates of interstitial tissue from rat testes (Murono and Payne, 1976), although 17-ketosteroid reductase activity associated with the seminiferous tubules did show activation by testosterone (Murono and Payne, 1976). In addition, 17β-hydroxysteroid dehydrogenase solubilized from human erythrocytes was inhibited by androstenedione (Mulder et al., 1972). The reason for these discrepancies is not yet clear.

The 17-ketosteroid reductase from rat interstitial tissue is inhibited by 5α-androstane-3α,17β-diol, 17β-estradiol, and dihydrotestosterone (Murono and Payne, 1976). Both 5α-androstane-3α,17β-diol and 17β-estradiol act by competitive inhibition. The potential *in vivo* significance of these inhibitions is uncertain and again depends upon the concentration of these steroids in the SER of the Leydig cells. Both 5α-androstane-3α,17β-diol and 17β-estradiol are, however, metabolites of testosterone, and both steroids may play a role in feedback inhibition of testosterone production *in vivo*.

Results from our laboratory (Bogovich and Payne, 1980) have shown that rat testicular 17-ketosteroid reductase and 17β-hydroxysteroid dehydrogenase are distinct enzymes. 17-Ketosteroid reductase was purified and found to have no 17β-hydroxysteroid dehydrogenase activity, and partially purified 17β-hydroxysteroid dehydrogenase was free of 17-ketosteroid reductase activity. These results are consistent with observations in cases of male pseudohermaphroditism due to testicular 17-ketosteroid reductase deficiency in both the rat and human. Testes from pseudohermaphrodite rats and men are unable to reduce androstenedione to testosterone or dehydroepiandrosterone to androstenediol, although the reverse reaction is either normal or greater than normal (Goldman and Klingele, 1974; Goebelsmann *et al.*, 1975).

The 17-ketosteroid reductase activity was measured in the three populations of Leydig cells using intact cell preparations. Cells were incubated for 1 hour at 34°C in the presence of 10 μM [³H]androstenedione, and production of testosterone and dihydrotestosterone was measured (O'Shaughnessy *et al.*, 1981). As shown in Table IV, 17-ketosteroid reductase activity did not differ markedly among the three populations, although activity in population IA was slightly less than in populations IB and II. During sexual maturation of the male rat, the

TABLE IV

17-Ketosteroid Reductase Activity in Different Populations of Leydig Cells[a]

Cell population	Products formed (nmol/10⁶ Leydig cells)[b]		Total 17-ketosteroid reductase activity (nmol/10⁶ Leydig cells·hr)[c]
	Testosterone	Dihydrotestosterone	
IA	4.15 ± 0.15	0.76 ± 0.06	4.92 ± 0.16
IB	5.43 ± 0.25	0.87 ± 0.10	6.29 ± 0.35
II	6.15 ± 0.02	0.23 ± 0.05	6.34 ± 0.02

[a] From O'Shaughnessy *et al.*, 1981.
[b] Mean ± SE of duplicate independent incubations.
[c] 17-Ketosteroid reductase activity was determined as the sum of testosterone and dihydrotestosterone formed.

increase in testicular 17-ketosteroid reductase activity closely parallels the ability of the testis to produce testosterone *in vitro* (Payne *et al.*, 1977). These results suggested that 17-ketosteroid reductase may be rate limiting in the immature rat. From results reported here, however, it can be seen that, although activity in population IA is lower than in populations IB and II, the magnitude of the difference is small and unlikely to be of physiological importance. This observation would suggest, therefore, that 17-ketosteroid reductase is not rate limiting in the mature rat testis.

D.   5α-Reductase

The principal pathway of testosterone metabolism in the rat testis is via 5α-reduction of the 4–5 double bond to form dihydrotestosterone and the 5α-androstanediols. In addition, testosterone is metabolized via 19-hydroxylation and aromatization to 17β-estradiol. Age-dependent differences in activity and the intratesticular localization of the 5α-reductase enzyme are described later in this chapter (Section VI,C). Dihydrotestosterone is a cellular mediator of androgenic effects in many target organs, and much of the characterization of 5α-reductase has been done using steroid target tissue such as the rat prostate. The original characterization of 5α- and 5β-reductases was by Tomkins and co-workers using the liver (Tomkins, 1957; McGuire and Tomkins, 1959; McGuire *et al.*, 1960). 5α-Reductases are found in the SER (Forchielli and Dorfman, 1956; Forchielli *et al.*, 1958), with varying amounts found in nuclei, depending upon the tissue under investigation (Moore and Wilson, 1972). In the testis, only a small percentage of activity appears to be associated with nuclei (Oshima *et al.*, 1970; Yoshizaki *et al.*, 1978). The enzyme requires NADPH as cofactor and in the prostate has an apparent pH optimum between 6.5 and 7 (Frederiksen and Wilson, 1971; Nozu and Tamaoki, 1974). 5α Reduction appears to involve a hybrid transfer from the β position of NADPH to the 5α position of the steroid (Abul-Hajj, 1972). The enzyme is inhibited by certain divalent cations; no evidence of product inhibition has been shown (Frederiksen and Wilson, 1971); but estrogens can inhibit the reaction in a competitive manner (Shimaziki *et al.*, 1972; Bonne and Raynaud, 1973; Nozu and Tamaoki, 1974).

The apparent 5α-reduction of testosterone to dihydrotestosterone, shown in Table IV, seemed to be higher in population IA and IB than in population II. It is possible, therefore, that the lower hCG-stimulated testosterone production in populations IA and IB compared to population II (shown in Fig. 13) may be partly due to increased testosterone

TABLE V

5α-Reductase Activity in Different Populations of Leydig Cells

Cell population	Products formed (nmol/10⁶ Leydig cells)[a]		Total 5α-reductase activity (nmol/10⁶ Leydig cells·hr)[c]
	Dihydrotestosterone	5α-Diols[b]	
IA	ND[d]	1.07 ± 0.03	1.07 ± 0.03
IB	0.22 ± 0.01	0.49 ± 0.15	0.71 ± 0.16
II	0.47 ± 0.01	0.05 ± 0.01	0.52 ± 0.01

[a] Mean ± SE of duplicate independent incubations.

[b] 5α-Diols represent both 5α-androstane-3α,17β-diol and 5α-androstane-3β,17β-diol. No attempt was made to separate these compounds.

[c] 5α-Reductase activity was determined as the sum of dihydrotestosterone and 5α-diols formed.

metabolism. To investigate this possibility, cells from each population were incubated with 10 μM [³H]testosterone at 34°C for 2 hours. As shown in Table V, 5α-reductase activity was significantly higher in populations IA and IB than in population II, with population IA showing higher activity than population IB. These data are consistent with the possibility that the lower observed capacity for testosterone production in population IA may be a result of higher 5α-reductase activity. Whether population IA produces significant amounts of 5α-reduced products from endogenous precursors needs to be determined.

E. Aromatase

The estrogens estrone and 17β-estradiol are synthesized from the precursors androstenedione and testosterone. The first step in the reaction is accepted to be 19-hydroxylation, catalyzed by a mixed-function oxidase in the presence of NADPH and molecular oxygen (Ryan, 1958, 1959). The aromatase enzyme is also a cytochrome P-450-dependent monooxygenase (Canick and Ryan, 1976). (For a recent review of the mechanism of aromatase action, see Brodie, 1980).

It has been known for some time that the testis is capable of estrogen synthesis and secretion (Rabinowitz, 1956; Baggett et al., 1959), although there has been considerable controversy over the intratesticular site of aromatization. Dorrington and co-workers have reported that cultured Sertoli cells from immature rats, maintained in the presence of FSH and testosterone, have the capacity to synthesize estradiol (Dorrington et al., 1978). However, results from our laboratory (Valladares and Payne, 1979a) and from Canick *et al.* (1979) have shown that treatment of immature or adult rats with LH or hCG *in vivo* results in induction of aromatase activity in the interstitial tissue. In addition, we have shown acute *in vitro* hCG and dibutyryl cAMP stimulation of aromatase activity in Leydig cells isolated from rats 25 days of age and 60 to 70 days of age (Valladares and Payne, 1979b, 1981). Leydig cells from 15-day-old rats also have the capacity to aromatize testosterone *in vitro,* but this activity cannot be acutely stimulated by dibutyryl cAMP or hCG (Valladares and Payne, 1981).

It was considered of interest to determine the relative capacity for aromatization of the two populations of Leydig cells in the mature rat, because differences in estradiol production may be related to sensitivity of the Leydig cell populations to large desensitizing doses of hCG (see Section V,B). No attempt was made in this study to separate population I Leydig cells into subpopulations IA and IB.

Population I and population II Leydig cells were incubated with a saturating concentration of [³H]testosterone (0.6 μ*M*) (Valladares and Payne, 1979b) and various concentrations of hCG (0.3–100 p*M*). The amount of [³H]estradiol produced during a 4-hour incubation was measured as previously described (Valladares and Payne, 1979b). Aromatization by population II Leydig cells was stimulated by hCG, with

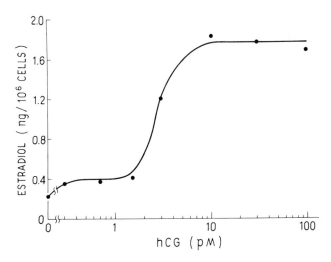

Fig. 14. Effect of increasing concentrations of hCG on *in vitro* aromatization by population II Leydig cells. Approximately 3×10^5 cells were incubated for 4 hours at 34°C under 95% O_2/5% CO_2 with 0.6 μ*M* [³H]testosterone and indicated concentrations of hCG. Each value represents the mean of duplicate incubations.

maximal production of 1.8 ng of estradiol per 10^6 cells observed at 10 pM hCG (Fig. 14). Aromatase activity was not detectable in population I Leydig cells in the absence or in the presence of hCG.

These data show that aromatization of testosterone to estradiol by rat Leydig cells is specific to population II Leydig cells. In addition, it appears that hCG is acting acutely to stimulate aromatase activity rather than simply increasing the substrate concentration, because its action is apparent in the presence of a saturating concentration of testosterone. As discussed earlier, population II Leydig cells are markedly desensitized by a single injection of a high dose of LH (150 μg), whereas population I Leydig cells are relatively unaffected. Because population II Leydig cells alone appear to have the capacity to aromatize testosterone, this differential effect of *in vivo* LH treatment may be related to estrogen production by population II.

VI. LEYDIG CELLS DURING SEXUAL MATURATION

Two generations of Leydig cells have been distinguished in the rat testis by histological, histochemical, and ultrastructural means: a "fetal" or "perinatal" generation that appears as early as the seventeenth fetal day and disappears during the second postnatal week, and an "adult" generation that begins to develop during the second or third postnatal week (Roosen-Runge and Anderson, 1959; Niemi and Ikonen, 1963; Lording and de Kretser, 1972). This section will review current information concerning changes in the "adult" generation of Leydig cells during sexual maturation in the rat.

A. Numbers of Leydig Cells

The total number of Leydig cells (identified by morphological and histochemical criteria) has been shown to increase by approximately 10-fold between approximately 3 and 8 weeks of age (Clegg, 1966; Knorr *et al.*, 1970; Lording and de Kretser, 1972; Pahnke *et al.*, 1975). In our laboratory, we have investigated changes in the distribution of Leydig cells between the two populations in relation to the increase in the total number of Leydig cells that occurs during sexual maturation (Payne *et al.*, 1981; Chase and Payne, 1981). Because the LH/hCG-binding capacity per Leydig cell is essentially the same in both populations and at all ages from 25 to at least 55 days (see Section VI,B, below), this could be accomplished by monitoring changes in ^{125}I-labeled hCG binding in the two populations after complete collagenase dissociation of whole testes

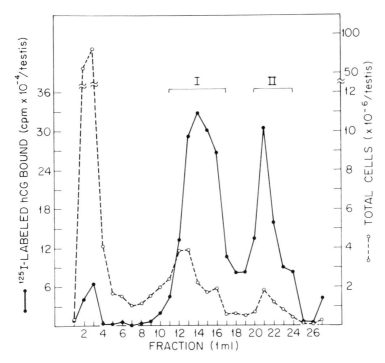

Fig. 15. Profile of ^{125}I-labeled hCG binding and total cell number in fractions collected after Metrizamide gradient centrifugation of dispersed testicular cells from 44-day-old rats. Testes were completely dissociated with collagenase and dispersed cells were centrifuged in a discontinuous gradient of Metrizamide. Specific binding of ^{125}I-labeled hCG (●) and total cell number (○) were determined for individual 1-ml fractions. Results are normalized to represent one testis. Fractions 11–17 represent population I and fractions 20–24 represent population II Leydig cells.

and separation of the dispersed cells by Metrizamide gradient centrifugation. In initial experiments, profiles of hCG binding and total cell number in individual gradient fractions were obtained at different ages. Figure 15 is a profile for testes from 44-day-old rats. It is representative of profiles obtained at all ages from 25 to approximately 44 days and shows considerably more binding in fractions representing population I than in fractions representing population II. Figure 16 is a profile for testes from 55-day-old rats. It is representative of profiles obtained after about 50 days of age and shows considerably more binding in fractions representing population II than in fractions representing population I. Between approximately 44 and 50 days of age, profiles of hCG binding appeared to be intermediate between the two illustrated here. These initial profiles revealed a pronounced shift in the distribution of Leydig

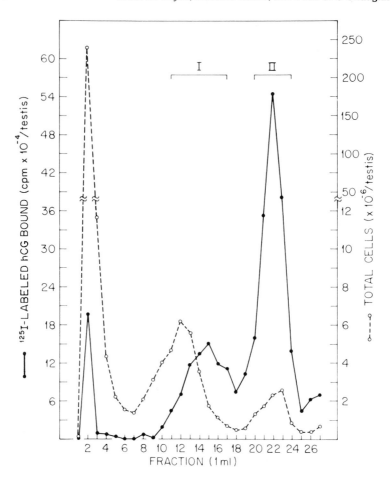

Fig. 16. Profile of ^{125}I-labeled hCG binding (●) and total cell number (○) in fractions collected after Metrizamide gradient centrifugation of dispersed testicular cells from 55-day-old rats. See legend to Fig. 15 for procedural details.

cells between the two populations during sexual maturation. To examine this shift further, cells from completely dissociated testes were centrifuged in Metrizamide gradients, and fractions were combined as indicated by the horizontal bars in Figures 15 and 16 representing populations I and II. Figure 17 illustrates changes in hCG binding (expressed as femtomoles per testis) in the two populations of Leydig cells from 25 to 55 days of age. Binding in both populations of Leydig cells increased markedly from 25 to approximately 40 days of age. Binding in population I then decreased through 55 days of age, whereas

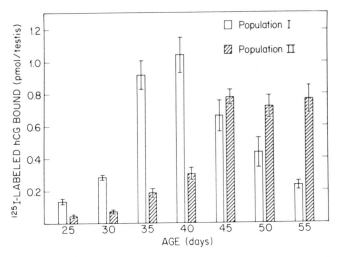

Fig. 17. Binding of ^{125}I-labeled hCG by populations I and II Leydig cells from rats from 25 to 55 days of age. Procedures were as described in the legend to Fig. 15, except that ^{125}I-labeled hCG binding was determined in pooled gradient fractions representing the two populations of Leydig cells.

binding in population II continued to increase until approximately 45 days of age and remained relatively constant thereafter. Thus, early in sexual maturation, most of the Leydig cells in the rat testis are in population I. The increase in the total number of Leydig cells that occurs before puberty results from increases in the numbers of Leydig cells in both of the populations. Later in sexual maturation, although the total number of Leydig cells no longer increases, the number in population II continues to increase while the number in population I decreases. These latter changes seem to happen rather abruptly and cause a shift in the relative abundance of Leydig cells in the two populations so that most of the Leydig cells in the testis after sexual maturity are in population II. That the number of Leydig cells in population II increases concomitantly with a decrease in the number in population I provides circumstantial evidence for the hypothesis that population II Leydig cells are derived from population I Leydig cells.

B. LH Receptors

Numerous studies of binding of ^{125}I-labeled LH and hCG by testicular homogenates have shown that the content of LH receptors in the rat testis increases during sexual maturation (Sharpe *et al.*, 1973; Desjardins *et al.*, 1974; Frowein and Engel, 1975; Pahnke *et al.*, 1975;

Thanki and Steinberger, 1976; Odell and Swerdloff, 1976; Ketelslegers *et al.*, 1978). We have observed a similar increase in ^{125}I-labeled hCG binding by cell suspensions from completely dissociated testes from rats between 25 and 55 days of age (Payne *et al.*, 1981; Chase and Payne, 1981). Scatchard analyses of LH binding by testicular homogenates have indicated that the affinity of the receptors for LH remains essentially constant throughout maturation (Thanki and Steinberger, 1976; Ketelslegers *et al.*, 1978). In general, the reported increases in testicular LH/hCG-binding capacity could be accounted for by the concurrent increase in the number of Leydig cells, suggesting that the number of LH receptors per Leydig cell does not change appreciably during sexual maturation. Our developmental studies of the two populations of Leydig cells have supported this suggestion, as we have consistently found that hCG-binding capacity varies only slightly around a mean value of approximately 100 fmoles per 10^6 Leydig cells in both populations and at all ages from 25 to 55 days.

C. Steroidogenesis

A variety of investigations have indicated that the major products of testicular androgen synthesis change during sexual maturation in the rat: Whereas testosterone is the predominant product in the mature testis, 5α-reduced androgens (especially 5α-androstane-3α,17β-diol) predominate during much of sexual maturation. These investigations have included (1) measurements of androgen concentrations in testes (Podestá and Rivarola, 1974; Corpéchot *et al.*, 1981), peripheral blood (Podestá and Rivarola, 1974; Moger, 1977; Moger and Murphy, 1977; Foldesy and Leathem, 1980; Corpéchot *et al.*, 1981), and testicular venous blood (Foldesy and Leathem, 1980); (2) determinations of basal and LH- or hCG-stimulated production of androgens *in vitro* from endogenous precursors by whole testes and "Leydig cell-enriched" suspensions of collagenase-dispersed testicular cells (Lacroix *et al.*, 1975, 1977; Moger, 1979; Purvis *et al.*, 1978a, 1980); and (3) studies of the products of conversion of exogenous cholesterol and C_{21}–C_{19} steroid precursors by various testicular preparations (Nayfeh *et al.*, 1966; Inano *et al.*, 1967; Steinberger and Ficher, 1968, 1971; Strickland *et al.*, 1970; Coffey *et al.*, 1971; Ficher and Steinberger, 1971; Folman *et al.*, 1972, 1973; Rivarola *et al.*, 1972, 1975; Matsumoto and Yamada, 1973; Tsang *et al.*, 1973; Goldman and Klingele, 1974; van der Molen *et al.*, 1975; Yoshizaki *et al.*, 1978). Although there have been reports that 5α-reductase activity in the immature testis is localized predominantly in the seminiferous tubules (Rivarola *et al.*, 1972, 1975), it is generally accepted that the pattern of testicular androgen production observed during sexual maturation reflects changes in the steroidogenic activity of the Leydig cells (Folman *et al.*, 1973; van der Molen *et al.*, 1975; Yoshizaki *et al.*, 1978; Purvis *et al.*, 1978a, 1980; Moger, 1979). Changes in production of testosterone and 5α-reduced androgens in the two populations of Leydig cells during sexual maturation remain to be determined.

The activities of essentially all key steroidogenic enzymes have been shown to change in the rat testis during sexual maturation, but in most cases changes in the activities of these enzymes in individual Leydig cells cannot be firmly established from the available data, because the number of Leydig cells increases during maturation and the necessary studies with isolated Leydig cells have not been done. Cholesterol side-chain cleavage activity increases throughout maturation (Kobayashi and Ishii, 1967), whereas the activities of Δ^5-3β-hydroxysteroid dehydrogenase–isomerase, 17α-hydroxylase, and C_{17}–C_{20} lyase increase dramatically from approximately 20 to 35 days of age and remain quite constant thereafter, at least until maturity (Inano *et al.*, 1967; Goldman and Klingele, 1974; Payne *et al.*, 1977). These increases in enzyme activities are presumably involved in the increase in testicular capacity to produce androgens that occurs early in sexual maturation (discussed further later). However, like the increase in testicular capacity to produce androgens, they probably result largely from the concurrent increase in the number of Leydig cells that occurs during maturation. Indeed, the activities of all of these enzymes, except perhaps cholesterol side-chain cleavage, may actually decrease per Leydig cell during the latter part of sexual maturation, as their activities per testis seem to stop increasing before the number of Leydig cells reaches its maximum. The activity of 17β-hydroxysteroid dehydrogenase also increases markedly early in maturation but declines just before maturity (Goldman and Klingele, 1974), whereas the activity of 17-ketosteroid reductase remains low until approximately 40 days of age and then increases dramatically during the latter part of sexual maturation (Inano *et al.*, 1967; Goldman and Klingele, 1974; Payne *et al.*, 1977). This temporal separation of these two enzyme activities provides additional evidence that (as discussed in Section V,C) they are associated with two distinct enzymes. The increase in testicular 17-ketosteroid reductase activity precedes by several days and closely parallels the increase in LH-stimulated testicular testosterone production that occurs late in sexual maturation (Payne *et al.*, 1977); this increase in enzyme activity may involve an increase in activity per Leydig cell, as it continues after the number of Leydig cells reaches its maximum. Testicular 5α-reductase activity increases early in maturation, reaches maximum levels from approximately 25 to 45 days of age, and declines thereafter (see precursor–product studies of testicular steroidogenesis cited in Section VI,C). These changes in 5α-reductase activity are responsible for the change discussed earlier in the major product(s) of testicular androgen synthesis (from 5α-reduced androgens to testosterone) that occurs during the latter part of sexual maturation. The decline in testicular 5α-reductase activity late in maturation must involve a decrease in enzyme activity per Leydig cell, as it starts at about the time that the number of Leydig cells is reaching its maximum. Further insight into the changes suggested here in the activities of key steroidogenic enzymes in individual Leydig cells will, of course, require studies using isolated Leydig cell suspensions (or homogenates). Such studies of the various enzyme activities in the two populations of Leydig cells during sexual maturation will be particularly important.

It has been proposed that testicular responsiveness—and, by inference, Leydig cell responsiveness—to LH increases during sexual maturation in the rat (Odell et al., 1973, 1974; Odell and Swerdloff, 1975, 1976). Evidence supporting this proposal can be found in the initial studies of the acute elevation of circulating testosterone following injection of LH (Odell et al., 1974; Moger and Armstrong, 1974; see also Moger, 1977) and in subsequent studies of testosterone production in vitro by whole testes in response to LH or hCG (Payne et al., 1977; Purvis et al., 1978a; Sharpe and Fraser, 1978; Moger, 1979). The increase in testicular testosterone production during maturation observed in these studies is not entirely due to the concurrent increase in the number of Leydig cells in the testis, as hCG-stimulated testosterone production by isolated Leydig cells in vitro also increases during sexual maturation (Purvis et al., 1978a, 1980). However, results of the few studies that considered 5α-reduced androgens in addition to testosterone have indicated that the preceding increases in LH- or hCG-stimulated testosterone production during sexual maturation result largely from a decrease in 5α-reductase activity rather than an increase in steroidogenic potential. In the only such in vivo study, circulating "total androgen" concentrations after injections of maximal doses of LH were no higher in 60- than in 40-day-old rats and only slightly higher in those animals than in 33-day-old rats (Moger, 1977). In vitro studies have indicated that production of total androgens or "17β-hydroxy androgens" by whole testes in response to LH or hCG increases somewhat during sexual maturation (Purvis et al., 1978a; Moger, 1979). These increases are much less dramatic than those for testosterone alone and seem to result largely from the concurrent increase in the number of

Leydig cells in the testis, as production of 17β-hydroxy androgens by isolated Leydig cells *in vitro* in response to hCG is greatest quite early in sexual maturation—between approximately 30 and 45 days of age (Purvis *et al.*, 1980; see also Purvis *et al.*, 1978a). Thus, the magnitudes of Leydig cell responses to LH or hCG, evaluated as production of 5α-reduced androgens as well as testosterone, seem to be greatest well before sexual maturity and to decline during the latter part of sexual maturation. Furthermore, the sensitivity of Leydig cells to stimulation by LH or hCG also appears to be greatest very early in sexual maturation (Purvis *et al.*, 1980; see also Sharpe and Fraser, 1978). It remains to be determined whether responsiveness to LH/hCG stimulation in the two populations of Leydig cells changes during sexual maturation.

D. Hormonal Regulation of Leydig Cell Function during Sexual Maturation

The number of Leydig cells in the testis has been reported to increase under the influence of repeated administration of hCG both in immature rats (Chemes *et al.*, 1976) and in mature rats (Christensen and Peacock, 1980). It is generally accepted that new Leydig cells can arise by differentiation from fibroblast-like precursor cells and by mitosis of existing Leydig cells (Christensen, 1975). These two mechanisms were not distinguished in the study with mature rats, but both seemed to be involved in the hCG-induced increases in Leydig cell numbers in immature rats. Although these results are suggestive, it remains to be established whether LH is normally involved in the increase in the number of Leydig cells that occurs during sexual maturation. The possibility that other hormones may also be involved in this process cannot be excluded.

In the immature rat, as in the mature rat, it is clear that the steroidogenic capacity of Leydig cells is greatly reduced by hypophysectomy and is, therefore, normally maintained by pituitary hormones. However, neither the mechanisms by which hypophysectomy reduces and pituitary hormones maintain steroidogenic capacity of Leydig cells nor the identities of the hormones involved in these effects have been clearly and unequivocally established.

Hypophysectomy of immature rats markedly reduces both basal and LH- or hCG-stimulated androgen production by Leydig cells *in vitro* (van Beurden *et al.*, 1976, 1978a,b; Purvis *et al.*, 1978b, 1980), as well as basal and LH-stimulated production of pregnenolone in the presence of inhibitors of 3β-hydroxysteroid dehydrogenase (cyanoketone) and 17α-hydroxylase (SU-10603) (van Beurden *et al.*, 1978b). In addition, van Beurden *et al.* (1978a) have reported that hypophysectomy reduces cAMP production by Leydig cells in response to LH (both in the presence and in the absence of methyl isobutyl xanthine), suggesting that the reduction of Leydig cell steroidogenic capacity caused by hypophysectomy may be mediated, at least in part, by a reduction in LH-binding capacity and/or LH-stimulable adenylate cyclase activity. However, Purvis *et al.* (1978b) have reported that hypophysectomy also reduces androgen production by Leydig cells in response to dibutyryl cAMP but has relatively little effect on Leydig cell LH receptors. These latter data suggest that the reduction of the steroidogenic capacity of Leydig cells caused by hypophysectomy is mediated mainly by mechanisms distal to the LH receptor–adenylate cyclase system, such as reduction of steroidogenic enzyme activities. This possibility is consistent with the evidence that the activities of essentially all key steroidogenic enzymes are reduced by hypophysectomy and/or stimulated by gonadotropin administration (e.g., Samuels and Helmreich, 1956; Shikita and Hall, 1967; Menon *et al.*, 1967; Purvis *et al.*, 1973; Murono and Payne, 1979; Shaw *et al.*, 1979).

In contrast to steroidogenic capacity, which is greatly reduced by hypophysectomy, sensitivity of Leydig cells to stimulation of androgen production by hCG or dibutyryl cAMP seems to be increased somewhat by hypophysectomy in the immature rat (Purvis *et al.*, 1978b, 1980; see also van Beurden *et al.*, 1976).

Although it is generally agreed that FSH by itself is incapable of acutely stimulating androgen production in the rat, several studies have suggested that FSH can enhance responsiveness of androgen production to acute LH stimulation in the immature rat. Treatment of immature rats, hypophysectomized at 20–25 days of age, with FSH for 5–10 days has been reported to increase subsequent LH-stimulated *in vivo* testosterone secretion (Odell and Swerdloff, 1975, 1976; Selin and Moger, 1977) and *in vitro* testosterone production by whole decapsulated testes (Chen *et al.*, 1976, 1977) and isolated Leydig cells (van Beurden *et al.*, 1976, 1978a,b). Enhancement of steroidogenic responsiveness of Leydig cells by FSH was also apparent when production of 17β-hydroxy androgens and production of pregnenolone (in the presence of inhibitors of 3β-hydroxysteroid dehydrogenase and 17α-hydroxylase) were used as indices of acute *in vitro* responses to LH (van Beurden *et al.*, 1978b). The effects of FSH on responsiveness to LH did not seem to be due to LH contamination, as they were not duplicated by treatment with LH at doses as high as 10 times the amounts contaminating the effective doses of FSH (Chen *et al.*, 1976; van Beurden *et al.*, 1976). However, contradictory results have been reported from experiments in which immature rats, hypophysectomized at 29 days of age, were treated for 5 days with various gonadotropin preparations prior to determinations of *in vitro* 17β-hydroxy androgen production by isolated Leydig cells in response to hCG (Purvis *et al.*, 1979). The evidence from these experiments, including the fact that pretreatment of an effective FSH preparation with anti-LH serum abolished its effects on responsiveness, suggested that the effects of FSH preparations on responsiveness to LH were due to LH contamination rather than to intrinsic FSH activity. The most likely explanation for the results of Purvis *et al.* (1979) is that by 29 days of age Leydig cells have already been exposed to large amounts of endogenous FSH, as circulating FSH concentrations begin to increase markedly as early as 20 days of age (Negro-Vilar *et al.*, 1973; Payne *et al.*, 1977). Because of the high endogenous FSH concentrations prior to 29 days of age, administration of exogenous FSH to rats hypophysectomized at that age may no longer have the ability to increase Leydig cell responsiveness. In contrast, repeated administration of LH may be able to increase responsiveness in rats older than 29 days of age as it has been shown to do in rats 55 days of age or older (Payne *et al.*, 1980b; see also Zipf *et al.*, 1978a,b).

The possibility that FSH can enhance Leydig cell responsiveness to LH stimulation in immature rats hypophysectomized between 20 and 25 days of age and may, therefore, help to maintain Leydig cell responsiveness during normal sexual maturation is worthy of further investigation. If FSH does have such an effect, it could be mediated by several mechanisms. Several of the studies cited earlier indicated that FSH treatment can increase testicular LH-binding capacity in immature hypophysectomized rats (Odell and Swerdloff, 1975, 1976; Chen *et al.*, 1976, 1977). FSH has also been reported to increase 17-ketosteroid reductase activity and, to a lesser extent, 3β-hydroxysteroid dehydrogenase activity in testes of hypophysectomized immature rats (Murono and Payne, 1979) and to synergize with LH in stimulating 3β-hydroxysteroid dehydrogenase activity in testes of hypophysectomized adult rats (Shaw *et al.*, 1979). The observed effects of FSH on Leydig cells in immature rats are probably mediated by some other cell type in the testis (e.g., Sertoli cells), as there is no evidence that Leydig cells possess FSH receptors.

Very little information is available on effects of LH and hCG on LH receptors and steroidogenic responsiveness in the immature rat. Purvis *et al.* (1979) reported that, in immature rats hypophysectomized at 29 days of age, twice daily injections of 1 μg of LH for 5 days increased maximal 17β-hydroxy androgen production by isolated Leydig cells in response to hCG; this treatment seemed to reduce Leydig cell LH-binding capacity slightly, but probably not significantly. Somewhat different results were reported by Sharpe and Fraser (1978) from experiments in which intact 23- to 36-day-old rats were treated with much higher doses of LH or hCG in several different regimens. Both gonadotropins consistently reduced testicular hCG-binding capacity, and treatment with hCG was also able to increase basal and reduce hCG-stimulated *in vitro* testicular testosterone production. These few data indicate that in the immature rat, as in the mature rat (see Section IV), the effects of LH/hCG on Leydig cell LH receptors and steroidogenic responsiveness depend on the gonadotropin that is used and the dose and regimen in which it is administered. If the reported effects of FSH on responsiveness to LH/hCG in immature rats are entirely due to LH contamination, as suggested by the experiments of Purvis *et al.* (1979) with rats hypophysectomized at 29 days of age, then extremely small amounts of LH (equivalent to doses of 15–25 ng per injection) may be capable of increasing Leydig cell responsiveness, at least in rats older than about 30 days. This would suggest that extremely low circulating concentrations of endogenous LH may be able to increase Leydig cell responsiveness early in normal sexual maturation when, as discussed in (Section VI,C), responsiveness seems to be maximal, and to maintain responsiveness thereafter. Such actions of LH could be mediated by effects on steroidogenic enzymes, as discussed earlier. The elevated activity of 5α-reductase, responsible for the predominance of 5α-reduced androgens among the products of steroidogenesis, early in sexual maturation may also be due to the action of LH (Nayfeh *et al.*, 1975; Murono and Payne, 1979). The cause of the declines in 5α-reductase activity and in steroidogenic responsiveness that occur during the latter part of sexual maturation remains to be determined.

Prolactin has been reported to increase the number of Leydig cell LH receptors but to have no effect on maximum 17β-hydroxy androgen production by Leydig cells in response to hCG or on sensitivity of Leydig cells to hCG in hypophysectomized immature rats (Purvis *et al.*, 1978b). Prolactin has also been shown to increase the concentration of LH receptors in interstitial tissue homogenates in intact immature rats (Morris and Saxena, 1980). These results are similar to those observed in sexually mature rats (Zipf *et al.*, 1978b) and consistent with the suggestion (based on experiments involving bromoergocriptine-induced hypoprolactinemia) that normal circulating concentrations of prolactin are essential for the increase in testicular LH-binding capacity that occurs during sexual maturation (Huhtaniemi and Catt, 1981).

Leydig cells in the rat testis have been shown to contain receptors for androgens (Sar *et al.*, 1975; Wilson and Smith, 1975), estrogens (Mulder *et al.*, 1974), and glucocorticoids (Evain *et al.*, 1976). Several studies have indicated that all of these types of steroid hormones can alter Leydig cell LH receptor concentration and responsiveness to LH in immature rats by actions that are not mediated by the pituitary gland.

Chen *et al.* (1977) reported that, in hypophysectomized immature rats, neither testosterone nor estradiol appreciably altered testicular hCG-binding capacity, but both steroids reduced testicular testosterone production in response to LH *in vitro*. In addition, testosterone enhanced the effect of FSH on testicular hCG-binding capacity but not on responsiveness, whereas estradiol had no effect on the FSH-induced increase in binding capacity but completely suppressed the enhancement of responsiveness. Similar observations have been reported from studies in which LH-binding capacity and production of testosterone and 17β-hydroxy androgens in response to LH or hCG were evaluated using isolated Leydig cells from hypophysectomized immature rats treated with testosterone or estradiol (van Beurden *et al.*, 1976, 1978a,b; Purvis *et al.*, 1978b). The effect of testosterone treatment on Leydig cell responsiveness in hypophysectomized immature rats was also apparent when 17β-hydroxy androgen production was assessed in response to dibutyryl cAMP (Purvis *et al.*, 1978b), suggesting that the effect of testosterone is at the level of steroidogenic enzyme activities. Experiments with intact and hypophysectomized animals have suggested that the effects of estradiol on Leydig cell responsiveness in the immature rat are on the magnitude of the response, not on sensitivity to LH or hCG, and include inhibition of 17α-hydroxylase activity (van Beurden *et al.*, 1978b; Purvis *et al.*, 1978b). Glucocorticoids may under certain conditions also be capable of reducing the number of LH receptors on Leydig cells, the sensitivity of Leydig cells to LH/hCG and dibutyryl cAMP, and the magnitudes of androgen responses of Leydig cells to LH/hCG in the immature rat (Purvis *et al.*, 1978b; Bambino and Hsueh, 1981).

It is clear from the preceding discussion that a number of hormones can alter Leydig cell function in the immature rat, but the ways in which these hormones interact to regulate normal Leydig cell development and function during sexual maturation remain to be elucidated. Future studies designed to accomplish this purpose should take into account the existence of more than one population of Leydig cells that differ and change in their relative abundance throughout maturation and that may also differ in function and in susceptibility to hormonal modulation of their function at any given time in sexual maturation.

VII. CONCLUSION

Regulation of testicular steroidogenesis is considerably more complicated than originally envisaged. The demonstration of the existence of more than one population of Leydig cells that differ in their capacities to produce testosterone, in the activities of certain key steroidogenic enzymes, and in their responses to *in vivo* gonadotropin treatments, and that change in relative abundance during sexual maturation has major implications for our understanding of factors that regulate testicular steroidogenesis.

Our observation that population I Leydig cells are dislodged from the testis more easily by collagenase treatment than population II Leydig cells suggests that the two populations of Leydig cells may be localized in different areas of the interstitial tissue. Separation of the two populations by centrifugation in different density gradients indicates an apparent difference in the densities of Leydig cells in each population. Whether the two populations of Leydig cells differ in size or shape has not been established.

The change in the distribution of Leydig cells during sexual maturation, from population I predominating before the total number of Leydig cells has become maximal to population II predominating thereafter, may reflect the final stage in the differentiation of Leydig cells. With the use of [³H]thymidine to label Leydig cell DNA during the time when the total number of Leydig cells is increasing most rapidly (between 30 and 40 days of age), we hope to determine whether population II Leydig cells are derived from population I Leydig cells.

The morphological and biochemical changes that occur during the shift of Leydig cells from population I to population II during the latter part of sexual maturation are not known at present.

The role of FSH in increasing testicular LH receptors and androgen production during sexual maturation (Odell and Swerdloff, 1975, 1976; Chen *et al.*, 1976, 1977; van Beurden *et al.*, 1976, 1978a,b) may only be a reflection of an increase in the number and a change in the distribution of Leydig cells in the two populations and not an effect of FSH on the number of LH receptors and androgen production per Leydig cell. Our demonstration that the number of LH receptors per Leydig cell is the same in both populations and at all ages between 25 and 55 days is consistent with the suggestion that FSH may regulate the total number of Leydig cells and/or the distribution of Leydig cells between the two populations rather than increasing the number of receptors or responsiveness to LH of individual Leydig cells.

The role of pituitary and other hormones in regulating Leydig cell development and function must be reevaluated, taking into consideration the existence of different populations of Leydig cells.

ACKNOWLEDGMENTS

This work was supported by research grants HD-04064 and HD-08358 from the National Institute of Child Health and Human Development. David J. Chase is supported by

Training Grant 5T23-HD-07048 from the National Institute of Child Health and Human Development. Peter J. O'Shaughnessy was supported by Ford Foundation Training Grant 700-0635B.

REFERENCES

Abul-Hajj, Y. J. (1972). Stereospecificity of hydrogen transfer from NADPH by steroid Δ⁴-5α- and Δ⁴-5β-reductase. *Steroids* **20**, 215–222.

Ascoli, M., and Puett, D. (1978a). Degradation of receptor-bound human choriogonadotropin by murine Leydig tumor cells. *J. Biol. Chem.* **253**, 4892–4899.

Ascoli, M., and Puett, D. (1978b). Gonadotropin binding and stimulation of steroidogenesis in Leydig tumor cells. *Proc. Natl. Acad. Sci. U.S.A.* **75**, 99–102.

Baggett, B., Engel, L. L., Balderas, L., Lanman, G., Savard, K., and Dorfman, R. I. (1959). Conversion of C^{14}-testosterone to C^{14}-estrogenic steroids by endocrine tissues. *Endocrinology (Baltimore)* **64**, 600–608.

Bambino, T. H., and Hsueh, A. J. W. (1981). Direct inhibitory effect of glucocorticoids upon testicular luteinizing hormone receptor and steroidogenesis *in vivo* and *in vitro*. *Endocrinology (Baltimore)* **108**, 2142–2148.

Basch, R. S., and Finegold, M. J. (1971). 3β-hydroxysteroid dehydrogenase activity in the mitochondria of rat adrenal homogenates. *Biochem. J.* **125**, 983–989.

Betz, G., and Michels, D. (1973). The effect of metyrapone on the 17,20 lyase from rat testis microsomes. *Biochem. Biophys. Res. Commun.* **50**, 134–139.

Betz, G., Tsai, P., and Weakley, R. (1975). Participation of cytochrome P-450 in the steroid 17α-hydroxylase of testis microsomes. *Steroids* **25**, 791–798.

Betz, G., Tsai, P., and Weakley, R. (1976). Heterogeneity of cytochrome P-450 in the rat testis microsomes. *J. Biol. Chem.* **251**, 2839–284.

Betz, G., Tsai, P., and Hales, D. (1980). Reconstitution of steroid 17,20 lyase activity after separation and purification of cytochrome P-450 and its reductase from rat testis microsomes. *Endocrinology (Baltimore)* **107**, 1055–1060.

Bogovich, K., and Payne, A. H. (1980). Purification of rat testicular microsomal 17-ketosteroid reductase. Evidence that 17-ketosteroid reductase and 17β-hydroxysteroid dehydrogenase are distinct enzymes. *J. Biol. Chem.* **255**, 5552–5559.

Bonne, C., and Raynaud, J.-P. (1973). Inhibition of 5α-reductase activity of rat prostate by estradiol derivatives. *Biochimie* **55**, 227–229.

Brodie, A. M. H. (1980). Recent advances in studies on estrogen biosynthesis. *J. Endocrinol. Invest.* **2**, 445–460.

Browning, J. Y., D'Agata, R., and Grotjan, H. E., Jr. (1981). Isolation of purified rat Leydig cells using continuous Percoll gradients. *Endocrinology (Baltimore)* **109**, 667–669.

Canick, J. A., and Ryan, K. J. (1976). Cytochrome P-450 and the aromatization of 16α-hydroxtestosterone and androstenedione by human placental microsomes. *Mol. Cell. Endocrinol.* **6**, 105–115.

Canick, J. A., Makris, A., Gunsalus, G. L., and Ryan, K. J. (1979). Testicular aromatization in immature rats: Localization and stimulation after gonadotropin administration *in vivo*. *Endocrinology (Baltimore)* **104**, 285–288.

Catt, K. J., Harwood, J. P., Clayton, R. N., Davies, T. F., Chan, V., Katikineni, M., Nozu, K., and Dufau, M. L. (1980). Regulation of peptide hormone receptors and gonadal steroidogenesis. *Recent Prog. Horm. Res.* **36**, 557–622.

Chasalow, F. (1979). Mechanism and control of rat testicular steroid synthesis. *J. Biol. Chem.* **254**, 3000–3005.

Chasalow, F., Marr, H., Haour, F., and Saez, J. M. (1979). Testicular steroidogenesis after human chorionic gonadotropin desensitization in rats. *J. Biol. Chem.* **254**, 5613–5617.

Chase, D. J., and Payne, A. H. (1981). Developmental changes in numbers of Leydig cells in two populations in the rat. *Biol. Reprod.* **24**, Suppl. 1, 101A.

Chemes, H. E., Rivarola, M. A., and Bergadá, C. (1976). Effect of hCG on the interstitial cells and androgen production in the immature rat testis. *J. Reprod. Fertil.* **46**, 279–282.

Chen, C. C. C., Lin, T., Murono, E., Osterman, J., Cole, B. T., and Nankin, H. (1981). The aging Leydig cell. II. Two distinct populations of Leydig cells and the possible site of defective steroidogenesis. *Steroids* **37**, 63–72.

Chen, Y.-D. I., Payne, A. H., and Kelch, R. P. (1976). FSH stimulation of Leydig cell function in the hypophysectomized immature rat. *Proc. Soc. Exp. Biol. Med.* **153**, 473–475.

Chen, Y.-D. I., Shaw, M. J., and Payne, A. H. (1977). Steroid and FSH action on LH receptors and LH-sensitive testicular responsiveness during sexual maturation of the rat. *Mol. Cell. Endocrinol.* **8**, 291–299.

Christensen, A. K. (1975). Leydig cells. *Handb. Physiol. Sect. 7: Endocrinol.* **5**, 57–94.

Christensen, A. K., and Peacock, K. C. (1980). Increase in Leydig cell number in testes of adult rats treated chronically with an excess of human chorionic gonadotropin. *Biol. Reprod.* **22**, 383–391.

Cigorraga, S. B., Dufau, M. L., and Catt, K. J. (1978). Regulation of luteinizing hormone receptors and steroidogenesis in gonadotropin-desensitized Leydig cells. *J. Biol. Chem.* **253**, 4297–4304.

Cigorraga, S. B., Sorrell, S., Bator, J., Catt, K. J., and Dufau, M. L. (1980). Estrogen dependence of a gonadotropin-induced steroidogenic lesion in rat testicular Leydig cells. *J. Clin. Invest.* **65**, 699–705.

Clegg, E. J. (1966). Pubertal growth in the Leydig cells and accessory reproductive organs of the rat. *J. Anat.* **100**, 369–379.

Coffey, J. C., French, F. S., and Nayfeh, S. N. (1971). Metabolism of progesterone by rat testicular homogenates. IV. Further studies of testosterone formation in immature testis *in vitro*. *Endocrinology (Baltimore)* **89**, 865–872.

Conn, P. M., Tsuruhara, T., Dufau, M., and Catt, K. J. (1977). Isolation of highly purified Leydig cells by density gradient centrifugation. *Endocrinology (Baltimore)* **101**, 639–642.

Cooke, B. A., Dix, C. J., and Magee-Brown, R. (1981a). Lutropin receptors in normal and tumour Leydig cells. *Biochem. Soc. Trans.* **9**, 40–42.

Cooke, B. A., Magee-Brown, R., Golding, M., and Dix, C. J. (1981b). The heterogeneity of Leydig cells from mouse and rat testes—evidence for a Leydig cell cycle? *Int. J. Androl.* **4**, 355–366.

Corpéchot, C., Baulieu, E.-E., and Robel, P. (1981). Testosterone, dihydrotestosterone, and androstanediols in plasma, testes, and prostates of rats during development. *Acta Endocrinol. (Copenhagen)* **96**, 127–135.

Cowan, R. A., Giles, C. A., and Grant, J. K. (1974). The intramitochondrial distribution of the 3β-hydroxysteroid dehydrogenase-oxosteroid isomerase. A probable redistribution artifact. *J. Steroid Biochem.* **5**, 604–608.

Desjardins, C., Zeleznik, A. J., Midgley, A. R., Jr., and Reichert, L. E., Jr. (1974). *In vitro* binding and autoradiographic localization of human chorionic gonadotropin and follicle stimulating hormone in rat testes during development. *In* "Hormone Binding and Target Cell Activation in the Testis" (M. L. Dufau and A. R. Means, eds.), pp. 221–235. Plenum, New York.

Dorrington, J. H., Fritz, I. B., and Armstrong, D. T. (1978). Control of testicular estrogen synthesis. *Biol. Reprod.* **18**, 55–64.

Dufau, M. L., Mendelson, C. R., and Catt, K. J. (1974). A highly sensitive *in vitro* bioassay for luteinizing hormone and chronic gonadotropin: Testosterone production by dispersed Leydig cells. *J. Clin. Endocrinol. Metab.* **39**, 610–613.

Dufau, M. L., Horner, K. A., Hayashi, K., Tsuruhara, T., Conn, P. M., and Catt, K. J. (1978). Actions of choleragen and gonadotropin in isolated Leydig cells. *J. Biol. Chem.* **253**, 3721–3729.

Dufau, M. L., Cigorraga, S., Baukal, A. J., Sorrell, S., Bator, J. M., Neubauer, J. F., and Catt, K. J. (1979). Androgen biosynthesis in Leydig cells after testicular desensitization by luteinizing hormone-releasing hormone and human chorionic gonadotropin. *Endocrinology (Baltimore)* **105**, 1314–1321.

Edwards, D. P., O'Conner, J. L., Bransome, E. D., Jr., and Braselton, W. E., Jr. (1976). Human placental 3β-hydroxysteroid dehydrogenase:Δ5-isomerase. Demonstration of an intermediate in the conversion of 3β-hydroxypregn-5-en-20-one to pregn-4-ene-3,20-dione. *J. Biol. Chem.* **251**, 1632–1638.

Evain, D., Morera, A. M., and Saez, J. M. (1976). Glucocorticoid receptors in interstitial cells of the rat testis. *J. Steroid Biochem.* **7**, 1135–1139.

Ewald, W., Werbin, H., and Chaikoff, I. L. (1964). Evidence for two substrate-specific Δ5-3-ketosteroid isomerases in beef adrenal glands, and their separation from 3β-hydroxysteroid dehydrogenase. *Biochim. Biophys. Acta* **81**, 199–201.

Ficher, M., and Steinberger, E. (1971). *In vitro* progesterone metabolism by rat testicular tissue at different stages of development. *Acta Endocrinol. (Copenhagen)* **68**, 285–292.

Foldesy, R. G., and Leathem, J. H. (1980). Simultaneous measurements of testosterone and three 5α-reduced androgens in the venous effluent of immature rat testes *in situ*. *Steroids* **35**, 621–631.

Folman, Y., Sowell, J. G., and Eik-Nes, K. B. (1972). The presence and formation of 5α-dihydrotestosterone in rat testes *in vivo* and *in vitro*. *Endocrinology (Baltimore)* **91**, 702–710.

Folman, Y., Ahmad, N., Sowell, J. G., and Eik-Nes, K. B. (1973). Formation *in vitro* of 5α-dihydrotestosterone and other 5α-reduced metabolites of ³H-testosterone by the seminiferous tubules and interstitial tissue from immature and mature rat testes. *Endocrinology (Baltimore)* **92**, 41–47.

Forchielli, E., and Dorfman, R. I. (1956). Separation of Δ4-5α- and Δ4-5β-hydrogenases from rat liver homogenates. *J. Biol. Chem.* **223**, 443–448.

Forchielli, E., Brown-Grant, K., and Dorfman, R. I. (1958). Steroid Δ4hydrogenases of rat liver. *Proc. Soc. Exp. Biol. Med.* **99**, 443–448.

Ford, H. C., and Engel, L. L. (1976). Purification and properties of the Δ5-3β-hydroxysteroid dehydrogenase-isomerase system of sheep adrenal cortical microsomes. *J. Biol. Chem.* **249**, 1363–1368.

Frederiksen, D. W., and Wilson, J. D. (1971). Partial characterization of the nuclear reduced nicotinamide adenine dinucleotide phosphate: Δ4-3-ketosteroid 5α-oxidoreductase of rat prostate. *J. Biol. Chem.* **246**, 2584–2593.

Frowein, J., and Engel, W. (1975). Binding of human chorionic gonadotropin by rat testis: Effect of sexual maturation, cryptorchidism, and hypophysectomy. *J. Endocrinol.* **64**, 59–66.

Gallay, J., Vincent, M., DePaillerets, C., and Alfren, A. (1978). Solubilization and separation of Δ5-3β-hydroxysteroid dehydrogenase and 3-oxosteroid-Δ4-Δ5-isomerase from bovine adrenal cortex microsomes. *Biochim. Biophys. Acta* **529**, 79–87.

Geynet, P. (1977). Heterogeneity of membrane-bound Δ^5-3-oxosteroid isomerase. Studies on bovine adrenocortical microsomes. *Biochim. Biophys. Acta* **486**, 369–377.

Gibb, W., and Hagerman, D. D. (1976). The specificity of the 3β-hydroxysteroid dehydrogenase activity of bovine ovaries toward dehydroepiandrosterone and pregnenolone: Evidence for multiple enzymes. *Steroids* **28**, 31–41.

Goebelsmann, U., Hall, T. D., Paul, W. L., and Stanczyk, F. Z. (1975). In vitro steroid metabolic studies in testicular 17β-reduction deficiency. *J. Clin. Endocrinol. Metab.* **41**, 1136–1143.

Goldman, A. S., and Klingele, D. A. (1974). Developmental defects of testicular morphology and steroidogenesis in the male rat pseudohermaphrodite and response to testosterone and dihydrotestosterone. *Endocrinology (Baltimore)* **94**, 1–16.

Hauger, R. L., Chen, Y.-D. I., Kelch, R. P., and Payne, A. H. (1977). Pituitary regulation of Leydig cell function in the adult male rat. *J. Endocrinol.* **74**, 57–66.

Hochberg, R. B., McDonald, P. D., Ladany, S., and Lieberman, S. (1975). Transient intermediates in steroidogenesis. *J. Steroid Biochem.* **6**, 323–327.

Hochberg, R. B., Ladany, S., and Lieberman, S. (1976). Conversion of a C-20-deoxy-C_{21} steroid, 5-Pregnen-3β-ol into testosterone by rat testicular microsomes. *J. Biol. Chem.* **251**, 3320–3325.

Hosaka, M., Oshima, H., and Troen, P. (1980). Studies of the human testis. XIV. Properties of C_{17}–C_{20} lyase. *Acta Endocrinol. (Copenhagen)* **94**, 389–396.

Hsueh, A. J. W., Dufau, M. L., and Catt, K. J. (1977). Gonadotropin-induced regulation of luteinizing hormone receptors and desensitization of testicular 3′:5′-cyclic AMP and testosterone responses. *Proc. Natl. Acad. Sci. U.S.A.* **74**, 592–595.

Huhtaniemi, I. T., and Catt, K. J. (1981). Induction and maintenance of gonadotropin and lactogen receptors in hypoprolactinemic rats. *Endocrinology (Baltimore)* **109**, 483–490.

Huhtaniemi, I. T., Katikineni, M., Chan, V., and Catt, K. J. (1981). Gonadotropin-induced positive regulation of testicular luteinizing hormone receptors. *Endocrinology (Baltimore)* **108**, 58–65.

Inano, H., and Tamaoki, B.-I. (1974). Purification and properties of NADP-dependent 17β-hydroxysteroid dehydrogenase solubilized from porcine-testicular microsomal fraction. *Eur. J. Biochem.* **44**, 13–23.

Inano, H., Hori, Y., and Tamaoki, B.-I. (1967). Effect of age on testicular enzymes related to steroid bio-conversion. *Ciba Found. Colloq. Endocrinol. Proc.* **16**, 105–117.

Janszen, F. H. A., Cooke, B. A., van Driel, M. J. A., and van der Molen, H. J. (1976). Purification and characterization of Leydig cells from rat testes. *J. Endocrinol.* **70**, 345–359.

Ketelslegers, J.-M., Hetzel, W. D., Sherins, R. J., and Catt, K. J. (1978). Developmental changes in testicular gonadotropin receptors: Plasma gonadotropins and plasma testosterone in the rat. *Endocrinology (Baltimore)* **103**, 212–222.

Knorr, D. W., Vanha-Perttula, T., and Lipsett, M. B. (1970). Structure and function of rat testis through pubescence. *Endocrinology (Baltimore)* **86**, 1298–1304.

Kobayashi, S., and Ishii, S. (1967). The effect of age on the activity of cholesterol side-chain cleavage in rat testis. *Endocrinol. Jpn.* **2**, 134–137.

Kremers, P. (1976). Progesterone and pregnenolone 17α-hydroxylase: Substrate specificity and selective inhibition by 17α-hydroxylated products. *J. Steroid Biochem.* **7**, 571–575.

Lacroix, E., Eechaute, W., and Leusen, I. (1975). Influence of age on the formation of 5α-androstanediol and 7α-hydroxytestosterone by incubated rat testes. *Steroids* **25**, 649–661.

Lacroix, E., Eechaute, W., and Leusen, I. (1977). The influence of gonadotropin (hCG) treatment on the steroidogenesis by incubated rat testis. *J. Steroid Biochem.* **8**, 269–275.

Lording, D. W., and de Kretser, D. M. (1972). Comparative ultrastructural and histochemical studies of the interstitial cells of the rat testis during fetal and postnatal development. *J. Reprod. Fertil.* **29**, 261–269.

McGuire, J. S., Jr., and Tomkins, G. M. (1959). The effects of thyroxin administration on the enzymic reduction of Δ^4-3-ketosteroids. *J. Biol. Chem.* **234**, 791–794.

McGuire, J. S., Jr., Hollis, V. W., and Tomkins, G. M. (1960). Some characteristics of the microsomal steroid reductases (5α) of rat liver. *J. Biol. Chem.* **235**, 3112–3117.

McMurty, R. J., and Hagerman, D. D. (1972). Carbon monoxide inhibition of progesterone hydroxylation and side-chain cleavage catalyzed by rat testis microsomes. *Steroids Lipids Res.* **3**, 8–13.

Matsumoto, K., and Samuels, L. T. (1969). Influence of steroid distribution between microsomes and soluble fraction on steroid metabolism by microsomal enzymes. *Endocrinology (Baltimore)* **85**, 402–409.

Matsumoto, K., and Yamada, M. (1973). 5α-reduction of testosterone *in vitro* by rat seminiferous tubules and whole testes at different stages of development. *Endocrinology (Baltimore)* **93**, 253–255.

Matsumoto, K., Mahajan, D. K., and Samuels, L. T. (1974). The influence of progesterone on the conversion of 17-hydroxyprogesterone to testosterone in the mouse testis. *Endocrinology (Baltimore)* **94**, 808–814.

Menon, K. M. J., Dorfman, R. I., and Forchielli, E. (1967). Influence of gonadotropins on the cholesterol side-chain cleavage reaction by rat testis mitochondrial preparations. *Biochim. Biophys. Acta* **148**, 486–494.

Moger, W. H. (1977). Serum 5α-androstane-3α,17β-diol, androsterone, and testosterone concentrations in the male rat. Influence of age and gonadotropin stimulation. *Endocrinology (Baltimore)* **100**, 1027–1032.

Moger, H. H. (1979). Production of testosterone, 5α-androstane-3α,17β-diol, and androsterone by dispersed testicular interstitial cells and whole testes *in vitro*. *J. Endocrinol.* **80**, 321–332.

Moger, W. H., and Armstrong, D. T. (1974). Changes in serum testosterone levels following acute LH treatment in immature and mature rats. *Biol. Reprod.* **11**, 1–6.

Moger, W. H., and Murphy, P. R. (1977). Serum 5α-androstane-3α,17β-diol, androsterone, and testosterone concentrations in the immature male rat: Influence of time of day. *J. Endocrinol.* **75**, 177–178.

Moore, R. J., and Wilson, J. D. (1972). Localization of the reduced nicotinamide adenine dinucleotide phosphate:Δ^4-3-ketosteroid 5α-oxidoreductase in the nuclear membrane of the rat ventral prostate. *J. Biol. Chem.* **247**, 958–967.

Mori, H., and Christensen, A. K. (1980). Morphometric analysis of Leydig cells in the normal rat testis. *J. Cell Biol.* **84**, 340–354.

Morris, P. L., and Saxena, B. B. (1980). Dose- and age-dependent effects of prolactin (PRL) on luteinizing hormone- and PRL-binding sites in rat Leydig cell homogenates. *Endocrinology (Baltimore)* **107**, 1639–1645.

Moyle, W. R., and Ramachandran, J. (1973). Effect of LH on steroidogenesis and cyclic AMP accumulation in rat Leydig cell preparations and mouse tumor Leydig cells. *Endocrinology (Baltimore)* **93**, 127–134.

Mulder, E., Lamers-Stahlhofen, G. J. M., and van der Molen, H. J. (1972). Isolation and characterization of 17β-hydroxysteroid dehydrogenase from human erythrocytes. *Biochem J.* **127**, 649–659.

Mulder, E., van Beurden-Lamers, W. M. O., de Boer, W., Brinkman, A. O., and van der Molen, H. J. (1974). Testicular estradiol receptors in the rat. In "Hormone Binding and Target Cell Activation in the Testis" (M. L. Dufau and A. R. Means, eds.), pp. 343–355. Plenum, New York.

Murono, E. P., and Payne, A. H. (1976). Distinct testicular 17-ketosteroid reductates, one in interstitial tissue and one in seminiferous tubules. Differential modulation by testosterone and metabolites of testosterone. Biochim. Biophys. Acta 450, 89–100.

Murono, E. P., and Payne, A. H. (1979). Testicular maturation in the rat. In vivo effect of gonadotropins on steroidogenic enzymes in the hypophysectomized immature rat. Biol. Reprod. 20, 911–917.

Nakajin, S., and Hall, P. F. (1981). Microsomal cytochrome P-450 from neonatal pig testis. Purification and properties of a C_{21} steroid side-chain cleavage system (17α-hydroxylase-$C_{17,20}$ lyase). J. Biol. Chem. 256, 3871–3876.

Nakajin, S., Hall, P. F., and Onoda, M. (1981a). Testicular microsomal cytochrome P-450 for C_{21} steroid side chain cleavage. Spectral and binding studies. J. Biol. Chem. 256, 6134–6139.

Nakajin, S., Shively, J. E., Yuan, P.-M., and Hall, P. F. (1981b). Microsomal cytochrome P-450 from neonatal pig testis: Two enzymatic activities (17α-hydroxylase and $C_{17,20}$ lyase) associated with one protein. Biochemistry 20, 4037–4042.

Nayfeh, S. N., Barefoot, S. W., Jr., and Baggett, B. (1966). Metabolism of progesterone by rat testicular homogenates. II. Changes with age. Endocrinology (Baltimore) 78, 1041–1048.

Nayfeh, S. N., Coffey, J. C., Hansson, V., and French, F. S. (1975). Maturational changes in testicular steroidogenesis: Hormonal regulation of 5α-reductase. J. Steroid Biochem. 6, 329–335.

Negro-Vilar, A., Krulich, L., and McCann, S. M. (1973). Changes in serum prolactin and gonadotropins during sexual development of the male rat. Endocrinology (Baltimore) 93, 660–664.

Neher, R., and Kahnt, F. W. (1965). On the biosynthesis of testicular steroids in vitro and its inhibition. Experientia 21, 310–312.

Neville, A. M., and Engel, L. L. (1968). Steroid Δ-isomerase of the bovine adrenal gland: Kinetics, activation by NAD and attempted solubilization. Endocrinology (Baltimore) 83, 864–872.

Neville, A. M., Orr, J. C., and Engel, L. L. (1969). The $Δ^5$-3β-hydroxysteroid dehydrogenase of bovine adrenal microsomes. J. Endocrinol. 43, 599–608.

Niemi, M., and Ikonen, M. (1963). Histochemistry of the Leydig cells in the postnatal prepubertal testis of the rat. Endocrinology (Baltimore) 72, 443–448.

Nozu, K., and Tamoaki, B.-I. (1974). Characteristics of the nuclear and microsomal steroid $Δ^4$-5α-hydrogenase of the rat prostate. Acta Endocrinol. (Copenhagen) 76, 608–624.

Odell, W. D., and Swerdloff, R. S. (1975). The role of testicular sensitivity to gonadotropins in sexual maturation of the male rat. J. Steroid Biochem. 6, 853–857.

Odell, W. D., and Swerdloff, R. S. (1976). Etiologies of sexual maturation: A model system based on the sexually maturing rat. Recent Prog. Horm. Res. 32, 245–288.

Odell, W. D., Swerdloff, R. S., Jacobs, H. S., and Hescox, M. S. (1973). FSH induction of sensitivity to LH: One cause of sexual maturation in the male rat. Endocrinology (Baltimore) 92, 160–165.

Odell, W. D., Swerdloff, R. S., Bain, J., Wollesen, F., and Grover, P. K. (1974). The effect of sexual maturation on testicular response to LH stimulation of testosterone secretion in the intact rat. Endocrinology (Baltimore) 95, 1380–1384.

Onoda, M., and Hall, P. F. (1981). Inhibition of testicular microsomal cytochrome P-450

(17α-hydroxylase/$C_{17,20}$ lase) by estrogens. *Endocrinology (Baltimore)* **109**, 763–767.

O'Shaughnessy, P. J., Wong, K.-L., and Payne, A. H. (1981). Differential steroidogenic enzyme activities in different populations of rat Leydig cells. *Endocrinology (Baltimore)* **109**, 1061–1066.

O'Shaughnessy, P. J. and Payne, A. H. (1982). Differential effects of single and repeated administration of gonadotropins on testosterone production and steroidogenic enzymes in Leydig cells. *J. Biol. Chem.* **257** (in press).

Oshima, H., and Ochiai, K. (1973). On testicular 17β-hydroxysteroid oxidoreductase product activation of testosterone formation from androstenedione *in vitro*. *Biochim. Biophys. Acta* **306**, 227–237.

Oshima, H., Sarada, T., Ochiai, K., and Tamaoki, B.-I. (1970). Δ⁴-5α-hydrogenase in immature rat testes: Its intracellular distribution, enzyme kinetics, and influence of administered gonadotrophin and testosterone propionate. *Endocrinology (Baltimore)* **80**, 1215–1224.

Oshima, H., Paraska, L., Yoshida, K.-I., and Troen, P. (1977). Studies of the human testis. VIII. Product activation of 17β-hydroxysteroid oxidoreductase for testosterone. *J. Clin. Endocrinol. Metab.* **45**, 1097–1099.

Oshima, H., Yoshida, K.-I., and Troen, P. (1980). A further study of 17β-hydroxysteroid oxidoreductase in the human testis: Mechanism of *in vitro* activation. *Endocrinol. Jpn.* **27**, 107–115.

Pahnke, V. G., Leidenberger, F. A., and Künzig, H. J. (1975). Correlation between hCG)LH)-binding capacity, Leydig cell number, and secretory activity of rat testis throughout pubescence. *Acta Endocrinol. (Copenhagen)* **79**, 610–618.

Payne, A. H., and Zipf, W. B. (1978). Regulation of Leydig cell function by prolactin, growth hormone, and luteinizing hormone. *Int. J. Androl. Suppl. No. 2*, pp. 329–344.

Payne, A. H., Kelch, R. P., Murono, E. P., and Kerlan, J. T. (1977). Hypothalamic, pituitary, and testicular function during sexual maturation of the male rat. *J. Endocrinol.* **72**, 17–26.

Payne, A. H., Downing, J. R., and Wong, K.-L. (1980a). Luteinizing hormone receptors and testosterone synthesis in two distinct populations of Leydig cells. *Endocrinology (Baltimore)* **106**, 1424–1429.

Payne, A. H., Wong, K.-L., and Vega, M. M. (1980b). Differential effects of single and repeated administrations of gonadotropins in luteinizing hormone receptors and testosterone synthesis in two populations of Leydig cells. *J. Biol. Chem.* **255**, 7118–7122.

Payne, A. H., O'Shaughnessy, P. J., Chase, D. H., Dixon, G. E. K., and Christensen, A. K. (1981). LH receptors and steroidogenesis in distinct populations of Leydig cells. *Ann. N. Y. Acad. Sci.*, **383**, 174–203.

Podestá, E. J., and Rivarola, M. A. (1974). Concentration of androgens in whole testis, seminiferous tubules, and interstitial tissue of rats at different stages of development. *Endocrinology (Baltimore)* **95**, 455–461.

Preslock, J. P., and Steinberger, E. (1979). Product-inhibition of testicular steroidogenic enzymes in the marmoset *Saguinus oedipus*. *J. Steroid Biochem.* **11**, 1151–1157.

Purvis, J. L., Canick, J. A., Latif, S. A., Rosenbaum, J. H., Hologgita, J., and Menard, R. H. (1973). Lifetime of microsomal cytochrome P-450 and steroidogenic enzymes in rat testis as influenced by human chorionic gonadotropin. *Arch. Biochem. Biophys.* **159**, 39–49.

Purvis, K., Clausen, O. P. F., and Hansson, V. (1978a). Age-related changes in responsiveness of rat Leydig cells to hCG. *J. Reprod. Fertil.* **52**, 379–386.

Purvis, K., Clausen, O. P. F., and Hansson, V. (1978b). Regulation of Leydig cell sensitivity and responsiveness to LH/hCG. *Int. J. Androl. Suppl. No. 2*, pp. 247–263.

Purvis, K., Clausen, O. P. F., and Hansson, V. (1979). LH contamination may explain FSH effects on rat Leydig cells. *J. Reprod. Fertil.* **56**, 657–665.

Purvis, K., Clausen, O. P. F., and Hansson, V. (1980). Effects of age and hypophysectomy on responsiveness of rat Leydig cells to hCG. *J. Reprod. Fertil.* **60**, 77–86.

Quinn, P. G., Dombrausky, L. J., Chen, Y.-D. I., and Payne, A. H. (1981). Serum lipoproteins increase testosterone production in hCG-desensitized Leydig cells. *Endocrinology (Baltimore)* **109**, 1790–1792.

Rabinowitz, J. L. (1956). The biosynthesis of radioactive 17β-estradiol. II. Synthesis by testicular and ovarian homogenates. *Arch. Biochem. Biophys.* **64**, 285–290.

Rivarola, M. A., Podestá, E. J., and Chemes, H. E. (1972). *In vitro* testosterone-^{14}C metabolism by rat seminiferous tubules at different stages of development: Formation of 5α-androstanediol at meiosis. *Endocrinology (Baltimore)* **91**, 537–542.

Rivarola, M. A., Podestá, E. J., Chemes, H. E., and Cigorraga, S. (1975). Androgen metabolism in the seniniferous tubules. *In* "Hormonal Regulation of Spermatogenesis" (F. S. French, V. Hansson, E. M. Ritzen, and S. N. Nayfeh, eds.), pp. 25–35. Plenum, New York.

Roosen-Runge, E. C., and Anderson, D. (1959). The development of the interstitial cells in the testis of the albino rat. *Acta Anat.* **37**, 125–137.

Ryan, K. J. (1958). Conversion of androstenedione to estrone by placental microsomes. *Biochim. Biophys. Acta* **27**, 658–659.

Ryan, K. J. (1959). Biological aromatization of steroids. *J. Biol. Chem.* **234**, 268–272.

Saez, J. M., Haour, F., and Cathiard, A. M. (1978). Early hCG-induced desensitization in Leydig cells. *Biochem. Biophys. Res. Commun.* **81**, 552–558.

Samuels, L. T., and Helmreich, M. L. (1956). The influence of chorionic gonadotropin on the 3β-ol dehydrogenase activity of testes and adrenals. *Endocrinology (Baltimore)* **58**, 435–442.

Sar, M., Stumpf, W. E., McLean, W. S., Smith, A. A., Hansson, V., Nayfeh, S. N., and French, F. S. (1975). Localization of androgen target cells in the rat testis: Autoradiographic studies. *In* "Hormonal Regulation of Spermatogenesis" (F. S. French, V. Hansson, E. M. Ritzen, and S. N. Nayfeh, eds.), pp. 311–319. Plenum, New York.

Schumacher, M., Schäfer, G., Holstein, A. F., and Hilz, H. (1978). Rapid isolation of mouse Leydig cells by centrifugation in Percoll density gradients with complete retention of morphological and biochemical integrity. *FEBS. Lett.* **91**, 333–338.

Selin, L. K., and Moger, W. H. (1977). The effect of FSH on LH induced testosterone secretion in the immature hypophysectomized male rat. *Endocr. Res. Commun.* **4**, 171–182.

Sharpe, R. M., and Fraser, H. M. (1978). The influence of sexual maturation and immunization against LH-RH on testicular sensitivity to gonadotrophin stimulation *in vitro. Int. J. Androl.* **1**, 501–508.

Sharpe, R. M., and McNeilly, A. S. (1978). Gonadotrophin-induced reduction in LH-receptors and steroidogenic responsiveness of the immature rat testis. *Int. J. Androl. Suppl. No. 2*, pp. 264–275.

Sharpe, R. M., Hartog, M., Ellwood, M. G., and Brown, P. S. (1973). Age-dependent differences in the binding of ^{131}I-LH by rat testis homogenates. *J. Reprod. Fertil.* **35**, 529–532.

Shaw, M. J., Georgopoulos, L. E., and Payne, A. H. (1979). Synergistic effect of follicle-stimulating hormone and luteinizing hormone on testicular Δ[5]-3β-hydroxysteroid dehydrogenase-isomerase: Application of a new method for the separation of testicular compartments. *Endocrinology (Baltimore)* **104**, 912–918.

Shikita, M., and Hall, P. F. (1967). Action of human chorionic gonadotropin *in vivo* upon microsomal enzymes in testes of hypophysectomized rats. *Biochim. Biophys. Acta* **141**, 433–435.

Shimazaki, J., Ohki, Y., Koya, A., and Shida, K. (1972). Inhibition of nuclear testosterone 5α-reductase in rat ventral prostate by estrogens and antiandrogens. *Endocrinol. Jpn.* **19**, 585–588.

Steinberger, E., and Ficher, M. (1968). Conversion of progesterone to testosterone by testicular tissue at different stages of maturation. *Steroids* **11**, 351–368.

Steinberger, E., and Ficher, M. (1971). Formation and metabolism of testosterone in testicular tissue of immature rats. *Endocrinology (Baltimore)* **89**, 679–684.

Strickland, A. L., Nayfeh, S. N., and French, F. S. (1970). Conversion of cholesterol to testosterone and androstanediol in testicular homogenates of immature and mature rats. *Steroids* **15**, 373–387.

Thanki, K. H., and Steinberger, A. (1976). ^{125}I-LH binding to rat testes at various ages and posthypophysectomy. *Endocr. Res. Commun.* **3**, 49–62.

Tomkins, G. M. (1957). The enzymatic reduction of Δ4-3-ketosteroids. *J. Biol. Chem.* **225**, 13–24.

Tsang, W. N., Lacy, D., and Collins, P. M. (1973). Leydig cell differentiation, steroid metabolism by the interstitium *in vitro*, and the growth of the accessory sex organs in the rat. *J. Reprod. Fertil.* **34**, 351–355.

Tsuruhara, T., Dufau, M. L., Cigorraga, S., and Catt, K. J. (1977). Hormonal regulation of testicular luteinizing hormone receptors. *J. Biol. Chem.* **252**, 9002–9009.

Valladares, L.E., and Payne, A. H. (1979a). Induction of testicular aromatization by luteinizing hormone in mature rats. *Endocrinology (Baltimore)* **105**, 431–436.

Valladares, L. E., and Payne, A. H. (1979b). Acute stimulation of aromatization in Leydig cells by human chorionic gonadotropin *in vitro*. *Proc. Natl. Acad. Sci. U.S.A.* **76**, 4460–4463.

Valladares, L. E., and Payne, A. H. (1981). Effects of hCG and cyclic AMP on aromatization in purified Leydig cells of immature and mature rats. *Biol. Reprod.*, **25**, 752–758.

van der Molen, H. J., Grootegoed, J. A., de Greef-Bijleveld, M. J., Rommerts, F. F. G., and van der Vusse, G. J. (1975). Distribution of steroids, steroid production, and steroid metabolizing enzymes in rat testis. *In* "Hormonal Regulation of Spermatogenesis" (F. S. French, V. Hansson, E. M. Ritzen, and S. N. Nayfeh, eds.), pp. 3–23. Plenum, New York.

van Beurden, W. M. O., Roodnat, B., de Jong, F. H., Mulder, E., and van der Molen, H. J. (1976). Hormonal regulation of LH stimulation of testosterone production in isolated Leydig cells of immature rats: The effect of hypophysectomy, FSH, and estradiol-17β. *Steroids* **28**, 847–866.

van Beurden, W. M. O., Roodnat, B., Mulder, E., and van der Molen, H. J. (1978a). Further characterization of the effects of hypophysectomy, FSH, and estrogen on LH stimulation of testosterone production in Leydig cells isolated from immature rats. *Steroids* **31**, 83–98.

van Beurden, W. M. O., Roodnat, B., and van der Molen, H. J. (1978b). Effects of oestrogens and FSH on LH stimulation of steroid production by testis Leydig cells from immature rats. *Int. J. Androl. Suppl. No. 2*, pp. 374–383.

Wilson, E. M., and Smith, A. A. (1975). Localization of androgen receptors in rat testis: Biochemical studies. *In* "Hormonal Regulation of Spermatogenesis" (F. S. French, V. Hansson, E. M. Ritzen, and S. N. Nayfeh, eds.), pp. 281–286. Plenum, New York.

Yoshizaki, K., Matsumoto, K., and Samuels, L. T. (1978). Localization of Δ4-5α-reductase in immature rat testis. *Endocrinology (Baltimore)* **102**, 918–925.

Zipf, W. B., Payne, A. H., and Kelch, R. P. (1978a). Dissociation of lutropin-induced loss of testicular lutropin receptors and lutropin-induced desensitization of testosterone synthesis. *Biochim. Biophys. Acta* **540**, 330–336.

Zipf, W. B., Payne, A. H., and Kelch, R. P. (1978b). Prolactin, growth hormone, and luteinizing hormone in the maintenance of testicular luteinizing hormone receptors. *Endocrinology (Baltimore)* **103**, 595–600.

Zirkin, B. R., Ewing, L. L., Kromann, M., and Cochran, R. L. (1980). Testosterone secretion by rat, rabbit, guinea pig, dog, and hamster testes perfused *in vitro:* Correlation with Leydig cell ultrastructure. *Endocrinology (Baltimore)* **107**, 1867–1874.

12

Regulation of Steroid Production in Adrenal, Gonadal, and Placental Tumor Cells

MARIO ASCOLI

I. INTRODUCTION

There are four mammalian tissues that produce steroid hormones: adrenals, ovaries, testes, and placenta.

409

In three of these tissues, the production of steroids is controlled by polypeptide hormones produced by the pituitary. Adrenocorticotropin (ACTH) regulates glucocorticoid production from the adrenals, and luteinizing hormone (LH) controls the production of androgens by the testes and progestins and estrogens by the ovary. In the pregnant human female, ovarian steroid production is controlled by human choriogonadotropin (hCG), a polypeptide hormone (analogous to LH) produced by the placenta. Placental steroid production, on the other hand, does not appear to be regulated by trophic hormones. In this tissue, steroidogenesis may be regulated by substrate availability.

Our increased understanding about the biochemistry of steroid biosynthesis and its regulation has been aided by the availability of cultured tumor cells derived from these steroidogenic tissues. In this chapter, an attempt has been made to summarize our knowledge about the origin and steroidogenic properties of cell lines derived from adrenal, gonadal, and placental tumor cells. Where appropriate, this chapter also covers data obtained with normal tissues. Because of the volume of data available and its complexity, the reader is also referred to reviews that deal more extensively with some of the specific topics discussed here (Kowal, 1970; Garren et al., 1971; Hall and Shikita, 1974; Moyle and Greep, 1974; Gill et al., 1978, 1980; Brown et al., 1979; Simpson, 1979; Bedin et al., 1980; Schimmer, 1980; Simpson and MacDonald, 1981; Chapter 11).

II. ORIGIN AND GENERAL CHARACTERISTICS OF STEROID-SECRETING TUMORS

A. Adrenal Tumors

The model system most widely used to study steroid production by adrenal cells is the Y-1 cell line. This cell line is a clonal strain of adrenocortical cells established in culture by Sato and colleagues (Buonassisi et al., 1962; Stollar et al., 1964; Yasumura et al., 1966) from a transplantable tumor of the LAF1 mouse (Cohen et al., 1957).

The Y-1 cells have a doubling time of 30–40 hours and a nearly diploid karyotype (modal number of chromosomes = 39) (Yasumura et al., 1966; Schimmer, 1979). This cell line is available from the American Type Culture Collection (No. CCL-79).

The major steroids synthesized by the Y-1 cells are 20α-hydroxyprogesterone and 11β,20α-dihydroxyprogesterone (Pierson,

TABLE I

Cultured Lines of Adrenocortical Tumor Cells

| | | | Steroidogenic response | | | |
| | | | | Cholera | | |
Cell line	Species	Major steroids[a]	ACTH	toxin	cAMP	Reference
Y-1	Mouse	20-OHP 11,20-diOHP	+	+	+	*f*
Y-6[b]	Mouse	20-OHP 11,20-diOHP	−	+	+	*g*
OS-3[b]	Mouse	20-OHP 11,20-diOHP	−[c]	+	+	*h*
Cyc 101–103[b]	Mouse	20-OHP 11,20-diOHP	−[d]	N.T.[e]	+	*i*
Kin 1, 2, 4, 7, 8[b]	Mouse	20-OHP 11,20-diOHP	−[d]	N.T.[e]	−[d]	*i*

[a] 20-OHP, 20α-Hydroxyprogesterone; 11,20-OHP, 11β,20α-hydroxyprogesterone.

[b] Variant cell lines isolated from the Y-1 cells.

[c] No increase in steroid production is observed at concentrations of ACTH 5000 times higher than those required to induce maximal steroidogenesis in the Y-1 cells.

[d] Steroidogenic responses to these agents are drastically impaired but not entirely lost.

[e] N.T., Not tested.

[f] Yasumura *et al.*, 1966; Wolff *et al.*, 1973; Donta *et al.*, 1973.

[g] Schimmer, 1969, 1972; Rae *et al.*, 1979a, 1980.

[h] Donta, 1974b; Schimmer, 1969, 1972; Wolff and Hope Cook, 1975; Rae *et al.*, 1979a, 1980.

1967; Kowal and Fiedler, 1968). Steroid production is stimulated by ACTH, cholera toxin, and cAMP (or analogs thereof) (Buonassisi *et al.*, 1962; Yasumura *et al.*, 1966; Wolff *et al.*, 1973; Donta *et al.*, 1973; Donta, 1974a,b; Wolff and Hope Cook, 1975). Several stable variants of the Y-1 cells have been isolated (reviewed by Schimmer *et al.*, 1979). These include clones with altered ACTH-sensitive adenylate cyclase (Schimmer, 1969, 1972; Rae *et al.*, 1979a, 1980), altered hypoxanthine phosphorybosyltransferase activity (Schimmer *et al.*, 1977a), and altered cAMP-dependent protein kinase activity (Schimmer *et al.*, 1977b; Rae *et al.*, 1979b).

The general properties of the Y-1 cells and variants are listed in Table I. The methodology used in maintaining these cells has been reviewed by Schimmer (1979).

B.   Gonadal Tumors

Most of the work on the regulation of steroid production in gonadal tumors has been done on transplantable Leydig cell tumors and derived cell lines. Some potentially useful ovarian tumors have been reported (Roth et al., 1972; Cole et al., 1973; Rice et al., 1975; Kammerman et al., 1977). Unfortunately, their steroidogenic properties have not been investigated in detail, and, therefore, they will not be reviewed here.

Shin and colleagues were the first to establish two clonal lines of cultured Leydig tumor cells (Shin, 1967; Shin et al., 1968). These cell lines, designated I-10 and R2C, are available from the American Type Culture Collection (Nos. CCL-83 and CCL-97, respectively).

The I-10 cells originated from a mouse Leydig cell tumor (Shin, 1967). They are nearly diploid (modal number of chromosomes = 41) and have a doubling time of approximately 3.5 days. The major steroids produced are progesterone and 20α-hydroxyprogesterone. Steroid production is increased by cAMP and cholera toxin but not by LH or hCG (Shin, 1967; Wolff and Hope Cook, 1975).

The R2C cells originated from a rat tumor. They are heteroploid (modal number of chromosomes = 73) and produce progesterone and 20α-hydroxyprogesterone. Steroid production cannot be increased with LH, hCG, or cAMP (Shin et al., 1968).

One of the most widely used Leydig cell tumors is designated M5480. This is a mouse tumor that was adapted to serial transplantation by W. F. Dunning and that has been studied in several laboratories including ours. The growth, morphology, and composition of the tumor have been studied by Neaves (1973, 1975a,b) and Yang et al. (1974). Its steroidogenic properties were originally studied by Moyle and co-workers (Moyle and Armstrong, 1970; Moudgal et al., 1971; Moyle et al., 1971, 1973a,b; Pokel et al., 1972; Moyle and Ramachandran, 1973; Moyle and Greep, 1974) and later by us (Ascoli, 1978, 1979, 1980, 1981a,b,c, 1982; Ascoli and Puett, 1978a,b,c; Albert et al., 1980; Lacroix et al., 1980; Freeman and Ascoli, 1981; Segaloff and Ascoli, 1981; Segaloff et al., 1981a,b).

Two variants of the M5480 tumor have been identified: One, designated M5480A, synthesizes progesterone and testosterone; the other, designated M5480P, synthesizes mainly progesterone (Ascoli and Puett, 1978a; Lacroix et al., 1980). Steroid production in freshly isolated Leydig tumor cells can be increased by LH, hCG, cholera toxin, and cAMP (Moyle and Ramachandran, 1973; Ascoli and Puett, 1978a; Ascoli, 1978; Segaloff et al., 1981a).

TABLE II

Cultured Lines of Leydig Tumor Cells

Cell line	Species	Major steroids[a]	Steroidogenic response			References
			LH/hCG	Cholera toxin	cAMP	
I-10	Mouse	P, 20-OHP	−	+	+	d
R2C	Rat	P, 20-OHP	−	+	−	e
LC-540	Rat	T, E$_2$	N.T.[b]	N.T.[b]	N.T.[b]	f
MA-10, 12	Mouse	P, 20-OHP	+	+	+	g
MA-14, 18, 19	Mouse	P, 20-OHP	−[c]	+	+	g

[a] P, Progesterone; 20-OHP, 20α-hydroxyprogesterone; T, testosterone; E$_2$, 17β-estradiol.

[b] N.T., Not tested.

[c] Response is drastically reduced but not entirely lost.

[d] Shin, 1967; Wolff and Hope Cook, 1975.

[e] Shin et al., 1968.

[f] Steinberger et al., 1970.

[g] Ascoli, 1981a.

I was able to establish several clonal lines of cultured Leydig tumor cells from the M5480P tumor (Ascoli, 1981a). The major steroids produced by these cells are progesterone and 20α-hydroxyprogesterone. Steroid production can be increased by LH, hCG, cholera toxin, and cAMP in two of the lines (designated MA-10 and MA-12), and by cholera toxin and cAMP, but not by LH or hCG, in the other three lines (designated MA-14, MA-18, and MA-19). These cells are heteroploid with modal chromosome numbers of 98–106 and a doubling time of approximately 24 hours (M. Ascoli, 1981a,b and unpublished observations).

Another potentially useful Leydig cell tumor (designated H-540) has been studied by Cooke et al. (1979). This is a rat tumor originally adapted to serial transplantation by Jacobs and Huseby (1968). Freshly isolated H-540 cells synthesize testosterone and at least two other unidentified steroids. Steroid production is increased with LH or cAMP (Cooke et al., 1979). The same tumor appears to have been used to establish (Steinberger et al., 1970) another line of cultured Leydig tumor cells (designated LC-540) available from the American Type Culture Collection (No. CCL-43). These cultured cells are reported to synthesize testosterone and estradiol (Steinberger et al., 1970). It is not known, however, whether steroid production is stimulated by hormones or cyclic nucleotides.

A summary of the characteristics of cultured Leydig tumor cells is presented in Table II.

C. Placental Tumors

The first line of cultured malignant trophoblastic cells was established by Patillo and Gey (1968) from a human choriocarcinoma adapted to serial transplantation in the cheek pouch of the hamster (Hertz, 1959). This cell line is designated BeWo and is available from the American Type Culture Collection (No. CCL-98). The cells are heteroploid (modal number of chromosomes = 86) and show a doubling time of approximately 24 hours (Patillo et al., 1970a).

Kohler and co-workers (Kohler and Bridson, 1971; Kohler et al., 1971) established six clonal lines of cultured choriocarcinoma cells (designated JEG 1, 2, 3, 4, 7, and 8) from the same tumor used to establish the BeWo cells. A third line of cultured human choriocarcinoma cells (designated Jar) was established directly from a trophoblastic tumor removed by biopsy (Patillo et al., 1970b).

All three lines synthesize polypeptide [hCG and human placental lactogen (hPL)] and steroid hormones (progesterone and several estrogens) (Huang et al., 1969; Patillo et al., 1970a,b, 1972; Kohler and Bridson, 1971; Bellino et al., 1978; Bahn et al., 1981).

A summary of the properties of these cell lines is shown in Table III.

III. STEROIDOGENIC PATHWAYS

A. Biosynthesis of Cholesterol

The normal adrenals, ovaries, testes, and placenta have the ability to synthesize cholesterol from acetate (Savard et al., 1959; Morris and Chaikoff, 1959; Villee et al., 1966; Andersen and Dietschy, 1978). Likewise, the Y-1 adrenocortical cells (Kowal, 1970; Faust et al., 1977), M5480 Leydig cells (Moyle and Armstrong, 1970; Albert et al., 1980; Ascoli, 1981d), MA-10 cells (M. Ascoli, unpublished observations), and choriocarcinoma (BeWo and JEG) cells (Simpson et al., 1978b; Bahn et al., 1980) have been shown to incorporate radiolabeled acetate into cholesterol and cholesteryl esters and/or to have measurable levels of hydroxymethyl glutaryl-CoA (HMG-CoA) reductase activity.

Thus, all steroidogenic tissues can synthesize cholesterol de novo and, therefore, may use it as a source of substrate for steroid production. Further discussion of the role of this pathway in the stimulation of steroidogenesis is presented in Section IV,B.

TABLE III

Cultured Lines of Choriocarcinoma Cells

Cell line	Species	Steroids[a]	Reference
BeWo	Human	P,E	Patillo and Gey, 1968
JEG	Human	P,E	Kohler and Bridson, 1971
Jar	Human	P,E	Patillo et al., 1970

[a] P, Progesterone; E, estrogen.

B. Pregnenolone Biosynthesis

The early steps of the pathways involved in the conversion of cholesterol to steroid hormones are similar in all steroidogenic tissues. Thus, pregnenolone and progesterone are obligatory intermediates in the biosynthesis of glucocorticoids, androgens, and estrogens. The final products synthesized by different steriodogenic tissues are dictated by the presence of different enzymes involved in the metabolism of pregnenolone.

The conversion of cholesterol to pregnenolone occurs in the mitochondria and is catalyzed by an enzyme system called cholesterol side-chain cleavage. This system is composed of three proteins: a cytochrome P-450 (designated P-450 scc), an FAD-containing flavoprotein, and an iron–sulfur protein. Like other reactions catalyzed by mixed-function oxidases, it requires O_2 and NADPH (Shikita and Hall, 1974; Simpson, 1979).

This reaction is of particular importance in the control of steroidogenesis because it is the rate-limiting step of the pathway (Stone and Hechter, 1954) and because it has been shown to be under hormonal control in the adrenals (Simpson and Boyd, 1967a,b; Koritz and Kumar, 1970; Mrotek and Hall, 1977) and testes (Van der Wusse et al., 1975; Cooke et al., 1979). Its involvement in the hormonal control of steroid biosynthesis is discussed in Section IV,B.

C. Late Steps of the Steroidogenic Pathway

1. Y-1 Adrenocortical Cells

The major glucocorticoid produced by the mouse adrenal cortex is corticosterone (Bloch and Cohen, 1960). This steroid is synthesized by two hydroxylations of progesterone (in positions 11 and 21), catalyzed by two "adrenal-specific" enzymes named 11β- and 21α-hydroxylase, respectively (Fig. 1).

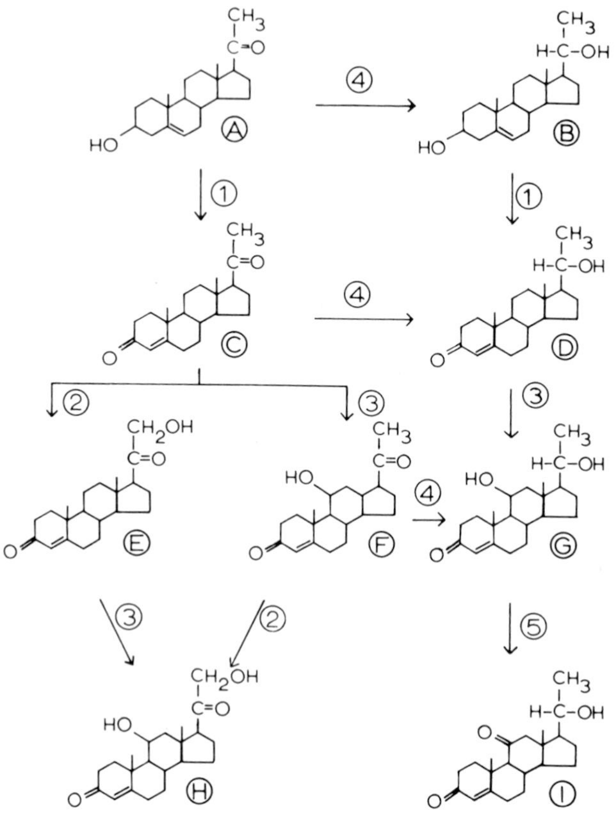

Fig. 1. Biosynthesis of steroids in normal mouse adrenocortical cells and Y-1 adrenocortical tumor cells. The numbers denote the following enzymes: (1) Δ^5-3β-hydroxysteroid dehydrogenase/Δ^5–Δ^4-isomerase complex; (2) 21α-hydroxylase; (3) 11β-hydroxylase; (4) 20α-hydroxylase; (5) 11β-reductase. The letters denote the following steroids: (A) pregnenolone; (B) 20α-hydroxypregnenolone; (C) progesterone; (D) 20α-hydroxyprogesterone; (E) 11-deoxycorticosterone; (F) 11β-hydroxyprogesterone; (G) 11β,20α-dihydroxyprogesterone; (H) corticosterone; (I) 11-keto-20α-hydroxyprogesterone. Corticosterone (H) is the major steroid produced by normal adrenocortical cells because of the low activity of 20α-hydroxylase (4). 20α-Hydroxyprogesterone (D) and 11β,20α-hydroxyprogesterone (G) are the major steroids produced by the Y-1 adrenal cells because of low 21α-hydroxylase (2) and high 20α-hydroxylase (4) activities (Pierson, 1967; Kowal and Fiedler, 1968).

The major steroids produced by the Y-1 cells are 20α-hydroxyprogesterone and 11β-hydroxy-20α-hydroxyprogesterone (Pierson, 1967; Kowal and Fiedler, 1968). These steroids are products of the action of 20α-hydroxylase on progesterone and 11β-hydroxyprogesterone, respectively (Fig. 1).

The difference in the steroids produced by the normal mouse adrenals and Y-1 cells is due to changes in the activities of two enzymes: (1) 21-Hydroxylase activity is low in the Y-1 cells. This reduction (or loss) in enzyme activity occurred while the adrenocortical tumor cells were being maintained by serial transplantation into animals (Bloch and Cohen, 1960). As a result of this, the tumor cells lost their ability to synthesize 11-deoxycorticosterone (a precursor of corticosterone; Fig. 1) and to convert 11β-hydroxyprogesterone to corticosterone. (2) 20α-Hydroxylase activity is high in the Y-1 cells. This enzyme activity is low in the normal mouse adrenals (Ertel and Unger, 1968) and in cells freshly isolated from the transplantable adrenocortical tumor used to establish the Y-1 adrenal cells (Pierson, 1967). When these cells are cultured, however, the enzyme activity increases 60-fold (Pierson, 1967). As a consequence of this change and the loss of 21-hydroxylase activity described earlier, the Y-1 adrenal cells synthesize the 20α-hydroxylated derivatives of pregnenolone, progesterone, and 11β-hydroxyprogesterone (Fig. 1). Another minor product of the Y-1 adrenal cells (11-keto-20α-hydroxyprogesterone) arises from the reduction of 11β,20α-dihydroxyprogesterone (Kowal and Fiedler, 1968).

2. Leydig Tumor Cells

The major steroid synthesized by normal mouse Leydig cells is testosterone (De la Torre *et al.*, 1976; Lacroix *et al.*, 1980). In this species, testosterone biosynthesis occurs predominantly via the Δ^4 pathway (Fig. 2).

Cells freshly isolated from the M5480 tumor were first reported to synthesize mainly testosterone (Moyle and Armstrong, 1970; Moyle and Ramachandran, 1973). At some point during serial transplantation, however, some of the tumors lost their ability to synthesize testosterone, and progesterone became the most predominant steroid (Ascoli and Puett, 1978a; Lacroix *et al.*, 1980; Ascoli, 1981a). This finding led to the identification of two tumor variants, designated M5480A and M5480P (Ascoli and Puett, 1978a; Lacroix *et al.*, 1980). The MA cell lines were established from the M5480P variant (Ascoli, 1981a).

A comparison of the levels of several intermediate steroids produced by freshly isolated M5480P cells and normal mouse Leydig cells suggests that the M5480P cells have reduced 17α-hydroxylase and 17β-

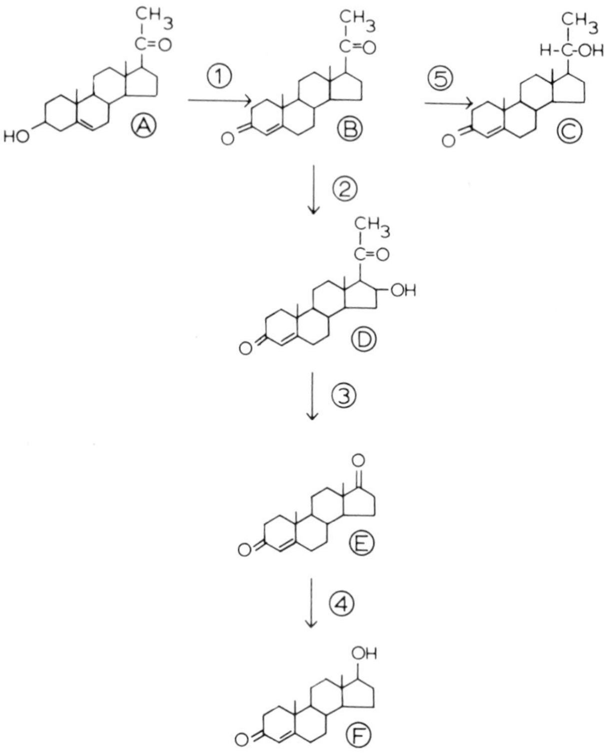

Fig. 2. Biosynthesis of steroids in normal mouse Leydig cells and cultured mouse Leydig tumor cells. The numbers denote the following enzymes: (1) Δ^5-3β-hydroxysteroid dehydrogenase/Δ^5–Δ^4-isomerase complex; (2) 17α-hydroxylase; (3) 17,20-desmolase; (4) 17β-hydroxysteroid dehydrogenase; (5) 20α-hydroxylase. The letters denote the following steroids: (A) pregnenolone; (B) progesterone; (C) 20α-hydroxyprogesterone; (D) 17α-hydroxyprogesterone; (E) androstenedione; (F) testosterone. Testosterone (F) is the major steroid produced by normal Leydig cells. Cultured Leydig tumor cells (MA-10, MA-14, I-10, R2C) produce progesterone (B) and 20α-hydroxyprogesterone (C). This is presumably due to a decrease in 17α-hydroxylase activity (2) and an increase in 20α-hydroxylase activity (5) (Lacroix *et al.*, 1980; Ascoli, 1981a).

hydroxysteroid dehydrogenase activities (Lacroix *et al.*, 1980). As a result of these changes (see Fig. 2), the major steroids produced under basal conditions are androstenedione and progesterone. When steroidogenesis is stimulated, however, progesterone becomes the predominant steroid.

A similar analysis carried out with the MA-10 and MA-14 cells indicates that the apparent reduction in 17α-hydroxylase activity becomes more pronounced when the cells are cultured. Moreover, the cultured cells also appear to have increased levels of 20α-hydroxylase activity (Ascoli, 1981a). As a result of these changes, the major steroids synthesized by the MA-10 and MA-14 cells are progesterone and 20α-hydroxyprogesterone (Fig. 2). It is of interest to note that these are also the major steroids synthesized by the I-10 and R2C Leydig tumor cells (Shin, 1967; Shin *et al.*, 1968). It is not known, however, if these changes arose during transplantation or culture.

3. Choriocarcinoma Cells

The human placenta synthesizes and secretes progesterone and three estrogens: estriol (E_3), estradiol (E_2), and estrone (E_1) (Diczfalusy, 1969). Progesterone is synthesized from cholesterol, whereas the estrogens are synthesized from C_{19}-steroid precursors obtained from the maternal or fetal compartment (Baulieu and Dray, 1963; Siiteri and MacDonald, 1963, 1966; Bolte *et al.*, 1964). The trophoblast does not have the enzymes (i.e., 17α-hydroxylase and 17,20-desmolase, see Fig. 2) necessary to convert C_{21} steroids to C_{19} steroids. Thus, during pregnancy, the conversion of C_{21} steroids (i.e., progesterone) produced by the placenta into C_{19} steroids (i.e., dehydroepiandrosterone and dehydroepiandrosterone sulfate) occurs in the fetal adrenal. These C_{19} steroids are then converted to estrogens in the trophoblast. These pathways are shown in Fig. 3. Further information may be obtained in the reviews by Diczfalusy (1969), Bedin *et al.* (1980), and Simpson and MacDonald (1981).

Cultured choriocarcinoma cells retain the same steroidogenic pathway of the normal trophoblast. Huang *et al.* (1969) have shown that BeWo cells convert radiolabeled pregnenolone to progesterone. Likewise, Bahn *et al.* (1981) showed that in the absence of serum, the major steroids produced by the three different lines of cultured choriocarcinoma cells are progesterone and pregnenolone. These cells were also shown to produce relatively low amounts of 17α-hydroxylated derivatives of progesterone and pregnenolone, suggesting the absence of 17α-hydroxylase activity. The absence of this enzyme and of the 17,20-desmolase is also supported by the inability of the cells to convert progesterone, pregnenolone, and their 17α-hydroxylated derivatives to estradiol (Bahn *et al.*, 1981).

Choriocarcinoma cells, however, have the ability to convert C_{19} steroids to estrogens. Thus, E_2 and E_1 are synthesized by choriocarcinoma cells from the following substrates: androstenedione, dehydroepiandrosterone, dehydroepiandrosterone sulfate, androstenediol, and testosterone (Kohler *et al.*, 1971; Patillo *et al.*, 1972; Bahn *et al.*, 1981).

The normal human placenta is also capable of converting 16α-hy-

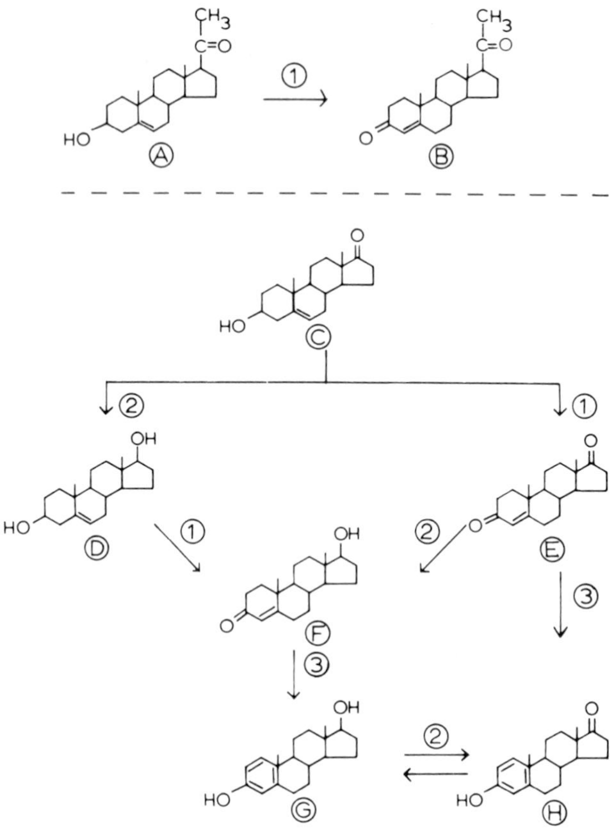

Fig. 3. Biosynthesis of steroids in normal placenta and cultured choriocarcinoma cells. The numbers denote the following enzymes: (1) Δ^5-3β-hydroxysteroid dehydrogenase/Δ^5–Δ^4-isomerase complex; (2) 17β-hydroxysteroid dehydrogenase; (3) aromatase. The letters denote the following steroids: (A) pregnenolone; (B) progesterone; (C) dehydroepiandrosterone; (D) androstenediol; (E) androstenedione; (F) testosterone; (G) estradiol; (H) estrone.

droxydehydroepiandrosterone sulfate (derived from the fetal adrenal and liver) to estriol (Siiteri and MacDonald, 1966). The aromatization of this precursor or of other 16α-hydroxylated steroids by choriocarcinoma cells has not been studied.

IV. HORMONAL CONTROL OF STEROIDOGENESIS

The biosynthesis of steroids in the adrenal cortex and gonads is acutely regulated by the tropic hormones ACTH and LH/hCG, respectively. Because of the similarities of the steroidogenic pathways, the mechanism of action of these hormones can be considered to be analogous. The specificity of action and the kinds of steroids produced are determined by the presence of specific hormone receptors and the enzymatic machinery of the cells, respectively.

ACTH and LH/hCG appear to stimulate steroidogenesis in these tissues by activating the adenylate cyclase/protein kinase pathway (see Schimmer, 1980, for a comprehensive review). The study of the hormonal stimulation of steroidogenesis is rewarding because one can measure several of these early steps involved in hormone action. Thus, the presence of hormone receptors, adenylate cyclase activity, increased synthesis of cAMP, and protein kinase activities can be determined and

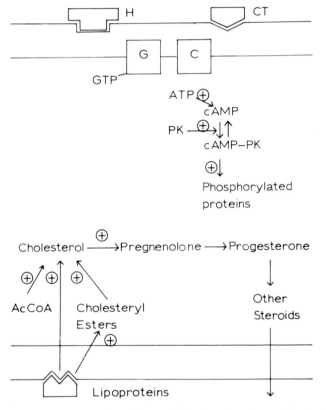

Fig. 4. Hormonal control of steroidogenesis in adrenal and gonadal cells. The arrows denote metabolic pathways. The (+)'s denote pathways that are stimulated by the appropriate hormone (H), cholera toxin (CT), or cAMP. G and C, The regulatory and catalytic subunits of adenylate cyclase; PK, protein kinases.

correlated with steroid production. Moreover, this pathway can also be activated by a nonhormonal protein (cholera toxin) that activates adenylate cyclase activity or by cAMP (or analogs thereof).

The activation of the adenylate cyclase/protein kinase pathway leads (presumably by phosphorylation of specific proteins) to the stimulation of steroid production via the activation of one or more of the following steps of the steroidogenic pathway (Fig. 4): (1) biosynthesis of cholesterol; (2) uptake of lipoproteins; (3) hydrolysis of intracellular cholesteryl esters; (4) transport of cholesterol into the mitochondria; and (5) conversion of cholesterol to pregnenolone.

A. Hormone Receptors, Adenylate Cyclase, and Protein Kinases

The stimulation of steroidogenesis by LH/hCG or ACTH in gonadal and adrenal cells is believed to be mediated by cAMP. Evidence for this hypothesis comes from the findings that these hormones stimulate adenylate cyclase activity in target cell membranes (Grahame-Smith *et al.*, 1967; Birnbaumer *et al.*, 1976; Dufau *et al.*, 1980) and increase the intracellular concentrations of cAMP in their target cells (Grahame-Smith *et al.*, 1967; Moyle and Ramachandran, 1973; Schumacher *et al.*, 1979; Sala *et al.*, 1979; Segaloff and Ascoli, 1981). Moreover, their effects can be mimicked by activating the adenylate cyclase with cholera toxin or by the addition of exogenous cAMP (Sandler and Hall, 1966; Haynes *et al.*, 1969; Wolff *et al.*, 1973; Sato *et al.*, 1975; Ascoli, 1978, 1981a; Segaloff *et al.*, 1981a).

Tumor cells provide a valuable tool to study these processes because of the potential availability of mutants. Thus, variant cell lines derived from adrenal and Leydig cell tumors that are deficient in hormone receptors, hormone-sensitive adenylate cyclase, and cAMP-dependent protein kinases have been isolated and can be used to study the role of hormone receptors and cAMP in the stimulation of steroidogenesis.

Mutations of the differentiated function of endocrine tumor cells can be "spontaneous" (i.e., resulting from malignant transformation or culture conditions) or purposely induced by mutagens (see Section III,C).

Three clonal lines of Leydig tumor cells (designated MA-14, -16, and -18; see Table II) isolated in this laboratory show reduced hCG binding activity and steroidogenic responses to hCG (Ascoli, 1981a). These lines, however, have a normal steroidogenic response to cholera toxin or 8-Br-cAMP (Ascoli, 1981a) and normal levels of receptors for another hormone (epidermal growth factor, or EGF) (Ascoli, 1981b). Thus, the inability of hCG to stimulate steroid production can be attributed to the low levels of hCG receptors. Furthermore, the presence of a steroidogenic response to cholera toxin and 8-Br-cAMP suggest that their adenylate cyclase and protein kinase(s) are normal. The reason for the low hCG binding activity of these cells is not clear. Because these cells were isolated by cloning mass cultures of Leydig tumor cells, it is possible that the original culture (and/or tumors) were heterogeneous (i.e., composed of cells with different levels of hCG binding activity) or that culture conditions led to a loss of hCG binding activity. The second possibility is unlikely because hCG binding activity is not increased when the MA-14 cells are reinjected into isogenic mice (Ascoli, 1981a).

The I-10 Leydig tumor cells are also hCG insensitive but show steroidogenic responses to cholera toxin and cAMP (Table II). Because these cells have not been tested for hCG binding activity, it is not known whether the defect is due to the lack of hormone binding or to a defect in the coupling of the receptor-bound hormone with adenylate cyclase. The R2C Leydig tumor cells are insensitive to LH/hCG and cAMP. Thus, a defect must exist either at the protein kinase level and/or in one or more steps of the steroidogenic pathway.

Some cultured adrenocortical cells derived from the Y-1 line (Table I) have reduced ACTH responsiveness but are responsive to cholera toxin and cAMP. These variants arose spontaneously (Y6 and OS-3) (Schimmer, 1969, 1972) or were selected by their resistance to cAMP-induced growth arrest following mutagenesis (*cyc* variants) (Schimmer *et al.*, 1977b; Rae *et al.*, 1979b). Membranes prepared from these variants show basal adenylate cyclase activities comparable to that present in the wild-type cells. This activity is also sensitive to fluoride, guanyl nucleotides, and cholera toxin, but not to ACTH. These results suggest that the regulatory and catalytic units of adenylate cyclase are intact (Schimmer *et al.*, 1979). These cell lines have not been tested for ACTH binding. Thus, it is not clear if the defect is due to reduced hormone binding activity or to the "coupling" between the receptor-bound hormone and adenylate cyclase (Rae *et al.*, 1979a, 1980).

A set of ACTH-insensitive adrenal tumor cells (designated Kin⁻, see Table I) are deficient in cAMP-dependent protein kinases (Schimmer *et al.*, 1977b; Gutman *et al.*, 1978; Rae *et al.*, 1979b). These clones were isolated (from the Y-1 line) by their resistance to 8-Br-cAMP-induced growth arrest following mutagenesis. Their basal adenylate cyclase activity is comparable to wild-type cells and is sensitive to fluoride and ACTH. These cells, however, show a reduced steroidogenic response to ACTH or 8-Br-cAMP (Schimmer *et al.*, 1977b; Schimmer *et al.*, 1979; Rae *et al.*, 1979b).

cAMP-dependent protein kinases have been identified in bovine (Gill and Garren, 1970; Steiss and Finn, 1979), rat (Shima *et al.*, 1974), and human (Evain *et al.*, 1977) adrenocortical cells, as well as in the Y-1 cells (Gutman *et al.*, 1978).

The Kin⁻ cells, like Y-1 cells, have two chromatographically distinct cAMP-dependent protein kinases. The defect in the Kin⁻ cells appears to be localized to the type I kinase only. The apparent K_d's for activation of protein kinase I by cAMP are 4 and 58 times higher in the Kin-1 and Kin-8 clones, respectively, than in the wild-type cells. The apparent K_d's for activation of protein kinase II by cAMP are identical in the two variants and the wild-type cells (Rae *et al.*, 1979b; Schimmer *et al.*, 1979).

The stimulation of protein kinase activity with ACTH or cAMP has been shown to stimulate phosphorylation of several ribosomal proteins in the Y-1 cells (Ross, 1973).

Normal rat Leydig cells and cells isolated from the H-540 Leydig cell tumor have been shown to have type I and type II cAMP-dependent protein kinases (Cooke *et al.*, 1976, 1979). The type I isozyme predominates in both tissues. Cooke and co-workers (Cooke *et al.*, 1976, 1979) have shown that in normal rat Leydig cells LH induces the phosphorylation of three endogenous proteins with apparent molecular weights of 14,000, 57,000, and 76,000. In the H-540 cells, however, only two proteins with apparent molecular weights of 14,000 and 57,000 are phosphorylated. The involvement of these proteins in the activation of steroidogenesis is suggested by the rapid time course of phosphorylation and the similarities between the dose responses for phosphorylation and steroid production.

There is little information about the identity and/or role of these phosphorylated proteins in the mechanism of action of ACTH or the gonadotropins. It appears likely, however, that protein phosphorylation may be involved in the activation of some enzymes that are involved in the biosynthesis of steroids. Several investigators have shown that a cholesteryl ester hydrolase purified from the bovine adrenal cortex is phosphorylated and activated by cAMP-dependent protein kinase (Becket and Boyd, 1977; Nagshineh *et al.*, 1978). Also, the activity of a reconstituted cholesterol side-chain cleavage system from the corpus luteum was reported to be increased when reconstituted with phosphorylated cytochrome P-450 (Caron *et al.*, 1975). Other investigators, however, have found that phosphorylation has no effect on the cholesterol side-chain cleavage system in acetone powders of rat adrenal mitochondria (Hoffman *et al.*, 1978). Another enzyme that may be regulated by phosphorylation is HMG-CoA reductase. This mechanism has not been investigated in steroidogenic tissues, but in hepatocytes Beg and co-workers (1978, 1979, 1980) have shown that the activity of this enzyme is reduced when phosphorylated by a cAMP-dependent protein kinase.

B. Mobilization of Cholesterol

1. Intracellular and Extracellular Cholesterol as Substrates for Steroidogenesis

It has been known for many years that a single injection of ACTH results in a considerable reduction in the adrenal content of free and esterified cholesterol (reviewed by Garren et al., 1971). This observation led to the hypothesis that adrenal cells use intracellular cholesterol for their acute steroidogenic response to ACTH. This hypothesis is also supported by the unequivocal ability of ACTH to stimulate steroidogenesis in isolated adrenal cells incubated in media devoid of extracellular cholesterol (Sayers et al., 1972; Mrotek and Hall, 1975; Vahouny et al., 1978; Gwyne and Hess, 1980). Gwyne and Hess (1980) showed that over a short time period (0–8 hours) the steroidogenic response of freshly isolated rat adrenocortical cells to ACTH was identical whether the cells were incubated with or without an extracellular source of cholesterol [high-density lipoprotein (HDL) or low-density lipoprotein (LDL)]; by 24 hours of incubation, however, the presence of HDL caused a significant increase in steroid production. These results provide direct evidence that, during the acute steroidogenic response to ACTH, adrenocortical cells do not need an extracellular source of cholesterol.

Adrenocortical cells contain both free and esterified cholesterol and may use these stores, or newly synthesized cholesterol, as a source of free cholesterol for steroid production under acute hormonal stimulation. For example, the mouse and rat adrenal cortex seem to rely primarily on cholesteryl esters. In these species, most (80–90%) of the adrenal cholesterol is present in the esterified form (Garren, 1971; Balasubramanian et al., 1977; Brecher and Hyun, 1978; Kovanen et al., 1980), and a single injection of ACTH leads to a drastic reduction in the content of adrenal cholesteryl esters. A reduction in cholesteryl esters has also been demonstrated during short (2 hours) ACTH exposure of freshly isolated rat adrenocortical cells (Vahouny et al., 1978). On the other hand, hamster adrenals (Lehoux and Preiss, 1980), cultured bovine adrenocortical cells (Kovanen et al., 1979a), and Y-1 adrenal cells (Kowal, 1970; Faust et al., 1977) contain more free cholesterol than cholesteryl esters. These cells may use preformed free cholesterol or newly synthesized cholesterol for steroid biosynthesis during acute hormonal stimulation. Kowal (1970) showed that during short-term incubations (2–6 hours), ACTH stimulated the incorporation of radiolabeled acetate, but not radiolabeled mevalonate, into cholesterol and steroids in the Y-1 adrenal cells. The incorporation of radioactivity into steroids, however, was more marked than the incorporation into cholesterol, suggesting that the cells used mainly newly synthesized cholesterol for steroid biosynthesis.

During prolonged (24–48 hours) exposure to ACTH, the steroidogenic response of the Y-1 cells is enhanced by the presence of LDL (Gwyne and Hess, 1980). In a series of experiments, it was shown that Y-1 cells (Faust *et al.*, 1977; Hall and Nakamura, 1979) and cultured bovine adrenocortical cells (Kovanen *et al.*, 1979a) possess the LDL pathway (Goldstein and Brown, 1976). They have specific cell-surface receptors for LDL that mediate the uptake of this lipoprotein. The uptake of LDL is followed by the lysosomal hydrolysis of its protein and cholesteryl ester moieties. As in other cell types, the free cholesterol liberated during this process regulates cholesterol biosynthesis, cholesterol esterification, and the synthesis of the LDL receptors. Morever, the Y-1 cells use this cholesterol for steroid biosynthesis when the intracellular supply of cholesterol is low. Thus, if the Y-1 adrenal cells are depleted of cholesterol by incubation with ACTH for 24–48 hours in lipoprotein-deficient medium, they will fail to respond to freshly added hormone unless LDL is also added. Under these conditions, as much as 75% of the steroids produced are synthesized from lipoprotein–cholesterol (Faust *et al.*, 1977). Similar observations have been made using cultured bovine adrenocortical cells (Kovanen *et al.*, 1979a; Simonian *et al.*, 1979) and freshly isolated rat adrenocortical cells (Gwyne and Hess, 1980).

Adrenocortical cells from different species have receptors for different lipoproteins. The Y-1 adrenal cells and cultured bovine adrenocortical cells have receptors for LDL, but not for HDL (Faust *et al.*, 1977; Kovanen *et al.*, 1979a,b; Simonian *et al.*, 1979; Hall and Nakamura, 1979; Gwyne and Hess, 1980). On the other hand, mouse and rat adrenocortical cells have both LDL and HDL receptors (Gwyne *et al.*, 1976; Balasubramanian *et al.*, 1977; Gwyne and Hess, 1978, 1980; Kovanen *et al.*, 1979c, 1980). The relative importance of HDL and LDL in providing cholesterol for steroid biosynthesis in these species is controversial (Gwyne *et al.*, 1976; Kovanen *et al.*, 1979c; Gwyne and Hess, 1980).

Further evidence for the role of LDL in the steroidogenic response of the Y-1 and normal bovine adrenocortical cells is provided by the finding that ACTH stimulates the uptake of this lipoprotein. As early as 5 minutes after the addition of ACTH to the Y-1 cells, an increase in the internalization of LDL is observed (Hall and Nakamura, 1979). Upon prolonged (24–48 hours) exposure to ACTH, increases in the amount of surface-bound, internalized, and degraded LDL are observed (Faust *et al.*, 1977; Kovanen *et al.*, 1979a). This effect can also be induced with cholera toxin and may be due to the increase in the number of LDL receptors mediated by cholesterol depletion (resulting from the activation of steroidogenesis), rather than a direct effect of ACTH on the activity of the receptor.

These studies have led to the following proposal about the source of cholesterol for adrenal steroidogenesis (Brown *et al.*, 1979): Under basal conditions, the output of free intracellular cholesterol is dictated by the basal amount of steroids produced and cholesterol esterification. The input of free cholesterol comes from *de novo* synthesis, lipoprotein uptake, and the hydrolysis of cholesteryl esters. Under acute hormonal stimulation, the cholesterol needed for steroid biosynthesis comes from intracellular pools and/or *de novo* synthesis (a process that is activated by ACTH; see earlier). The intracellular pools utilized under these conditions may vary within different species. If the stimulation of steroidogenesis continues, the processes mentioned earlier cannot satisfy the demand for cholesterol, and the enhanced output of free cholesterol is balanced mainly by increased uptake of lipoproteins. This enhanced uptake occurs as a result of an increase in the number of lipoprotein receptors. When hormonal stimulation ceases, the intracellular pools of cholesterol are replenished by the enhanced uptake of lipoproteins and *de novo* synthesis. As a result of the increased levels of intracellular cholesterol, the synthesis of the LDL receptor is suppressed and the system returns to the basal state.

The source of cholesterol used for steroid biosynthesis in Leydig tumor cells has not been investigated in great detail. The M5480 Leydig tumor cells have been reported to contain variable amounts of free and esterified cholesterol. Pokel *et al.* (1972) reported that the ratio of esterified to free cholesterol was 1.3. Neaves (1976) reported a ratio of approximately 2, whereas our studies showed a ratio of approximately 0.5 (Albert *et al.*, 1980; Segaloff *et al.*, 1981b; Ascoli, 1981c). A single injection of LH or hCG into mice bearing the M5480 tumor was shown to reduce the content of cholesteryl esters and to produce no change or increase the content of free cholesterol (Pokel *et al.*, 1972; Ascoli, 1981c). The decrease in cholesteryl esters cannot be observed *in vitro* by direct measurements of cholesterol content (Segaloff *et al.*,

1981b). When the cholesteryl ester fraction was prelabeled (*in vivo*) with radiolabeled cholesterol or arachidonic acid, however, *in vitro* exposure of the cells to hCG, LH, or cAMP caused a decrease in the radioactivity associated with cholesteryl esters (Moyle *et al.*, 1973a; Albert *et al.*, 1980). Moreover, exposure of freshly isolated M5480P cells to hCG caused a 2- to 3-fold stimulation of cholesteryl esterase activity (Albert *et al.*, 1980).

In vitro exposure of freshly isolated Leydig tumor cells to gonadotropins may also affect cholesterol biosynthesis and esterification. Thus, LH or hCG have been reported to decrease the incorporation of acetate into cholesteryl esters (Moyle and Armstrong, 1970; Albert *et al.*, 1980) and to reduce (Moyle and Armstrong, 1970) acetate incorporation into free cholesterol (Moyle and Armstrong, 1970; Albert *et al.*, 1980; M. Ascoli, unpublished observations).

Studies in this laboratory (Ascoli, 1981c) have shown that drug-induced hypocholesterolemia in mice bearing the M5480P tumor has no effect on the amount of tumor cholesterol (free and esterified), on the incorporation of radiolabeled acetate into cholesterol or cholesteryl esters, and on the amount of steroid produced by the cells under basal or stimulated conditions. Chronic hCG treatment of normal or hypocholesterolemic mice bearing the M5480P tumor also failed to change the levels of tumor cholesterol but increased acetate incorporation into cholesterol and cholesteryl esters.

These data suggest that, in contrast to adrenocortical cells, the Leydig tumor cells may rely primarily on intracellular cholesterol pools and/or newly synthesized cholesterol to synthesize steroids under acute and prolonged hormonal stimulation. Nevertheless, it appears that lipoproteins may also play a role in testicular steroidogenesis, because lipoprotein receptors have been identified in bovine, rat, and porcine testes (Kovanen *et al.*, 1979b; Chen *et al.*, 1980; Benahmed *et al.*, 1981). Moreover, lipoproteins have been shown to affect cholesterol metabolism in hypocholesterolemic rats that have been chronically treated with hCG (Andersen and Dietschy, 1978).

2. Transport of Cholesterol into the Mitochondria and Pregnenolone Formation

The rate-limiting process of steroidogenesis in adrenal and gonadal cells appears to lie between cholesterol and pregnenolone (Stone and Hechter, 1954; Hall and Shikita, 1974). The conversion of cholesterol to pregnenolone occurs in the mitochondria and is catalyzed by a cytochrome P-450-dependent enzyme called the cholesterol side-chain cleavage enzyme (reviewed by Simpson, 1979). Current evidence suggests that the rate-limiting step of steroidogenesis is the availability of mitochondrial cholesterol rather than the actual conversion of cholesterol to pregnenolone.

Several years ago, Mahaffee *et al.* (1974) showed that the increased formation of pregnenolone observed in adrenal mitochondria isolated from ACTH-treated rats was associated with an increase in the amount of free cholesterol present in the mitochondria. The ACTH-induced accumulation of cholesterol was enhanced when the cholesterol side-chain cleavage enzyme was inhibited with aminoglutethimide. These results were later reproduced by Mrotek and Hall (1977) and Nakamura *et al.* (1980) using the Y-1 adrenal cells.

The ACTH-induced accumulation of cholesterol into the mitochondria of the Y-1 cells appears to be mediated by a mechanism involving microfilaments, because it is inhibited by liposomes containing anti-actin (Hall *et al.*, 1979a). The importance of this process in the stimulation of steroidogenesis is supported by the finding that cytochalasin B and liposomes containing anti-actin inhibit the stimulatory effects of ACTH on steroidogenesis (Mrotek and Hall, 1975, 1977; Hall *et al.*, 1979a). Moreover, cytochalasin B has been shown to have no direct effect on the cholesterol side-chain cleavage enzyme or on the metabolism of pregnenolone (Mrotek and Hall, 1977). Similar observations have been made by Crivello and Jefcoate (1978, 980), who showed that cytochalasin B and vinblastine inhibited the ACTH-stimulated cholesterol transport (to the mitochondria) and steroid production in freshly isolated rat adrenocortical cells.

Different results on the effects of cytochalasin B and colchicine on steroid production by the Y-1 adrenal cells and the I-10 Leydig cells have been reported by Temple and Wolff (1973) and Cortese and Wolff (1978). These authors showed that colchicine, vinblastine, and podophyllotoxin stimulated steroid production in the Y-1 and I-10 cells after a lag period of 6–9 hours. Moreover, D_2O inhibited the ability of ACTH, cAMP, and colchicine to stimulate steroidogenesis in the Y-1 cells (Temple and Wolff, 1973). The authors concluded that the stimulatory effects of anti-microtubular agents on steroid production were exerted at the same loci as the stimulatory effects of ACTH (i.e., prior to pregnenolone formation) because both were inhibited by aminoglutethimide or cycloheximide. Moreover, neither ACTH nor these agents stimulated the metabolism of pregnenolone (Temple and Wolff, 1973).

The apparent discrepancy between these results and those of Crivello and Jefcoate (1978, 1980) may be explained by the differences in the time frame during which the experiments were performed. Likewise, the stimulatory effect of cytochalasin B on basal steroid production by the Y-1 adrenal cells reported by Cortese and Wolff (1978) and the lack of effect reported by Mrotek and Hall (1975) is apparently due to the presence of serum in the former experiments (Cortese and Wolff, 1978).

Other experiments utilizing normal rat Leydig cells have shown that LH stimulates the transport of cholesterol into the mitochrondria by a process that seems to involve microfilaments (Hall *et al.*, 1979b). Further discussion about the involvement of cytoskeletal elements in the hormonal control of steroidogenesis can be found in Chapter 6.

There is clear evidence that isolated adrenal mitochondria from rats treated with ACTH or testicular mitochrondria from rats treated with LH have a capacity to synthesize pregnenolone greater than that of mitochondria isolated from control rats (Koritz and Kumar, 1970; Mahaffee *et al.*, 1974; Van der Wusse *et al.*, 1975; Simpson *et al.*, 1978a). This effect can be abolished by sonicating the mitochondria (Johnson *et al.*, 1973) or by cycloheximide treatment (Arthur *et al.*, 1976; Simpson *et al.*, 1978b); and it can be enhanced by the addition of cholesterol and/or calcium (Van der Wusse *et al.*, 1975; Mason *et al.*, 1978; Simpson *et al.*, 1978b). Other experiments have shown that mitochondria isolated from stimulated cells contain an increased amount of cholesterol bound to the cholesterol side-chain cleavage system and that the binding of cholesterol to the enzyme is blocked by cycloheximide (Brownie *et al.*, 1973; Alfano *et al.*, 1973; Simpson *et al.*, 1978b; Nakamura *et al.*, 1980).

Thus, it appears that the increased conversion of cholesterol to pregnenolone observed during hormonal stimulation may be due to the stimulation of one or more of the following steps: (1) availability of intracellular cholesterol; (2) transport of cholesterol into the mitochondria; and (3) binding of cholesterol to the side-chain cleavage enzyme. Further discussion about the relative importance of these processes can be found in a review by Simpson (1979).

C. Morphological Correlates of Steroid Production

The stimulation of steroidogenesis in cultured Y-1 adrenocortical cells (Yasumura *et al.*, 1966), normal rat adrenocortical cells (Slavinski *et al.*, 1976), and Leydig tumor cells of the MA series (Ascoli, 1981a) results in a dramatic change in cellular morphology (Fig. 5).

This change can be induced by the appropriate hormone (i.e., ACTH or hCG), cholera toxin, or cAMP and can be correlated with the steroidogenic response of the cells. Thus, variants that do not have hormone receptors or hormone-sensitive adenylate cyclase change morphology in response to cholera toxin or cAMP, but not to the appro-

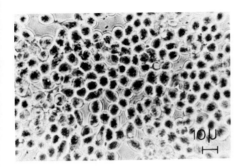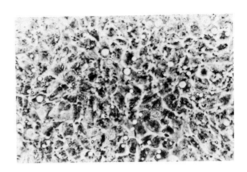

Fig. 5.   Morphological appearance of the MA-10 cells. Cells were incubated with (left panel) or without (right panel) 8-Br-cAMP (1 mM) for 4 hours. Phase contrast; ×800).

priate hormone (Donta, 1974a; Ascoli, 1981a). Likewise, variants of the Y-1 line that are deficient in cAMP-dependent protein kinases do not change morphology in response to cAMP (Schimmer et al., 1977b; Rae et al., 1979b).

In the Y-1 cells, Wolff and co-workers (Temple and Wolff, 1973; Cortese and Wolff, 1978) have shown that cytochalasin B, which in their studies stimulates steroidogenesis, induces the same kinds of morphological changes observed with ACTH. Furthermore, D_2O was shown to inhibit both cAMP-stimulated steroidogenesis and any morphological changes. These results suggest that the change in morphology is associated with increased steroid synthesis and/or release.

D.   Trophic Responses to Hormonal Stimulation

ACTH and LH are generally believed to have important trophic effects on the adrenal cortex and testes, respectively.

Prolonged treatment of the Y-1 cells with ACTH has been shown to induce cellular hypertrophy (Gill and Weidman, 1977; Weidman and Gill, 1977) and to increase the levels of 11β-hydroxylase, cytochrome P-450, and NADPH–cytochrome c reductase activities (Kowal, 1969; Kowal et al., 1970; Asano and Harding, 1976). The increase in cytochrome P-450 and 11β-hydroxylase activities have also been observed in cultures of normal bovine adrenocortical cells (Hornsby, 1980; DuBois et al., 1981).

ACTH (and 8-Br-cAMP) has also been shown to inhibit DNA synthesis and cell multiplication in the Y-1 cells (Masui and Garren, 1971; Gospodarowicz and Handley, 1975; Armelin et al., 1977; Gill and Weidman, 1977; Weidman and Gill, 1977) and in normal bovine adrenocortical cells (reviewed by Gill *et al.*, 1978, 1980). Fibroblast growth factor stimulated DNA synthesis and cell multiplication in the Y-1 cells, whereas epidermal growth, factor, angiotensin II, and hydrocortisone were without effect (Gospodarowicz and Handley, 1975; Armelin *et al.*, 1977; Gospodarowicz *et al.*, 1977). Glucocorticoids have also been reported to inhibit DNA synthesis, cellular proliferation, and steroidogenesis in the Y-1 cells (Saito *et al.*, 1979).

In the cultured Leydig tumor cells of the MA lines, epidermal growth factor and fibroblast growth factor are not mitogenic (Ascoli, 1981b). In the MA-10 cells, epidermal growth factor reduces the number of hCG receptors and has a modest stimulatory effect on the conversion of progesterone to 20α-hydroxyprogesterone (Ascoli, 1981b). Prolonged exposure of the MA-10 cells to hCG (in the presence of phosphodiesterase inhibitors), cholera toxin, or 8-Br-cAMP inhibits cell multiplication and ultimately leads to cell death (M. Ascoli, unpublished observations).

Prolonged hormonal stimulation of mice bearing the M5480 tumor has also been shown to result in increases in cell size and content of smooth endoplasmic reticulum (Neaves, 1973, 1975b, 1976).

V. CONTROL OF STEROIDOGENESIS BY SUBSTRATE AVAILABILITY: CHORIOCARCINOMA CELLS

A. Progesterone Biosynthesis

In the absence of any C_{19} steroid precursors, the major steroid produced by choriocarcinoma cells is progesterone (Bahn *et al.*, 1981). Although the pathway involved in the conversion of cholesterol to progesterone in these cells is similar to that in the adrenals, ovaries, and testes (Simpson and Miller, 1978), there is no evidence that placental progesterone biosynthesis is under hormonal control.

The concentration of cytochrome $P\text{-}450_{SCC}$ present in placental mitochondria is approximately one-tenth of the cytochrome $P\text{-}450_{SCC}$ concentration in adrenal mitochondria, but the activity of the enzyme is about the same in placental mitochondria as it is in adrenal mitochondria isolated from ACTH-treated rats (Simpson and Miller, 1978). This finding suggests that the side-chain cleavage enzyme in the placenta is operating at its maximal rate and that the supply of cholesterol to the mitochondria is rate limiting in the biosynthesis of progesterone.

In a series of studies, Simpson and co-workers (Simpson *et al.*, 1978b,

1979; Winkel *et al.*, 1980) showed that the biosynthesis of progesterone in the BeWo choriocarcinoma cells and in primary cultures of normal human trophoblastic cells is controlled by plasma lipoproteins. When these cells are cultured in the presence of LDL, they bind, internalize, and degrade the lipoprotein (Simpson *et al.*, 1979). The cholesterol derived from these processes decreases the *de novo* synthesis of cholesterol, stimulates cholesterol esterification, and is used for the biosynthesis of pregnenolone and progesterone (Simpson *et al.*, 1978b; Winkel *et al.*, 1980; Simpson and Burkhart, 1980a,b).

Thus, under these conditions, the cells preferentially use lipoprotein-derived cholesterol for steroid biosynthesis. The importance of lipoproteins in providing cholesterol for steroid biosynthesis is also supported by the finding that the amounts of pregnenolone and progesterone produced by these cells is higher when they are cultured in the presence of lipoproteins than in the absence of lipoproteins (Simpson *et al.*, 1978b; Winkel *et al.*, 1980).

Because high concentrations of progesterone have been shown to inhibit cholesterol esterification in human fibroblasts (Goldstein *et al.*, 1978), choriocarcinoma cells (Simpson and Burkhart, 1980a), and human placental microsomes (Simpson and Burkhart, 1980b), it is possible that the progesterone produced by these cells serves as a feedback inhibitor of cholesterol esterification, thus providing more free cholesterol for steroid biosynthesis. This effect of progesterone and the rapid utilization of cholesterol for steroid synthesis may provide an explanation for the low levels of cholesterol esters found in the placenta (Simpson and Burkhart, 1980a).

Further support for the hypothesis that progesterone biosynthesis is regulated by the supply of cholesterol is provided by the data of Bahn *et al.* (1980). These authors showed that EGF produced a 2- to 3-fold stimulation of radiolabeled acetate incorporation into free cholesterol and a 2- to 3-fold stimulation of progesterone production by the JEG 3 cells.

B. Estrogen Biosynthesis

As already mentioned (see Section II,C), the human placenta and choriocarcinoma cells are capable of metabolizing C_{19} steroids to estrogens. This reaction is catalyzed by a cytochrome P-450-dependent enzyme system (called aromatase) localized in the microsomes (see Simpson and MacDonald, 1981, for a review). In choriocarcinoma cells (Jar), the activity of this enzyme and the cytochrome P-450 content are increased by cAMP and/or theophylline (Bellino *et al.*, 1978; Bellino and Hussa, 1978), suggesting that this step may be under hormonal control.

The hormones responsible for the stimulation of estrogen biosynthesis may include hCG and/or some prostaglandins. hCG has been shown to increase cAMP levels (Demers *et al.*, 1973; Menon and Jaffe, 1978) and the conversion of C_{19} steroids to estrogens (Cedard *et al.*, 1970) in the human placenta. Likewise, prostaglandins also increase the conversion of C_{19} steroids to estrogens in the human placenta (Alsat and Cedard, 1973). Similar studies have not been done in the choriocarcinoma cells.

VI. CONCLUSIONS

Our understanding of the mechanisms involved in the regulation of steroid production by the adrenals, gonads, and placenta has reached a point where detailed studies on the biochemical and molecular processes involved are now possible.

The availability of cultured tumor cells derived from steroidogenic tissues offer suitable model systems in which these phenomena can be studied. Although some differences do exist between normal cells and cells derived from tumors, they do not appear to be more pronounced than differences between normal cells derived from different species.

The study of steroidogenesis in these systems offers the advantage of using two different experimental approaches: conventional biochemical measurements and genetic manipulations.

ACKNOWLEDGMENTS

I wish to thank Dr. Deborah Segaloff for helpful suggestions in preparing the manuscript. Unpublished observations from the author's laboratory were supported by grants from the National Cancer Institute (CA-23603) and the American Cancer Society (BC-343).

REFERENCES

Albert, D. H., Ascoli, M., Puett, D., and Coniglio, J. G. (1980). Lipid composition and gonadotropin-mediated lipid metabolism of the M5480 murine Leydig cell tumor. *J. Lipid Res.* **21,** 862–867.

Alfano, J., Brownie, A. C., Orme-Johnson, W. H., and Beinert, H. (1973). Adrenal mitochondrial cytochrome P-450 and cholesterol side chain cleavage activity. *J. Biol. Chem.* **248,** 7860–7864.

Alsat, E., and Cedard, L. (1973). The stimulatory action of prostaglandins on the production of oestrogens by the human placenta perfused *in vitro*. *Prostaglandins* **3**, 145–153.

Andersen, J. M., and Dietschy, J. M. (1978). Relative importance of high and low density lipoproteins in the regulation of cholesterol synthesis in the adrenal gland, ovary, and testis of the rat. *J. Biol. Chem.* **253**, 9024–9032.

Armelin, M. C. S., Gambarini, A. G., and Armelin, H. A. (1977). On the regulation of DNA synthesis in a line of adrenocortical tumor cells: Effect of serum, adrenocorticotropin and pituitary factors. *J. Cell Physiol.* **93**, 1–10.

Arthur, J. R., Mason, J. I., and Boyd, G. S. (1976). The effect of calcium ions on the metabolism of exogenous cholesterol by rat adrenal mitochondria. *FEBS Lett.* **66**, 206–209.

Asano, K., and Harding, B. (1976). Biosynthesis of adrenodoxin in mouse adrenal tumor cells. *Endocrinology (Baltimore)* **99**, 977–987.

Ascoli, M. (1978). Demonstration of a direct effect of inhibitors of the degradation of receptor-bound human choriogonadotropin on the steroidogenic pathway. *J. Biol. Chem.* **253**, 7839–7843.

Ascoli, M. (1979). Inhibition of the degradation of receptor bound human choriogonado-tropin by leupeptin. *Biochim. Biophys. Acta* **586**, 608–614.

Ascoli, M. (1980). Degradation of the subunits of receptor-bound human choriogonadotropin by Leydig tumor cells. *Biochim. Biophys. Acta* **629**, 409–417.

Ascoli, M. (1981a). Characterization of several clonal lines of cultured Leydig tumor cells: Gonadotropin receptors and steroidogenic responses. *Endocrinology (Baltimore)* **108**, 88–95.

Ascoli, M. (1981b). Regulation of gonadotropin receptors and gonadotropin responses in a clonal strain of Leydig tumor cells by epidermal growth factor. *J. Biol. Chem.* **256**, 179–183.

Ascoli, M. (1981c). Effects of hypocholesterolemia and chronic hormonal stimulation on sterol and steroid metabolism in a Leydig cell tumor. *J. Lipid Res.* **22**, 1247–1253.

Ascoli, M. (1982). Receptor-mediated uptake and degradation of human choriogonado-tropin: Fate of the hormone subunits. *Ann. N. Y. Acad. Sci.* **383**, 151–173.

Ascoli, M., and Puett, D. (1978a). Gonadotropin binding and stimulation of steroid-ogenesis in Leydig tumor cells. *Proc. Natl. Acad. Sci. U.S.A.* **75**, 99–102.

Ascoli, M., and Puett, D. (1978b). Degradation of receptor-bound human choriogonado-tropin by Leydig tumor cells. *J. Biol. Chem.* **253**, 4892–4899.

Ascoli, M., and Puett, D. (1978c). Inhibition of the degradation of receptor-bound human choriogonadotropin by lysosomotropic agents, protease inhibitors, and metabolic inhibitors. *J. Biol. Chem.* **253**, 7832–7838.

Bahn, R. S., Speeg, K. V., Jr., Ascoli, M., and Rabin, D. (1980). Epidermal growth factor stimulates production of progesterone in cultured human choriocarcinoma cells. *Endocrinology (Baltimore)* **107**, 2121–2123.

Bahn, R. S., Worsham, A., Speeg, K. V., Jr., Ascoli, M., and Rabin, D. (1981). Characterization of steroid production in cultured human choriocarcinoma cells. *J. Clin. Endocrinol. Metab.* **52**, 447–450.

Balasubramanian, S., Goldstein, J. L., Faust, J. R., Brunschede, G. Y., and Brown, M. S. (1977). Lipoprotein-mediated regulation of 3-hydroxy-3-methylglutaryl coenzyme A reductase activity and cholesterol ester metabolism in the adrenal gland of the rat. *J. Biol. Chem.* **252**, 1771–1779.

Baulieu, E. E., and Dray, F. (1963). Conversion of ^{3}H-dehydroisoandrosterone(3β-hy-droxy-Δ^5-androsten-17-one) sulfate to ^{3}H-estrogens in normal pregnant women. *J. Clin. Endocrinol. Metab.* **23**, 1298–1301.

Becket, G. J., and Boyd, G. S. (1977). Purification and control of bovine adrenal cortical cholesterol ester hydrolase and evidence for the activation of the enzyme by a phosphorylation. *Eur. J. Biochem.* **72**, 223–233.

Bedin, M., Ferre, F., Alsat, E., and Cedard, L. (1980). Regulation of steroidogenesis in the human placenta. *J. Steroid Biochem.* **12**, 17–24.

Beg, Z. H., Stonik, J. A., and Brewer, H. B., Jr. (1978). 3-Hydroxy-3-methylglutaryl coenzyme A reductase: Regulation of enzymatic activity by phosphorylation and dephosphorylation. *Proc. Natl. Acad. Sci. U.S.A.* **75**, 3678–3682.

Beg, Z. H., Stonik, J. A., and Brewer, H. B., Jr. (1979). Characterization and regulation of reductase kinase, a protein kinase that modulates the enzymatic activity of 3-hydroxy-3-methylglutaryl-coenzyme A reductase. *Proc. Natl. Acad. Sci. U.S.A.* **76**, 4375–4379.

Beg, Z. H., Stonik, J. A., and Brewer, H. B., Jr. (1980). *In vitro* and *in vivo* phosphorylation of rat liver 3-hydroxy-3-methyl glutaryl Coenzyme A reductase and its modulation by glucagon. *J. Biol. Chem.* **255**, 8541–8545.

Bellino, F. L., and Hussa, R. O. (1978). Trophoblastic estrogen synthetase stimulation by dibutyryl cAMP and theophylline: Increase in cytochrome P-450 content. *Biochem. Biophys. Res. Commun.* **85**, 1588–1595.

Bellino, F. L., Hussa, R. O., and Osawa, Y. (1978). Estrogen synthetase in the choriocarcinoma cell culture: Stimulation by dibutyryl cyclic adenosine monophosphate and theophylline. *Steroids* **32**, 37–44.

Benahmed, M., Dellamonica, C., Haour, F., and Saez, J. M. (1981). Specific low density lipoprotein receptors in pig Leydig cells: Role of this lipoprotein in cultured Leydig cells steroidogenesis. *Biochem. Biophys. Res. Commun.* **99**, 1123–1130.

Birnbaumer, L., Yang, P.-C., Hunzicker-Dunn, M., Bockaert, J., and Duran, J. M. (1976). Adenylyl cyclase activities in ovarian tissues. I. Homogenization and conditions of assay in Graafian follicles and corpora lutea of rabbits, rats, and pigs: Regulation by ATP, and some comparative properties. *Endocrinology (Baltimore)* **99**, 163–185.

Bloch, E., and Cohen, A. I. (1960). Steroid production *in vitro* by normal and adrenal tumor-bearing male mice. *J. Natl. Cancer Inst.* **24**, 97–107.

Bolte, E., Mancuso, S., Eriksson, G., Wiqvist, N., and Dickzfalusy, E. (1964). Studies on the aromatization of neutral steroids in pregnant women. I. Aromatization of C-19 steroids by placentas perfused *in situ*. *Acta Endocrinol. (Copenhagen)* **45**, 535–549.

Brecher, P. I., and Hyun, Y. (1978). Effect of 4-aminopyrazolopyrimidine and aminoglutethimide on cholesterol metabolism and steroidogenesis in the rat adrenal. *Endocrinology (Baltimore)* **102**, 1404–1413.

Brown, M. S., Kovanen, P. T., and Goldstein, J. L. (1979). Receptor-mediated uptake of lipoprotein-cholesterol and its utilization for steroid biosynthesis in the adrenal cortex. *Rec. Prog. Horm. Res.* **35**, 215–257.

Brownie, A. C., Alfano, J., Jefcoate, C. R., Orme-Johnson, W. H., Beinert, H., and Simpson, E. R. (1973). Effect of ACTH on adrenal mitochondrial cytochrome P-450 in the rat. *Ann. N. Y. Acad. Sci.* **212**, 344–360.

Bryson, M. J., and Sweat, M. L. (1968). Cleavage of cholesterol side chain associated with cytochrome P-450, flavoprotein, and non-HEME iron-protein derived from the bovine adrenal cortex. *J. Biol. Chem.* **243**, 2799–2804.

Buonassisi, V., Sato, G., and Cohen, A. I. (1962). Hormone-producing cultures of adrenal and pituitary tumor origin. *Proc. Natl. Acad. Sci. U.S.A.* **48**, 1148–1190.

Caron, M. G., Goldstein, S., Savard, K., and Marsh, J. M. (1975). Protein kinase stimulation of a reconstituted cholesterol side chain cleavage enzyme system in the bovine corpus luteum. *J. Biol. Chem.* **250**, 5137–5143.

Cedard, L., Alsat, E., Urtasun, M. J., and Varaugot, J. (1970). Studies on the mode of action of luteinizing hormone and chorionic gonadotropin on estrogenic biosynthesis and glycogenolysis by human placenta perfused *in vitro*. *Steroids* **16**, 361–375.

Chen, Y.-D. I., Kraemer, F. B., and Reaven, G. M. (1980). Identification of specific high density lipoprotein-binding sites in rat testis and regulation of binding by human choriogonadotropin. *J. Biol. Chem.* **255**, 9162–9167.

Cohen, A. I., Bloch, E., and Cellozi, E. (1957). *In vitro* response of functional experimental adrenal tumors to corticotropin. *Proc. Soc. Exp. Biol. Med.* **95**, 304–309.

Cole, F. E., Davis, K., Huseby, R. A., and Rice, B. F. (1973). Gonadotropin receptor of a mouse luteoma: Interactions with luteinizing hormone (LH) and its α and β subunits. *Biol. Reprod.* **8**, 550–559.

Cooke, B. A., Lindh, L. M., and Janszen, F. H. A. (1976). Correlation of protein kinase activation and testosterone production after stimulation of Leydig cells with luteinizing hormone. *Biochem. J.* **160**, 439–446.

Cooke, B. A., Lindh, L. M., Janszen, F. H. A., Van Driel, M. J. A., Bakker, C. P., Van der Plank, M. P. I., and Van der Molen, H. J. (1979). A Leydig cell tumour: A model for the study of lutropin action. *Biochim. Biophys. Acta* **583**, 320–331.

Cortese, F., and Wolff, J. (1978). Cytochalasin-stimulated steroidogenesis from high density lipoproteins. *J. Cell Biol.* **77**, 507–516.

Crivello, J. F., and Jefcoate, C. R. (1978). Mechanism of corticotropin action in rat adrenal cells. I. The effects of inhibitors of protein synthesis and of microfilaments formation on corticosterone synthesis. *Biochim. Biophys. Acta* **542**, 315–329.

Crivello, J. F., and Jefcoate, C. R. (1980). Intracellular movement of cholesterol in rat adrenal cells: Kinetics and effects of inhibitors. *J. Biol. Chem.* **255**, 8144–8151.

De la Torre, B., Benagiemo, G., and Diczfalusy, E. (1976). Pathways of testosterone biosynthesis in decapsulated testes of mice. *Acta Endocrinol. (Copenhagen)* **81**, 170–184.

Demers, L. M., Gabbe, S. G., Villee, C., and Greep, R. O. (1973). Human choriogonadotropin mediated glycogenolysis in human placenta. *Biochim. Biophys. Acta* **313**, 202–210.

Diczfalusy, E. (1969). Steroid metabolism in the foeto-placental unit. *In* "The Foeto-Placental Unit" (A. Pecile and C. Finzi, eds.), pp. 65–109. Excerpta Medica, Amsterdam.

Donta, S. T. (1974a). Comparison of the effects of cholera enterotoxin and ACTH on adrenal cells in tissue culture. *Am. J. Physiol.* **227**, 109–113.

Donta, S. T. (1974b). Differentiation between the steroidogenic effects of cholera enterotoxin and adrenocorticotropin through use of a mutant adrenal cell line. *J. Infect. Dis.* **129**, 728–731.

Donta, S. T., King, M., and Sloper, K. (1973). Induction of steroidogenesis in tissue culture by cholera enterotoxin. *Nature (London)* **243**, 246–247.

DuBois, R. N., Simpson, E. R., Kramer, R. E., and Waterman, M. R. (1981). Induction of synthesis of cholesterol side chain cleavage cytochrome P-450 by adrenocorticotropin in cultured bovine adrenocortical cells. *J. Biol. Chem.* **256**, 7000–7005.

Dufau, M. L., Baukal, A. J., and Catt, K. J. (1980). Hormone-induced guanyl nucleotide binding and activation of adenylate cyclase in the Leydig cell. *Proc. Natl. Acad. Sci. U.S.A.* **77**, 5837–5841.

Ertel, R. J., and Unger, F. (1968). 20α-Hydroxysteroid dehydrogenase and reductive pathways in mouse adrenal glands *in vitro*. *Endocrinology (Baltimore)* **82**, 527–534.

Evain, D., Riou, J. P., and Saez, J. M. (1977). Adenosine $3',5'$-monophosphate-dependent protein kinase from normal human adrenal. *Mol. Cell. Endocrinol.* **6**, 191–201.

Faust, J. R., Goldstein, J. L., and Brown, M. S. (1977). Receptor-mediated uptake of low density lipoprotein and utilization of its cholesterol for steroid synthesis in cultured mouse adrenal cells. *J. Biol. Chem.* **252**, 4861–4871.

Freeman, D. A., and Ascoli, M. (1981). Desensitization to gonadotropins in cultured Leydig tumor cells involves both loss of gonadotropin receptors and decreased capacity for steroidogenesis. *Proc. Natl. Acad. Sci. U.S.A.* **78**, 6309–6313.

Garren, L. D., Gill, G. N., Masui, H., and Walton, G. M. (1971). On the mechanism of action of ACTH. *Recent Prog. Horm. Res.* **27**, 433–478.

Gill, G. N., and Garren, L. D. (1970). A cyclic-3′,5′-adenosine monophosphate dependent protein kinase from the adrenal cortex: Comparison with a cAMP binding protein. *Biochem. Biophys. Res. Commun.* **39**, 335–343.

Gill, G. N., and Weidman, E. R. (1977). Hormonal regulation of initiation of DNA synthesis and of differentiated function in Y-1 adrenal cortical cell. *J. Cell Physiol.* **92**, 65–76.

Gill, G. N., Hornsby, P. J., Ill, C. R., Simonian, M. H., and Weidman, R. E. (1978). Regulation of adrenocortical cell growth. *In* "Endocrine Function of the Human Adrenal Cortex" (V. H. T. James, M. Serio, G. Giusti, and L. Martini, eds.), pp. 207–228. Academic Press, New York.

Gill, G. N., Hornsby, P. J., and Simonian, M. H. (1980). Hormonal regulation of the adrenocortical cell. *J. Supramol. Struct.* **14**, 353–369.

Goldstein, J. L., and Brown, M. S. (1976). The LDL pathway in human fibroblasts: A receptor-mediated mechanism for the regulation of cholesterol metabolism. *Curr. Top. Cell. Regul.* **11**, 147–182.

Goldstein, J. L., Faust, J. R., Dygos, J. H., Chorvat, R. J., and Brown, M. S. (1978). Inhibition of cholesteryl ester formation in human fibroblasts by an analogue of 7-ketocholesterol and by progesterone. *Proc. Natl. Acad. Sci. U.S.A.* **75**, 1877–1881.

Gospodarowicz, D., and Handley, H. H. (1975). Stimulation of division of Y-1 adrenal cells by a growth factor isolated from bovine pituitary glands. *Endocrinology (Baltimore)* **97**, 102–107.

Gospodarowicz, D., Ill, C. R., Hornsby, P. J., and Gill, G. N. (1977). Control of bovine adrenal cortical cell proliferation by fibroblast growth factor: Lack of effect of epidermal growth factor. *Endocrinology (Baltimore)* **100**, 1080–1089.

Grahame-Smith, D. G., Butcher, R. W., Ney, R. L., and Sutherland, E. W. (1967). Adenosine 3′,5′-monophosphate as the intracellular mediator of the action of adrenocorticotropic hormone on the adrenal cortex. *J. Biol. Chem.* **242**, 5535–5541.

Gutman, N. S., Rae, P. A., and Schimmer, B. P. (1978). Altered cyclic AMP-dependent protein kinase activity in a mutant adrenocortical tumor cell line. *J. Cell. Physiol.* **97**, 451–460.

Gwyne, J. T., and Hess, B. (1978). Binding and degradation of human ^{125}I-LDL by rat adrenocortical cells. *Metabolism* **27**, 1593–1600.

Gwyne, J. T., and Hess, B. (1980). The role of high density lipoproteins in rat adrenal cholesterol metabolism and steroidogenesis. *J. Biol. Chem.* **255**, 10875–10883.

Gwyne, J. T., Mahaffee, D., Brewer, H. B., Jr., and Ney, R. L. (1976). Adrenal cholesterol uptake from plasma lipoproteins: Regulation by corticotropin. *Proc. Natl. Acad. Sci. U.S.A.* **73**, 4329–4333.

Hall, P. F., and Nakamura, M. (1979). The influence of adrenocorticotropin on transport of a cholesteryl linoleate-low density lipoprotein complex into adrenal tumor cells. *J. Biol. Chem.* **254**, 12547–12554.

Hall, P. F., and Shikita, M. (1974). The role of cytochrome P-450 in the side chain cleavage of cholesterol. *In* "Gonadotropins and Gonadal Function" (N. R. Moudgal, ed.), pp. 403–410. Academic Press, New York.

Hall, P. F., Lewis, J. L., and Lipson, E. D. (1975). The role of mitochondria cytochrome P-450 from bovine adrenal cortex in side chain cleavage of 20,22R-dihydro-cholesterol. *J. Biol. Chem.* **250**, 2283–2286.

Hall, P. F., Charponnier, C., Nakamura, M., and Gabbiani, G. (1979a). The role of microfilaments in the response of adrenal tumor cells to adrenocorticotropin hormone. *J. Biol. Chem.* **254**, 9080–9084.

Hall, P. F., Charponnier, C., Nakamura, M., and Gabbiani, G. (1979b). The role of microfilaments in the response of Leydig cells to luteinizing hormone. *J. Steroid Biochem.* **11**, 1361–1366.

Haynes, R. C., Jr., Koritz, S. B., and Peron, F. G. (1969). Influence of adenosine 3′,5′-monophosphate on corticoid production by rat adrenal glands. *J. Biol. Chem.* **234**, 1421–1423.

Hertz, R. (1959). Choriocarcinoma of women maintained in serial passage in hamster and rat. *Proc. Soc. Exp. Biol. Med.* **102**, 77–80.

Hoffman, K., Kim, J. J., and Finn, F. M. (1978). The role of protein kinases in ACTH stimulated steroidogenesis. *Biochem. Biophys. Res. Commun.* **84**, 1136–1143.

Hornsby, P. J. (1980). Regulation of cytochrome P-450-supported 11β-hydroxylation of deoxycortisol by steroids, oxygen, and antioxidants in adrenocortical cell cultures. *J. Biol. Chem.* **255**, 4020–4027.

Huang, W. Y., Patillo, R. A., Delfs, E., and Mattingly, R. F. (1969). Progesterone synthesis in the pure trophoblasts of human choriocarcinoma. *Steroids* **14**, 755–763.

Jacobs, B. B., and Huseby, R. A. (1968). Transplantable Leydig cell tumors in Fischer rats: Hormone responsivity and hormone production. *J. Natl. Cancer Inst.* **41**, 1141–1153.

Johnson, L. R., Ruhmann-Wennhold, A., and Nelson, D. H. (1973). The *in vivo* effect of ACTH on utilization of reducing energy for pregnenolone synthesis by adrenal mitochondria. *Ann. N. Y. Acad. Sci.* **212**, 307–318.

Kammerman, S., Demopoulous, R. I., and Ross, J. (1977). Gonadotropin receptors in experimentally induced ovarian tumors in mice. *Cancer Res.* **37**, 2578–2582.

Kohler, P. O., and Bridson, W. E. (1971). Isolation of hormone-producing clonal lines of human choriocarcinoma. *J. Clin. Endocrinol. Metab.* **32**, 683–687.

Kohler, P. O., Bridson, W. E., Hammond, J. M., Weintraub, B., Kirschner, M. A., and Van Thiel, D. H. (1971). Clonal lines of human choriocarcinoma cells in culture. *Acta Endocrinol. (Copenhagen) Suppl.* **153**, 137–153.

Koritz, S. B., and Kumar, A. M. (1970). On the mechanism of action of the Adrenocorticotropin hormone. The stimulation of the activity of enzymes involved in pregnenolone synthesis. *J. Biol. Chem.* **245**, 152–159.

Kovanen, P. T., Faust, J. R., Brown, M. S., and Goldstein, J. L. (1979a). Low density lipoprotein receptors in bovine adrenal cortex. I. Receptor-mediated uptake of low density lipoprotein and utilization of its cholesterol for steroid synthesis in cultured adrenocortical cells. *Endocrinology (Baltimore)* **104**, 599–609.

Kovanen, P. T., Basu, S. K., Goldstein, J. L., and Brown, M. S. (1979b). Low density lipoprotein receptors in bovine adrenal cortex. II. Low density lipoprotein binding to membranes prepared from fresh tissue. *Endocrinology (Baltimore)* **104**, 610–616.

Kovanen, P. T., Schneider, W. J., Hillman, G. M., Goldstein, J. L., and Brown, M. S. (1979c). Separate mechanisms for the uptake of high and low density lipoproteins by mouse adrenal gland *in vivo*. *J. Biol. Chem.* **255**, 5498–5505.

Kovanen, P. T., Goldstein, J. L., Chappell, D. A., and Brown, M. S. (1980). Regulation of low density lipoprotein receptors by adrenocorticotropin in the adrenal gland by tissue and rats *in vivo. J. Biol. Chem.* **255,** 5591–5598.

Kowal, J. (1969). Adrenal cells in tissue culture. III. Effects of adrenocorticotropin and 3′,5′-cyclic adenosine monophosphate on 11β-hydroxylase and other steroidogenic enzymes. *Biochemistry* **8,** 1821–1831.

Kowal, J. (1970). ACTH and the metabolism of adrenal cell cultures. *Recent Prog. Horm. Res.* **26,** 623–676.

Kowal, J., and Fiedler, R. (1968). Adrenal cells in tissue culture. I. Assay of steroid products; steroidogenic responses to peptide hormones. *Arch. Biochem. Biophys.* **128,** 406–421.

Kowal, J., Simpson, E. R., and Estabrook, R. W. (1970). Adrenal cells in tissue culture. V. On the specificity of the stimulation of 11β-hydroxylation by adrenocorticotropin. *J. Biol. Chem.* **245,** 2438–2443.

Lacroix, A., Ascoli, M., Puett, D., and McKenna, T. J. (1980). Steroidogenesis in hCG-responsive Leydig cell tumor variants. *J. Steroid Biochem.* **10,** 669–675.

Lehoux, J.-G., and Preiss, B. (1980). Regulation of hamster adrenal 3-hydroxy-3-methylglutaryl coenzyme A reductase activity. *Endocrinology (Baltimore)* **107,** 215–223.

McIntosh, E. N., Mitani, F., Uzgiris, V. I., Alonso, C., and Salhanick, H. A. (1973). Comparative studies on mitochondria and partially purified bovine corpus luteum cytochrome P-450. *Ann. N. Y. Acad. Sci.* **212,** 392–405.

Mahaffee, D., Reitz, R. C., and Ney, R. L. (1974). The mechanism of action of adrenocorticotropic hormone. The role of mitochondrial cholesterol accumulation in the regulation of steroidogenesis. *J. Biol. Chem.* **249,** 227–233.

Mason, J. I., Arthur, J. R., and Boyd, G. S. (1978). Regulation of cholesterol metabolism in rat adrenal mitochondria. *Mol. Cell. Endocrinol.* **10,** 209–223.

Masui, H., and Garren, L. D. (1971). Inhibition of replication in functional mouse adrenal tumor cells by adrenocorticotropin hormone mediated by adenosine 3′:5′-cyclic monophosphate. *Proc. Natl. Acad. Sci. U.S.A.* **68,** 3206–3210.

Menon, K. M. J., and Jaffe, R. B. (1973). Chorionic gonadotropin sensitive adenylate cyclase in human placenta. *J. Clin. Endocrinol. Metab.* **39,** 440–442.

Morriss, M. D., and Chaikoff, J. L. (1959). The origin of cholesterol in liver, small intestine, adrenal gland, and testis of the rat: Dietary versus endogenous contributions. *J. Biol. Chem.* **234,** 1095–1097.

Moudgal, N. R., Moyle, W. R., and Greep, R. O. (1971). Specific binding of luteinizing hormone to Leydig tumor cells. *J. Biol. Chem.* **246,** 4983–4986.

Moyle, W. R., and Armstrong, D. T. (1970). Stimulation of testosterone biosynthesis by luteinizing hormone in transplantable mouse Leydig cell tumors. *Steroids* **15,** 681–693.

Moyle, W. R., and Greep, R. O. (1974). Steroid secreting tumors as models in endocrinology. *In* "Hormones and Cancer" (K. W. McKerns, ed.), pp. 329–361. Academic Press, New York.

Moyle, W. R., and Ramachandran, J. (1973). Effect of LH on steroidogenesis and cyclic AMP accumulation in rat Leydig cell preparations and mouse tumor Leydig cells. *Endocrinology (Baltimore)* **93,** 127–134.

Moyle, W. R., Moudgal, N. R., and Greep, R. O. (1971). Cessation of steroidogenesis in Leydig cell tumors after removal of luteinizing hormone and adenosine cyclic 3′,5′-monophosphate. *J. Biol. Chem.* **246,** 4978–4982.

Moyle, W. R., Jungas, R. L., and Greep, R. O. (1973a). Influence of luteinizing hormone and adenosine 3′:5′-cyclic monophosphate on the metabolism of free and esterified cholesterol in mouse Leydig-cell tumours. *Biochem. J.* **134,** 407–413.

Moyle, W. R., Jungas, R., and Greep, R. O. (1973b). Metabolism of free and sterified cholesterol by Leydig-cell tumour mitochondria. *Biochem. J.* **134**, 415–424.

Mrotek, J. J., and Hall, P. F. (1975). The influence of cytochalasin B on the response of adrenal tumor cells to ACTH and cyclic AMP. *Biochem. Biophys. Res. Commun.* **64**, 891–896.

Mrotek, J. J., and Hall, P. F. (1977). Response of adrenal tumor cells to adrenocorticotropin: Site of inhibition by cytochalasin B. *Biochemistry* **16**, 3177–3181.

Nagshineh, S., Treadwell, C. R., Gallo, L. L., and Vahouny, G. V. (1978). Protein kinase-mediated phosphorylation of a purified sterol ester hydrolase from bovine adrenal cortex. *J. Lipid Res.* **19**, 561–569.

Nakamura, M., Watanuki, M., Tilley, B. E., and Hall, P. F. (1980). The effect of ACTH on intracellular cholesterol transport. *J. Endocrinol.* **84**, 179–188.

Neaves, W. B. (1973). Ultrastructural transformation of a murine Leydig cell tumor after gonadotropin administration. *J. Natl. Cancer Inst.* **50**, 1069–1073.

Neaves, W. B. (1975a). Growth and composition of a transplantable murine Leydig cell tumor. *J. Natl. Cancer Inst.* **55**, 623–631.

Neaves, W. B. (1975b). Gonadotropin-induced proliferation of endoplasmic reticulum in an androgenic tumor and its relation to elevated plasma testosterone levels. *Cancer Res.* **35**, 2663–2669.

Neaves, W. B. (1976). Cytologic correlates of testosterone production. *In* "Regulatory Mechanisms of Male Reproductive Physiology" (C. H. Spilman, ed.), pp. 35–43. Excerpta Medica, Amsterdam.

Patillo, R. A., and Gey, G. O. (1968). The establishment of a cell line of human hormone-synthesizing trophoblastic cells *in vitro*. Cancer Res. **28**, 1231–1236.

Patillo, R. A., Hussa, R. O., Delfs, E., Garancis, J., Bernstein, R., Ruckert, A. C. F., Huang, W. Y., Gey, G. O., and Mattingly, R. F. (1970a). Control mechanisms for gonadotropic hormone production *in vitro*. *In Vitro* **6**, 205–214.

Patillo, R. A., Ruckert, A., Hussa, R., Bernstein, R., and Delfs, E. (1970b). The Jar cell line—continuous human multihormone production and control. *In Vitro* **6**, 398 (Abstr. No. 101).

Patillo, R. A., Hussa, R., Huang, W. Y., Delfs, E., and Mattingly, R. F. (1972). Estrogen production by trophoblastic tumors in tissue culture. *J. Clin. Endocrinol. Metab.* **34**, 59–61.

Pierson, R. W., Jr. (1967). Metabolism of steroid hormones in adrenal cortex tumor cells. *Endocrinology (Baltimore)* **81**, 693–707.

Pokel, J. D., Moyle, W. R., and Greep, R. O. (1972). Depletion of esterified cholesterol in mouse testes and Leydig cell tumors by luteinizing hormone. *Endocrinology (Baltimore)* **91**, 323–325.

Rae, P. A., Tsao, J., and Schimmer, B. P. (1979a). Evaluation of receptor function in ACTH-responsive and ACTH-insensitive adrenal tumor cells. *Can. J. Biochem.* **57**, 509–516.

Rae, P. A., Gutmann, N. S., Tsao, J., and Schimmer, B. P. (1979b). Mutations in cyclic AMP-dependent protein kinase and corticotropin (ACTH)-sensitive adenylate cyclase affect adrenal steroidogenesis. *Proc. Natl. Acad. Sci. U.S.A.* **76**, 1896–1900.

Rae, P. A., Zinman, H., Ramachandran, J., and Schimmer, B. P. (1980). Responses of Y-1 adrenocortical tumor cells to o-nitrophenyl sulfenyl ACTH. *Mol. Cell. Endocrinol.* **17**, 171–179.

Rice, B. F., Roth, L. M., Cole, F. E., MacPhee, A. A., Davis, K., Ponthier, R. L., and Sternberg, W. H. (1975). Hypercalcemia and neoplasia: Biological, biochemical, and ultrastructural studies of a hypercalcemia-producing Leydig cell tumor of the rat. *Lab. Invest.* **33**, 428–439.

Ross, B. A. (1973). ACTH and cAMP stimulation of adrenal ribosomal protein phosphorylation. *Endocrinology (Baltimore)* **94**, 685–690.

Roth, L. M., Sternberg, W. H., Huseby, R. A., MacPhee, A. A., Cole, F. E., and Rice, B. F. (1972). Transplantable luteoma of the mouse: An ultrastructural and biochemical study. *Lab. Invest.* **27**, 115–122.

Saito, E., Mukai, M., Muraki, T., Ichikawa, Y., and Homma, M. (1979). Inhibitory effects of corticosterone on cell proliferation and steroidogenesis in the mouse adrenal tumor cell line Y-1. *Endocrinology (Baltimore)* **104**, 487–492.

Sala, G. B., Dufau, M. L., and Catt, K. J. (1979). Gonadotropin actions in isolated ovarian luteal cells. The intermediate role of adenosine 3':5'-monophosphate in hormonal stimulation of progesterone synthesis. *J. Biol. Chem.* **254**, 2077–2083.

Sandler, R., and Hall, P. F. (1966). Stimulation *in vitro* by adenosine-3',5'-cyclic monophosphate of steroidogenesis in rat testis. *Endocrinology (Baltimore)* **79**, 647–649.

Sato, K., Mijachi, Y., Ohsawa, N., and Kosaka, K. (1975). *In vitro* stimulation of steroidogenesis in rat testis by cholera enterotoxin. *Biochim. Biophys. Res. Commun.* **62**, 696–703.

Savard, K., Marsh, J. M., and Rice, B. F. (1965). Gonadotropins and ovarian steroidogenesis. *Recent Prog. Horm. Res.* **21**, 285–365.

Sayers, G., Beall, R. J., and Seelig, S. (1972). Isolated adrenal cells: Adrenocorticotropic hormone, calcium, steroidogenesis, and cyclic adenosine monophosphate. *Science* **175**, 1131–1133.

Schimmer, B. P. (1969). Phenotypically variant adrenal tumor cell cultures with biochemical lesions in the ACTH-stimulated steroidogenic pathway. *J. Cell. Physiol.* **74**, 115–122.

Schimmer, B. P. (1972). Adenylate cyclase activity in adrenocorticotropic hormone-sensitive and mutant adrenocortical tumor cell lines. *J. Biol. Chem.* **247**, 3134–3138.

Schimmer, B. P. (1979). Adrenocortical Y1 cells. *Methods Enzymol.* **58**, 570–574.

Schimmer, B. P. (1980). Cyclic nucleotides in hormonal regulation of adrenocortical function. *Adv. Cyclic Nucleotide Res.* **13**, 181–214.

Schimmer, B. P., Tsao, J., and Cheung, N. H. (1977a). Regulation of adenylate cyclase activity in glial-adrenal hybrid cells. *Nature (London)* **269**, 162–163.

Schimmer, B. P., Tsao, J., and Knapp, M. (1977b). Isolation of mutant adrenocortical tumor cells resistant to cyclic nucleotides. *Mol. Cell. Endocrinol.* **8**, 135–145.

Schimmer, B. P., Rae, P. A., Gutman, N. S., Matt, V. M., and Tsao, J. (1979). Genetic dissection of ACTH action in adrenal tumor cells. *In* "Hormones and Cell Culture" (G. H. Sato and R. Ross, eds.), pp. 281–297. Cold Spring Harbor Lab., Cold Spring Harbor, New York.

Schumacher, M., Schafer, G., Lichtenberg, V., and Hilz, H. (1979). Maximal steroidogenic capacity of mouse Leydig cells. Kinetic analysis and dependence on protein kinase activation and cAMP accumulation. *FEBS Lett.* **107**, 398–402.

Segaloff, D. L., and Ascoli, M. (1981). Removal of the surface-bound human choriogonadotropin results in the cessation of hormonal responses in cultured Leydig tumor cells. *J. Biol. Chem.* **256**, 11420–11423.

Segaloff, D. L., Puett, D., and Ascoli, M. (1981a). The dynamics of the steroidogenic response of perifused Leydig tumor cells to human chorionic gonadotropin, ovine luteinizing hormones, cholera toxin, and adenosine 3',5'-cyclic monophosphate. *Endocrinology (Baltimore)* **108**, 632–638.

Segaloff, D. L., Ascoli, M., and Puett, D. (1981b). Characterization of the desensitized state of Leydig tumor cells. *Biochim. Biophys. Acta* **675**, 351–358.

Shikita, M., and Hall, P. F. (1974). The stoichiometry of the conversion of cholesterol and hydroxycholesterols to pregnenolone catalysed by adrenal cytochrome P-450. *Proc. Natl. Acad. Sci. U.S.A.* **71**, 1441–1445.

Shima, S., Mitsunaga, M., Kawashima, Y., Taguchi, S., and Nakao, T. (1974). Studies on cyclic nucleotides in the adrenal gland. IV. Effects of ACTH on cyclic nucleotides-dependent protein kinases in the adrenal gland. *Endocrinology (Baltimore)* **104**, 588–595.

Shin, S. (1967). Studies on interstitial cells in tissue culture: Steroid biosynthesis in monolayers of mouse testicular interstitial cells. *Endocrinology (Baltimore)* **81**, 440–448.

Shin, S., Yasumura, Y., and Sato, G. H. (1968). Studies on interstitial cells in tissue culture. II. Steroid biosynthesis by a clonal line of rat testicular interstitial cells. *Endocrinology (Baltimore)* **82**, 614–616.

Siiteri, P. K., and MacDonald, P. C. (1963). The utilization of circulating dehydro-isoandrosterone sulfate for estrogen synthesis during human pregnancy. *Steroids* **2**, 713–730.

Siiteri, P. K., and MacDonald, P. C. (1966). Placental estrogen biosynthesis during human pregnancy. *J. Clin. Endocrinol. Metab.* **26**, 751–761.

Simonian, M. H., Hornsby, P. J., Ill, C. R., O'Hare, M. J., and Gill, G. N. (1979). Characterization of cultured bovine adrenocortical cells and derived clonal lines: Regulation of steroidogenesis and culture life span. *Endocrinology (Baltimore)* **105**, 99–105.

Simpson, E. R. (1979). Cholesterol side chain cleavage, cytochrome P-450, and the control of steroidogenesis. *Mol. Cell. Endocrinol.* **13**, 213–227.

Simpson, E. R., and Boyd, G. S. (1967a). The cholesterol side-chain cleavage system of bovine adrenal cortex. *Eur. J. Biochem.* **2**, 275–285.

Simpson, E. R., and Boyd, G. S. (1967b). Partial resolution of the mixed-function oxidase involved in the cholesterol side-chain cleavage reaction in bovine adrenal mitochondria. *Biochem. Biophys. Res. Commun.* **28**, 945–950.

Simpson, E. R., and Burkhart, M. F. (1980a). Acyl CoA cholesterol acyl transferase activity in human placental microsomes: Inhibition by progesterone. *Arch. Biochem. Biophys.* **200**, 79–85.

Simpson, E. R., and Burkhart, M. F. (1980b). Regulation of cholesterol metabolism by human choriocarcinoma cells in culture: Effect of lipoproteins and progesterone on cholesteryl ester synthesis. *Arch. Biochem. Biophys.* **200**, 86–92.

Simpson, E. R., and MacDonald, P. C. (1981). Endocrine physiology of the placenta. *Annu. Rev. Physiol.* **43**, 163–188.

Simpson, E. R., and Miller, D. A. (1978). Cholesterol side-chain cleavage, cytochrome P-450, and iron-sulfur protein in human placental mitochondria. *Arch. Biochem. Biophys.* **190**, 800–808.

Simpson, E. R., McCarthy, J. L., and Peterson, J. A. (1978a). Evidence that the cyclohex-imide-sensitive site of adrenocorticotropin hormone action is in the mitochondria. Changes in pregnenolone formation, cholesterol content, and the electron paramagnetic resonance spectra of cytochrome P-450. *J. Biol. Chem.* **253**, 3135–3139.

Simpson, E. R., Porter, J. C., Milewich, L., Bilheimer, D. W., and MacDonald, P. C. (1978b). Regulation by plasma lipoproteins of progesterone biosynthesis and 3-hydroxy-3-methyl-glutaryl coenzyme A reductase activity in cultured human choriocarcinoma cells. *J. Clin. Endocrinol. Metab.* **47**, 1099–1105.

Simpson, E. R., Bilheimer, D. W., MacDonald, P. C., and Porter, J. C. (1979). Uptake and degradation of plasma lipoproteins by human choriocarcinoma cells in culture. *Endocrinology (Baltimore)* **104,** 8–16.

Slavinski, E. A., Tull, J. W., and Aversperg, N. (1976). Steroidogenic pathways and trophic response to adrenocorticotropin of cultured adrenocortical cells in different states of differentiation. *J. Endocrinol.* **69,** 385–394.

Steinberger, E., Steinberger, A., and Ficher, M. (1970). Study of spermatogenesis and steroid metabolism in cultures of mammalian testes. *Recent Prog. Horm. Res.* **26,** 547–588.

Steiss, R. G., and Finn, F. M. (1979). Bovine adrenal cortical protein kinases: isolation of the type II catalytic subunit. *Biochem. Biophys. Res. Commun.* **89,** 1245–1252.

Stollar, V., Buonassisi, V., and Sato, G. (1964). Studies on hormone secreting adrenocortical tumor in tissue culture. *Exp. Cell Res.* **35,** 608–616.

Stone, D., and Hechter, O. (1954). Studies on ACTH action in perfused bovine adrenals: The site of action of ACTH in corticosteroidogenesis. *Arch. Biochem. Biophys.* **51,** 457–469.

Temple, R., and Wolff, J. (1973). Stimulation of steroid secretion by antimicrotubular agents. *J. Biol. Chem.* **248,** 2691–2698.

Vahouny, G. V., Chanderbhan, R., Hinds, R., Hodges, V. A., and Treadwell, C. R. (1978). ACTH induced hydrolysis of cholesteryl esters in rat adrenal cells. *J. Lipid Res.* **19,** 570–577.

Van der Wusse, G. J., Kalkman, M. L., Van Winsen, M. P. I., and Van der Molen, H. J. (1975). On the regulation of rat testicular steroidogenesis. Short term effects of luteinizing hormone and cycloheximide *in vivo* and Ca^{+2} *in vitro* on steroid production in cell-free systems. *Biochim. Biophys. Acta* **398,** 28–38.

Villee, C. A., Van Leusden, H., and Zelewski, L. (1966). The regulation of the biosynthesis of sterols and steroids in the placenta. *Adv. Enzyme Regul.* **4,** 161–179.

Weidman, E. R., and Gill, G. N. (1977). Differential effects of ACTH or 8-Br-cAMP on growth and replication in a functional adrenal tumor cell lines. *J. Cell Physiol.* **90,** 91–104.

Winkel, G. A., Snyder, J. M., MacDonald, P. C., and Simpson, E. R. (1980). Regulation of cholesterol and progesterone synthesis in human placental cells in culture by serum lipoproteins. *Endocrinology* **106,** 1054–1060.

Wolff, J., and Hope Cook, G. (1975). Choleragen stimulates steroidogenesis and adenylate cyclase in cells lacking functional hormone receptors. *Biochim. Biophys. Acta* **413,** 283–290.

Wolff, J., Temple, R., and Hope Cook, G. (1973). Stimulation of steroid secretion in adrenal tumor cells by choleragen. *Proc. Natl. Acad. Sci. U.S.A.* **70,** 2741–2744.

Yang, W. H., Jones, A. L., and Li, C. H. (1974). The effects of interstitial cell-stimulating hormone, prolactin, and bovine growth hormone on the transplantable Leydig cell tumor in the mouse. *Cancer Res.* **34,** 2440–2450.

Yasumura, Y., Buonassisi, V., and Sato, G. (1966). Clonal analysis of differentiated function in animal cell cultures. I. Possible correlated maintenance of differentiated function and the diploid karyotype. *Cancer Res.* **26,** 529–535.

13

Possible Regulatory Roles of Calmodulin and Myosin Light Chain Kinase in Secretion

JAMES G. CHAFOULEAS, VINCE GUERRIERO, JR., AND
ANTHONY R. MEANS

I. INTRODUCTION

All living cells have the ability to respond to extracellular stimuli. Implicit in this property is the requirement to transduce an extracellular signal into an intracellular action. Although the external signal may be a change in pH, temperature, or osmolarity, perhaps the best-studied examples involve hormone action on target tissues. Although there are a vast number of hormones eliciting an equally large number of responses, one common aspect of all peptide hormone action is the key role of Ca^{2+} in the signal transduction. Over the past 5 years it has become evident that most, if not all, of the Ca^{2+}-regulated events in the eukaryotic cell are mediated by the intracellular Ca^{2+}-binding protein calmodulin (for reviews, see Wang and Waissman, 1979; Means and Dedman, 1980; Cheung, 1980). Although this protein is involved in many different aspects of hormone action, it will be the purpose of this chapter to focus on its regulation of one enzyme—

445

CELLULAR REGULATION OF SECRETION AND RELEASE

myosin light chain kinase—and the possible role of this enzyme in regulation of nonmuscle motility and secretion.

II. CALMODULIN

Calmodulin is a heat-stable, 17,000-M_r, multifunctional, Ca^{2+}-binding protein that meets all the criteria set forth for a Ca^{2+} receptor. It contains four equivalent Ca^{2+}-binding sites that have a K_d of 2.4 × 10^{-6} M and do not bind Mg^{2+} under physiological conditions (Dedman *et al.*, 1977). Ca^{2+} binding induces a more α-helical conformation of the protein, which precedes activation of the calmodulin-dependent phosphodiesterase (Dedman *et al.*, 1977). It is now established that the Ca^{2+} binding exposes lipophilic regions on the molecule that àre the sites of association with the regulated enzymes (LaPorte *et al.*, 1980; Tanaka and Hidaka, 1980). In addition, it is to these lipophilic sites that the phenothiozine antipsychotic and naphthalenesulfonamide drugs bind, thus inhibiting calmodulin-mediated regulation.

Calmodulin has been shown to mediate the calcium regulation of a large number of fundamental intracellular enzyme systems. These enzymes include a calcium-dependent form of phosphodiesterase (Kakiuchi and Yamagaki, 1970; Cheung, 1970), brain adenylate cyclase (Lynch *et al.*, 1976; Brostrom *et al.*, 1977), human erythrocyte membrane Ca^{2+}, Mg^{2+}-ATPase (Gopinath and Vincenzi, 1977; Luthra *et al.*, 1977; Jarrett and Penniston, 1977), myosin light chain kinase (Dabrowska *et al.*, 1977b; Yagi *et al.*, 1978; Hathaway and Adelstein, 1979), skeletal muscle phosphorylase kinase (Cohen *et al.*, 1978), glycogen synthase (Srivastava *et al.*, 1979; Soderling *et al.*, 1979), human phospholipase A_2 (Wong and Cheung, 1979), and pea NAD kinase (Anderson and Cormier, 1978). Calmodulin has also been reported to be the calcium-binding protein regulating calcium transport in the sarcoplasmic reticulum (Katz and Remtulla, 1978; LePeuch *et al.*, 1979) and autophosphorylation of membrane proteins (Schulman and Greengard, 1977, 1978; DeLorenzo *et al.*, 1979). In addition, immunofluorescence studies on a variety of cultured cells have demonstrated that calmodulin is localized on the actomyosin-containing stress fibers in interphase and is a dynamic component of the mitotic apparatus (Welsh *et al.*, 1978; Dedman *et al.*, 1978b; Anderson *et al.*, 1978). In this regard, this protein has been shown to regulate the calcium-dependent assembly–disassembly of microtubules *in vitro* (Marcum *et al.*, 1978).

Calmodulin has been demonstrated to be ubiquitous in eukaryotes (Kakiuchi *et al.*, 1974; Waissman *et al.*, 1975; Chafouleas *et al.*, 1979).

The highly conserved nature of this protein has been suggested by studies that demonstrate that the amino acid sequence of calmodulin is relatively invariant in the cow, rat (Dedman *et al.,* 1978a; Vanaman, 1980), and sea pansy, *R. reniformis* (Vanaman, 1980), differing by no more than six conservative amino acid substitutions. Moreover, each of these proteins contains four internally homologous calcium-binding domains, and only one of the substitutions (in *R. reniformis*) occurs in these highly conserved regions. The extent to which this protein is conserved in eukaryotes was demonstrated by Chafouleas *et al.* (1979). Employing a radioimmunoassay for the protein, they demonstrated that calmodulin from representative species of primitive algae, slime mold, and coelenterate to the more advanced plants and mammals exhibited immunological identity. Taken together, these data suggest that calmodulin is one of the most highly conserved, as well as widely dispersed, proteins studied.

III. CALMODULIN AND HORMONE ACTION

Because calmodulin is a component of virtually every intracellular compartment as well as the plasma membrane, efforts have been made to determine whether cell surface-acting agents promote an alteration in the distribution of calmodulin. Distinct anatomical regions of the central nervous system such as the corpus striatum contain dopamine receptors that seem to be coupled to adenylate cyclase (Hanbauer *et al.,* 1979a). Calmodulin has been suggested to mediate dopamine action because phosphorylation of membrane proteins promotes the apparent release of calmodulin from membrane-bound to soluble form (Gnegy and Lau, 1980a). Because a soluble calmodulin-dependent phosphodiesterase exists, it has been proposed that long-term stimulation of dopamine receptors is associated with an increase in the soluble calmodulin content, thereby activating phosphodiesterase and decreasing receptor responsiveness. Similar data suggest interneuronal pathways also exist where opiates increase soluble calmodulin via a release of dopamine and thus act as indirect dopamine agonists (Hanbauer and Phyall, 1980). Smoake and Solomon (1980) have reported altered calmodulin distribution in liver cells from rats with streptozotocin-induced diabetes. These authors conclude that such changes might play a role in the alteration of cAMP metabolism known to exist in such pathological states.

The difficulties with interpretation of most calmodulin distribution studies is that the protein is assayed by its ability to stimulate a calmodulin-dependent enzyme. Because all such assays are Ca^{2+} dependent and because other calmodulin-binding proteins are likely to be present in each subcellular fraction, it is difficult to obtain quantitative values for calmodulin. This difficulty is circumvented when a radioimmunoassay is employed because the assay can be performed in the presence of EGTA and is therefore Ca^{2+} independent (Chafouleas *et al.*, 1979). The radioimmunoassay has been utilized to determine the quantity and subcellular distribution of calmodulin in the rat pituitary gonadotrophe before and during GnRH-induced LH release (Conn *et al.*, 1981a). Indeed the distribution of calmodulin does change in response to GnRH. There is an initial rise in the percentage of calmodulin that is associated with the plasma membrane and that appears concomitantly with the depletion of cytoplasmic calmodulin. These changes occur temporally in concert with secretion of LH. As the calmodulin begins to be cleared from the plasma membrane, its level increases first in the secretory granule and microsomal fractions before finally replenishing the cytoplasm. The magnitude of the changes that occur between plasma membrane and cytoplasmic content of calmodulin are related to the dose of GnRH. Calmodulin redistribution is also hormone specific because analogs such as des[1] GnRH(2–10), which has no efficacy in promoting LH secretion, did not alter intracellular changes in calmodulin. Finally, a budget of calmodulin content in all subcellular fractions revealed that GnRH did not increase total calmodulin, and greater than 95% of the cellular calmodulin was recovered (see also Chapter 14).

The preceding data suggest that calmodulin may be important in the regulation of protein secretion but provide little information concerning the mechanism. At this juncture it is impossible to predict whether calmodulin redistribution is a cause or consequence of the secretory process. In the red blood cell (Hinds *et al.*, 1978), pancreatic islet (Pershadsingh *et al.*, 1980), and adipocyte (Pershadsingh and McDonald, 1980), calmodulin-activated ATPases are found in the plasma membrane, and, at least in the adipocyte, the enzyme appears to be hormonally regulated. Plasma membranes from islet cells also have been reported to contain a calmodulin-stimulated adenylate cyclase activity (Valverde *et al.*, 1979). Calmodulin is also a major component of postsynaptic membranes (Grab *et al.*, 1979; Lin *et al.*, 1980; Wood *et al.*, 1980), has been proposed to mediate the Ca^{2+} effects on synaptic transmission (Hanbauer *et al.*, 1979a,b; Gnegy and Lau, 1980a,b), and accordingly may play a role in neurotransmitter release (DeLorenzo *et al.*, 1979). Finally, as mentioned earlier, trifluoperazine and naphthalenesulfonamides are drugs that bind to calmodulin and inhibit many of its actions. These drugs also inhibit the receptor-mediated secretory process in a variety of systems.

Receptor-mediated endocytosis is also a Ca^{2+}-dependent process and also involves clathrin-coated vesicles (Goldstein *et al.*, 1979; Salisbury *et al.*, 1980). Although internalization of GnRH does not appear to be required for the LH release process, the gonadotrophe response to this releasing hormone does include the pattern of patching, capping, and internalization observed for many cell surface-mediated ligand systems (Conn *et al.*, 1981b; and Chapter 1 and 14). This receptor redistribution pattern in the gonadotrophe is mimicked by changes found in calmodulin that is associated with the plasma membrane (when assessed by indirect immunofluorescence microscopy). Recruitment of clathrin-coated vesicles to the plasma membrane of human lymphoblastoid cells occurs following stimulation with multivalent anti-IgM antibodies (Salisbury *et al.*, 1980). This recruitment is inhibited by the presence of anti-calmodulin drugs, and calmodulin is a component of such vesicles. Thus, the appearance of calmodulin at the plasma membrane may be associated with the accumulation of coated pits involved in the receptor internalization process. Insulin, which also is internalized, following cap formation, promotes the translocation of glucose transport activity from the microsomal or Golgi fractions to the plasma membrane (Cushman and Wardzala, 1980; Suzuki and Kono, 1980). Actin and myosin have also been reported to co-cap with several cell surface receptors (Bourguignon *et al.*, 1978; Flanagan and Koch, 1978), and actin-containing matrices have been isolated from *Dictyostellium discoideum* (Condeelis, 1979), murine tumor cells, and lymphocyte plasma membranes (Mescher *et al.*, 1981) associated with various receptors. Thus, the phenomenon of redistribution of new activities to the plasma membrane may be a generalized occurrence for plasma membrane receptor-mediated events. This redistribution suggests a mechanism by which calmodulin-regulated events could be affected without the requirement for new protein synthesis. It is likely that calmodulin redistribution is secondary to alterations in the net flux or distribution of Ca^{2+} within the cell.

IV. MYOSIN LIGHT CHAIN KINASE

The structural basis of motility in smooth and nonmuscle cells involves the cellular cytoskeleton. The cytoskeleton is composed of a few specific proteins. The structural elements can be regulated by a wide variety of molecules, one of which is Ca^{2+}. The component of the cytoskeleton most intimately involved with contractility and force generation required for endo- or exocytosis is the actin-based microfilament (Dedman *et al.*, 1979).

Many of the muscle contractile proteins have been found in nonmuscle cells (see Gröshel-Stewart, 1980, for a review). These proteins are physically and biochemically similar to the same proteins found in smooth muscle. For this reason, smooth muscle contraction can be used as a model system to study nonmuscle motility. The mechanism by which Ca^{2+} regulates smooth muscle motility has been extensively studied. Contraction results from the interaction of actin and myosin. Myosin is composed of two high-molecular-weight subunits (200,000 each) and four low-molecular-weight subunits (two each of 20,000 and 17,000). Native myosin has a coiled tail region and a globular head region. The tail regions of myosin molecules interact to form thick filaments. The globular head of this bipolar molecule contains an actin-binding site and the ATPase activity. The light chain subunits are associated with the globular head.

The release of Ca^{2+} into the sarcoplasm is the initial event in excitation–contraction coupling of muscle. The mechanism of regulation of the smooth muscle contractile systems occurs via Ca^{2+}-regulated phosphorylation at the 20,000-MW regulatory or P light chain of myosin (Chacko *et al.*, 1977; Sherry *et al.*, 1978; Lebowitz and Conti, 1979; Chacko, 1981; deLanerolle and Stull, 1980; Barron *et al.*, 1980). The Ca^{2+}–calmodulin-dependent enzyme myosin light chain kinase (MLCK) catalyzes the transfer of the γ-phosphate of ATP to the regulatory light chain of myosin. This phosphorylation is obligatory for the stimulation of smooth muscle actin-activated myosin ATPase. The result is tension development and motility. The dephosphorylation of the light chain is catalyzed by a myosin light chain phosphatase.

MLCK has been purified from smooth (Dabrowska *et al.*, 1977a; Adelstein and Klee, 1981; Guerriero *et al.*, 1981) skeletal (Pires and Perry, 1977; Blumenthal and Stull, 1980; Crouch *et al.*, 1981), and cardiac muscle (Walsh *et al.*, 1979; Wolf and Hofmann, 1980). The reported molecular weights of the enzymes from these tissues range from 80,000 to 130,000, depending on both the tissue and the procedure used for purification. It has been suggested either that there are multiple forms of MLCK in these tissues (Yamauchi and Fujisawa, 1980; Stull, 1980) or that the smaller-molecular-weight proteins are proteolytic fragments of the native enzyme (Walsh *et al.*, 1980). A study by Guerriero *et al.* (1981) addressed this question. An antibody against chicken gizzard MLCK was produced. This probe and the protein transfer technique of Towbin *et al.* (1979) were used to determine the molecular weight of the enzyme in a variety of chicken tissues. The MW was found to be 130,000. These data suggest that some proteolysis of the native enzyme may occur during purification.

MLCK activity has been demonstrated to be present in several non-muscle cell types including brain, platelets, alveolar macrophages, and baby hamster kidney cells (BHK-21) (Adelstein and Conti, 1975; Dabrowska and Hartshorne, 1978; Trotter and Adelstein, 1979; Yerna *et al.*, 1979; Hathaway *et al.*, 1981a). As in smooth muscle, phosphorylation of the regulatory light chain in these tissues results in an increase in actin-activated myosin ATPase activity. These results, then, support the view that the Ca^{2+}–calmodulin complex is capable of regulating myosin–actin interactions and therefore motility in non-muscle cells.

Enzymes that dephosphorylate the regulatory light chain of myosin have been purified from skeletal (Morgan *et al.*, 1976) and smooth muscle (Pato and Adelstein, 1980). Dephosphorylation of smooth muscle myosin results in a form of myosin ATPase that cannot be activated by actin. The removal of the phosphate from the regulatory light chain, then, leads to smooth muscle relaxation.

The second messenger cAMP can also regulate smooth muscle contraction. Turkey gizzard MLCK was phosphorylated by the catalytic subunit of cAMP-dependent protein kinase (Adelstein *et al.*, 1978; Conti and Adelstein, 1981). Phosphorylation of the enzyme in the absence of calmodulin resulted in phosphate incorporation into two sites on the molecule. The phosphorylated enzyme required a 10- to 20-fold increase in the amount of calmodulin needed for 50% activation of enzyme activity. Also, cAMP and its dependent protein kinase inhibited phosphorylation of myosin light chains in bovine aortic actomyosin (Silver and DiSalvo, 1979). Anderson *et al.* (1981) have provided further support for cAMP involvement in smooth muscle relaxation by measuring ^{32}P incorporation into cultured vascular smooth muscle cells in response to angiotensin. The regulatory light chain of myosin was specifically phosphorylated in response to this hormone. Myosin light chain phosphorylation was greatly reduced following exposure of the cells to cAMP. These results are consistent with a mechanism by which cAMP can affect smooth muscle contraction. Following stimulation of β-receptors by epinephrine, there is an increase in adenylate cyclase activity and therefore the production of cAMP. The binding of cAMP to the regulatory subunit liberates the catalytic subunit that can now phosphorylate myosin light chain kinase. The phosphorylated enzyme is less active, leading to a decrease in regulatory light chain phosphorylation. Actin will not interact with myosin if the light chains are not phosphorylated, resulting in a relaxation of the muscle.

A similar mechanism involving cAMP regulation of actin–myosin interaction exists in platelets (Hathaway *et al.*, 1981b). Platelet myosin light chain kinase can serve as a substrate for the catalytic subunit of cAMP-dependent protein kinase. As in smooth muscle, the phosphorylated MLCK has decreased activity. The phosphorylation of myosin light chain kinase by cAMP-dependent protein kinase is a mechanism by which cAMP can potentially regulate contractile activity in nonmuscle cells.

The machinery exists for actin–myosin regulation of secretion in nonmuscle cells, as discussed earlier. To determine if MLCK phosphorylation of the regulatory light chain of myosin triggers the production of the motive force needed to move secretory granules to the plasma membrane, various groups have studied secretagogue-induced serotonin release in blood platelets. Treatment of platelets with thrombin causes an increase in the phosphorylation of a 20,000-dalton protein identified as the regulatory light chain by gel electrophoresis (Nishikawa *et al.*, 1980; Daniel *et al.*, 1981). Low temperature (0°C) causes microtubule depolymerization and shape changes in platelets. Bennett and Lynch (1980) have shown that two proteins of 20,000 and 40,000 M_r become phosphorylated in response to this low-temperature shape change preceding serotonin release. The smaller protein is thought to be the light chain of myosin. The possibility exists then that the phosphorylation is triggered by microtubule disassembly.

To better understand the role of myosin light chain kinase in nonmuscle motility, antibodies to the smooth muscle enzyme have been produced and used to localize MLCK in tissue culture cells (de-Lanerolle *et al.*, 1981; Guerriero *et al.*, 1981). These studies have revealed that MLCK is found associated with the actin–myosin-containing stress fibers. Similar localization of calmodulin on these fibers (Dedman *et al.*, 1978b; Guerriero *et al.*, 1981) is consistent with the hypothesis that calmodulin regulates Ca^{2+}-dependent motility in nonmuscle cells.

V. CONCLUSION

There is little doubt that calmodulin occupies a central regulatory role in hormone action. The association of MLCK and calmodulin with the stress fibers and the correlation between secretion and the phosphorylation of the regulatory light chain of myosin are in agreement with an actin–myosin-based system providing the motile force needed for secretion. Microtubules may provide a system of fibers that give directionality for the movement of secretory granules toward the plasma membrane. The microfilaments, then, would provide force needed to move the granules along the microtubule network. Both Ca^{2+} and cAMP would be potential regulators of the system. An increase in Ca^{2+} concentration via secretogogue stimulation would result in the formation of a Ca^{2+}–calmodulin complex. This complex can now bind to and activate MLCK. The activated MLCK phosphorylates the regulatory light chain of myosin, resulting in actin-activated myosin ATPase and motility. Inhibitors of secretion that elevate cAMP levels activate the catalytic subunit of cAMP-dependent protein kinase, which can phosphorylate MLCK. The phosphorylated enzyme is less active, leading to an inhibition of light chain phosphorylation and therefore secretion.

REFERENCES

Adelstein, R. S., and Conti, M. A. (1975). Phosphorylation of platelet myosin increases actin-activated myosin ATPase activity. *Nature (London)* **256,** 597–598.
Adelstein, R. S., and Klee, C. B. (1981). Purification and characterization of smooth muscle myosin light chain kinase. *J. Biol. Chem.* **256,** 7501–7509.
Adelstein, R. S., Conti, M. A., and Hathaway, D. R. (1978). Phosphorylation of smooth muscle myosin light chain kinase by the catalytic subunit of adenosine 3':5'-monophosphate-dependent protein kinase. *J. Biol. Chem.* **253,** 8347–8350.
Anderson, B., Osborn, M., and Weber, K. (1978). Specific visualization of the distribution of the calcium-dependent regulatory protein of cyclic nucleotide phosphodiesterase (modulator protein) in tissue culture cells by immunofluorescence microscopy: Mitosis and intercellular bridge. *Eur. J. Cell Biol.* **17,** 354–364.
Anderson, J. M., and Cormier, M. J. (1978). Calcium-dependent regulator of NAD kinase. *Biophys. Biochem. Res. Commun.* **84,** 595–602.
Anderson, J. M., Gimbrone, M. A., Jr., and Alexander, R. W. (1981). Angiotensin II stimulates phosphorylation of the myosin light chain cultured vascular smooth muscle cells. *J. Biol. Chem.* **256,** 4693–4696.
Barron, J. T., Bárány, M., Bárány, K., and Storti, R. V. (1980). Reversible phosphorylation and dephosphorylation of the 20,000 dalton light chain of myosin during the contraction-relaxation-contraction cycle of arterial smooth muscle. *J. Biol. Chem.* **255,** 6238–6244.
Bennett, W. F., and Lynch, G. (1980). Low-temperature induction of calcium-dependent protein phosphorylation in blood platelets. *J. Cell Biol.* **86,** 280–285.
Blumenthal, D. F., and Stull, J. T. (1980). Activation of skeletal muscle myosin light chain kinase by calcium (2+) and calmodulin. *Biochemistry* **19,** 5608–5614.
Bourguignon, L. Y. W., Tokuyasu, K. T., and Singer, S. J. (1978). The capping of lymphocytes and other cells studied by an improved method of immunofluorescence staining of frozen sections. *J. Cell. Physiol.* **95,** 239–258.

Brostrom, C. O., Brostrom, M. A., and Wolff, D. J. (1977). Calcium-dependent adenylate cyclase from rat cerebral cortex. *J. Biol. Chem.* **252,** 5677–5685.

Chacko, S. (1981). Effects of phosphorylation, calcium ion, and tropomyosin on actin-activated adenosine 5′-triphosphatase activity of mammalian smooth muscle myosin. *Biochemistry* **20,** 702–707.

Chacko, S., Conti, M. A., and Adelstein, R. S. (1977). Effect of phosphorylation of smooth muscle myosin on actin activation and Ca^{++} regulation. *Proc. Natl. Acad. Sci. U.S.A.* **74,** 129–133.

Chafouleas, J. G., Dedman, J. R., Munjaal, R. P., and Means, A. R. (1979). Calmodulin: Development and application of a sensitive radioimmunoassay. *J. Biol. Chem.* **254,** 10262–10267.

Cheung, W. Y. (1970). Cyclic 3′,5′-nucleotide phosphodiesterase: demonstration of an activator. *Biochem. Biophys. Res. Commun.* **38,** 533–538.

Cheung, W. Y. (1980). Calmodulin plays a pivotal role in cellular regulation. *Science* **207,** 19–27.

Cohen, P., Burchell, A., Foulkes, J. G., Cohen, P. T. W., Nairn, A., and Vanaman, T. (1978). Identification of the Ca^{2+}-dependent modulator protein as the fourth subunit of rabbit skeletal muscle phosphorylase kinase. *FEBS Lett.* **92**(2), 287–293.

Condeelis, J. S. (1979). Isolation of concanavalin A caps during various stages of formation and their association with actin and myosin. *J. Cell Biol.* **80,** 751–758.

Conn, P. M., Chafouleas, J. G., Rogers, D., and Means, A. R. (1981a). Gonadotropin releasing hormone stimulates calmodulin redistribution in rat pituitary. *Nature (London)* **292,** 264–265.

Conn, P. M., Marian, J., McMillian, M., Stern, J. E., Rogers, D. R., Hamby, M., Penna, A., and Grant, E. (1981b). Gonadotropin releasing hormone action in the pituitary: A three step mechanism. *Endocr. Rev.* **2,** 174–185.

Conti, M. A., and Adelstein, R. S. (1981). The relationship between calmodulin binding and phosphorylation of smooth muscle myosin kinase by the catalytic subunit of 3′:5′-cAMP-dependent protein kinase. *J. Biol. Chem.* **256,** 3178–3181.

Crouch, T. H., Holroyde, M. J., Collins, J. H., Solaro, R. J., and Potter, J. D. (1981). Interaction of calmodulin with skeletal muscle myosin light chain kinase. *Biochemistry* **20,** 6318–6325.

Cushman, S. W., and Wardzala, L. J. (1980). Potential mechanism of insulin action on glucose transport in the isolated rat adipose cell. *J. Biol. Chem.* **255,** 4758–4762.

Dabrowska, R., and Hartshorne, D. J. (1978). A Ca^{2+}- and modulator-dependent myosin light chain kinase from non-muscle cells. *Biochem. Biophys. Res. Commun.* **85,** 1352–1359.

Dabrowska, R., Aromatorio, D., Sherry, J. M. F., and Hartshorne, D. J. (1977a). Composition of the myosin light chain kinase from chicken gizzard. *Biochem. Biophys. Res. Commun.* **78,** 1263–1272.

Dabrowska, R., Sherry, J. M. F., Aromatorio, D. K., and Hartshorne, D. J. (1977b). Modulator protein as a component of the myosin light chain kinase from chicken gizzard. *Biochemistry* **17,** 253–258.

Daniel, J. L., Molish, I. R., and Holmsen, H. (1981). Myosin phosphorylation in intact platelets. *J. Biol. Chem.* **256,** 7510–7514.

Dedman, J. R., Brinkley, B. R., Means, A. R. (1979). Regulation of microfilaments and microtubules by calcium and cyclic AMP. *Adv. Cyclic Nucleotide Res.* **11,** 131–174.

Dedman, J. R., Jackson, R. L., Schreiber, W. E., and Means, A. R. (1978a). Sequence homology of the CA^{2+}-dependent regulator of cyclic nucleotide phosphodiesterase from rat testis with other Ca^{2+}-binding proteins. *J. Biol. Chem.* **253,** 343–346.

Dedman, J. R., Potter, J. D., Jackson, R. L., Johnson, J. D., and Means, A. R. (1977). Physiochemical Properties of rat testis Ca^{2+}-dependent regulator protein of cyclic nucleotide phosphodiesterase: relationship of Ca^{2+} binding, conformational changes and phosphodiesterase activity. *J. Biol. Chem.* **252,** 8415–8422.

Dedman, J. R., Welsh, M. J., and Means, A. R. (1978b). Ca^{2+}-dependent regulator: Production and characterization of a monospecific antibody. *J. Biol. Chem.* **253,** 7515–7521.

deLanerolle, P., and Stull, J. T. (1980). Myosin phosphorylation during contraction and relaxation of tracheal smooth muscle. *J. Biol. Chem.* **255,** 9993–10000.

deLanerolle, P., Adelstein, R. S., Feramisco, J. R., and Burridge, K. (1981). Characterization of antibodies to smooth muscle myosin kinase and their use in localizing myosin kinase in non-muscle cells. *Proc. Natl. Acad. Sci. U.S.A.* **78,** 4738–4742.

DeLorenzo, J. R., Freedman, S. D., Yohe, W. B., and Maurer, S. C. (1979). Stimulation of Ca^{2+}-dependent neurotransmitter release and presynaptic nerve terminal protein phosphorylation by calmodulin and a calmodulin-like protein isolated from synaptic vesicles. *Proc. Natl. Acad. Sci. U.S.A.* **76,** 1838–1842.

Flanagan, J., and Koch, G. L. E. (1978). Cross-linked surface Ig attaches to actin. *Nature (London)* **273,** 278–281.

Gnegy, M. E., and Lau, Y. S. (1980a). Effects of chronic and acute treatment of antipsychotic drugs on calmodulin release from rat striatal membranes. *Neuropharmacology* **19,** 319–323.

Gnegy, M. E., and Lau, Y. S. (1980b). Calmodulin release from striatal membranes after acute and chronic treatment with Butaclamol. *Adv. Biochem. Psychopharmacol.* **24,** 147–151.

Goldstein, J. L., Anderson, R. G. W., and Brown, M. S. (1979). Coated pits, coated vesicles, and receptor-mediated endocytosis. *Nature (London)* **279,** 679–685.

Gopinath, R. M., and Vincenzi, F. F. (1977). Phosphodiesterase protein activator of $(Ca^{2+} + Mg^{2+})$ ATPase. *Biochem. Biophys. Res. Commun.* **77,** 1203–1209.

Grab, D. J., Berzins, K., Cohen, R. S., and Siekevitz, P. (1979). Presence of calmodulin in postsynaptic densities isolated from canine cerebral cortex. *J. Biol. Chem.* **254,** 8690–8696.

Gröschel-Stewart, U. (1980). Immunochemistry of cytoplasmic contractile protein. *Int. Rev. Cytobiol.* **65,** 195–254.

Guerriero, V., Jr., Rowley, D. R., and Means, A. R. (1981). Production and characterization of an antibody to myosin light chain kinase and intracellular localization of the enzyme. *Cell* **27,** 449–458.

Hanbauer, I., and Phyall, W. (1980). Involvement of calmodulin in the modulation of dopamine receptor function. *Adv. Biochem. Psychopharmacol.* **24,** 133–138.

Hanbauer, I., Gimble, J., and Lovenberg, W. (1979a). Changes in soluble calmodulin following activation of dopamine receptors in rat striatal slices. *Neuropharmacology* **18,** 851–857.

Hanbauer, I., Gimble, J., Sankaran, K., and Sherard, R. (1979b). Modulation of striatal cyclic nucleotide phosphodiesterase by calmodulin: Regulation by opiate and dopamine receptor activation. *Neuropharmacology* **18,** 859–864.

Hathaway, D. R., and Adelstein, R. S. (1979). Human platelet myosin light chain kinase requires the calcium-binding protein calmodulin for activity. *Proc. Natl. Acad. Sci. U.S.A.* **76,** 1653–1657.

Hathaway, D. R., Adelstein, R. S., and Klee, C. B. (1981a). Interaction of calmodulin with myosin light chain kinase and cAMP-dependent protein kinase in bovine brain. *J. Biol. Chem.* **256,** 8183–8189.

Hathaway, D. R., Eaton, C. R., and Adelstein, R. S. (1981b). Regulation of human platelet myosin light chain kinase by the catalytic subunit of cyclic AMP-dependent protein kinase. *Nature (London)* **291,** 252–254.

Hinds, T. R., Larsen, F. L., and Vincenzi, F. F. (1978). Plasma membrane Ca^{2+} transport: Stimulation by soluble proteins. *Biochem. Biophys. Res. Commun.* **81,** 455–461.

Jarrett, H. W., and Penniston, J. T. (1977). Partial purification of the Ca^{2+}-Mg^{2+} ATPase activator from human erythrocytes: Its similarity to the activator of 3′:5′-cyclic nucleotide phosphodiesterase. *Biochem. Biophys. Res. Commun.* **77,** 1210–1216.

Kakiuchi, S., and Yamagaki, R. (1970). Calcium-dependent phosphodiesterase activity and its activating factor (PAF) from brain. Studies on cyclic 3′,5′-nucleotide phosphodiesterase (III). *Biochem. Biophys. Res. Commun.* **41,** 1104–1110.

Kakiuchi, S., Yamagaki, R., Teshima, Y., and Miyamoto, E. (1974). Multiple cyclic nucleotide phosphodiesterase activities from rat tissues and occurrences of a calcium-plus magnesium-ion-dependent phosphodiesterase and its protein activator. *Biochem. J.* **146,** 109–120.

Katz, S., and Remtulla, M. A. (1978). Phosphodiesterase protein activator stimulates calcium transport in cardiac microsomal preparations enriched in sarcoplasmic reticulum. *Biochem. Biophys. Res. Commun.* **88,** 1373–1379.

LaPorte, D. C., Wierman, B. M., and Storm, D. R. (1980). Calcium-induced exposure of a hydrophobic surface on calmodulin. *Biochemistry* **19,** 3814–3819.

Lebowitz, E. A., and Conti, R. (1979). Phosphorylation of uterine smooth muscle myosin permits actin-activation. *J. Biochem.* **85,** 1489–1494.

LePeuch, C., Haiech, J., and Demaille, J. G. (1979). Concerted regulation of cardiac sarcoplasmic reticulum calcium transport by cyclic adenosine monosphosphate-dependent and calcium-calmodulin-dependent phosphorylations. *Biochemistry* **18,** 5150–5157.

Lin, C. T., Dedman, J. R., Brinkley, B. R., and Means, A. R. (1980). Localization of calmodulin in rat cerebellum by immunoelectron microscopy. *J. Cell Biol.* **85,** 473–480.

Luthra, M. G., Au, K. S., and Hanahan, D. J. (1977). Purification of an activator of human erythrocyte membrane (Ca^{2+} + Mg^{2+})ATPase. *Biochem. Biophys. Res. Commun.* **77,** 678–687.

Lynch, T. J., Tallant, E. A., and Cheung, W. Y. (1976). Ca^{++}-dependent formation of brain adenylate cyclase-protein activator complex. *Biochem. Biophys. Res. Commun.* **68**(2), 616–625.

Marcum, M., Dedman, J. R., Brinkley, B. R., and Means, A. R. (1978). Regulation of microtubule polymerization by rat testis calcium-dependent regulator protein. *Proc. Natl. Acad. Sci. U.S.A.* **75,** 3771–3775.

Means, A. R., and Dedman, J. R. (1980). Calmodulin—an intracellular calcium receptor. *Nature (London)* **285,** 73–77.

Mescher, M. F., Jose, M. J. L., and Balk, S. P. (1981). Actin-containing matrix associated with the plasma membrane of murine tumor and lymphoid cells. *Nature (London)* **289,** 139–144.

Morgan, M., Perry, S. V., and Ottaway, J. (1976). Myosin light chain phosphatase. *Biochem. J.* **157,** 687–697.

Nishikawa, M., Tanak, T., and Hidaka, H. (1980). Ca^{2+}-calmodulin-dependent phosphorylation and platelet secretion. *Nature (London)* **287,** 863–865.

Pato, M. D., and Adelstein, R. S. (1980). Dephosphorylation of the 20,000-dalton light chain of myosin by two different phosphatases from smooth muscle. *J. Biol. Chem.* **255**, 6535–6538.

Pershadsingh, H. A., and McDonald, J. M. (1980). A high affinity calcium-stimulated magnesium-dependent adenosine triphosphatease in rat adipocyte plasma membranes. *J. Biol. Chem.* **255**(9), 4087–4093.

Pershadsingh, H. A., McDaniel, M. L., Landt, M., Bry, C. G., Lacy, P. E., and McDonald, J. M. (1980). Ca^{2+}-activated ATPase and ATP-dependent calmodulin-stimulated Ca^{2+} transport in islet cell plasma membrane. *Nature (London)* **288**, 492–495.

Pires, E. M. V., and Perry, S. V. (1977). Purification and properties of myosin light chain kinase from fast skeletal muscle. *Biochem. J.* **167**, 137–146.

Salisbury, J. L., Condeelis, J. S., and Satir, P. (1980). Role of coated vesicles, microfilaments, and calmodulin in receptor-mediated endocytosis by cultured B lymphoblastoid cells. *J. Cell Biol.* **87**, 132–141.

Schulman, H., and Greengard, P. (1977). Stimulation of brain membrane protein phosphorylation by calcium and an endogeous heat-stable protein. *Nature (London)* **271**, 478–479.

Schulman, H., and Greengard, P. (1978). Ca^{2+}-dependent protein phosphorylation system in membranes from various tissues, and its activation by "calcium-dependent regulator." *Proc. Natl. Acad. Sci. U.S.A.* **75**, 5432–5436.

Sherry, J. M. F., Gorecko, A., Aksoy, M. O., Dabrowska, R., and Hartshorne, D. J. (1978). Roles of calcium and phosphorylation in the regulation of the activity of gizzard myosin. *Biochemistry* **17**, 4411–4418.

Silver, P. J., and DiSalvo, J. (1979). Adenosine 3':5'-monophosphate-mediated inhibition of myosin light chain phosphorylation in bovine aortic actomyosin. *J. Biol. Chem.* **254**, 9951–9954.

Smoake, J. A., and Solomon, S. S. (1980). Subcellular shifts in cyclic AMP phosphodiesterase and its calcium-dependent regulator in liver: Role of diabetes. *Biochem. Biophys. Res. Commun.* **94**, 242–430.

Soderling, T. R., Sheorain, V. S., and Ericsson, L. H. (1979). Phosphorylation of glycogen synthase by phosphorylase kinase. *FEBS Lett.* **106**, 181–184.

Srivastava, A. K., Waisman, D. M., Brostrom, C. O., and Socerling, T. R. (1979). Stimulation of glycogen synthase phosphorylation by calcium-dependent regulator protein. *J. Biol. Chem.* **254**, 583–586.

Stull, J. T. (1980). Phosphorylation of contractile proteins in relation to muscle function. *Adv. Cyclic Nucleotide Res.* **13**, 39–93.

Suzuki, K., and Kono, T. (1980). Evidence that insulin causes translocation of glucose transport activity to the plasma membrane from an intrcellular storage site. *J. Biol. Chem.* **77**, 2542–2545.

Tanaka, T., and Hidaka, H. (1980). Hydrophobic regions function in calmodulin enzyme(s) interactions. *J. Biol. Chem.* **255**, 11078–11080.

Towbin, H., Staehelin, T., and Gordon, J. (1979). Electrophoretic transfer of proteins from polyacrylamide gels to nitrocellulose sheets: Procedure and some applications. *Proc. Natl. Acad. Sci. U.S.A.* **76**, 4350–4554.

Trotter, J. A., and Adelstein, R. S. (1979). Macrophage myosin: Regulation of actin-activated ATPase activity by phosphorylation of the 20,000 dalton light chain. *J. Biol. Chem.* **254**, 8781–8785.

Valverde, I., Vandermeers, A., Anjaneyulu, R., and Malaisse, W. J. (1979). Calmodulin activation of adenylate cyclase in pancreatic islets. *Science* **206**, 225–227.

Vanaman, T. C. (1980). Structure, function and evolution of calmodulin. *Calcium Cell Funct.* **1**(3), 41–58.

Walsh, M. D., Vallet, B., Autric, F., and Demaille, J. G. (1979). Purification and characterization of bovine cardiac calmodulin-dependent myosin light chain kinase. *J. Biol. Chem.* **254**, 12136–12144.

Walsh, M. P., Cavadore, J. C., Vallet, B., and Demaille, J. G. (1980). Calmodulin-dependent myosin light chain kinase from cardiac and smooth muscle: A comparative study. *Can. J. Biochem.* **58**, 299–308.

Waissman, D. M., Stevens, F. C., and Wang, J. H. (1975). The distribution of the Ca^{++}-dependent protein activator of cyclic nucleotide phosphodiesterase in invertebrates. *Biochem. Biophys. Res. Commun.* **65**, 975–982.

Wang, J. H., and Waissman, D. M. (1979). Calmodulin and its role in the second messenger system. *Curr. Top. Cell Regul.* **15**, 47–107.

Welsh, M. J., Dedman, J. R., Brinkley, B. R., and Means, A. R. (1978). Calcium-dependent regulator protein: Localization in mitotic apparatus of eucaryotic cells. *Proc. Natl. Acad. Sci. U.S.A.* **75**, 1867–1871.

Wolf, H., and Hofmann, F. (1980). Purification of myosin light chain kinase from bovine cardiac muscle. *Proc. Natl. Acad. Sci. U.S.A.* **77**, 5852–5855.

Wong, P. Y. K., and Cheung, W. Y. (1979). Calmodulin stimulates human platelet phospholipase A_2. *Biochem. Biophys. Res. Commun.* **90**, 473–480.

Wood, J. G., Wallace, R. W., Whitaker, J. N., and Cheung, W. Y. (1980). Immunocytochemical localization of calmodulin and a heat-labile calmodulin-binding protein (CaM-BP$_{80}$) in basal ganglia of mouse brain. *J. Cell Biol.* **84**, 66–76.

Yagi, K., Yazawa, M., Kakiuchi, S., Ohshima, M., and Uenishi, K. (1978). Identification of an ativator protein for myosin light chain kinase as the Ca^{2+}-dependent modulator protein. *J. Biol. Chem.* **253**, 1338–1340.

Yamauchi, T., and Fujisawa, H. (1980). Evidence for three distinct forms of calmodulin-dependent protein kinase from rat brain. *FEBS Lett.* **116**, 141–144.

Yerna, M.-J., Dabrowska, R., Hartshorne, D. J., and Goldman, R. D. (1979). Calcium-sensitive regulation of actin-myosin interaction in baby hamster kidney (BHK-21) cells. *Proc. Natl. Acad. Sci. U.S.A.* **76**, 184–188.

14

Gonadotropin-Releasing Hormone Stimulation of Pituitary Gonadotropin Release: A Model System for Receptor-Mediated, Ca²⁺-Dependent Secretion

P. MICHAEL CONN

459

I. INTRODUCTION

Gonadotropin-releasing hormone (GnRH*) is released from the hypothalamus, circulates through a portal system, and stimulates pituitary gonadotropin [luteinizing hormone (LH) and follicle-stimulating hormone (FSH)] release to the peripheral circulation. Recent advances have enabled characterization of the pituitary GnRH receptor, and considerable information is now available and has been assembled into a working model of the postreceptor events that result in increased gonadotropin release. For simplicity, we proposed (Conn *et al.*, 1981b) a "Three-Step" model for the mechanism of GnRH action in the pituitary. In this model, which remains consistent with extant experimental observations, GnRH action is viewed as being divided into three sequential steps: (1) interaction of GnRH with a specific plasma membrane receptor; (2) mobilization of ionic calcium (Ca^{2+}); and (3) expulsion of the contents of the gonadotropin secretory granule to the extracellular space. This molecular "outline" is used in the present chapter to describe the information available about the mechanism of GnRH action. The detail of the model has been increased to reflect recently obtained information about the relationship between receptor occupancy and responses and about the apparent involvement of calmodulin in mediating the response mechanism.

II. DISTRIBUTION, CHARACTERIZATION, AND MOLECULAR BIOLOGY OF THE GNRH RECEPTOR

A. Localization and Binding Characteristics

The first step in the mechanism of GnRH action is binding of the releasing hormone to its receptor. Morphological evidence (Hopkins and Gregory, 1977) indicates that such receptors are localized on the

---

*GnRH is variously referred to as luteinizing hormone-releasing hormone (LHRH) and luteinizing hormone-releasing factor (LRF). Because its status as a hormone is unquestionable and because it functionally stimulates release of both LH and FSH, the abbreviation GnRH (gonadotropin-releasing hormone) is used in the present chapter.

(A) Authentic GnRH: pyroGlu[1]-His[2]-Trp[3]-Ser[4]-Tyr[5]-Glu[6]-Leu[7]-Arg[8]-Pro[9]-Gly[10]-NH$_2$
      (Blocked "N" terminus)   (Blocked "C" terminus)

(B) Buserelin: pyroGlu[1]-His[2]-Trp[3]-Ser[4]-Tyr[5]-D-Ser(tBU)[6]-Leu[7]-Arg[8]-Pro[9]-ethyla-mide

(C) D-Lys[6]-GnRH: pyroGlu[1]-His[2]-Trp[3]-Ser[4]-Tyr[5]-D-Lys[6]-Leu[7]-Arg[8]-Pro[9]-Gly[10]-NH$_2$

(D) Lys[6]   *(Fujino)-GnRH* pyroGlu[1]-His[2]-Trp[3]-Ser[4]-Tyr[5]-D-Lys[6]-Leu[7]-Arg[8]-Pro[9]-ethylamide

Fig. 1. Chemical structure of GnRH and some useful GnRH analogs. GnRH is blocked at both termini. It contains a Tyr[5] that may be labeled by chloramine-T radioiodination as described in the text. Buserelin (B) is blocked with a D-amino acid at its principal degradation site and, accordingly, is more metabolically stable than GnRH itself. The presence of a Pro[9] increases the binding affinity to the receptor. Compounds C and D contain a D-Lys[6], which may be chemically modified without loss of efficacy.

plasma membrane, and, consistent with this view, GnRH-binding activity is found in plasma membrane fractions prepared from rat (Spona, 1974a, 1974b; Marshall *et al.*, 1975; Marian *et al.*, 1981) and sheep (Berault *et al.*, 1974) pituitaries. Some evidence is available suggesting that GnRH is also found bound to sites on granules within the cytoplasm (Sternberger and Petrali, 1975) or associated in some other way with the granules (Bauer *et al.*, 1981). Although the significance of this observation is unclear, a possible explanation is presented in Section II,E.

A reliable radioligand assay for the GnRH receptor took many years to develop. It was obvious that a good probe should have high specific activity with a high percentage of specific binding to the GnRH receptor. It was possible to label authentic GnRH (Fig. 1) either by tritiation or by iodination (a Tyr[5] is present). Both labeled compounds were highly susceptible to proteolytic degradation by enzymes in the pituitary (Kochman *et al.*, 1975), blood (Benuck and Marks, 1976), and hypothalamus (Griffiths and Kelly, 1979). Thus, the concentration of intact GnRH present in binding assays might be expected to change with time and complicate the reaction kinetics. The tritiated derivatives had lower specific activities (16–25 Ci/mmol, Perrin *et al.*, 1980) than the iodinated ones (1000 Ci/mmol, Clayton *et al.*, 1979; Marian and Conn, 1980), although tritiation had the advantage of not introducing any atoms not present in the native molecule. Problems in development of assays were further complicated because GnRH dissociated rapidly (minutes) from its receptor.

A major step in the development of the radioligand assay came from the observation that insertion of D-amino acids at the principal degradation site in the GnRH molecule provided a relatively stable radioligand (Clayton *et al.*, 1979). In native GnRH, the bonds adjacent to the sixth amino acid appear to be preferentially cleaved by endopeptidases.

(Koch et al., 1974). A carboxyamide peptidase has also been characterized; it cleaves the Pro^9-Gly^{10}-NH_2 bond (Marks, 1970). Thus, substitution of six-position D-amino acids (often D-Leu^6, D-Trp^6, D-Ala^6, D-(t-butyl)Ser^6, or D-Lys^6) offers considerable protection against degradation during the assay. Removal of the C terminus (which is actually blocked by Gly-amide in native GnRH) and termination by Pro^9-ethylamide (the so-called "Fujino modification") (Fujino et al., 1974) has been found to result in a superagonist. Because agonists that contain the D-amino $acid^6$ with or without the Fujino modification can be conveniently radioiodinated (Clayton et al., 1979; Marian and Conn, 1980; Marian et al., 1981; Conn and Hazum, 1981; Conn et al., 1981d), these have served as useful probes of the GnRH receptor.

For reasons of superagonist activity and enhanced metabolic stability, we have chosen Buserelin [a trade name of Hoescht Pharmaceuticals for D-$Ser(t$-butyl$)^6$-des^{10}-Pro^9-ethylamide-GnRH; see Fig. 1] for the preparation of the radioligand used in studies of the GnRH receptor. Radioiodination of this GnRH analog was done (Marian and Conn, 1980) in a reaction mixture that contained 5 µg analog in 10 µl 0.1 M phosphate buffer, pH 7.5, 1 mCi ^{125}I, and 250 ng chloramine-T in 0.1 M phosphate. The reaction mixture was stopped by dilution in 2 mM ammonium acetate, pH 4.5, after 2 minutes at room temperature and the mixture was applied to a 3.0-ml carboxymethyl-cellulose column (0.7 meq/gm, fine mesh) previously equilibrated in 2 mM ammonium acetate, pH 4.5. The column was washed first with the equilibration buffer to remove unbound iodide, then with 60 mM ammonium acetate, pH 4.5, to elute the labeled analog. Typical specific activity was 850–1250 µCi/µg (assessed by self-displacement), and maximum binding ranged from 30 to 50% in different batches. This procedure has been useful for labeling a large number of GnRH analogs. Readers who attempt to use this method should note that elevation of the concentration of the elution buffer to 200 mM acetate is used to elute other GnRH analogs containing D-Lys^6 substitutions (Conn et al., 1981d; Conn and Hazum, 1981). We have also found that equimolar HEPES or phosphate (buffers) may be substituted without loss of yield when acetate cannot be tolerated for a particular experiment.

The competitive binding characteristics of the radioligand assay are shown in Figs. 2 and 3. Binding occurs with high affinity (Fig. 2) and high specificity (Fig. 3) to pituitary and ovarian membranes. No specific binding was found in heart, lung, spleen, adrenal, kidney, or cerebral cortex. Section V contains a discussion of extrapituitary actions of GnRH. The ovarian receptor has been characterized by Jones et al. (1980).

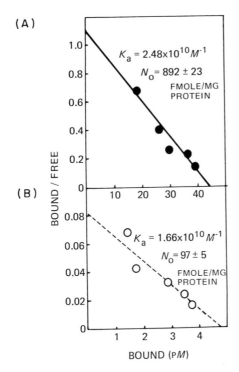

Fig. 2. Scatchard analyses of ^{125}I-labeled Buserelin binding to ovarian and pituitary membrane fractions from young precycling female rats. The affinity constant (K_a) and number of binding sites per milligram protein (N_0) were established by linear regression analysis. Although the target of hypothalamic GnRH is clearly the pituitary, a limited number of other binding sites for cross-reactive molecules have been described and are summarized in Section V. Figure from Marian *et al.* (1981), reproduced by permission of the American Society for Pharmacology and Experimental Therapeutics. (A) Pituitary membranes; (B) ovarian membranes.

These labeled superactive analogs have been used by us (Marian *et al.*, 1981) and others (Savoy-Moore *et al.*, 1980; Clayton and Catt, 1980) to characterize GnRH levels in the pituitary during the rat estrous cycle. The results of these studies from three different laboratories are nearly identical; they indicate a low concentration of GnRH receptors on the morning of estrus and a gradual increase to a plateau on the afternoon of diestrus II through proestrus (time of the LH surge). There is no marked change in receptor affinity for the radioligand (in our own study the range was $K_a = 1.6$–$2.7 \times 10^{10} \, M^{-1}$). These observations suggest that GnRH receptors may be important in regulation of LH release.

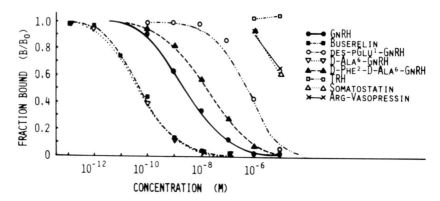

Fig. 3. Hormone and GnRH analog specificity of the radioligand–receptor assay. Increasing concentrations of the competing peptides were added to 25μg rat membrane protein and ^{125}I-labeled Buserelin (40,000 cpm). Following a 2-hour equilibration on ice, samples were centrifuged, and radioactivity in pellets was determined. B is the amount of radioactivity in the indicated pellet and B_0 is the amount of radioactivity in the absence of added competing peptide. Figure from Marian *et al.* (1981), reproduced by permission of the American Society for Pharmacology and Experimental Therapeutics.

B.   Changes Following Ovariectomy and Steroid Replacement

In addition, we assessed the contribution of estrogen *in vivo* to the regulation of the GnRH receptor in ovariectomized rats (Marian *et al.,* 1981). Rats 24 days old, which had been ovariectomized at 14 days of age, had twice the number of pituitary GnRH receptors as sham-operated rats of the same age. Receptor affinity did not vary significantly $(K_a = 1.1–1.9 \times 10^{10} \, M^{-1})$. Within 3 hours of administration of 10 μg estradiol benzoate (in oil, sc), receptor number returned sham levels, and LH serum concentration dropped 86% from nontreated ovariectomized rats. Twelve hours after the initial estradiol injection, both receptor number and LH serum concentration were again above sham levels, although not as high as nontreated ovariectomized rats. Marshall's group (Frager *et al.,* 1981) has provided convincing evidence that administration of antiserum to GnRH concomitant with castration inhibits the rise in both GnRH receptor number and LH release that follow castration. They have shown that changes in pituitary GnRH receptors parallel previously demonstrated changes in hypothalamic secretion of GnRH. The authors have suggested that GnRH probably regulates its own receptor *in vivo* and gonadal steroids may influence pituitary GnRH receptors by changing hypothalamic GnRH secretion.

C. Ontogeny of the GnRH Receptor

A comprehensive study of pituitary and gonadal GnRH receptors in the rat has been presented by Marshall's group (Dalkin *et al.*, 1981). They used the nondegradable agonist D-Ala^6-des-Gly^{10}-ethylamide-GnRH and found that receptor-binding affinities did not change throughout maturation and were similar in the pituitary, testes, and ovaries. Pituitary GnRH receptor concentration (fmol/mg protein) increased 2-fold in both sexes. In females, the peak values (720 ± 52 fmole/mg protein) occurred at 20 days of age, and in males the peak value (594 ± 54) occurred at 30 days. The changes in receptor correlated well with plasma follicle-stimulating hormone (FSH). Age-dependent changes in gonadal receptors were also noted and were maximal (271 ± 25) on day 20 in females and in males (256 ± 13) on day 40, despite the undetectable levels at day 30. These studies further substantiate the key role of the receptor in regulating tissue responsiveness and suggest that substances that cross-react with the GnRH receptor may be important in regulating steroidogenesis at puberty. The gonadal GnRH receptor is one of the extrapituitary GnRH receptors, which are discussed more fully in Section V,B.

D. Changes during Normal Aging

Because of the marked reproductive changes associated with aging (for review, Smith and Conn, 1982), we also examined receptor number and binding affinity in pituitaries from pseudopregnant (PP) and constant-estrus (CE) rats (20–24 months) in comparison to 30-day-old pups (Marian *et al.*, 1981). Because these old animals differ from weanlings both in age and in endocrine status, 6- and 12-month spontaneously CE rats (controls for endocrine status) were also examined. For all ages of CE rats, receptor binding was dramatically decreased compared to weanling females. A similar decrease was observed for old PP rats. Receptor affinity was not different between the groups, whereas receptor concentration in the CE and old animals was 18–24% of that in the young. It was observed that the number of GnRH receptors in lactating rats (when LH levels are low) were also diminished compared with nonlactating animals. Accordingly, it appeared that alterations in GnRH receptor, but not binding affinity, occur during different endocrine states. Because functional receptor levels can effectively alter target cell sensitivity and because relatively elevated receptor levels appear necessary for elevated serum LH, the possibility remains that gonadotrope sensitivity is regulated in part by altered receptor levels.

E.   Occupancy of the GnRH Receptor Leading to Patching, Capping, and Internalization

We have found chemical properties in a number of GnRH agonists that make them particularly useful for determining some of the biological characteristics of the GnRH receptor. Because of the free epsilon amino group in D-Lys^6-GnRH, it was possible to prepare a rhodamine derivative of this compound (Hazum *et al.*, 1980). The presence of the D-amino acid has the advantage of adding stability against proteolytic degradation. The rhodamine-D-Lys^6-GnRH derivative retained high affinity (3 n*M*) binding to the GnRH receptor. This derivative, then, was suitable for visualization and localization of GnRH receptors in cultured cells, using the technique of image intensification. Photographs of this can be found in Chapter 1 in this volume. The fluorescently labeled receptors were initially distributed on the cell surface and formed patches that subsequently internalized (at 37°C) into endocytic vesicles. These processes were dependent on specific binding sites for the peptide and conceivably could be the vesicular, intracellular binding sites of GnRH reported previously (Sternberger and Petrali, 1975). An independent report (Noar *et al.*, 1981) subsequently confirmed the sequence of events described earlier using the identical technique. Duello and Nett (1980) have used autoradiography to show internalization of GnRH and its analogs. They indicated that uptake and length of retention correlate well with biological potency. Although the intracellular target for the GnRH–receptor complex is still unknown, movement to the lysosomal compartment, followed by degradation, is consistent with observations made in other systems.

F.   GnRH Internalization Is Not a Requirement for Stimulation of Gonadotropin Release

Our interest in internalization of the GnRH–receptor complex was based on the idea that this phenomenon might be involved in the mechanism by which GnRH stimulates gonadotropin release. In order to determine whether patching, capping, and internalization were involved, we examined gonadotropin release under circumstances in

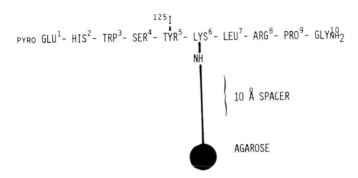

Fig. 4. Drawing of the agarose derivative of D-Lys^6-GnRH. Although only a single molecule per agarose bead is shown for clarity, many are present. The agarose bead is sufficiently large so that the derivative cannot enter cells.

which internalization was blocked (either by GnRH analog immobilization or by incubation in the presence of vinblastine) or when the cells were stimulated under conditions in which only internalized GnRH was available. In one approach (Conn *et al.*, 1981d), the GnRH analog D-Lys^6-GnRH (Fig. 1) was coupled by its epsilon amino group with an *N*-hydroxysuccinimide ester; then, through a 10 Å spacer arm, to a cross-linked agarose matrix (Fig. 4). Exposure of the product to proteases, soaps, detergents, solvents, chaotropic agents, or cell cultures resulted in dissociation of at most < 0.28% biologically active releasing hormone. Although the apparent potency of the immobilized analog was one-fourth that of the free form, it was still capable of evoking a full LH secretory response. In other covalent immobilization studies, the more potent agonist D-Lys^6-des^{10}-Pro^9-ethylamide-GnRH (Fig. 1) was prepared with a high ratio of agonist to bead. This resulted in a derivative that stimulated LH release with full efficacy. Because of the increased potency of this compound and the increased molar coupling ratio, the quantity of LH release was restricted by the number of beads added at concentrations of releasing hormone sufficient to evoke release (Fig. 5). This finding was interpreted as added evidence that the immobilization of the agonist was stable during the bioassay and indicated that LH release could be stimulated with full efficacy without the requirement for GnRH internalization.

In order to confirm these findings by an independent means, a comparative study (Conn and Hazum, 1981) was undertaken using image-intensified microscopy and the cell culture bioassay. The detailed use of this technique in several systems is described in Chapter 1 in this volume. With this technique, it was possible to show that 100 μ*M*

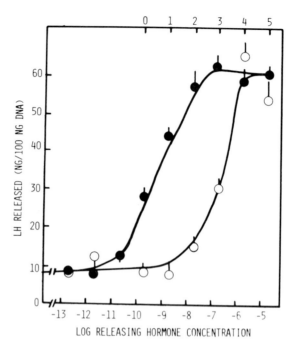

Fig. 5. Stimulation of LH release from pituitary cell cultures by D-Lys[6]-des-Gly[10]-Pro[9]-ethylamide-GnRH. Cell cultures were incubated for 3 hours with the GnRH agonist in free solution (solid symbol) or immobilized on agarose (open symbol). LH release is normalized for the number of cells present by DNA determination. The upper horizontal axis gives an upper estimate of the number of hormone-containing agarose beads present in each assay. From Conn and Hazum (1981), reprinted by permission of The Endocrine Society.

vinblastine markedly inhibited large-scale patching and capping of the GnRH receptor (viewed by image intensification) but did not alter the EC_{50} or efficacy of LH release stimulated by GnRH or by the agonist described earlier. Another approach demonstrated that exposure of cells to GnRH evoked LH release, which underwent prompt extinction following removal of GnRH from the incubation medium (Fig. 6). Accordingly, a continuous supply of externally applied GnRH appeared to be required for stimulation of LH release. These observations indicated that internalization as well as large-scale patching and capping of the GnRH receptor are not required for LH release. They did not exclude the possibility that microaggregation (small numbers of receptors; too small to be seen by image intensification) are involved in the mechanism of action of GnRH.

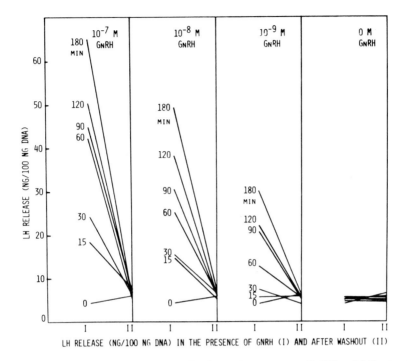

Fig. 6. LH release from pituitary cell cultures in response to GnRH and following its washout. Cultures were incubated with 10^{-7}, 10^{-8}, or 10^{-9} M or with no GnRH for the indicated period of time (0, 15, 30, 60, 90, 120, or 180 minutes, incubation I). After this period, the cells were washed in GnRH-free medium, then returned to medium for 3 hours (incubation II). LH (ng/100 ng DNA) was determined in the extracellular fluid from incubations I and II by radioimmunoassay SEM's ($\leq 10\%$ of the indicated means) were not added to the figures for the sake of clarity. Reprinted from Conn and Hazum (1981), by permission of The Endocrine Society.

G. Possible Microaggregation of the GnRH Receptor

Although large-scale patching, capping, and internalization of the GnRH receptor do not appear to be needed for the release process, microaggregation (possibly dimerization) of the receptor has not yet been rigorously ruled out. This would be too small a signal to observe by image intensification, which has a sensitivity of approximately 40–50 molecules of hormone.

Several lines of evidence indicate that microaggregation of plasma membrane receptors is sufficient for activation of some plasma membrane-regulated systems. This event occurs prior to large-scale patching and capping and is a distinct process. In the case of epidermal growth factor (EGF) stimulation of mitogenesis in 3T3 cells (fibro-blasts, Schecter *et al.*, 1979), it has been shown that cyanogen bromide treatment of EGF results in a molecule (CN-EGF) that binds to the EGF receptor but does not elicit mitogenesis. Addition of divalent anti-EGF antibody to cultures previously exposed to CN-EGF results in activation of mitogenesis. Because stimulation is not observed when a monovalent form (papain digest) of the antibody is used, these authors concluded, with additional support from video-intensified microscopy, that CN-EGF occupied the receptor but did not allow microaggrega-tion. They inferred that addition of the divalent antibody promoted microaggregation of the receptor–CN-EGF complex and led to activa-tion of mitogenesis. Other laboratories have suggested (Davies *et al.*, 1980) that microaggregation may result from receptor cross-linking by transglutaminases, and both this event and the response are inhibited by dansylcadaverine and low-molecular-weight amines (methyl-, eth-yl-, propyl-, and butyl-).

For insulin receptors, the importance of microaggregation has been suggested by the observation that anti-insulin receptor antibodies stimulate insulin-like functions in target tissues (Jacobs *et al.*, 1978). Divalent antibodies are required for such stimulation (Kahn *et al.*, 1978).

Additional studies will be required before this process can be impli-cated in or excluded from the mechanism of action of GnRH.

III. CALCIUM AS A SECOND MESSENGER FOR GNRH

Early studies with hemipituitaries and pituitary slices (Samli and Geschwind, 1968) suggested that the ionic makeup of the incubation medium, especially with regard to Ca^{2+}, influenced the release of pituitary hormones. Although these studies were not conclusive be-cause they relied upon crude hypothalamic extracts (synthetic releas-ing hormones were not yet available), they indicated the importance of calcium (Vale *et al.*, 1967; Geschwind, 1969; McCann, 1971). It was shown (Samli and Geschwind, 1968) that although Ca^{2+} was required for optimal release of LH, changes in extracellular Ca^{2+} levels did not alter the pattern of incorporation of [^{14}C]leucine into pituitary LH. In addition, metabolic inhibitors (dinitrophenol and oligomycin), at con-centrations sufficient to inhibit 75% of the leucine incorporation into LH, did not alter gonadotropin release. These observations suggested that LH biosynthesis and LH release are distinct processes and that Ca^{2+} was involved in pituitary LH release but not in its biosynthesis.

Wakabayashi *et al.* (1969) showed that optimal stimulation of pituitary LH release in response to hypothalamic extract required extracellular Ca^{2+} and that ethylenediaminetetraacetic acid (EDTA) inhibited release. Although these studies demonstrated that Ca^{2+} was needed for the release process, its status as a second messenger was not established. We proposed (Marian and Conn, 1979) criteria that would have to be fulfilled to establish Ca^{2+} as a second messenger of GnRH action. First, removal of Ca^{2+} from its site of action must block LH release in response to GnRH. Second, as a direct consequence of stimulation with GnRH, it should be possible to demonstrate the movement of Ca^{2+} (either from internal stores or from the extracellular spaces) into a site that can be linked directly to LH release. Third, any manipulation that results in movement of Ca^{2+} to this site should evoke LH release that is independent of stimulation by GnRH.

A. The Locus of Calcium Action Subsequent to GnRH Recognition

The first criterion that was fulfilled in order to implicate Ca^{2+} in the mechanism of GnRH action was the demonstration that GnRH did not stimulate gonadotropin release in the absence of extracellular Ca^{2+} or in the presence of drugs that blocked Ca^{2+} entry from the extracellular medium (Marian and Conn, 1979; Conn *et al.*, 1980b; Stern and Conn, 1981). This requirement has been fulfilled in rat (Marian and Conn, 1979; Stern and Conn, 1981), pig (Hopkins and Walker, 1978), and sheep (Adams and Nett, 1979). In the rat cell culture system, we have demonstrated that return of Ca^{2+} to the medium of cells preincubated without Ca^{2+} serves to restore responsiveness to GnRH (Conn and Rogers, 1979). Because the Ca^{2+} requirement for responsiveness could reflect a permissive action for the binding of GnRH to its plasma membrane receptor, we examined (Marian and Conn, 1980) the ionic requirements for binding. In these studies, we employed the superactive, degradation-resistant GnRH analog Buserelin (Hoechst Pharmaceutical Company). This molecule (fully described in Section II,A) can be derivatized with ^{125}I to high specific activity (approximately 250,000 cpm/ng) with retention of approximately 30–50% binding (Marian *et al.*, 1981). Ca^{2+} did not exert a permissive effect for binding of the analog to this site; in fact, at high concentrations (> 10 mM), it actually inhibited specific binding due to an effect on affinity, which dropped from $4 \times 10^9\ M^{-1}$ at $< 10^{-6}\ M\ Ca^{2+}$ to $9 \times 10^8\ M^{-1}$ at 10 m$M\ Ca^{2+}$. Accordingly, the Ca^{2+} requirement for GnRH-stimulated release cannot be explained simply by a permissive effect at the receptor, as clearly demonstrated by the inverse correlation between the Ca^{2+} requirement for GnRH-stimulated LH release and the effect at the receptor. The inhibitory effects observed with Ca^{2+} are not specific for this ion because inhibition of receptor binding is also seen with Ba^{2+}, Mn^{2+}, Co^{2+}, Mg^{2+}, Na^+, and La^{3+}. Although all of the ions listed decrease specific binding to the GnRH receptor, their effects upon GnRH-stimulated LH release are markedly different. At the concentration used, Ba^{2+} acts as a secretogogue, Mg^{2+} has no effect, and La^{3+}, Mn^{2+}, and Co^{2+} are inhibitory. Thus, these studies suggest that the specific action of Ca^{2+} occurs at a locus after the initial recognition of GnRH by its receptor.

B. Evidence for Calcium Flux as the First Measurable Event after GnRH Binding

The second criterion for Ca^{2+} as an intracellular mediator for GnRH action required demonstration of movement of Ca^{2+} into an active site prior to release of LH. Technical problems make direct demonstration of $^{45}Ca^{2+}$ uptake difficult (Putney, 1979), although it has been possible to do so in some cases (Hopkins and Walker, 1978) by relying on special manipulations. By preloading cells with $^{45}Ca^{2+}$ and using the efflux of this isotope to measure channel activity, Williams (1976) first used a perifusion system of hemipituitaries to demonstrate that opening of a Ca^{2+} channel could be seen at an early time following administration of GnRH. Ovariectomy appears to enhance the magnitude of the Ca^{2+} flux relative to the background. The samples were not collected at small enough intervals, however, to determine the precise temporal relation between LH release and Ca^{2+} flux. Although there was a dose–response relation between GnRH and Ca^{2+} flux, the flux was not shown to be a specific action of GnRH. We have confirmed (Conn *et al.*, 1981b) Williams' observations and extended them by demonstrating that Ca^{2+} mobilization actually *precedes* LH release and is a specific function of GnRH. Release of $^{45}Ca^{2+}$ from preloaded cells was measured at short intervals following addition of either GnRH or an inactive analog [des^1-GnRH(2–10)] to the pituitary slices (Conn *et al.*, 1981b). LH was determined in aliquots taken at the same times. Our results extend Williams' findings and suggest that (1) GnRH specifically stimulates efflux of $^{45}Ca^{2+}$ from preloaded gonadotropes; (2) flux occurs rapidly (< 1.5 minutes) after GnRH administration, preceding measurable LH release; and (3) $^{45}Ca^{2+}$ flux and LH release cannot be uncoupled.

C. LH Release Evoked by Increases in Intracellular Calcium

The third requirement that implicated Ca^{2+} as a mediator of GnRH action was the observation that compounds that themselves stimulated increased Ca^{2+} levels in the cytosol also stimulated LH release. We showed that this occurs even in the absence of GnRH. Thus, the connection may be made between Ca^{2+} mobilization itself and LH release, even in the absence of GnRH receptor occupancy. Three approaches to assessing Ca^{2+} mobilization have been useful. Cytosolic Ca^{2+} can be increased by (1) addition of bacterial ionophores, (2) insertion by liposome fusion, or (3) activation of endogenous ion channels by membrane depolarizing agents.

We have used the three calcium ionophores that are currently available; all are bacterial products that bind Ca^{2+} and, because of their hydrophobic nature, insert themselves into the plasma membrane to provide a specific conduit for Ca^{2+}. When ionophore A23187 (Lilly) was added to the pituitary cultures in the presence of 1 mM Ca^{2+}, the cells responded with release of LH (Conn et al., 1979b). This response was dose and time dependent and required extracellular Ca^{2+}. Ionomycin (Squibb; Conn et al., 1980a) and X537A (Roche; Conn et al., 1979b) also stimulated LH release, but in contrast to A23187 and ionomycin, X537A did not require extracellular Ca^{2+}. A series of experiments suggested that X537A may have released Ca^{2+} from intracellular pools (such as those in the mitochondria; Conn et al., 1979b).

Liposomes (lipid vesicles) have the increasing characteristic of inserting their contents into living cells and, accordingly, have been used for insertion of drugs, messenger RNA, and ions. We showed that Ca^{2+}-bearing liposomes, but neither Mg^{2+}-bearing nor monovalent ion-containing liposomes, successfully evoked LH release from pituitary cells (Conn et al., 1979b). Thus, it appeared that in addition to a Ca^{2+} requirement for GnRH-stimulated LH release, insertion of Ca^{2+}, even in the absence of GnRH, was sufficient to stimulate LH release.

In order to explore possible routes of ion entry into the gonadotrope, we used drugs that exert direct effects on ion channels and determined their effects on the release of LH. Veratridine, which activates the Na^+ channel of electrically excitable cells and upon depolarization allows extracellular Ca^{2+} to enter, stimulated LH release from the cultures (Conn and Rogers, 1980). The response was measurable 15 minutes after the addition of veratridine and was maximal at 180 minutes, displaying an efficacy similar to that for GnRH. The time course for veratridine-stimulated LH release was similar to that seen in response to GnRH or ionophoretic Ca^{2+} mobilization and was consistent with the view that the rate-limiting step in stimulated LH release from these cells occurs after Ca^{2+} mobilization. Veratridine-stimulated LH release was blocked by tetrodotoxin (TTX, 10^{-5} M), by chelation of Ca^{2+} with EGTA, by low Na^+-containing medium, or by D600. Both GnRH- and veratridine-stimulated LH release required extracellular Ca^{2+}; however, GnRH was not blocked by TTX or low Na^+.

In addition to veratridine, aconitine and batrachotoxin produced TTX-sensitive LH release that required Ca^{2+} and Na^+. This suggests that the site of action for all these agents is similar to that reported in nervous tissue. Veratridine appears to stimulate LH release via Ca^{2+} mobilization resulting from activation of the Na^+ channel, whereas GnRH-stimulated Ca^{2+} mobilization is not mediated via the Na^+ channel. Indeed, the ability of D600 (which blocks the Ca^{2+} channels) to block GnRH action suggests that the GnRH receptor may be functionally coupled to a distinct Ca^{2+} channel. In addition to providing a method for Ca^{2+} mobilization by stimulation of endogenous ion channels, these results suggest considerable functional homology between the pituitary gonadotrope and neural tissue, which also contain these channels.

D.   Excitability of Pituitary Cells

The requirements for release of trophic hormones from the pituitary resemble those for release of catecholamines from the adrenal chromaffin cell. Because release from chromaffin cells is associated with electrical excitability, several laboratories have sought to measure electrical activity in (nongonadotrope) pituitary-derived tumor cells and to determine whether hypothalamic factors or steroids (which mediate pituitary responsiveness in several cell types) could alter the pattern of this activity. These studies were conducted by impalement with microelectrodes. In several instances, there appears to be a Ca^{2+}-dependent component of excitability.

Biales et al. (1977) examined action potentials in GH3 cells (rat neoplastic pituitary cells) and in cells derived from an acidoma (presumably secreting growth hormone). They concluded that these potentials resulted from combined Na^+- and Ca^{2+}-dependent mechanisms, because tetrodotoxin (which blocks Na^+ channels) could be used to inhibit Na^+ spikes whereas Mn^{2+} (5 mM) and Co^{2+} (7.5 mM) blocked the Ca^{2+}-dependent spike. Ozawa and Miyazaki (1979) also have explored the electrical excitability of the GH3 cell. They measured a mean resting potential of -48.0 ± 1.1 mV in saline and determined Na^+- and Ca^{2+}-dependent components of the action potential. The importance of Ca^{2+} in maintaining a resting potential was shown by substitution of Ba^{2+} for Ca^{2+}, which shifted the membrane potential to -6.1 ± 1.1 mV.

Lactotropes (prolactin-secreting cells) also show action potentials that indicate Ca^{2+} influx (Kidokoro, 1975; Taraskevich and Douglas, 1977). Taraskevich and Douglas (1978) examined the influence of TRH (thyrotropin-stimulating hormone-releasing hormone, which also evokes prolactin release) and catecholamines (which inhibit prolactin release) on the evoked action potential, taking advantage of the alewife fish (*Alosa pseudoharengus*), which has a clearly defined region of prolactin-secreting cells. Although TTX reversibly depressed the amplitude of the action potentials (which indicated that they resulted from altered Na^+ conductance), a Ca^{2+}-dependent component was also present. When tetraethylammonium chloride (TEA) was added to the solution already containing TTX, large regenerative potentials occurred and could be inhibited reversibly by replacement of medium Ca^{2+} with Mn^{2+}, thus indicating the importance of both Na^+ and Ca^{2+} in this process. Addition of catecholamines (dopamine, norepinephrine) inhibited firing, and arrest occurred at concentrations of $10^{-6} M$, within seconds of the addition to the medium. In other studies (Dufy *et al.*, 1979), using GH3/B6 cells (a prolactin-secreting line), it could be shown that 17β-estradiol and TRH induced Ca^{2+}-dependent action potentials in less than 1 minute. This was preceded by a progressive increase of the input resistance without any change in the resting membrane potential. Thus, it appears that pituitary cells have Ca^{2+}-dependent action potentials that can be influenced by physiological stimuli. This finding correlates well with the biochemical observation (Tashjian *et al.*, 1978) that Ca^{2+} is an essential cation in mediating the actions of K^+ (as a depolarant) and TRH on the release of prolactin by GH4C1 cells.

It is clear that some aspects of the mechanism of GnRH action in the pituitary bear resemblance to neural tissue characteristics. Indeed, as indicated in Section V,a, there has been localization of GnRH in neural tissues. A related finding is that antigen for monoclonol antibody F12 A2B5 is found on the pituitary gonadotrope (Eisenbarth *et al.*, 1981). This antibody was generated by immunizing mice with chick retinal cells. It was shown to be highly specific for nerve cells and binds to a tetrasialic acid residue. Its presence on pituitary gonadotrope cells is indicative of chemical similarities between the pituitary and neural.

Furthermore, a nerve-specific isozyme of enolase (Schmeckel *et al.,* 1978) is found in the pituitary.

A detailed discussion of the significance of cellular excitability in secretion can be found in Chapter 4 in this volume.

E. Calmodulin as the Possible Site of Calcium Action in the Pituitary

One likely intracellular target for Ca^{2+} action is calmodulin, which is a ubiquitous intracellular Ca^{2+} receptor that has been shown to modulate many cellular processes including cyclic nucleotide and glycogen metabolism, protein phosphorylation, microtubule assembly and disassembly, and Ca^{2+} flux, as well as the activities of NAD kinase, tryptophan $5'$-monooxidase, and phospholipase A_2 (for reviews, see Chapter 13 in this volume). In order to explore this possibility, a specific and sensitive radioimmunoassay for calmodulin was used to determine its quantity and distribution in the gonadotrope before and during GnRH-stimulated LH release (Conn *et al.,* 1981a).

GnRH (10^{-2} to 2 µg/rat, as indicated, obtained from the National Pituitary Agency) was administered by subcutaneous injection to ovariectomized rats (Zivic-Miller, 5–7 weeks old, ovariectomized at 24 days). After 35 minutes (or as indicated in the time course study), the rats were killed by decapitation. Trunk blood was collected and serum LH determined by radioimmunoassay. The pituitary was removed, homogenized, and filtered through organza cloth. Nuclear, plasma membrane, mitochondrial/granular, microsomal, and cytosolic fractions were identified by marker enzymes (aldolase, glucose-6-phosphatase, malic dehydrogenase, NADH cytochrome *c* reductase, and $5'$-nucleotidase) and chemical analysis for DNA, protein, and LH using standard methods. These analyses indicated less than 10% cross-contamination between fractions. Aliquots of these fractions were stored at $-70°C$, then heat treated, and assayed for calmodulin by radioimmunoassay.

The distribution of calmodulin in the fractions was expressed as a percentage of the total immunoassayable activity in the homogenate. There was an initial rise (Fig. 7) in the percentage of calmodulin that is associated with the plasma membrane and that appears concomitantly with the depletion of the cytosolic calmodulin. The increase occurs with a similar time course to secretion of LH into the blood. As the calmodulin begins to be cleared from the plasma membrane fraction, its level increases first in the mitochondrial/granular and microsomal fractions and finally in the cytosol. There is also a dose–response relation be-

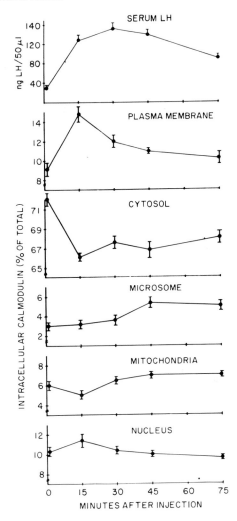

Fig. 7. Time course of LH release and subcellular calmodulin redistribution follow-ing a 2-μg injection of GnRH. Rats were killed at the indicated time. Subcellular frac-tions were prepared and assayed (radioimmunoassay) for calmodulin. Trunk blood was assayed for LH (radioimmunoassay). Reprinted from Conn *et al.* (1981a), with permis-sion of *Nature (London)*.

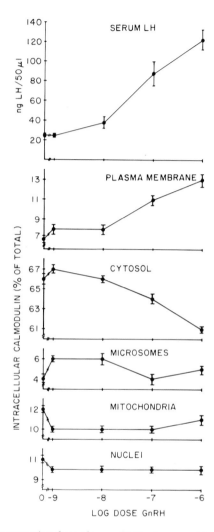

Fig. 8. GnRH concentration dependence of LH release and intracellular redistribution of calmodulin. GnRH (0.1 to 2 μg/rat, as indicated) was administered by subcutaneous injection. After 35 minutes, the rats were killed by decapitation. Trunk blood was collected and serum LH determined by radioimmunoassay. Subcellular fractions were prepared and assayed for calmodulin. The calmodulin concentration in the homogenate was 0.56 ± 0.04 ng/μg protein. The values shown are means ± SEM. Reprinted from Conn *et al.* (1981a), with permission of *Nature (London)*.

tween plasma membrane accumulation of calmodulin and its cytosolic depletion (Fig. 8). A chemically similar analog [des¹-GnRH(2–10)], which has no efficacy in stimulating LH release and which does not bind to the GnRH receptor (Marian et al., 1981), also did not stimulate calmodulin redistribution.

Because calmodulin synthesis is constitutive in all systems examined (including the GnRH-stimulated pituitary, Chafouleas et al., 1980), the possibility remains that the redistribution reported in the present work is caused by translocation between cellular compartments. The apparent initial accumulation at the plasma membrane may allow calmodulin to exert regulatory functions at that locus.

Although translocation of calmodulin has not been reported previously, there are observations in other systems that indicate that such an event occurs. In the red blood cell, islet cell, and adipocyte (Larsen and Vincenzi, 1979; Pershadsingh and McDonald, 1980), calmodulin-activated ATPases are located at the plasma membrane. In the case of the adipocyte, Ca^{2+}-ATPases appear to be hormonally regulated and activated in response to insulin. Although calmodulin redistribution may be either a cause or a consequence of the secretory process, a role for calmodulin seems to be emerging. Calmodulin has been found at the postsynaptic membrane and appears to mediate the Ca^{2+} effects on synaptic transmission (Grab et al., 1979; Iludian and Naftalin, 1979) and may, accordingly, have a role in the release of neurotransmitters.

F. Inhibition by Calmodulin Antagonists of GnRH-Stimulated LH Release at a Postreceptor and Post-Calcium Mobilization Locus

Additional support for the involvement of calmodulin in the mechanism of action of GnRH comes from the observation that pimozide is a noncompetitive antagonist of GnRH-stimulated LH release from pituitary cell cultures (Debeljuk et al., 1978; Conn et al., 1981e). For this and several other neurotropic agents (penfluridol, chlordiazepoxide, chlorpromazine), the concentration needed to inhibit 50% of LH release in response to GnRH correlated well with the ability to inhibit enzyme activation by calmodulin in vitro (Fig. 9; Conn et al., 1981c). Pimozide does not alter the K_a or N_0 of releasing hormone binding by the GnRH receptor. The additional observation that pimozide inhibits Ca^{2+} ionophore (A23187 and ionomycin)-stimulated LH release, suggests that the locus of pimozide action is after Ca^{2+} mobilization. Because pimozide is known to bind and inactivate the Ca^{2+}–calmod-

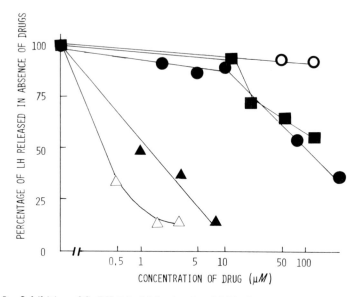

Fig. 9. Inhibition of GnRH (10^{-8} M) stimulated LH release from pituitary cultures by penfluridol (open triangle), pimozide (closed triangle), chlordiazepoxide (closed circle), chlorpromazine (closed square), and chlorpromazine sulfoxide (open circle). Pituitary cell cultures were incubated at 37°C in the presence of the indicated concentration of drug and 10^{-8} M GnRH. LH release was determined by radioimmunoassay. The standard error of the mean is less than 10% for all points. Reprinted from Conn *et al.* (1981c), with the permission of The Endocrine Society.

ulin complex and because Ca^{2+} is a second messenger for GnRH, it is likely that calmodulin is the target of action of these drugs. These observations may be useful, by indicating the basis for the clinical reports of inhibition of LH release in humans receiving pimozide (Ojeda *et al.*, 1974; Leppaluoto *et al.*, 1976) or other antipsychotics (DeWied, 1967).

G. Possible Sites of Calmodulin Action in the Gonadotrope

The observations that (1) calmodulin redistribution occurs in the pituitary following stimulation by GnRH (Conn *et al.*, 1981a) and (2) GnRH-stimulated LH release is inhibited by drugs that bind calmodulin (Conn *et al.*, 1981c) implicate calmodulin as the likely mediator of Ca^{2+} action in this system. This ubiquitous intracellular Ca^{2+} receptor has been shown to modulate many cellular processes, several of which deserve special mention.

1. Cyclic Nucleotides

GnRH stimulation of cAMP levels were initially reported in hemi-pituitaries in culture (Borgeat *et al.*, 1972). It does not appear that this cyclic nucleotide fulfills the requirements of a second messenger for the release process, however, because cAMP and stimulation of LH release can be clearly uncoupled in the cultured pituitary cell system. Conn *et al.* (1979a) showed that dibutyryl cAMP in saturating amounts (1 mM) did not stimulate LH release with an efficacy similar to that of GnRH nor did it potentiate LH release in response to GnRH. Similarly, choleragen (cholera toxin) and prostaglandin E$_1$, each of which stimulated cAMP production and its release, did not cause LH release from these cells. The occupancy of the protein kinase regulatory subunit (with cAMP) did not change following incubation of the cells with GnRH (although it did increase with choleragen and PGE$_1$) and 0.2 mM methylisobutylxanthine (MIX; an inhibitor of phosphodiesterase) did not alter the dose–response curve for GnRH-stimulated LH release. MIX, 2 mM, was actually inhibitory, probably because of the general toxic effect also seen in steroidogenic cells. Finally, treatment of cultured cells with a wide range of GnRH concentrations did not stimulate production of intra- or extracellular cAMP, even at acute time periods following GnRH administration. Consistent with these findings, it was shown that radioactive GnRH can be bound to pituitary plasma membranes in the absence of measurable adenylate cyclase stimulation (Theoleyre *et al.*, 1976; Clayton *et al.*, 1978). These findings suggested that although cAMP may be involved in regulation of GnRH-induced LH biosynthesis or other gonadotrope functions, it could be uncoupled readily from LH release. Accordingly, we do not propose further studies on the cyclic nucleotides.

Doubt has been cast on a role for cGMP in LH release by showing that blockade of its synthesis does not inhibit LH release in response to GnRH (Naor and Catt, 1980).

2. Phospholipase

This enzyme is (1) characterized as being stimulated by calmodulin (Wong and Cheung, 1980), although it has considerable activity in its absence; (2) localized largely at the plasma membrane (calmodulin redistributes to the plasma membrane following GnRH stimulation of the cells, see Section III,G; and (3) at least partially responsible for the metabolism of arachidonic acid.

The turnover of arachidonic acid appears to cause changes in membrane fluidity during accelerated secretion of lysosomal enzymes from rabbit neutrophils (Rubin *et al.*, 1981) and during adrenocorticotropin-stimulated release from the adrenal (Schrey and Rubin, 1979). Antagonists of arachidonic acid metabolism alter gonadotropin release from pituitary cultures (Conn *et al.*, 1980c). Changes in arachidonic acid release have been noted (Naor and Catt, 1981) during response to GnRH. Accordingly, there is circumstantial evidence for a role of phospholipase in response to GnRH-stimulated alterations in cell calcium distribution and subsequent gonadotropin release.

3. Ca^{2+}-ATPase

This enzyme is an attractive candidate for a target of calmodulin action. Reasons to suspect this enzyme include the observation (see Section III,B) that alterations in calcium flux occur in response to GnRH stimulation of the cells and appear to precede LH release. It is possible that alteration in the activity of this ATPase might be related either to the onset or extinction of gonadotropin release (i.e., pumping out of intracellular calcium). Calcium-ATPases are characterized as being calmodulin dependent and have been shown to be activated by some hormones (Larsen and Vincenzi, 1979; Pershadsingh and McDonald, 1980).

4. *Contractile Proteins*

Although microtubules are clearly important in other secretory cells (see Chapters 6 and 7 in this volume), there is little evidence regarding whether microtubules and microfilaments are involved in the mechanism of gonadotropin release, although clearly these can be regulated by calmodulin (see Chapter 13 in this volume). One study has indicated diminished release in the presence of colchicine (Khar *et al.*, 1979) but an extremely long incubation (7 hours total) in the presence of these inhibitors was needed. We have reported that vinblastine, an inhibitor of microtubules, inhibits patching and capping of the GnRH receptor in response to agonist occupancy. It does *not,* however, inhibit GnRH analog-stimulated LH release (Conn and Hazum, 1981).

IV. EXTRAPITUITARY SITES OF ACTION OF GNRH AND CROSS-REACTIVE SUBSTANCES

Although most of the work on the mechanism of action of GnRH and on its receptor has been done in the pituitary, it is apparent that GnRH (and substances that cross-react at its pituitary receptor) are present in gonadal, neural, and other tissues. Little information is available to indicate whether these compounds have similar mechanisms of action to GnRH in the pituitary; however, it is clear that nonpituitary tissues contain receptors that bind GnRH analogs with high affinity and specifity. Specific and direct biological effects can be attributed to occupancy of GnRH binding sites in several systems. GnRH of hypothalamic origin does not enter the circulation at concentrations that allow substantial occupancy of these receptors. Accordingly, it has been necessary to look for extrapituitary sites of synthesis of these compounds. The following section is presented to indicate the distribution of GnRH-like hormones and their binding sites.

A. Neural

Immunohistochemical studies have indicated that GnRH-containing axonal projections are present in many regions of the brain, including the main and accessory olfactory bulb, parolfactory region, nucleus of the diagonal band, medial and lateral septum, preoptic region, piriform cortex, hippocampus, amygdala, medial basal hypothalamus, interpeduncular nucleus, raphe nuclei, locus ceruleus, and central gray (Jennes and Stumpf, 1980a). Considerable quantities of GnRH are also found in contact with fenestrated capillaries in the organum vasculosum of the lamina terminalis (OVLT) (Pelletier *et al.*, 1976; Mazzuca, 1977). The target for GnRH released from the median eminence is the pituitary, whereas the site of action and the effects of GnRH released into the OVLT are not known. The pituitary may be excluded as a target, because no venous link exists between the OVLT and the median eminence (Amback *et al.*, 1975; Weindl and Schinko, 1975; Weindl and Sofroniew, 1978). The only efferent vessel from the OVLT is an artery that is connected to the preoptic artery or the anterior cerebral artery. It is not known whether the GnRH released in the OVLT reaches the peripheral circulation or remains in the pericommissural capillary system.

Another body fluid into which GnRH may be secreted is the cerebrospinal fluid (CSF), both within the ventricles and in the subarachnoid space (Jennes and Stumpf, 1980b). GnRH-immunoreactive fibers that contact the ventricular surface were noted in the septal part of the lateral ventricle, the ventral aspect of the hypothalamic third ventricle, the pineal recess, including the lamina intercalaris and habenular commissures, the subfornical organ, and the fovea centralis of the fourth ventricle (Burchanowski *et al.*, 1979; Jennes and Stumpf, 1980b). GnRH-containing nerve fibers contact the cerebrospinal fluid of the subarachnoid space on the surface of the brain in the region of the ventrocaudal aspect of the main olfactory bulb and the accessory olfactory bulb, and in the substantia perforata, the prechiasmatic area, and the interpeduncular recess (Jennes and Stumpf, 1980a,b).

GnRH has been measured in the CSF by radioimmunoassay. GnRH has been found under pathological conditions (Koch and Okon, 1979) in large quantities, but studies of GnRH under normal physiological conditions differ, with one group reporting it to be present (Joseph *et al.*, 1975) and another being unable to detect it in the CSF (Cramer and Barraclough, 1975).

Although the actual release of GnRH into the CSF has not yet been demonstrated, evidence exists in support of a physiological role for intra-CSF GnRH. Thus, intraventricular injections of GnRH are followed by an LH surge that is similar to that produced by intravenous injections but is of longer duration (Ondo *et al.*, 1973; Ben-Jonathan *et al.*, 1974). Autoradiographic studies following intraventricular injections of ^{125}I-labeled GnRH showed an accumulation of silver grains in the median eminence and the lateral recess, indicating a possible route for the transport of GnRH from the CSF to the portal system of the median eminence (Uemura *et al.*, 1975).

The route from nose to brain and pituitary via the subarachnoid space may play a role in the uptake of GnRH following application of nasal GnRH sprays (Happ, 1978a,b; Katzorke *et al.*, 1980). The estimated absorption of GnRH through the nose was initially thought to be on the order of 1.25–4% (London *et al.*, 1972; Dahlen *et al.*, 1974; Schally *et al.*, 1976; Katzorke *et al.*, 1980). However, one report indicates an absorption efficiency approaching that of an intravenous injection when GnRH analogs are administered pernasally (Katzorke *et al.*, 1980). This may be due to the resistance to degradation that is characteristic of GnRH analogs that have been modified at the 6 position. Thus, both anatomical and physiological studies have provided evidence that suggests a functional role of the CSF in the transport of exogenously administered GnRH.

Further evidence of the extrapituitary action of GnRH has come from immunohistochemical, electrophysiological, and behavioral studies, which have demonstrated that GnRH has effects within the brain itself. In addition to its neurohormonal action, this peptide may function as a neurotransmitter, that is, it may be secreted from the axon ending of one neuron, cross a synaptic cleft, and initiate a new electrical impulse in an adjacent neuron.

Terminal fields of GnRH axons, characterized by a distinct and anatomically well-restricted arborization of axons with terminal boutons, have been described in different regions of the telencephalon, diencephalon, and mesencephalon by immunohistochemistry. These GnRH-containing axon endings, which appear to be synaptoid, do not terminate upon blood vessels. They are present in the olfactory and septal–preoptic areas; in arcuate, interpeduncular, and raphe nuclei; and in the locus ceruleus and central gray region of the midbrain (Barry *et al.*, 1973, 1974; Silverman and Krey, 1978; Jennes and Stumpf, 1980a,b; Jennes and Croix, 1980). All these brain regions are known to influence behavior and/or GnRH secretion, and considerable evidence that suggests a direct effect of GnRH in these areas has accumulated. Infusions of GnRH into the ventrolateral midbrain central gray, preoptic, or arcuate/ventromedial areas significantly increase lordosis behavior in estrogen-primed ovariectomized rats (Moss and Foreman, 1976; Riskind and Moss, 1979). This effect of GnRH persists following hypophysectomy, (Pfaff, 1973) adrenalectomy, and ovariectomy (see Mauk *et al.*, 1980, for review), which indicates that this behavioral effect is due to a direct action of GnRH on the regions of the brain that control this behavior. This hypothesis is partly confirmed by electrophysiological studies that demonstrate that neurons in the midbrain central gray and hypothalamus altered their electrical activity following iontophoretic application of GnRH (Renaud *et al.*, 1976; Richard *et al.*, 1978). Behavioral changes have also been attributed to GnRH (Moss and McCann, 1975; Moss and Foreman, 1976).

B. Gonadal

It is clear that superactive analogs of GnRH exert direct effects on the gonads. Inhibition of steroidogenesis has been shown in hypophysectomized rats and in cultured granulosa cells. This area has been reviewed recently (Hsueh and Jones, 1981).

C. Other Tissues

1. *Adipose Tissue*

Murthy and Modesto (1974) examined the effects of GnRH and thyrotropin-releasing hormone on rabbit adipose tissue. GnRH increased [^{14}C]glucose oxidation and incorporation into fatty acids and had lipolytic activity at the same time, decreasing [^{14}C]glucose incorporation into glyceride–glycerol fractions. TRH has no significant effect on glucose oxidation or lipolysis but decreased [^{14}C]glucose incorporation into glyceride–glycerol fractions.

486

P. Michael Conn

2. Placenta

GnRH synthesis (Gibbons *et al.*, 1975) and storage (Siler-Khodr and Khodr, 1979) have been described in the placenta. Placental GnRH-like material is similar to hypothalamic GnRH in immunochemical, physicochemical, and biological properties. The placental content varies throughout gestation. A GnRH receptor is located in the plasma membrane fraction and binds ^{125}I-labeled GnRH with high affinity $(5.5 \times 10^{-7} M^{-1})$ and appears to be specific (Currie *et al.*, 1981). A similar receptor has been reported in the hydatiform mole (Currie *et al.*, 1981).

V. CONCLUSIONS

A large body of evidence from many laboratories suggests that (1) occupancy of the GnRH receptor leads to (2) mobilization of calcium

TABLE I

"Three-Step" Mechanism for GnRH-Stimulated LH Release

Steps	Reference[a]
1. GnRH binding to its plasma membrane receptor	
a. Receptor regulation by endocrine status of the animal	Marian *et al.* (1981)
b. Possible microaggregation	
c. Patching, capping, and internalization of the GnRH–receptor complex	Hazum *et al.* (1980)
d. Step 1b does not appear to be required for gonadotropin release	Conn *et al.* (1981d); Conn and Hazum (1981)
2. Calcium mobilization	
a. Increased calcium flux	Conn *et al.* (1981b)
Requirement for extracellular calcium	Marian and Conn (1979, 1980); Stern and Conn (1981)
Reversibility of depletion	Conn and Rogers (1979)
Gonadotropin release by ionophores, liposomes, and activators of endogenous ion channels	Conn *et al.* (1979b); Conn *et al.* (1980a); Conn and Rogers (1980)
b. Calcium action is postreceptor	Marian and Conn (1980)
c. Occupancy and redistribution of calmodulin	Conn *et al.* (1981a)
Block of stimulated release by anti-calmodulin drugs	Conn *et al.* (1981c)
d. Altered cellular function	
3. Release of gonadotropin via granule exocytosis	

[a] Representative references from the author's laboratory.

and (3) release of gonadotropin from preexisting storage granules. Although experimental evidence indicates that these steps are integrated, it is only within the past year that progress has been made to indicate the molecular basis of this integration. Recent findings regarding early events following hormone occupancy of the receptor indicate that, although patching, capping, and internalization occur as early steps in the mechanism of GnRH action, these are not requisite for stimulation of release (although they have not been excluded as having a role in biosynthesis or other processes). The observations that pituitary calmodulin redistribution follows pituitary stimulation with GnRH and that calmodulin-antagonistic drugs inhibit GnRH-stimulated release at a site of action after calcium mobilization indicate a possible role of calmodulin in this system. Accordingly, an updated version of the "three-step model" can be presented (Table I).

The three-step model provides a useful means to integrate extant information on the mechanism of stimulated gonadotropin release. It provides a potential mechanism for identifying the molecular site of action of hormones and drugs that alter pituitary gonadotrope responsiveness. In addition, it suggests postreceptor sites for potential clinical regulation of pituitary function for contraception and for management of altered regulation such as occur in precocious puberty and in infertility.

ACKNOWLEDGMENT

Work described from the author's laboratory was supported by NIH grant HD13220, RCDA HD00337, and the Mellon Foundation. Aging studies were supported by NIH AG1204.

REFERENCES

Adams, T. E., and Nett, T. M. (1979). Interaction of GnRH with anterior pituitary: Role of divalent cations, microtubules, and microfilaments in the GnRH activated gonadotroph. *Biol. Reprod.* **21**, 1073–1086.

Ambach, G., Horvath, S., and Palkovits, M. (1975). The arterial and venous blood supply of the septum pellucidum in the rat. *Acta Morphol. Acad. Sci. Hung.* **23**, 133–144.

Barry, J., Dubois, M. P., and Poulain, P. (1973). LRF producing cells of the mammalian hypothalmus: A fluorescent antibody study. *Z. Zellforsch. Mikrosk. Anat.* **146**, 351–366.

Barry, J., Dubois, M. P., and Carette, B. (1974). Immunofluorescence study of the preoptico-infundibular LRF neurosecretory pathway in the normal castrated or testosterone-treated male guinea pig. *Endocrinology (Baltimore)* **95**, 1416–1423.

Bauer, T. W., Moriarity, C. M., and Childs, G. V. (1981). Studies of immunoreactive gonadotropin releasing hormone (GnRH) in the rat anterior pituitary. *J. Histo-chem. Cytochem.* **29,** 1171–1178.

Ben-Jonathan, N., Mical, R. S., and Porter, J. C. (1974). Transport of LRF from CSF to hypophysial portal and systemic blood and the release of LH. *Endocrinology (Baltimore)* **95,** 18–25.

Benuck, M., and Marks, N. (1976). Differences in the degradation of hypothalamic releasing factors by rat and human serum. *Life Sci.* **19,** 1271–1276.

Berault, A., Theoleyre, M., and Jutisz, M. (1974). A simplified method for the preparation of plasma membranes from ovine anterior pituitary glands. *FEBS Lett.* **39,** 267–270.

Biales, B., Dichter, M. A., and Tischler, A. (1977). Sodium and calcium action potential in pituitary cells. *Nature (London)* **267,** 172–174.

Borgeat, P., Chavancy, G., Dupont, A., Labrie, F., Arimura, A., and Schally, A. V. (1972). Stimulation of adenosine 3':5'-cyclic monophosphate accumulation in anterior pituitary gland *in vitro* by synthetic luteinizing hormone-releasing hormone. *Proc. Natl. Acad. Sci. U.S.A.* **69,** 2677–2681.

Burchanowski, B. J., Knigge, K. M., and Rich, L. A. (1979). Ependymal investment of Luliberin (LHRH) fibers revealed immunocytochemically in an image like that from Golgi stain. *Proc. Natl. Acad. of Sciences U.S.A.* **76,** 6671–6674.

Chafouleas, J. G., Conn, P. M., Dedman, J. R., and Means, A. R. (1980). Regulation of calmodulin in endocrine tissues. *Endocrinology (Baltimore)* **106A,** 289. (Abstr.)

Clayton, R. N., and Catt, K. J. (1980). Receptor-binding affinity of gonadotropin releasing hormone analogs: Analysis by radioligand receptor assay. *Endocrinology (Baltimore)* **106,** 1154–1159.

Clayton, R. N., Shakespear, R. A., and Marshall, J. C. (1978). LHRH binding to purified pituitary plasma membranes: Absence of adenylate cyclase activation. *Mol. Cell. Endocrinol.* **11,** 63–78.

Clayton, R. N., Shakespear, R. A., Duncan, J. A., and Marshall, J. C. (1979). Radioiodinated nondegradable GnRH analogs: New probes for the investigation of pituitary GnRH receptors. *Endocrinology (Baltimore)* **105,** 1369–1376.

Conn, P. M., and Hazum, E. (1981). LH release and GnRH-receptor internalization: Independent actions of GnRH. *Endocrinology (Baltimore),* **109,** 2040–2045.

Conn, P. M., and Rogers, D. C. (1979). Restoration of responsiveness of gonadotropin releasing hormone (GnRH) in calcium depleted rat pituitary cells. *Life Sci.* **24,** 2461–2466.

Conn, P. M., and Rogers, D. C. (1980). Gonadotropin release from pituitary cultures following activation of endogenous ion channels. *Endocrinology (Baltimore)* **107,** 2133–2133.

Conn, P. M., Morrell, D. V., Dufau, M. L., and Catt, K. J. (1979a). Gonadotropin-releasing hormone action in cultured pituitary cells: Independence of luteinizing hormone release and adenosine 3',5'-monophosphate production. *Endocrinology (Baltimore)* **104,** 448–453.

Conn, P. M., Rogers, D. C., and Sandhu, F. S. (1979b). Alteration of intracellular calcium level stimulates gonadotropin release from cultured rat pituitary cells. *Endocrinology (Baltimore)* **105,** 1122–1127.

Conn, P. M., Kilpatrick, D., and Kirshner, N. (1980a). Ionophoretic Ca^{2+} mobilization in rat gonadotropes and bovine adrenomedullary cells. *Cell Calcium* **1,** 129–133.

Conn, P. M., Marian, J., McMillian, M., and Rogers, D. (1980b). Evidence for calcium mediation of gonadotropin releasing hormone action in the pituitary. *Cell Calcium* **1,** 7–20.

Conn, P. M., Whorton, R., and Lazar, J. (1980c). An inhibitor of arachidonic acid metabolism stimulates luteinizing hormone (LH) release from cultured cells. *Prostaglandins* 19, 873–879.

Conn, P. M., Chafouleas, J., Rogers, D., and Means, A. R. (1981a). Gonadotropin releasing hormone stimulates calmodulin redistribution in the rat pituitary. *Nature (London)* 292, 264–264.

Conn, P. M., Marian, J., McMillian, M., Stern, J. E., Rogers, D. R., Hamby, M., Penna, A., and Grant, E. (1981b). Gonadotropin releasing hormone action in the pituitary: A three step mechanism. *Endocr. Rev.* 2, 174–185.

Conn, P. M., Rogers, D. R., and Sheffield, T. (1981c). Inhibition of gonadotropin releasing hormone stimulated luteinizing hormone release by pimozide: Evidence for a site of action after calcium mobilization. *Endocrinology (Baltimore)* 109, 1122–1126.

Conn, P. M., Smith, R. G., and Rogers, D. C. (1981d). Stimulation of pituitary release does not require internalization of gonadotropin releasing hormone. *J. Biol. Chem.* 256, 1098–1091.

Cramer, O. M., and Barraclough, C. A. (1975). Failure to detect luteinizing hormone-releasing hormone in third ventricle cerebrospinal fluid under a variety of experimental conditions. *Endocrinology (Baltimore)* 96, 913–921.

Currie, A. J., Fraser, H. M., and Sharpe. (1981). Human placental receptors for luteinizing hormone releasing hormone. *Biochem. Biophys. Res. Commun.* 99, 332–338.

Dahlen, H. G., Keller, E., and Schneider, H. P. G. (1974). Linear dose dependent LH release following intranasally sprayed LRH. *Horm. Metab. Res.* 6, 510–513.

Dalkin, A. C., Bourne, G. A., Pieper, D. R., Regiani, S., and Marshall, J. C. (1981). Pituitary and gonadal GnRH receptors during sexual maturation in the rat. *Endocrinology (Baltimore)* 108, 1658–1663.

Davies, P. J. A., Davies, D. R., Levitzki, A., Maxfield, F. R., Milhaud, P., Willingham, M. C., and Pasten, I. H. (1980). Transglutaminase is essential in receptor mediate endocytosis of alpha2-macroglobulin and polypeptide hormones. *Nature (London)* 283, 162–167.

Debeljuk, L., Khar, A., and Jutisz, M. (1978). Effect of pimozide and sulpiride on the release of LH and FSH by pituitary cells in culture. *Mol. Cell. Endocrinol.* 10, 159–162.

DeWied, D. (1967). Chlorpromazine and endocrine function. *Pharmacol. Rev.* 19, 251–275.

Duello, T. M., and Nett, T. M. (1980). Uptake, localization, and retention of gonadotropin-releasing hormone and gonadotropin releasing hormone analogs in rat gonadotrophs. *Mol. Cell. Endocrinol.* 19, 101–112.

Dufy, B., Vincent, J. D., Fleury, H., duPasquier, P., Gourdji, D., Tixier-Vidal, A. (1979). Membrane effects of thyrotropin releasing hormone and estrogen shown by intracellular recording from pituitary cells. *Science* 204, 509–511.

Eisenbarth, G. S., Shimzu, K., Conn, P. M., Mittler, B., and Wells, S. (1981). Monoclonal antibody F12A2B5: Reaction with a plasma membrane antigen of vertebrate neurons and peptide-secreting endocrine cells. *In* "Monoclonal Antibodies Against Neural Antigens" (S. McKay, B. Raff, and P. Reichardt, eds.), Vol. 2, pp. 209–218.

Frager, M. S., Pieper, D. R., Tonetta, J. A., and Marshall, J. C. (1981). Pituitary GnRH receptors: Effects of castration, steroid replacement, and the role of GnRH in modulating receptors in the rat. *J. Clin. Invest.* 67, 615–621.

Fujino, M., Fukuda, T., Shinagawa, S., Kobayashi, S., Yamazaki, I., and Nakayama, R. (1974). Synthetic analogs of luteinizing hormone releasing hormone (LH-RH) substituted in position 6 and 10. *Biochem. Biophys. Res. Commun.* 60, 406–413.

Geschwind, I. I. (1969). Mechanism of action of releasing factors. In "Frontiers in Neu-roendocrinology" (L. Martini and W. F. Ganong, eds.), pp. 389–431. Oxford Univ. Press, London and New York.

Gibbons, J. M., Mitnick, M., and Chieffo, V. (1975). In vitro biosynthesis of TSH- and LH-releasing factors by the human placenta. Am. J. Obstet. Gynecol. 121, 127–131.

Grab, D. J., Berzins, K., Cohen, R. S., and Siekevitz, P. (1979). Presence of calmodulin in postsynaptic densities isolated from canine cerebral cortex. J. Biol. Chem. 254, 8690–8696.

Griffiths, E. C., and Kelly, J. A. (1979). Mechanism of inactivation of hypothalamic regulatory hormones. Mol. Cell. Endocrinol. 14, 3–17.

Happ, J., Hartmann, U., Weber, T., Cordes, U., and Beyer, J. (1978a). Gonadatropin and testosterone secretion in normal human males after stimulation with gonadatropin-releasing hormone (GnRH) or potent GnRH analogs using different modes of ap-plication. Fertil. Steril. 30, 666–673.

Happ, J., Hartmann, U., Weber, T., Cordes, U., and Beyer, J. (1978b). Gonadatropin and testosterone secretion in normal human males after stimulation with gonadatropin-releasing hormone (GnRH) or potent GnRH analogs using different modes of ap-plication. Fertil. Steril. 30, 666–673.

Hazum, E., Cuatrecasas, P., Marian, J., and Conn, P. M. (1980). Receptor mediated internalization of fluorescent gonadotropin releasing hormone by pituitary gonadotropes. Proc. Natl. Acad. Sci. U.S.A. 77, 6692–6695.

Hopkins, C. R., and Gregory, H. (1977). Topographical localization of the receptors for luteinizing hormone releasing hormone on the surface of dissociated pituitary cells. J. Cell Biol. 75, 528–540.

Hopkins, C. R., and Walker, A. M. (1978). Calcium as a second messenger in the stimula-tion of luteinizing hormone secretion. Mol. Cell. Endocrinol. 12, 189–208.

Hsueh, A. J. W., and Jones, P. B. C. (1981). Extrapituitary actions of GnRH. Endocr. Rev., 2, 437–461.

Ilundain, A., and Naftalin, R. J. (1979). Role of Ca^{2+} dependent protein in intestinal secretion. Nature (London) 279, 446–448.

Jacobs, S., Chang, K.-J., and Cuatrecasas, P. (1978). Antibodies to purified insulin receptor have insulin-like activity. Science 200, 1283–1284.

Jennes, L., and Croix, D. (1980). Changes in the LHRH-immunoreactivity of hypothalmic structures during late pregnancy and after parturition in the guinea pig. Cell Tissue Res. 205, 121–131.

Jennes, L., and Stumpf, W. E. (1980a). LHRH-systems in the brain of the golden ham-ster. Cell Tissue Res. 209, 239–256.

Jennes, L., and Stumpf, W. E. (1980b). LHRH-systems in the brain of the golden ham-ster. Cell Tissue Res. 209, 239–256.

Jones, P. B. C., Conn, P. M., Marian, J. M., and Hsueh, A. J. W. (1980). Binding of GnRH agonist to rat ovarian granulosa cells. Life Sci. 27, 2125–2132.

Joseph, S. A., Sorrentino, S., and Sundberg, D. K. (1975). Releasing hormones, LRF and TRF, in the cerbrospinal fluid of the third ventricle. Proc. Int. Symp. Brain-Endocr. Interact. II, pp. 306–312.

Kahn, C. R., Baird, K. L., Jarrett, D. B., and Flier, J. S. (1978). Direct demonstration that receptor crosslinking or aggregation is important in insulin action. Proc. the Natl. Acad. Sci. U.S.A. 75, 4209–4213.

Katzorke, T., Propping, D., Von der Ohe, M., and Tauber, P.F. (1980). Clinical evalua-tion of the effects of a new long-acting superactive lutenizing hormone-releasing hormone (LH-RH) analog, D-Ser(TBU)6-des-Gly10-EthylamideLH-RH, in women with secondary amenorrhea. Fertil. Steril. 33, 35–42.

Khar, A., Kunert-Radek, J., and Jutisz, M. (1979). Involvement of microtubule and microfilament system in the GnRH-induced release of gonadotropins by rat anterior pituitary cells in culture. *FEBS Lett.* **104,** 410–414.

Kidokoro, Y. (1975). Spontaneous calcium action potentials in a clonal pituitary cell line and their relationship to prolactin secretion. *Nature (London)* **258,** 741–742.

Koch, Y., and Okon, E. (1979). Localization of releasing hormones in the human brain. *Int. Rev. Exp. Pathol.* **19,** 45–62.

Koch, Y., Baram, T., Chobsieng, P., and Fridkin, M. (1974). *Enzymic degradation of LHRH by hypothalamic tissue. Biochem. Biophys. Res. Commun.* **61,** 95–103.

Kochman, K., Kerdelhue, B., Zor, U., and Jutisz, M. (1975). Studies of enzymatic degradation of LHRH by different tissues. *FEBS Lett.* **50,** 190–194.

Larsen, F. L., and Vincenzi, F. F. (1979). Calcium transport across the plasma membrane: Stimulation by calmodulin. *Science* **204,** 306–308.

Leppaluoto, J., Mannisto, P., Ranta, T., and Linnoila, M. (1976). Inhibition of mid-cycle gonadotrophin release in healthy women by pimozide and fusaric acid. *Acta Endocrinol. (Copenhagen)* **81,** 455–460.

London, D. R., Butt, W. R., Lynch, S. S., Marshall, J. C., Owusu, S., Robison, W. R., and Stephenson, J. M. (1973). Hormonal responses to intranasal LHRH. *J. Clin. Endocrinol. Metab.* **37,** 829–831.

McCann, S. M. (1971). Mechanism of action of hypothalamic-hypophyseal stimulatory and inhibitory hormones. *In* "Frontiers in Neuroendocrinology" (L. Martini and W. F. Ganong, eds.), pp. 209–235. Oxford Univ. Press, London and New York.

Marian, J., and Conn, P. M. (1979). GnRH stimulation of cultured pituitary cells requires calcium. *Mol. Pharmacol.* **16,** 196–201.

Marian, J., and Conn, P. M. (1980). The calcium requirement in GnRH-stimulated LH release is not mediated through a specific action on the receptor. *Life Sci.* **27,** 87–92.

Marian, J., Cooper, R., and Conn, P. M. (1981). Regulation of the rat pituitary GnRH-receptor. *Mol. Pharmacol.* **19,** 399–405.

Marks, N. (1970). Biodegradation of hormonally active peptides in the central nervous system. *In* "Subcellular Mechanisms in Reproductive Neuroendocrinology" (F. Naftolin, R. J. Ryan, and J. Davis, eds.), pp. 129–147. Elsevier, Amsterdam.

Marshall, J. C., Shakespear, R. A., and Odell, W. D. (1975). Pituitary plasma membrane luteining hormone releasing hormone binding: Evidence for the presence of specific sites in other tissues. *J. Endocrinol.* **67,** 38P.

Mauk, M. D., Olson, G. A., Kastin, A. J., and Olson, R. D. (1980). Behavioral effects of LH-RH. *Neurosci. Behav. Rev.* **4,** 1–8.

Mazzuca, M. (1977). Immunocytochemical and ultrastructural identification of luteinizing hormone-releasing hormone (LHRH)-containing neurons in the vascular organ of the lamina terminals (OVLT) of the squirrel monkey. *Neuroscience* **5,** 123–127.

Moss, R. L., and Foreman, M. M. (1976). Potentiation of lordosis behavior by intrahypothalmic infusion of synthetic luteinizing hormone-releasing hormone. *Neuroendocrinology* **20,** 176–186.

Moss, R. L., and McCann, S. M. (1975). Action of luteinizing hormone-releasing factor (LRF) in the initiation of lordosis behavior in the estrone-primes ovarietomized female rat. *Neuroendocrinology* **17,** 309–318.

Murthy, G. G., and Modesto, R. R. (1974). Effects of luteinizing hormone releasing hormone and thyrotrophin releasing hormone on rabbit adipose tissue. *J. Endocrinol.* **62,** 639–643.

Naor, Z., and Catt, K. J. (1980). Independent actions of GnRH upon cyclic GMP production and LH release. *J. Biol. Chem.* **255,** 342–344.

Naor, Z., and Catt, K. J. (1981). Mechanism of action of GnRH: Involvement of phospholipid turnover in LH release. *J. Biol. Chem.* **256**, 2226–2228.

Naor, Z., Atlas, A., Clayton, R. N., Forman, D. S., Amsterdam, A., and Catt, K. J. (1981). Interaction of fluorescent GnRH with receptors in pituitary cells. *J. Biol. Chem.* **256**, 3049–3052.

Ojeda, S. R., Harms, P. G., and McCann, S. M. (1974). Effect of blockade of dopaminergic receptors on prolactin and LH release: Median eminence and pituitary sites of action. *Endocrinology (Baltimore)* **94**, 1650–1660.

Ondo, J. G., Eskay, R. L., Mical, R. S., and Porter, J. C. (1973). Effect of synthetic LRF infused into a hypophysial portal vessel on gonadotropin release. *Endocrinology (Baltimore)* **93**, 205–209.

Ozawa, S., and Miyazaki, S. (1979). Electrical excitability in the rat clonal pituitary cell and its relation to hormone secretion. *Jpn. J. Physiol.* **29**, 411–426.

Pelletier, G., LeClerc, R., and Dube, D. (1976). Immunohistochemical localization of hypothalamic hormones. *J. Histochem. Cytochem.* **24**, 864–871.

Perrin, M. H., Rivier, J., and Vale, W. W. (1980). Radioligand Assay for gonadotropin-releasing hormone: Relative potencies of agonists and antagonists. *Endocrinology (Baltimore)* **106**, 1289–1296.

Pershadsingh, H. A., and McDonald, J. M. (1980). Calcium-activated ATPase and ATP-dependent calmodulin-stimulated calcium transport in islet cell plasma membranes. *Nature (London)* **281**, 495–497.

Pfaff, D. W. (1973). Luteinizing hormone-releasing factor potentiates lordosis behavior in hypophysectomized ovariectomized female rats. *Science* **182**, 1148–1149.

Putney, J. W. (1979). Stimulus-permiability coupling: Role of Ca^{2+} in the receptor regulation of membrane permability. *Pharmacol. Rev.* **30**, 209–245.

Renaud, L. P., Martin, J. B., and Brazeau, P. (1976). Hypothalamic releasing factors: Physiological evidence for a regulatory action on central neurons and pathways for their distribution in brain. *Pharmacol. Biochem. Behav.* **5**, 171–178.

Richard, P., Freund-Mercier, M. J., and Moos, F. (1978). Les neurones hypothalamiques ayant une fonction endocrine. Identification, localization, caracteristiques electrophysiologiques et controle hormonal. *J. Physiol. (Paris)* **5**, 61–112.

Riskind, P., and Moss, R. L. (1979). Midbrain central gray: LHRH infusion enhances lordotic behavior in estrogen-primed ovariectomized rats. *Brain Res. Bull.* **4**, 203–205.

Rubin, R. P., Sink, L. E., and Freer, R. J. (1981). On the relationship between formylmethionyl-leucyl-phenylalanine stimulation of arachidonyl phosphatidylinositol turnover and lysosomal enzyme secretion by rabbit neutrophils. *Mol. Pharmacol.* **19**, 31–37.

Samli, M. H., and Geschwind, I. I. (1968). Some effects of energy-transfer inhibitors and of Ca^{2+}-free and of K^+-enhanced media on the release of LH from the rat pituitary gland *in vitro*. *Endocrinology (Baltimore)* **82**, 225–231.

Savoy-Moore, R. T., Schwartz, N. B., Duncan, J. A., and Marshall, J. C. (1980). Pituitary gonadotropin-releasing hormone receptors during the rat estrous cycle. *Science* **209**, 942–944.

Schally, A. V., Kastin, A. J., and Coy, C. H. (1976). LH-releasing hormone and its analogues: Recent basic and clinical investigations. *Int. J. Fertil.* **21**, 1–30.

Schechter, Y., Hernaez, L., Schlessinger, J., and Cuatrecasas, P. (1979). Localization aggregation of hormone-receptor complexes is required for activation by epidermal growth factor. *Nature (London)* **278**, 835–838.

Schmechel, D., Marangos, P. J., and Brightman, M. (1978). Neurone-specific enolase is a molecular marker for peripheral and central neuroendocrine cells. *Nature (London)* **276**, 834–836.

Schrey, M. P., and Rubin, R. P. (1979). Characterization of a calcium-mediated activation of arachidonic acid turnover in adrenal phospholipids by corticotropin. *J. Biol. Chem.* **254**, 11234–11241.

Siler-Khodr, T. M., and Khodr, G. S. (1978). Content of luteinizing hormone-releasing factor in the human placenta. *Am. J. Obstet. Gynecol.* **130**, 216–219.

Silverman, A. J., and Krey, L. C. (1978). The luteinizing hormone releasing hormone (LH-RH) neuronal networks of the guinea pig brain. I. Intra- and extra-hypothalamic projections. *Brain Res.* **157**, 233–246.

Smith, W. A., and Conn, P. M. (1982). Causes and consequences of altered gonadotropin secretion in the aging rat. In "Clinical and Experimental Intervention in the Pituitary During Aging" (R. Walker and R. L. Cooper, eds.), in press.

Spona, J. (1974a). LHRH interaction with the pituitary plasma membrane is affected by sex steroids. *FEBS Lett.* **39**, 221–224.

Spona, J. (1974b). LHRH receptor interaction is inhibited by des-his-des-gly[10] LHRH-EA. *FEBS Lett.* **48**, 88–92.

Stern, J. E., and Conn, P. M. (1981). Requirements for GnRH stimulated LH release from perifused rat hemipituitaries. *Am. J. Physiol. (Endocrinol. Sect.)* **240**, 504–509.

Sternberger, L. A., and Petrali, J. P. (1975). Quantitative immunocytochemistry of pituitary receptors for LHRH. *Cell Tissue Res.* **162**, 141–176.

Taraskevich, P. S., and Douglas, W. W. (1977). Action potentials occur in cells of the normal anterior pituitary gland and are stimulated by the hypophysiotrophic peptide TRH. *Proc. Natl. Acad. Sci. U.S.A.* **74**, 4064–4067.

Taraskevich, P. S., and Douglas, W. W. (1978). Catecholamines of supposed inhibitory hypophysiotrophic functions suppress action potentials in prolactin cells. *Nature (London)* **276**, 832–834.

Tashjian, A. H., Lomedico, M. E., and Maina, D. (1978). Role of calcium in the TRH-stimulated release of prolactin from pituitary cells in culture. *Biochem. Biophys. Res. Commun.* **81**, 798–806.

Theoleyre, M., Berault, A., Garnier, J., and Jutisz, M. (1976). Binding of GnRH to the pituitary plasma membrane and the problem of adenylate cyclase stimulation. *Mol. Cell. Endocrinol.* **5**, 365–372.

Uemura, H., Asai, T., Nozaki, M., and Kobayashi, H. (1975). Ependymal absorption of luteinizing hormone-releasing hormone injected into the third ventricle of the rat. *Cell Tissue Res.* **160**, 443–452.

Vale, W., Burgus, R., and Guillemin, R. (1967). Presence of calcium ions as a requisite for the *in vitro* stimulation of TSH release by hypothalamic TRF. *Experientia* **23**, 853–859.

Wakabayashi, K., Kamberi, I. A., and McCann, S. M. (1969). *In vitro* response of the rat pituitary to gonadotropin releasing factors and to ions. *Endocrinology (Baltimore)* **85**, 1046–1056.

Weindl, A., and Schinko, I. (1975). Vascular and ventricular neurosecretion in the organum vasulosum of the lamina terminalis of the golden hamster. *Proc. Int. Symp. Brain-Endocrine Interact.* **II**, pp. 190–203.

Weindel, A., and Sofroniew, D. (1978). "Neurohormones and Circumventricular Organs," 117–137. Karger, Basel.

Williams, J. A. (1976). Stimulation of $^{45}Ca^{2+}$ efflux from rat pituitary by LHRH and other pituitary stimulators. *J. Physiol. (London)* **260**, 105–115.

Wong, P., and Cheung, W. Y. (1980). Calmodulin stimulates human platelet phospholipase A2. *Biochem. Biophys. Res. Commun.* **90**, 473–480.

15

Hormonal Modulation of LH and FSH Secretion by Cultured Pituitary Cells

AARON J. W. HSUEH AND ELI Y. ADASHI

I. INTRODUCTION

Luteinizing hormone (LH) and follicle-stimulating hormone (FSH) secretion by pituitary gonadotropes is under the control of hypothalamic gonadotropin-releasing hormone (GnRH) (Schally *et al.*, 1971; Amoss *et al.*, 1971; Chapter 14). After the identification of the structure of GnRH, many analogs of this decapeptide were synthesized to identify either agonists that are more potent and longer-lasting than GnRH or antagonists that are able to block the action of GnRH (Vale *et al.*, 1976; Sandow *et al.*, 1978).

495

Although the possibility of a separate hypothalamic factor specifically controlling FSH secretion cannot be excluded, the disparate secretion patterns of the gonadotropins during various physiological and pathological states may be explained by the differential modulatory actions of gonadal steroids and gonadal inhibin-like factor at the pituitary level. Ovarian steroids (estrogens, androgens, and progestins) are known to be involved in the regulation of gonadotropin releases. Estradiol has been shown to exert positive as well as negative feedback effects on gonadotropin release *in vivo,* and the effects appear to be dose and time dependent (Arimura and Schally, 1971; Kalra *et al.,* 1973; Yen *et al.,* 1974; Jaffe and Keyes, 1974). In contrast to estradiol, progesterone alone appears to have little effect on gonadotropin secretion in castrated animals (McCann, 1962; Nallar *et al.,* 1966). However, after estrogen priming, progesterone has been shown to exert both facilitatory and inhibitory effects on LH release *in vivo* (McCann, 1962; O'Dell and Swerdloff, 1968; Nillius and Wide, 1971; Lasley *et al.,* 1975).

Steroid hormones have been shown to bind to specific receptor molecules in the cytoplasmic fraction of cells before translocation to the nucleus (O'Malley and Means, 1974). Estrogen-binding sites have been studied in the anterior pituitary (Notides, 1970) and have been characterized in both cytoplasmic and nuclear fractions of the rat anterior pituitary (Anderson *et al.,* 1973). Androgen receptors have also been identified in the pituitary (Naess *et al.,* 1975). Studies of progesterone receptors in the pituitary are more difficult because of the possible binding of progesterone by circulating corticoid-binding globulin. However, *in vivo* uptake of [^{3}H]progesterone by the pituitary has been reported (Luttage and Wallis, 1973; Seiki and Hattori, 1973), and progesterone receptors have also been demonstrated in the pituitary of estrogen-treated animals through the use of a synthetic radiolabeled progestin ([^{3}H]R-5020) (Kato and Onouchi, 1977). These binding studies reinforced the notion that gonadal steroids act directly upon pituitary cells.

Although considerable attention has been given to the effects of gonadal steroids on gonadotropin secretion, the possible secretion of a nonsteroidal factor by the gonads in the regulation of gonadotropin production has also been explored. The presence of a nonsteroidal testicular inhibitor of FSH secretion was proposed as early as 1932 (McCullagh, 1932). Later, direct evidence for the presence of a testicular protein that suppresses FSH secretion was obtained (see review by Baker *et al.,* 1976). A nonsteroidal, water-soluble factor obtained from seminal plasma, rete testis fluid, and extracts of testicular tissue were all shown to exert differential inhibition of FSH production by the pituitary (Franchimont, 1972, Setchell and Jacks, 1974; Keogh *et al.*, 1976).

An ovarian inhibin-like factor that specifically suppresses FSH secretion in castrated male and female rats has also been found in extracts of bovine ovary and in follicular fluid obtained from both bovine and procine Graafian follicles (DeJong and Sharpe, 1976; Marder *et al.*, 1977). These studies indicated that a nonsteroidal, protein-like factor may be secreted by the ovary to preferentially suppress FSH secretion.

Earlier attempts to study the site of action of the gonadal modulators (steroids and inhibin-like factor) on pituitary gonadotropin production were complicated by the fact that these gonadal factors may also regulate the secretion of hypothalamic GnRH. The observation that treatment with GnRH can potentiate the responsiveness of pituitary gonadotropes to subsequent action of GnRH (Aiyer *et al.*, 1974) further complicated the attempts to dissociate between pituitary and hypothalamic actions of the gonadal factors *in vivo*.

To elucidate the direct modulatory actions of the gonadal factors on pituitary gonadotropin production, we used a primary culture of anterior pituitary cells (Vale *et al.*, 1972) and studied the actions of estrogens, antiestrogens, progestins, androgens, insulin, and ovarian inhibin-like factor on pituitary gonadotropin secretion. The agonistic and antagonistic actions of various synthetic analogs of GnRH on pituitary LH release were also studied.

II. EFFECT OF AGONISTIC AND ANTAGONISTIC ANALOGS OF GNRH ON GONADOTROPIN PRODUCTION

In order to elucidate the actions of various GnRH analogs on LH secretion, anterior pituitary glands were dissected free of the posterior and intermediate lobes. Each pituitary was cut into eight pieces and the pooled tissue was dispersed by an enzyme solution containing collagenase and 0.1% bovine serum albumin. The pituitary fragments were incubated at 37°C for 1.5 hours, during which time they were dissociated into a cell suspension by repeated pipetting every 30 minutes with a graded series of micropipets. At the end of the incubation period, anterior pituitary cells were collected by centrifugation at 250 g for 5 minutes, washed five times with HEPES/0.1% BSA buffer, and resuspended into a known volume of medium. Cell viability was consistently $\geq 90\%$.

Anterior pituitary cells were cultured in 35 × 10 mm Falcon tissue culture dishes in 2 ml McCoy's 5a medium supplemented with strep-

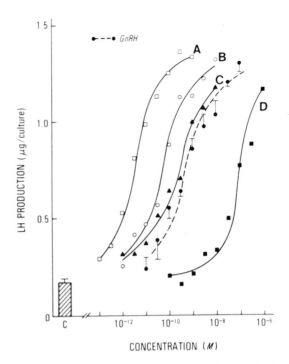

Fig. 1. Effects of various agonistic analogs of GnRH on LH release by cultured pituitary cells. Anterior pituitary cells (1×10^5 cells/dish) were cultured for 2 days at 37°C. After 2 days *in vitro*, the cells were washed 4 times and reincubated in 2 ml McCoy's 5a medium containing 1% serum and various concentrations of GnRH (●) or various GnRH agonists (A–D) for 3 hours. Medium LH content was measured by radioimmunoassay.

tomycin sulfate (100 μg/ml), penicillin (100 U/ml), L-glutamine (2 mM), 10% horse serum, and 2.5% fetal calf serum. Cell cultures were maintained for 2 days at 37°C under a water-saturated atmosphere in 5% CO_2 and 95% air without any treatment. The cells were then washed and treated with various concentrations of GnRH or its analogs in 2 ml McCoy's media for 3 hours. Medium concentration of LH was measured by radioimmunoassay. The various analogs were provided by Nicholas Ling (Salk Institute, CA) and Marvin Karten (NIC-HD, NIH). Some were originally synthesized by Coy *et al.* (1979) and Channabasavaiah *et al.* (1979).

As shown in Fig. 1, basal LH production was low, whereas treatment with increasing concentrations of GnRH or its agonistic analogs [A, des-Gly^{10},D-Ser(t-Bu)^6,Pro^9-NHEt-GnRH; B, des-Gly^{10},D-

Leu^6,(N^αMe)Leu^7,Pro^9-NHEt-GnRH; C, D-Lys^6-GnRH; D, des
Lys^6,(N^αMe)Leu^7,Pro^9-NHEt-GnRH] led to dose-dependent
in LH production. Based on the ED$_{50}$ values of GnRH and it
agonists, agonist D proved to be 143-fold less potent tha
whereas agonists C, B, and A were 1.8-, 12-, and 190-fold mo
than GnRH, respectively. These results indicated that subst
D-amino acid in position 6 and modification of the C terminus
enhances the releasing potency of GnRH analogs. In contra
troduction of a methyl group in position 7, along with D-lys
sixth position, significantly reduces LH releasing activity.

   To determine the abilities of several GnRH antagonists to
GnRH-stimulated production of LH, pituitary cells were cu
described, in the presence or absence of GnRH ($10^{-8}M$) wit
out increasing concentrations (10^{-9}–$10^{-6}M$) of antagonist

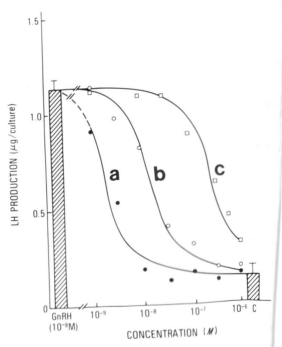

   Effects of various antagonistic analogs of GnRH on LH re   red
      terior pituitary cells were cultured for 2 days as de   g. 1.
         were treated with 10^{-8} M GnRH with or w   sing
             nRH antagonists for 3 hours. Medium LH   mea-
             say.

D-Trp³,⁶-GnRH; b, Ac-D-Ala¹,D-Phe²,D-thienyl-Ala³,⁶-
G,⁶-GnRH) (Fig. 2). Basal production of LH was low,
w nt with GnRH (10^{-8} M) brought about an 8-fold
i roduction. However, concomitant treatment with in-
c rations of GnRH antagonists led to dose-dependent
bl GnRH-stimulated production of LH [IDR₅₀ value
(G t): a = 0.17 ± 0.01; b = 1.6 ± 0.6; and c = 25 ± 3].
Th icated the potent antagonistic activity of GnRH ana-
lo o acid replacement at the second position. Further
m ositions 1 and 6 further enhanced the antagonistic
act

III. ESTROGENS AND CATECHOL ESTROGENS
TROPIN PRODUCTION

In idate the nature of the feedback actions of estrogens
on l the effect of estradiol, estrone, estriol, 2-hydroxy-
estr hydroxyestrone on pituitary cell responsiveness to
GnR tigated by adding different concentrations of these
ster cubation media before the addition of cells (Hsueh et
$al.$, ra used in the culture media were pretreated with
char b free steroids (Erickson and Hsueh, 1978). After 2
days t in $vitro$, the cell cultures were washed four times
with s of medium 199 and subsequently reincubated in
McC um containing increasing concentrations of the synthetic 12–$10^{-6}M$). After a 3-hour incubation period, media
were d stored at $-20°C$ until assayed for LH by radioim-
muno cate culture dishes were used for each GnRH dose
and d rminations were made for each culture dish by LH
radioi y.

The dent action of estradiol on GnRH-induced LH release
by cult ary cells is shown in Fig. 3. In control cultures, in-
creasin tions of GnRH caused a dose-dependent increase in
LH pro h 10^{-6} M GnRH causing a maximum increase in LH
product alf-maximal effective dose (ED₅₀) of GnRH in the
control as $1.9 ± 0.6 × 10^{-9}$ M. Pretreatment for 2 days with
estradio) caused an apparent increase in LH production, but
the incr not statistically significant ($p > 0.05$). At a higher
concentr radiol (10^{-9} M) sensitized the pituitary gonadotropes t s indicated by the marked decrease (approximately
10-fold) o value to $1.5 ± 0.2 × 10^{-10}$ M. Similar sensitizi

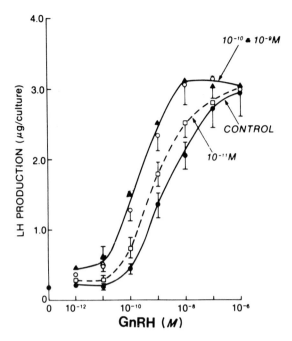

Fig. 3. Effects of various doses of estradiol (E_2) on GnRH-induced LH release in cultured pituitary cells. Pituitary cells (2×10^5 viable cells/dish) obtained from adult ovariectomized rats were cultured *in vitro* for 2 days in the absence (●, control cultures) or presence of E_2 (▲, 10^{-9} M; ○, 10^{-10} M; □, 10^{-11} M). At the end of the 2-day incubation, the pituitary cells were washed and reincubated for 3 hours with increasing concentrations of GnRH ($10^{-12}–10^{-6}$ M).

effects on GnRH-induced LH production were obtained with 10^{-10} M and 10^{-8} M estradiol.

Like estradiol, estrone also caused a sensitizing effect on pituitary gonadotropes. As shown in Fig. 4, estrone (10^{-10} and 10^{-8} M) increased pituitary sensitivity to GnRH and, at both concentrations, the ED_{50} value of GnRH was decreased to 1.2×10^{-10} M. The maximal production of LH was not significantly different between control and estrone-treated cultures ($p > 0.05$). In contrast, estriol at 10^{-10} and 10^{-8} M (Fig. 5) induced a slight but not statistically significant ($p > 0.05$) increase in LH production at all doses of GnRH.

The effect of two catechol estrogens on GnRH-induced LH release was also tested. At 10^{-8} M, 2-hydroxyestradiol (2-OHE$_2$; Fig. 6) sensitized pituitary gonadotropes to GnRH, as shown by a decrease in the ED_{50} value of GnRH to $2.5 \pm 0.5 \times 10^{-10}$ M; however, LH production in cultures treated with a lower dose of 2-OHE$_2$, (10^{-10} M) was not

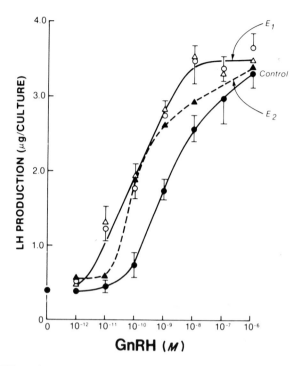

Fig. 4. Effect of estrone (E_1) on GnRH-induced LH release in cultured pituitary cells. Pituitary cells were cultured, as described in Fig. 3, either as controls (●) or treated with E_2 (▲, $10^{-9}\ M$) or E_1 (△, $10^{-8}\ M$; ○, $10^{-10}\ M$). Reprinted with permission from Hsueh *et al.* (1979).

different from controls ($p > 0.05$). In contrast, 2-hydroxyestrone (2-OHE_1) at $10^{-8}\ M$ (Fig. 6) showed no sensitizing effect. In neither case was a change in maximal LH production detected ($p > 0.05$). These results indicate that 2-OHE_2, but not 2-OHE_1, is estrogenic in nature.

These studies have demonstrated that estradiol, estrone, and 2-OHE_2, but not estriol and 2-OHE_1, sensitized pituitary gonadotropes to GnRH. The estradiol effect was shown to be dose dependent and confirms the results of Drouin *et al.* (1976), who reported that $10^{-9}\ M$ estradiol decreased the ED_{50} value from $3.0 \times 10^{-10}\ M$ in control cultures to $1.6 \times 10^{-10}\ M$ in estradiol-treated cultures.

Estrone was found to sensitize pituitary gonadotropes to GnRH equally as well as estradiol (Fig. 4). Although the physiological role of estrone in LH release is not known, plasma levels of estrone and LH are elevated in postmenopausal women and in women with polycystic ovarian syndrome (Gordon *et al.*, 1973; DeVane *et al.*, 1974). In view of

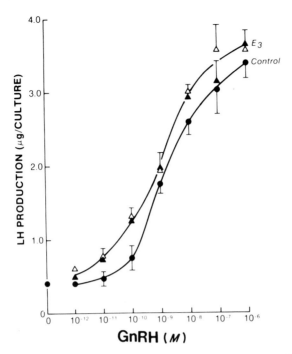

Fig. 5.   Effect of estriol (E_3) on GnRH-induced LH release by cultured pituitary cells. Pituitary cells were cultured, as described in Fig. 3, either as controls (●) or treated with E_3 (△, 10^{-8} M; ▲, 10^{-10} M). Reprinted with permission from Hsueh *et al.* (1979).

the present findings, the elevation of serum estrone in these conditions may sensitize the gonadotropes to GnRH, resulting in an increase in circulating LH. In contrast to estrone and estradiol, estriol did not sensitize pituitary cells to GnRH (Fig. 5). Estriol has been shown to be as potent as estradiol in inducing a uterotrophic response after multiple injections (Clark *et al.*, 1977). Because the pituitary gonadotropes were continuously exposed to estriol in the present culture conditions and because estriol was shown to be ineffective, our data suggest that the actions of estriol on the pituitary gonadotropes and the uterus may be different.

2-Hydroxylation is an important pathway of estrogen metabolism (Fishman, 1977). In the present experiments, 2-OHE$_2$ sensitized pituitary gonadotropes to GnRH, whereas 2-OHE$_1$ had no effect (Fig. 6). These results are consistent with earlier findings by Davies *et al.* (1975) in that 2-OHE$_2$ effectively competes with [^{3}H]estradiol for pituitary estrogen receptors, whereas 2-OHE$_1$ is less potent. Furthermore,

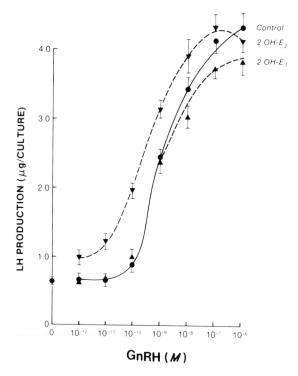

Fig. 6. Effects of 2-hydroxyestradiol (2-OHE$_2$) and 2-hydroxyestrone (2-OHE$_1$) on GnRH-induced LH release by cultured pituitary cells. Pituitary cells were cultured, as described in Fig. 3, either as control (●) or treated with 2-OHE$_2$ (▼, 10^{-8} M) or 2-OHE$_1$ (▲, 10^{-8} M). Reprinted with permission from Hsueh *et al.* (1979).

Martucci and Fishman (1977) have demonstrated that 2-OHE$_2$, but not 2-OHE$_1$, exhibits uterotrophic activity.

IV. EFFECT OF PROGESTINS ON GONADOTROPIN PRODUCTION AND THE ANTAGONISM OF ESTROGEN ACTION BY PROGESTINS

Compared to control cultures, incubation of pituitary cells with progesterone (10^{-8} and 10^{-6} M) did not significantly change LH production with GnRH doses ranging from 10^{-12} to 10^{-7} M. However, at 10^{-6} M GnRH, progesterone (10^{-6} M) caused a decrease in LH production ($p < 0.01$ compared to control), whereas progesterone at 10^{-8} M was not effective (Fig. 7).

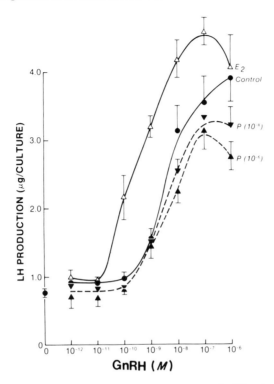

Fig. 7. Effects of estradiol (E_2) and progesterone (P) on GnRH-induced LH release by cultured pituitary cells. GnRH-induced LH release was measured in pituitary cells preincubated in the absence (●, control) or presence of E_2 (△) or P (▼, $10^{-8}\,M$; ▲, $10^{-6}\,M$). Reprinted with permission from Hsueh *et al.* (1979).

When pituitary cells were treated with a combination of progesterone ($10^{-6}\,M$) and estradiol ($10^{-9}\,M$), the estradiol-induced sensitization of the gonadotropes was completely inhibited. At all doses of GnRH, LH production of these cultures was comparable to that of the control cultures ($p > 0.05$; Fig. 8). Therefore, progesterone antagonized the estradiol-induced sensitization of gonadotropes. At a lower dose, progesterone ($10^{-8}\,M$) appeared to exert less inhibition on the estradiol-induced sensitization of gonadotropes (Fig. 8); however, LH production by these cultures was not significantly different from control cultures ($p > 0.05$).

As shown in Fig. 9, incubation of pituitary cells with 20α-hydroxyprogesterone (20α-OHP) ($10^{-6}\,M$) resulted in a significant decrease in the maximal LH production ($p < 0.01$) but did not significantly change the ED_{50} value for GnRH ($1.9 \pm 0.6 \times 10^{-9}\,M$ in control

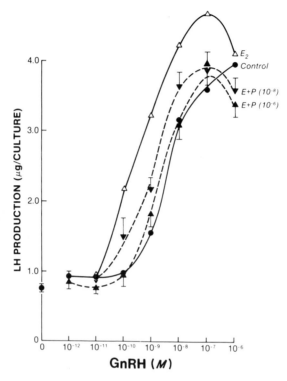

Fig. 8. Antagonistic effect of progesterone (p) on estradiol-induced sensitization of pituitary cells to GnRH stimulation. GnRH-induced LH release in cultured pituitary cells was measured in control cultures (●), cultures treated with E_2 (△), and with E_2 plus P (E + P; ▼, 10^{-9} M E_2 and 10^{-8} M P; ▲, 10^{-9} M E_2 and 10^{-6} M P). Experimental details are the same as described in Fig. 3. Reprinted with permission from Hsueh *et al.* (1979).

cultures and $1.8 \pm 0.8 \times 10^{-9}$ M in 20α-OHP-treated cultures). The sensitizing effect of estradiol (10^{-9} M) to GnRH was antagonized by 20α-OHP (Fig. 9). At all doses of GnRH, 20α-OHP exerted a significant inhibition of LH production when compared to estradiol-treated cultures ($p > 0.01$). The ED_{50} value was also increased from $1.5 \pm 0.2 \times 10^{-10}$ M in estradiol-treated cultures to $3.0 \pm 0.3 \times 10^{-10}$ M in cultures treated with estradiol plus 20α-OHP. Thus, 20α-OHP, like progesterone, antagonized the sensitizing effect of estradiol on pituitary gonadotropes.

The antagonizing effect of progestins on estradiol-induced sensitization of pituitary responsiveness is consistent with the *in vivo* observations by Greeley *et al.* (1975) in that progesterone inhibits estradiol-

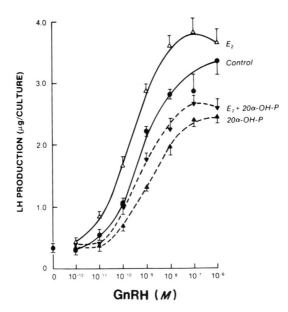

Fig. 9. Antagonistic effect of 20α-hydroxyprogesterone (20α-OHP) on estradiol-induced sensitization of pituitary cells to GnRH stimulation. GnRH-induced release of LH in cultured pituitary cells was measured in control cultures and cultures treated with E_2, 20α-OHP and E_2 plus 20α-OHP. (Experimental details are shown in Fig. 3). Reprinted with permission from Hsueh *et al.* (1979).

induced sensitization of pituitary responsiveness in ovariectomized, stalk-sectioned rats. A facilitatory effect of 20α-OHP on LH release in the rabbit has been postulated (Hilliard *et al.*, 1967); however, a subsequent study was not able to substantiate the hypothesis (Goodman and Neill, 1976). The present results exclude a facilitatory role of this steroid at the pituitary level.

V.   EFFECT OF ANTIESTROGENS ON GONADOTROPIN PRODUCTION

Since the original study of Greenblatt (1962), clomiphene citrate (Clomid) has been used successfully to induce ovulation in anovulatory conditions. The ovulation-inducing effect of Clomid is mediated through a transient increase in the pituitary release of LH and FSH, which in turn initiates follicular maturation and ovulation (Vaitukaitis *et al.*, 1971; Vandenberg and Yen, 1973). Although the mechanism of action of

Clomid is unknown, this substance has been reported to possess both antiestrogenic and estrogenic properties. Experimental studies of the pituitary, hypothalamus, and uterus have shown that Clomid competitively inhibits estradiol binding to estrogen receptors, suggesting an antiestrogenic action (Eisenfeld and Axelrod, 1967; Kato *et al.*, 1968; Kahwanago *et al.*, 1970; Roy *et al.*, 1970). On the other hand, the observation that Clomid stimulates uterine growth is suggestive of an estrogenic action (Clark *et al.*, 1974). We also tested the possible anti-estrogenic or estrogenic effects of Clomid on LH release *in vitro*, and demonstrated that Clomid, like 17β-estradiol, increases the responsiveness of pituitary gonadotropes to GnRH *in vitro* (Hsueh *et al.*, 1978; Adashi *et al.*, 1981a).

When pituitary cells were treated with Clomid ($10^{-8} M$), an increase in GnRH responsiveness was observed (Fig. 10). Compared to control

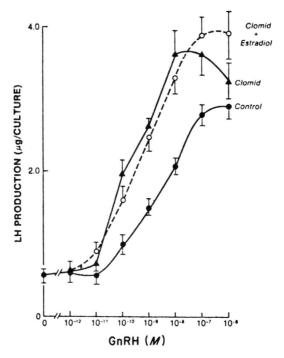

Fig. 10. Effects of Clomid and Clomid plus estradiol on GnRH-induced LH release *in vitro*. Experimental procedures are described in Fig. 3. Anterior pituitary cells were incubated for 2 days in media alone (control group, ●), media containing $10^{-9} M$ Clomid (▲), or media containing $10^{-9} M$ Clomid plus $10^{-9} M$ 17β-estradiol (○). Reprinted with permission from Hsueh *et al.* (1978).

cultures, Clomid lowered the ED_{50} value of GnRH from 3×10^{-9} to $1 \times 10^{-10} M$. A similar decrease in ED_{50} value was also observed when the pituitary cells were incubated with a combination of estradiol and Clomid.

As enclomiphene citrate (Enclomid; formerly called *cis*-clomiphene citrate) is believed to be the active component in the Clomid mixture, the effect of this isomer on cultured pituitary cells was also tested (Fig. 11). Similar to the effect of Clomid, treatment of pituitary cells with Enclomid yielded an ED_{50} value of $2.8 \times 10^{-10} M$, indicating a marked sensitization of the gonadotropes to GnRH by a factor of 7.5. These findings suggest that the Enclomid isomer is as effective as Clomid in sensitizing the gonadotropes to the action of GnRH.

To test the effect of another nonsteroidal "antiestrogen" on the responsiveness of the pituitary to GnRH, anterior pituitary cells were treated with Tamoxifen and/or estradiol. As shown in Fig. 12, the ED_{50} value of GnRH for control pituitary cells was $2.1 \times 10^{-9} M$. Treatment of pituitary cells with $10^{-9} M$ estradiol resulted in a marked decrease in the ED_{50} value of GnRH. In contrast, treatment with $10^{-7} M$ of Tamox-

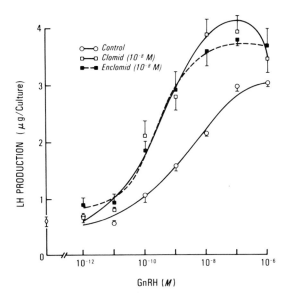

Fig. 11. The effect of treatment with Enclomid on the GnRH-stimulated release of LH. Pituitary cells were cultured as described in Fig. 3, either as controls or treated with Clomid ($10^{-8} M$) or Enclomid ($10^{-8} M$). Reprinted with permission from Adashi *et al.* (1981a).

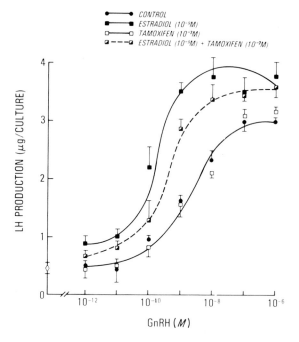

Fig. 12. The effects of treatment with estradiol (E_2) and/or Tamoxifen on the GnRH-stimulated release of LH. Pituitary cells were cultured as described in Fig. 3, either as controls or treated with E_2 (10^{-9} M), Tamoxifen (10^{-7} M), or E_2 (10^{-9} M) plus Tamoxifen (10^{-7} M). Reprinted with permission from Adashi *et al.* (1981a).

ifen did not result in a significant alteration in the sensitivity of the pituitary to GnRH. Furthermore, simultaneous treatment with Tamoxifen and estradiol led to an apparent increase in the ED_{50} value, representing a 2-fold reduction in pituitary sensitivity to GnRH as compared with estradiol-treated cells. However, the maximal and the overall release of LH for cells treated with estradiol and Tamoxifen did not differ significantly from that of estradiol-treated cells. These findings imply that Tamoxifen, unlike Clomid, does not exert an estrogenic effect on cultured pituitary cells.

To further study the ability of estradiol, Clomid, and Tamoxifen to interact with pituitary estrogen receptors and to correlate their binding affinity with physiological responses, the crude nuclear fraction obtained from anterior pituitaries of estradiol-treated rats was incubated with a saturating concentration of [^{3}H]estradiol in the presence or absence of increasing concentrations of estradiol, Clomid, or Tamoxifen. As shown in Fig. 13, all the compounds tested displayed a dose-depen-

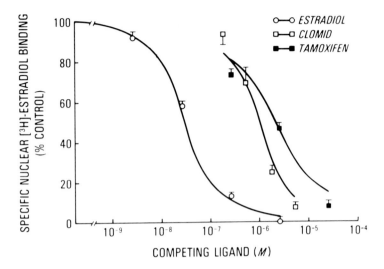

Fig. 13. Competition of specific [3H]estradiol binding to pituitary nuclear preparations by Clomid, Tamoxifen, and estradiol. The nuclear fraction of anterior pituitary obtained from estrogen-treated rats were incubated (37°C for 30 minutes) with 2.6 nM of [3H]estradiol in the presence or absence of various concentrations of either estradiol, Clomid, or Tamoxifen. The results are expressed as the percentage of the specific nuclear binding in the absence of the inhibitor. Reprinted with permission from Adashi *et al.* (1981a).

dent inhibition of [3H]estradiol binding. The apparent molar concentrations required to inhibit 50% of the specific [3H]estradiol binding were 30, 1000, and 2200 nM for estradiol, Clomid, and Tamoxifen, respectively. The relative affinity of Clomid and Tamoxifen for nuclear pituitary estrogen receptors was determined to be 33- and 73-fold lower than that of estradiol, respectively. These results suggest that the inability of 10^{-7} M Tamoxifen to affect GnRH action at the pituitary is not due to its inability to interact with pituitary estrogen receptors. Because Clomid, like estradiol, can competitively inhibit the binding of [3H]estradiol to pituitary nuclear preparations, these observations suggest that the effects of Clomid observed here are probably mediated through the estrogen receptors.

In view of the important role of FSH in Clomid-induced ovulation, the effects of treatment with either estradiol (10^{-9} M) or Clomid ($10^{-8}M$) on the GnRH-stimulated release of FSH were also studied. As shown in Fig. 14, treatment with increasing concentrations of GnRH resulted in dose-dependent increases in FSH release. The ED_{50} value of GnRH for control pituitary cells was $2.4 \pm 0.1 \times 10^{-9}$ M. Treatment with estradiol

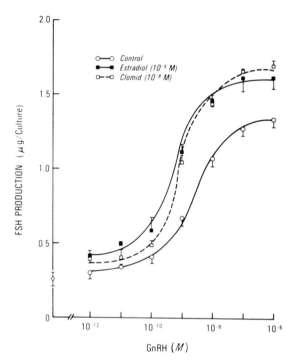

Fig. 14. The effects of treatment with estradiol or Clomid on the GnRH-stimulated release of FSH. Pituitary cells (3×10^5 viable cells/culture) were cultured as described in Fig. 3 either as controls or treated with estradiol ($10^{-9} M$) or Clomid ($10^{-8} M$). FSH released into the medium was measured by radioimmunoassay. Reprinted with permission from Adashi *et al.* (1981a).

($10^{-9} M$) or Clomid ($10^{-8} M$) resulted in a reduction in the ED_{50} value of GnRH to 5.8×10^{-10} and $7.5 \times 10^{-10} M$, respectively. These decreases in the ED_{50} values represent 4.3- and 3.3-fold increases in pituitary sensitivity to GnRH for estradiol- and Clomid-treated cells, respectively. These findings suggest that estradiol and Clomid are both capable of enhancing the GnRH-stimulated release of FSH.

The effects of co-incubating estradiol ($10^{-9} M$) and Clomid ($10^{-8} M$) on the GnRH-stimulated release of FSH are depicted in Fig. 15. Following concomitant treatment of pituitary cells with estradiol and Clomid, the ED_{50} value was decreased from $2.3 \times 10^{-9} M$ in control cells to $6.3 \times 10^{-10} M$. This represents a 3.6-fold increase in pituitary sensitivity to GnRH over controls. Both the overall and the maximal release of FSH following treatment with estradiol and Clomid were significantly ($p < 0.05$) increased as compared with controls. Thus, Clomid does not antag-

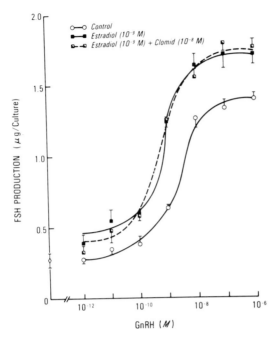

Fig. 15.   The effects of treatment with estradiol, Clomid, or their combination on the GnRH-stimulated release of FSH. Pituitary cells were treated with various steroids as shown in Fig. 3. Reprinted with permission from Adashi *et al.* (1981a).

onize the sensitizing effect of estradiol on the GnRH-stimulated release of FSH.

These results suggest that Clomid and its Enclomid isomer, unlike Tamoxifen, may exert a direct, estrogenic, rather than an anti-estrogenic, effect on rat anterior pituitary cells by enhancing the GnRH-stimulated release of gonadotropin. It is well established that the administration of Clomid to anovulatory female subjects is followed in short sequence by a rise in the circulating concentrations of both FSH and LH (Ross *et al.*, 1970). Nevertheless, it is the initial rise of FSH that is particularly critical for the initiation of folliculogenesis (Ross *et al.*, 1970). Of considerable interest was the finding that Clomid alone, like estradiol, is capable of augmenting the pituitary sensitivity to GnRH in terms of FSH release. However, because Clomid is usually given to estrogen-primed subjects *in vivo,* it became of interest to examine the combined effect of Clomid and estradiol on the GnRH-stimulated release of FSH. The finding that co-incubation of Clomid with estradiol did not affect the sensitizing effect of estradiol on the GnRH-stimulated release of LH and FSH is in keeping with the notion that Clomid acts as an estrogen, rather than an antiestrogen, at the pituitary level. The observation that estradiol (10^{-9} M) treatment induced a 4.3-fold increase in pituitary sensitivity in terms of FSH release extends the findings of Labrie *et al.* (1978).

Although Tamoxifen is almost as effective as Clomid in binding to pituitary estrogen receptors, our findings suggest that Tamoxifen (10^{-7} M) has little or no estrogenic activity in terms of its ability to enhance the GnRH-stimulated release of LH. These findings sharply contrast with those obtained for Clomid, suggesting that the estrogenic action of Clomid at the pituitary represents a unique feature of this compound and that Tamoxifen may indeed be devoid of estrogenic activity (Sutherland *et al.*, 1977) and hence a weak profertility agent (Klopper and Hall, 1971).

The possibility of a pituitary site of action for Clomid has previously been suggested by the *in vivo* studies of Döcke (1969), who was able to induce corpus luteum formation with Clomid in rats rendered anovulatory by electrolytic lesioning of the medial preoptic–suprachiasmatic regions of the hypothalamus. This notion is further supported by our observation (Adashi *et al.*, 1980) that Clomid treatment *in vivo* resulted in a prolonged retention of nuclear estrogen receptors and depletion of cytoplasmic estrogen receptors in the pituitary gland but not in the hypothalamus. Nevertheless, the present study does not rule out the possibility that, in addition to its action on the pituitary gonadotropes, Clomid may also affect hypothalamic release of GnRH.

VI. EFFECT OF ANDROGENS ON GONADOTROPIN PRODUCTION

The effect of a nonaromatizable androgen (dihydrotestosterone; DHT) on pituitary responsiveness to GnRH has also been tested. Anterior pituitary cells were treated for 1 day in media containing 10% serum to facilitate cell attachment. The cells were then washed and reincubated in serum-free culture media (Adashi *et al.*, 1981b) for 2 additional days with or without DHT. After androgen treatment, the cells were washed and treated with increasing concentrations of GnRH for 3 hours. As shown in Fig. 16, control cells responded to GnRH treatment and secreted LH in a dose-dependent fashion with an ED_{50} value of 1.8 × 10^{-10} M. In contrast, cells pretreated with DHT secreted 35% less LH in response to the maximal dose of GnRH. The ED_{50} value was also increased by DHT treatment to 8 × 10^{-10} M. These results indicated

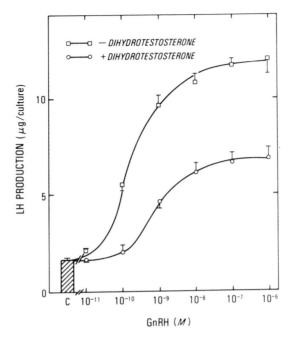

Fig. 16. Effect of treatment with dihydrotestosterone (DHT) on pituitary responsiveness to GnRH. Anterior pituitary cells were cultured for 1 day in serum-containing media and then washed and treated for 2 more days in McCoy's 5a medium with or without 10^{-7} M DHT. At the end of 2 days, media were changed and cells treated with various concentrations of GnRH for 3 hours. Media LH concentrations were determined by radioimmunoassay.

that DHT decreased the responsiveness and the capacity of gonadotropes to respond to GnRH, a finding consistent with earlier studies using serum-containing media (Drouin and Labrie, 1976).

VII. EFFECT OF OVARIAN INHIBIN-LIKE FACTOR ON GONADOTROPIN PRODUCTION

As discussed in a previous section, an inhibin-like factor has been identified in the follicular fluid from porcine and bovine Graafian follicles; however, the site of inhibin-like factor production in the ovary was unknown. It has been demonstrated that Sertoli cells in the testis produce an inhibin-like factor *in vitro*. Analogous to the testicular Sertoli cell, the granulosa cell in the ovary is known to possess FSH receptors and several FSH-inducible enzymes. We therefore hypoth-

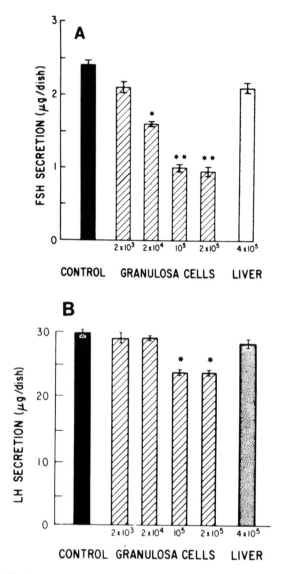

Fig. 17. FSH (A) and LH (B) release by cultured pituitary cells incubated with spent media from various numbers of rat granulosa cells obtained from preovulatory follicles. Pituitary cells were treated as described in the text. Reprinted with permission from Erickson and Hsueh (1978).

esized that ovarian granulosa cells may produce an inhibin-like factor. In order to test this hypothesis, we cultured various numbers of rat granulosa or liver cells *in vitro* and collected the media. The media were then treated with charcoal to strip endogenous steroids, and the effects of these media on gonadotropin production were studied in cultured pituitary cells.

Dispersed pituitary cells were cultured as described earlier. After a 3-day incubation, pituitary cells were washed twice with McCoy's medium and then reincubated for 3 additional days with charcoal-extracted spent media from cultured granulosa or liver cells. After the 3-day culture period, the amount of FSH and LH released by pituitary cells was measured.

Control pituitary cells released 2.4 and 30.1 μg/culture of FSH and LH, respectively, during the 3-day incubation (Fig. 17A and B). A significant inhibition of FSH release was observed when pituitary cells were incubated with spent media from granulosa cell cultures (Fig. 17A). The amount of FSH inhibition increased with increasing numbers of cultured granulosa cells and ranged from $14 \pm 3\%$ inhibition to $61 \pm 3\%$ inhibition. In contrast, no effect upon LH release by pituitary cells was observed with spent media from low concentrations of granulosa cells; however, culture media collected from higher concentrations of granulosa cells caused a moderate inhibition of LH secretion (Fig. 17B). No significant decrease in FSH or LH release was observed with spent media from rat liver cell cultures (Fig. 17A and B).

The present experiments support previous findings of an inhibin-like substance in ovarian follicular fluid and suggest (1) that granulosa cells are a source of the ovarian inhibin-like factor and (2) that the pituitary gonadotropes are a site of ovarian inhibin-like factor action. In view of these data, it is tempting to postulate that a closed-loop negative feedback mechanism exists between pituitary gonadotropes and developing granulosa cells in which FSH production is regulated by ovarian inhibin-like factor and, in turn, ovarian inhibin-like factor production may be controlled by pituitary FSH.

VIII. EFFECT OF INSULIN AND GROWTH FACTORS ON GONADOTROPIN PRODUCTION

Reproductive failure invariably accompanies experimentally induced diabetes in laboratory animals. Although the deleterious effect of insulin deficiency may be exerted at multiple levels, a decreased gonadotropic function constitutes a major feature of the insulin-defi-

cient state. The observed decrease in gonadotropin production is unrelated to decreased availability of hypothalamic GnRH or diminshed
pituitary stores of gonadotropins. Kirchick *et al.* (1978, 1979) reported
that anovulation in diabetic female rats treated with pregnant mare
serum gonadotropin was not related to a decreased ovarian secretion of
estradiol nor to a diminished hypothalamic release of GnRH, but rather
was due to a decrease in the responsiveness of the pituitary to GnRH. In
contrast, Paz *et al.* (1978) did not observe any change in pituitary
sensitivity in diabetic male rats. It therefore remains unclear whether
or not a pituitary component underlies the decreased serum

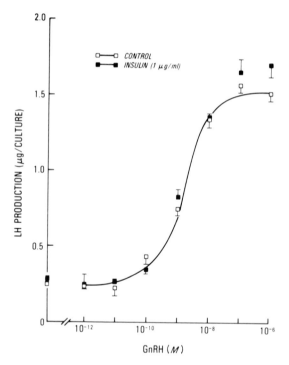

Fig. 18. The effects of treatment with insulin on basal and GnRH-stimulated release
of LH in a serum-supplemented medium. Anterior pituitary cells were obtained from
adult ovariectomized female rats. After culturing pituitary cells for 1 days *in vitro* in a
medium supplemented with 10% horse serum and 2.5% fetal calf serum, the medium was
changed and the cells reincubated for 2 additional days in the same serum-containing
medium in the presence or absence of insulin (1.0 μg/ml). At the end of the 2-day
incubation period, the cells were washed and then reincubated for 3 hours with increasing concentrations of GnRH (10^{-12}–10^{-6} M). The LH released into the medium was
assayed by radioimmunoassay. Reprinted with permission from Adashi *et al.* (1981b).

gonadotropin levels of the insulin-deficient state. We have performed *in vitro* experiments in which the role of insulin in the regulation of basal and GnRH-stimulated release of gonadotropins was studied in cultured rat anterior pituitary cells. This *in vitro* approach eliminated complicating variables of *in vivo* diabetes.

After incubation for 1 day in culutre media supplemented with 10% horse serum and 2.5% calf serum, pituitary cells were reincubated with or without insulin (1.0 μg/ml) for 2 additional days in a culture medium supplemented with the same serum. Insulin treatment did not result in a significant alteration of either the basal or the maximal release of LH as compared with control cells (Fig. 18). Similarly, no significant

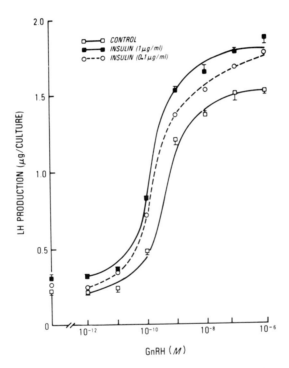

Fig. 19. The effects of treatment with insulin on basal and GnRH-stimulated release of LH in a serum-free medium. Anterior pituitary cells from adult ovariectomized rats were cultured as described in Fig. 18 for 1 day and then reincubated in the serum-free McCoy's media in the presence or absence of insulin (0.1 and 1.0 μg/ml). At the end of the 2-day incubation period, the cells were washed and then reincubated for 3 hours with increasing concentrations of GnRH (10^{-12}–10^{-6} M). The LH released into the medium was assayed by radioimmunoassay. Reprinted with permission from Adashi *et al.* (1981b).

change could be detected in the ED_{50} value ($1.7 \pm 0.2 \times 10^{-9}\ M$) of GnRH.

Because the serum-supplemented media may contain insulin and because serum may interfere with the action of insulin, we further tested the effect of insulin in serum-free media. Anterior pituitary cells were initially cultured in a serum-supplemented medium to allow maximal plating. One day later, the medium was changed and the attached cells reincubated for 2 additional days in a serum-free medium with or without insulin (Fig. 19). Treatment with GnRH caused a dose-dependent increase in LH release in control and insulin-treated cultures. In insulin-treated (0.1 μg/ml) cells, a significant increase in the basal, maximal, and overall release of LH was detected. The ED_{50} value of

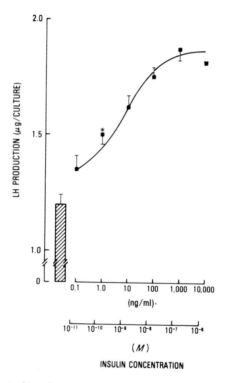

Fig. 20. The effect of insulin concentration on the GnRH-stimulated release of LH. Anterior pituitary cells were cultured as described in Fig. 19, in the presence or absence of various concentrations of insulin. A GnRH concentration of $3 \times 10^{-10}\ M$ was used during the 3 hours of the GnRH treatment period. The hatched bar represents LH release by cultures not treated with insulin. Reprinted with permission from Adashi *et al.* (1981b).

GnRH had decreased by 3.2-fold from the control level of $4.8 \pm 0.2 \times 10^{-10}\,M$ to $1.5 \pm 0.1 \times 10^{-10}\,M$. The minimal effective dose of GnRH in insulin-treated cells (defined as 2 SD above basal levels) was $4.8 \times 10^{-12}\,M$, i.e., 5.7 pg/ml. In contrast, given a lower dose of insulin (0.1 μg/ml), no significant alteration could be discerned for the basal release of LH, whereas the maximal as well as the overall release of LH was significantly increased over control.

Because the effects of insulin cannot be demonstrated when the cells are cultured in a serum-supplemented medium, it can be inferred that the presence of serum constituent(s) has an inhibitory effect on the function of the gonadotropes. As compared to cells cultured in serum-containing media, treatment of pituitary cells with insulin in a serum-free medium results in a significant decrease (3.2-fold in terms of LH release) in ED_{50} values for GnRH (Fig. 18 versus Fig. 19). It is apparent that the combined use of a serum-free medium and insulin treatment may decrease the ED_{50} value for GnRH by a factor of 10 or more, enabling the detection of concentrations of GnRH as low as 5 pg/ml. This observation can be applied to bioassay measurements of low concentrations of GnRH.

Figure 20 depicts the dose–response relationship for the effect of increasing concentrations of insulin on the GnRH-stimulated ($3 \times 10^{-10}\,M$) release of LH. Treatment of pituitary cells with a physiological concentration (1.0 ng/ml) of insulin resulted in significant increases in GnRH-stimulated release of LH when compared with controls. Additional dose-dependent increases in the GnRH-stimulated release of LH could be observed for higher concentrations of insulin, and the stimulatory effect of insulin appeared to plateau at supraphysiological concentrations (100–10,000 ng/ml) of insulin. Half maximal enhancement of the GnRH-stimulated release of LH occurred at an insulin concentration of 4.0 ng/ml.

Treatment of pituitary cells with insulin (1.0 μg/ml) for 2 days also resulted in significant increases in the basal, maximal, and the overall releases of FSH as compared with controls (Fig. 21). The ED_{50} value of GnRH was decreased by 6.3-fold from the control level of $5.8 \pm 0.2 \times 10^{-10}$ to $9.2 \pm 0.1 \times 10^{-11}\,M$.

Figure 22 depicts the dose–response relationship for the effect of increasing concentrations of insulin on the GnRH-stimulated ($3 \times 10^{-10}\,M$) release of FSH. Treatment of pituitary cells with a physiological concentration (1.0 ng/ml) of insulin led to a significant increase in the GnRH-stimulated release of FSH. The effect of insulin appeared to plateau when supraphysiological concentrations (100–10,000 ng/ml) of insulin were used. Half maximal enhancement of the GnRH-stimulated

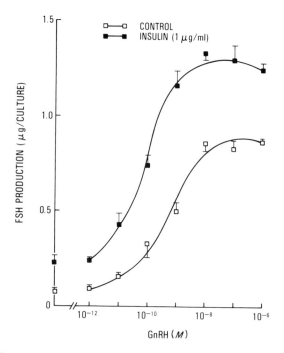

Fig. 21. The effects of treatment with insulin on basal and GnRH-stimulated release of FSH. Pituitary cells were cultured as described in Fig. 19 in the presence or absence of insulin (1.0 μg/ml). The FSH released into the medium was measured by radioimmunoassay. Reprinted with permission from Adashi *et al.* (1981b).

release of FSH occurred at an insulin concentration of 4.8 ng/ml. Because the circulating concentrations of insulin *in vivo* are known to fluctuate over a range of 1–4 ng/ml in the rat (Tannenbaum *et al.*, 1976; Isaksson *et al.*, 1978), the present findings are physiologically relevant.

To determine whether the effects of insulin on the gonadotrope are specific to this hormone, we investigated the effect of other "growth factors," i.e., epidermal growth factor (EGF) and fibroblast growth factor (FGF), on pituitary LH release *in vitro*. As shown in Table I, pretreatment with mouse EGF or bovine FGF (1 μg/ml) for 2 days did not significantly affect basal, maximal, or overall LH release. Furthermore, the ED_{50} values were comparable among the three groups, These results demonstrate the specificity of insulin action and suggest that these growth factors do not affect pituitary LH release.

Our findings suggest that the gonadotrope constitutes a target cell of insulin and that insulin may act directly on the anterior pituitary in the regulation of gonadotropin release. It is possible that the effect of insulin treatment on the GnRH-stimulated release of gonadotropins is

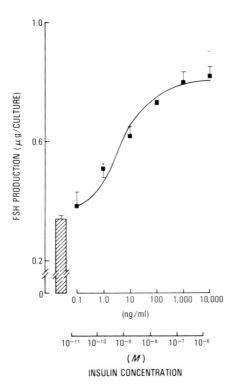

Fig. 22. The effect of insulin concentration on the GnRH-stimulated release of FSH. Anterior pituitary cells were cultured as described in Fig. 19 in the presence or absence of various concentrations of insulin. A GnRH concentration of 3×10^{-10} M was used during the 3 hours of the GnRH treatment period. The hatched bar represents FSH release by cultures not treated with insulin. Reprinted with permission from Adashi *et al.* (1981b).

due to an increase in the affinity and/or the number of pituitary GnRH receptors. Regardless of the mechanism, the interaction of insulin with the gonadotrope clearly results in profound effects on the secretory dynamics of the gonadotropes. Our findings suggest that insulin may play a physiological role in regulating the secretory activity of the gonadotrope and that insulin deficiency results in a state of hypo-gonadotropic anovulation.

IX. CONCLUSION

The present studies demonstrate the direct hormonal modulation of gonadotropin production in a primary culture of anterior pituitary cells.

TABLE I

Effect of Treatment with Epidermal Growth Factor and Fibroblast Growth Factor on Basal and GnRH-Stimulated Release of LH by Cultured Anterior Pituitary Cells

GnRH dose (M)	LH production (μg/culture)		
	Control	EGF	FGF
0	0.18 ± 0.02	0.12 ± 0.03	0.14 ± 0.03
10^{-11}	0.17 ± 0.04	0.22 ± 0.02	—
10^{-10}	0.83 ± 0.13	0.81 ± 0.05	0.57 ± 0.09
10^{-9}	1.31 ± 0.07	1.33 ± 0.04	1.24 ± 0.08
10^{-8}	1.90 ± 0.31	1.57 ± 0.12	1.63 ± 0.15
10^{-7}	1.94 ± 0.22	1.79 ± 0.10	1.75 ± 0.07
10^{-6}	2.00 ± 0.17	1.97 ± 0.21	1.79 ± 0.10

The releases of LH and FSH are under the diverse control of GnRH, various ovarian factors (i.e., steroids, inhibin-like factor) and insulin. Although these studies do not preclude hypothalamic involvement in the regulation of gonadotropin release, a distinct pituitary component is clearly operative. Further studies on the direct control of gonadotropin secretion by various hormones and their mechanism of action at the pituitary level should provide further insight into the control of gonadal functions under both physiological and pathological conditions. It is anticipated that the improved understanding of the regulation of pituitary gonadotropin release will provide a basis for elucidating the basic mechanism of cell secretion and release of peptides.

ACKNOWLEDGMENT

Work from this laboratory was supported by NIH Grant HD-14084 and HD-12303. A. J. W. Hsueh is the recipient of Research Career Development Award HD-00375. Eli Y. Adashi was a Research Fellow in Reproductive Endocrinology and is presently at the Department of Obstetrics and Gynecology, University of Maryland School of Medicine and Hospital, Baltimore, MD 21201. We thank Kayle Watts for typing the manuscript and Linda Tucker and Cheryl Fabics for technical help.

REFERENCES

Adashi, E., Hsueh, A. J. W., and Yen, S. S. C. (1980). Alterations induced by clomiphene in the concentrations of oestrogen receptors in the uterus, pituitary gland, and hypothalamus of female rats. *J. Endocrinol.* **87**, 383–392.

Adashi, E. Y., Hsueh, A. J. W., Bambino, T. H., and Yen, S. S. C. (1981a). Disparate effects of clomiphene and tamoxifen on pituitary gonadotropin release *in vitro*. *Am. J. Physiol: Endocrinol. Metab.* **240**, E125–E130.

Adashi, E. Y., Hsueh, A. J. W., and Yen, S. S. C. (1981b). Insulin enhancement of LH and FSH release by cultured pituitary cells. *Endocrinology (Baltimore)* **108**, 1441–1449.

Aiyer, M. S., Chiappa, S. A., and Fink, G. (1974). A priming effect of luteinizing releasing factor on the anterior pituitary gland in the female rat. *J. Endocrinol. (London)* **62**, 573–588.

Anderson, J. N., Clark, J. H., and Peck, E. J. (1973). Nuclear receptor estrogen complex: Accumulation, retention, and localization in the hypothalamus and pituitary. *Endocrinology (Baltimore)* **93**, 711–717.

Amoss, M., Burgus, R., Blackwell, R., Vale, W., Fellows, R., and Guillemin, R. (1971). Purification, amino acid composition, and N-terminus of the hypothalamic luteinizing hormone releasing factor of ovine origin. *Biochem. Biophys. Res. Commun.* **44**, 205–210.

Arimura, A., and Schally, A. V. (1971). Augmentation of pituitary responsiveness to LH-releasing hormone by estrogen. *Proc. Soc. Exp. Biol. Med.* **136**, 290–293.

Baker, H. W. G., Bremner, W. J., Burger, H. G., Dekretser, D. M., Dulmanis, A., Eddie, L. W., Hudson, B., Keogh, E. J., Lee, V. W. K., and Rennie, G. C. (1976). Testicular control of follicle-stimulating hormone secretion. *Recent Prog. Horm. Res.* **32**, 429–476.

Channabasavaiah, K., Alvarez, E., Stewart, J. M., and Bowers, C. Y. (1979). New potent agonist and antagonist analogs of luteinizing hormone releasing hormone. *Pept., Proc. Am. Pept. Symp., 6th*, pp. 803–806.

Clark, J. H., Anderson, J. N., and Peck, E. J. (1974). Oestrogen receptors and antagonism of steroid hormone action. *Nature (London)* **251**, 446–448.

Clark, J. H., Paszko, Z., and Peck, E. J. (1977). Nuclear binding and retention of the receptor estrogen complex: Relation to the agonistic and antagonistic properties of estriol. *Endocrinology (Baltimore)* **100**, 91–96.

Coy, D. H., Mezo, I., Pedroza, E., Nekola, Z., Vilchez, P., Piyachaturawat, P., Schally, A. V., Seprodi, J., and Teplan, I. (1979). LHRH antagonist with potent antiovulatory activity. *Pept., Proc. Am. Pept. Symp., 6th*, pp. 775–779.

Davies, J. I., Naftolin, F., Ryan, K. J., Fishman, J., and Siu, J. (1975). The affinity of catechol estrogens for estrogen receptors in the pituitary and anterior hypothalamus of the rat. *Endocrinology (Baltimore)* **97**, 554–557.

DeJong, F. H., and Sharpe, R. M. (1976). Evidence for inhibin-like activity in bovine follicular fluid. *Nature (London)* **263**, 71–72.

DeVane, G. M., Czekala, N. M., Judd, H. L., and Yen, S. S. C. (1974). Circulating gonadotropins, estrogens, and androgens in polycystic ovarian disease. *Am. J. Obstet. Gynecol.* **38**, 476–486.

Döcke, R (1969). Ovulation-inducing action of clomiphene citrate in the rat. *J. Reprod. Fertil.* **18**, 135–137.

Drouin, J., and Labrie, F. (1976). Selective effect of androgens on LH and FSH release in anterior pituitary cells in culture. *Endocrinology (Baltimore)* **98**, 1528–1534.

Drouin, J., Lagase, L., and Labrie, F. (1976). Estradiol induced increase of the LH responsiveness to LHRH in rat anterior pituitary cells in culture. *Endocrinology (Baltimore)* **99**, 1477–1483.

Eisenfeld, A. J., and Axelrod, J. (1967). Evidence for estradiol binding sites in the hypothalamus—effect of drugs. *Biochem. Pharmacol.* **16**, 1781–1785.

Erickson, G. F., and Hsueh, A. J. W. (1978). Secretion of "inhibin" by rat granulosa cells *in vitro*. *Endocrinology (Baltimore)* **103**, 1960–1963.

Fishman, J. (1977). The catechol estrogens. *Neuroendocrinology* **22**, 363–374.

Franchimont, P. (1972). Human gonadotropin secretion. *J. R. Coll. Physic. (London)* **6**, 283–298.

Goodman, A. L., and Neill, J. D. (1976). Ovarian regulation of postcoital gonadotropin release in the rabbit: Reexamination of a functional role for 20α-dihydroxy-progesterone. *Endocrinology (Baltimore)* **99**, 852–860.

Gordon, J. M., Sitteri, P. K., and MacDonald, P. C. (1973). Source of estrogen production in the postmenopausal woman. *J. Clin. Endocrinol. Metab.* **36**, 207–214.

Greeley, G., H., Allen, M. B., and Mahesh, V. B. (1975). Potentiation of luteinizing hormone release by estradiol at the level of the pituitary. *Neuroendocrinology* **18**, 233–241.

Greenblatt, R. B. (1962). Chemical induction of ovulation. *Fertil. Steril.* **12**, 402–404.

Hilliard, J., Penardi, R., and Sawyer, C. H. (1967). A functional role for 20α-dihydroxy-pregn-4-en-3-one in the rabbit. *Endocrinology (Baltimore)* **80**, 901–909.

Hsueh, A. J. W., Erickson, G. F., and Yen, S. S. C. (1978). Sensitisation of pituitary cells to luteinising hormone releasing hormone by clomiphene citrate *in vitro*. *Nature (London)* **273**, 57–59.

Hsueh, A. J. W., Erickson, G. F., and Yen, S. S. C. (1979). The sensitizing effect of estrogens and catechol estrogen on cultured pituitary cells to luteinizing hormone-releasing hormone: Its antagonism by progestins. *Endocrinology (Baltimore)* **104**, 807–813.

Isaksson, O., Nutting, D. F., Kostyo, J. L., and Reagan, C. R. (1978). Hourly variations in plasma concentrations of growth hormone and insulin and in amino acid uptake and incorporation into protein in diaphragm muscle of the rat. *Endocrinology (Baltimore)* **102**, 1420–1428.

Jaffe, R. B., and Keye, W. R. (1974). Estradiol augmentation of pituitary responsiveness to gonadotropin-releasing hormone in women. *J. Clin. Endocrinol. Metab.* **39**, 850–855.

Kahwanago, I., Heinrichs, W. L., and Hermann, W. L. (1970). Estradiol "receptors" in hypothalamus and anterior pituitary gland: Inhibition of estradiol binding by SH-group blocking agents and clomiphene citrate. *Endocrinology (Baltimore)* **86**, 1319–1326.

Kalra, P. S., Fawcett, C. P., Krulich, L., and McCann, S. M. (1973). The effects of gonadal steroids on plasma gonadotropins and prolactin in the rat. *Endocrinology (Baltimore)* **92**, 1256–1268.

Kato, J., and Dnouchi, T. (1977). Specific progesterone receptors in the hypothalamus and anterior hypophysis of the rat. *Endocrinology (Baltimore)* **101**, 920–928.

Kato, J., Kobáyashi, T., and Ville, C. (1968). Effect of clomiphene on the uptake of estradiol by the anterior hypothalamus and hypophysis. *Endocrinology (Baltimore)* **82**, 1049–1052.

Keogh, E. J., Lee, V. W. K., Rennie, G. C., Burger, H. G., Hudson, B., and Dekretser, D. M. (1976). Selective suppression of FSH by testicular extracts. *Endocrinology (Baltimore)* **98**, 997–1004.

Kirchick, H. J., Keyes, P. L., and Frye, B. E. (1978). Biology of anovulation in the immature alloxan-diabetic rat treated with pregnant mare's serum gonadotropin: Absence of the preovulatory luteinizing hormone surge. *Endocrinology (Baltimore)* **102**, 1867–1873.

Kirchick, H. J., Keyes, P. L., and Frye, B. E. (1979). An explanation for anovulation in immature alloxan-diabetic rats treated with pregnant mare's serum gonadotropin: Reduced pituitary response to gonadotropin-releasing hormone. *Endocrinology (Baltimore)* **105**, 1343–1349.

Klopper, A., and Hall, M. (1971). New synthetic agent for the induction of ovulation: Preliminary trials in women. *Br. Med. J.* **1**, 152–154.

Labrie, F., Drouin, J., Ferland, L., Lagace, L., Beaulieu, M., DeLean, A., Kelly, P. A., Caron, M. G., and Raymond, V. (1978). Mechanism of action of hypothalamic hormones in the anterior pituitary gland and specific modulation of their activity by sex steroids and thyroid hormones. *Recent Prog. Horm. Res.* **34**, 25–93.

Lasley, B. L., Wang, C. F., and Yen, S. S. C. (1975). The effects of estrogen and progesterone on the functional capacity of the gonadotrophs. *J. Clin. Endocrinol. Metab.* **41**, 820–831.

Luttage, W. G., and Wallis, C. J. (1973). *In Vitro* accumulation and saturation of ^{3}H-progestins in selected brain regions and in the adenohypophysis, uterus and pineal gland of the female rat. *Steroids* **22**, 493–502.

McCann, S. M., (1962). Effect of progesterone on plasma luteinizing hormone activity. *Am. J. Physiol.* **202**, 601–604.

McCullagh, G. R. (1932). Dual endocrine activity of the testes. *Science* **76**, 19–20.

Marder, M. L., Channing, C. P., and Schwartz, N. R. (1977). Suppression of serum follicle stimulating hormone in intact and acutely ovariectomized rats by porcine follicular fluid. *Endocrinology (Baltimore)* **101**, 1639–1642.

Martucci, C., and Fishman, J. (1977). Direction of estradiol metabolism as a control of its hormone action-uterotrophic activity of estradiol metabolites. *Endocrinology (Baltimore)* **101**, 1709–1715.

Naess, O., Attramadal, A., and Aakvaag, A. (1975). Androgen binding proteins in the anterior pituitary, hypothalamus, preoptic area, and brain cortex of the rat. *Endocrinology (Baltimore)* **96**, 1–9.

Nallar, R., Antunes-Rodriguez, J., and McCann, S. M. (1966). Effect of progesterone on the level of plasma luteinizing hormone in normal female rats. *Endocrinology (Baltimore)* **79**, 907–911.

Nillius, S. J., and Wide, L. (1971). Effects of progesterone on the serum levels of FSH and LH in postmenopausal women treated with estrogen. *Acta Endocrinol. (Copenhagen)* **67**, 362–370.

Notides, A. C. (1970). Binding affinity and specificity of the estrogen receptor of the rat uterus and anterior pituitary. *Endocrinology (Baltimore)* **87**, 987–992.

O'Dell, W. D., and Swerdloff, R. S. (1968). Progesterone induced luteinizing and follicle-stimulating hormone surge in postmenopausal women: A simulated ovulatory peak. *Proc. Natl. Acad. Sci. U.S.A.* **61**, 529–536.

O'Malley, B. W., and Means, A. R. (1974). Female steroid hormones and target cell nuclei. *Science* **183**, 610–620.

Paz, G., Homonnai, Z. T., Drasnin, N., Sofer, A., Kaplan, R., and Kraicer, P. F. (1978). Fertility of the streptozocin-diabetic male rat. *Andrologia* **10**, 127–136.

Ross, G. T., Cargille, C. M., Lipsett, M. B., Rayford, P. L., Marshall, J. R., Strott, C. A., and Rodbard, D. (1970). Pituitary and gonadal hormones in women during spontaneous and induced ovulatory cycles. *Recent Prog. Horm. Res.* **26**, 1–62.

Roy, S., Mahesh, V. B., and Greenblatt, R. B. (1970). Effects of clomiphene on the physiology of reproduction in the rat. *Acta Endocrinol. (Copenhagen)* **47**, 669–675.

Sandow, J., Konig, W., Geiger, R., Uhmann, R., and von Rechenberg, W. (1978). Structure-activity relationship in the LH-RH molecule. *In* "Control of Ovulation" (D. B. Crighton, G. R. Foxcroft N. B. Haynes, and G. E. Lamming, eds.), pp. 49–69. Butterworths, London.

Schally, A. V., Arimura, A., Kastin, A., Matsuo, H., Baba, Y., Redding, T., Nair, R., Debeljuk, L., and White, W. (1971). Gonadotropin releasing hormone with one polypeptide regulates secretion of luteinizing and follicle stimulating hormones. *Science* **173**, 1036–1038.

Seiki, K., and Hattori, M. (1973). *In vivo* uptake of progesterone by the hypothalamus and pituitary of the female ovariectomized rat and its relationship to cytoplasmic progesterone-binding protein. *Endocrinol. Jpn.* **20**, 111–119.

Setchell, B. P., and Jacks, F. (1974). Inhibin-like activity in rete testis fluid. *J. Endocrinol.* **62**, 675–676.

Sutherland, R., Mester, J., and Baulieu, E. M., (1977). Tamoxifen is a potent "pure" anti-oestrogen in chick oviduct. *Nature (London)* **267**, 434–435.

Tannenbaum, G. S., Martin, J. B., and Colle, E. (1976). Ultradian growth hormone rhythm in the rat: Effects of feeding, hyperglycemia, and insulin-induced hypoglycemia. *Endocrinology (Baltimore)* **99**, 720–727.

Vaitukaitis, J. L., Bermudez, J. A., Cargille, C. M., Lippsett, M. B., and Ross, G. T. (1971). New evidence for an anti-estrogenic action of clomiphene citrate in women. *J. Clin. Endocrinol. Metab.* **32**, 503–508.

Vale, W., Grant, G., Amoss, M., Blackwell, R., and Guillemin, R. (1972). Culture of enzymatically dispersed anterior pituitary cells: Functional validation of a method. *Endocrinology (Baltimore)* **91**, 562–572.

Vale, W., Rivier, C., Brown, M., Leppaluoto, J., Ling, N., Monahan, M., and Rivier, J. (1976). Pharmacology of hypothalamic regulatory peptides. *Clin. Endocrinol. (Oxford)* **5**, Suppl., 261s–273s.

Vandenberg, G., and Yen, S. S. C. (1973). Effect of anti-estrogenic action of clomiphene during the menstrual cycle: Evidence for a change in the feedback sensitivity. *J. Clin. Endocrinol. Metab.* **37**, 356–365.

Yen, S. S. C., Vandenberg, G., and Siler, T. M. (1974). Modulation of pituitary responsiveness to LRF by estrogen. *J. Clin. Endocrinol. Metab.* **39**, 170–177.

16

Mechanisms of Regulation of Prolactin Release

PRISCILLA S. DANNIES AND S. WILLIAM TAM

I. BASAL PROLACTIN RELEASE

Mechanisms that regulate prolactin release have been investigated using a variety of methods including morphological, biochemical, electrophysiological, and pharmacological studies. The results of some of these studies and the conclusions that can be drawn from them are discussed in this chapter, beginning with what we know about basal prolactin release.

A. Processing and Release of Prolactin

The anterior pituitary gland contains several different kinds of cells that secrete hormones; these cells were characterized first by chemical stains and later by morphology using the electron microscope (Far-

529

quhar, 1977). Prolactin cells contain rows of rough endoplasmic reticulum, a Golgi zone, and several morphologically distinct types of secretory granules: small granules, irregularly shaped larger granules, and large rounded granules. The size of these large granules has been used as a criterion for identifying prolactin-producing cells. These cells have the largest secretory granules of all the cells of the rat pituitary gland; the granules can range from 500 to 900 nm in diameter. Recently immunocytochemical stains for prolactin have been developed. Use of these stains has revealed that some smaller cells that lack the large granules also stain for prolactin, although large granules exist only in prolactin-producing cells (Baker, 1970; Tougard *et al.*, 1980). Therefore, mammotrophs in the pituitary gland show some heterogeneity of morphology.

Prolactin is synthesized on the membranes of the rough endoplasmic reticulum (Biswas and Tashjian, 1974). The hormone is made in a precursor form larger than the final product (Evans and Rosenfeld, 1976; Maurer *et al.*, 1976; Dannies and Tashjian, 1976a; see also Chapter 8). Prolactin is similar to most other secreted proteins in that the precursor is larger because it contains a leader sequence that inserts the nascent polypeptide chain into the membranes. (The structure and function of the signal peptide is discussed in Chapter 9 in this volume.) Blobel and his colleagues used the synthesis of prolactin as a model system to study the processing of proteins by membranes during synthesis. They found that if membranes are present while prolactin is synthesized in a cell-free system, then prolactin becomes resistant to degradation by trypsin, because it is transported through the membranes. Membranes added after prolactin is synthesized do not have this protective effect; therefore, transport cccurs only during synthesis (Lingappa *et al.*, 1977). Walter and Blobel (1980) demonstrated the presence of a factor that gives the membranes the capacity to translocate prolactin; removal of this factor from the membranes makes them inactive, and when added back, reconstitutes activity. In addition, the presence of microsomal fractions in a cell-free system processes preprolactin into the mature form (Jackson and Blobel, 1977; Lingappa *et al.*, 1977).

The precursor of prolactin is rapidly cleaved into prolactin in the intact cell, so that preprolactin is only detectable using short labeling periods, and the precursor form is not found in the secretory granules. Maurer and McKean (1978) found detectable preprolactin after only a 3-minute incubation with radioactive leucine, and most of the label is in prolactin even after this short time. Preprolactin accumulates in pituitary glands when they are incubated with the threonine analog βhydroxynorvaline (Hortin and Boime, 1980). Although preprolactin accumulates in the presence of this analog, only prolactin, and not preprolactin, is secreted from the cell. The substitution for threonine may simply slow down the processing of the prohormone enough to enable detection in the cell. Alternative explanations are that the polypeptides containing the analog are unstable and are selectively broken down before release or that the packaging may be selective so that only the mature form is processed for release, whereas the rest is eventually degraded.

The course of prolactin through the cell after synthesis on the membranes of the rough endoplasmic reticulum was studied by Farquhar *et al.* (1978), using autoradiographic studies of tritiated leucine incorporation. Pituitary glands from estrogen-treated rats incorporate radioactive amino acids primarily into prolactin, and cultured cells from such glands also incorporate amino acids primarily into prolactin (Hopkins and Farquhar, 1973). Therefore, the location in the cell of incorporated tritiated leucine is mainly the site of the newly synthesized prolactin. Farquhar *et al.* (1978) incubated dispersed cells from the glands of estrogen-treated female rats with radioactive leucine for 5 minutes, at which time the tritiated leucine is mainly associated with the rough endoplasmic reticulum. Fifteen minutes after this 5-minute labeling period, autoradiographic grains are located over elements of the Golgi zone, and there are a few grains in secretory granules. One hour after the 5-minute labeling period, the amount of radioactivity in the granules increases and continues to increase for the next 2 hours. Small granules and irregularly shaped granules have more radioactivity at early times; at later times (2 to 3 hours after the pulse), the large rounded granules are labeled, indicating that these are formed after the smaller granules.

Biochemical studies using continuous labeling give results that are consistent with the results of the autoradiographic studies. Labeled prolactin of primary cells in culture begins to appear in the medium after 1 hour of incubation and in large quantities after 2 hours (Dannies and Rudnick, 1980; Maurer, 1980). GH cells (clonal strains of rat pituitary tumor cells that secrete prolactin and growth hormone) (Tashjian *et al.*, 1970) contain only a few small secretory granules (Tixier-Vidal, 1975). Labeled prolactin is released from GH cells in large amounts more quickly than from normal cells under the same culture conditions; the labeled prolactin is secreted into the medium in large amounts beginning at 45 minutes after the addition of tritiated leucine (Dannies *et al.*, 1976; Kiino and Dannies, 1981). Newly synthesized prolactin can be secreted faster under some culture conditions;

Walker and Farquhar (1980) found that radioactive prolactin is released from normal cultures of cells after 15 minutes of exposure to the label, and Stachura (1982a) found that radioactive prolactin is released from perfused GH cells within 15 minutes. Variations in culture conditions, not yet identified, may account for changes in time of transit through the cell.

Swearingen (1971) showed that pituitary glands that incorporate [^{3}H]leucine secrete prolactin with a higher specific activity than that of the prolactin that remains in the glands, indicating that newly synthesized prolactin is preferentially released. These results have been repeated using ^{3}H and ^{14}C labels in addition to specific activity to distinguish newly synthesized prolactin from older prolactin (Walker and Farquhar, 1980). Therefore, biochemical studies showed that some of the prolactin synthesized by the cells is secreted within a few hours, and some is stored. What determines whether the newly synthesized prolactin is stored or secreted is not known. We showed in GH cells that the amount of prolactin stored can be increased by insulin and estrogen, independently of effects on prolactin synthesis (Kiino and Dannies, 1981), indicating that the amount of storage can be regulated.

Cells obviously do not have to process prolactin into the large round granules to release the hormone because GH cells do not have this granular form and because, as previously mentioned, not all prolactin-producing cells in the pituitary gland have these types of granules. The large granules appear to be a form of stored prolactin that accumulates when cells are not secreting at a rapid rate. Rats that are continually suckling and therefore releasing large amounts of prolactin do not contain many mature large granules in the cells. If secretion is stopped by eliminating suckling, the large forms accumulate (Smith and Farquhar, 1966; Shiino et al., 1972).

Heterogeneity in the incorporation of tritiated leucine into prolactin also has been seen, in addition to the morphological heterogeneity already mentioned. Walker and Farquhar (1980) counted the total number of grains over each cell and found that the distribution of grains does not correspond to a single rate of leucine incorporation. Thirty minutes after a 5-minute labeling period, the cells fall into three groups: a lightly labeled group, an intermediate group, and a heavily labeled group. Two and three hours after the labeling period, there are only the lightly labeled and the intermediate cells. There are several possible explanations for this heterogeneity. First, one group of cells may synthesize more prolactin than the other cells and release most of it; this group would be the heavily labeled group at 30 minutes and would disappear by 2 hours. The intermediate and lightly labeled cells would store most of what they synthesize. Second, all cells may release prolactin, but only the cells that are more actively synthesizing prolactin store the hormone. In this model, all three groups of cells lose label after incorporation; the lightly labeled cells lose all of the label, and the heavy and intermediate group become more lightly labeled. Third, the cells may synthesize and release prolactin at similar rates but may differ in the transport of leucine or in the size of the intracellular leucine pools which would cause the specific activity of intracellular leucine to vary from cell to cell.

These models can be distinguished if the heterogeneous cells can be physically separated. Hymer *et al.* (1974) reported sedimentation profiles of mammotrophs in concentration gradients of bovine serum albumin. The sedimentation properties vary, depending on the source of the pituitary glands. Cells from lactating rats that have not suckled for 10 hours, and therefore should contain more large secretory granules, sediment faster than cells from rats that have been constantly suckling, and therefore should be depleted of granules. Snyder *et al.* (1976) showed that mammotrophs from different fractions of the gradient do not secrete the same amounts of prolactin when put into culture. It will be of interest to see whether there is a consistent variation in the morphology of these fractions and whether the rate of prolactin synthesis, the time of its release, and the response to various releasing factors vary with the morphology. Denef (1980) reported differences in the responses of gonadotropin fractions and proposed that these differences may correlate with various morphological types found among the gonadotropin cells. Similar events may occur in prolactin-producing cells.

Prolactin is tightly packaged in the mature forms of the secretory granules; Farquhar *et al.* (1978) estimate that prolactin in the mature granules is 50–150 times more concentrated than prolactin in the rough endoplasmic reticulum, based on relative grain density after autoradiography. Once packaged, the contents of the granules are relatively stable; the inner cores remain visible by electron microscopy after the surrounding membranes are removed by detergent treatment, and intact and membraneless granules are stable at low pH (Giannattasio *et al.*, 1975). Purified prolactin granules contain macromolecules that were labeled with [^{35}S]sulfate and digested with proteolytic enzymes (Giannattasio and Zanini, 1976). These molecules are associated with the inner core of the granules after the membrane is removed and so appear to be different from the membrane components (Giannattasio and Zanini, 1976; Slaby and Farquhar, 1980). The function of these molecules and the mechanisms by which prolactin is concentrated in the granules are not yet understood.

Prolactin granules are released from the cell membrane by exocytosis, that is, fusion of the granule membrane to the outer membrane of the cells to release the contents. This process has been observed by electron microscopy by a number of laboratories (see Farquhar, 1977, for a review). If the granules are not released, they may be digested by lysosomes—a process termed crinophagy. This process was demonstrated by Smith and Farquhar (1966). Suckling rats, which synthesize large amounts of prolactin, show a sudden drop in the release of prolactin when deprived of their young. Mature secretory granules accumulate in the prolactin-producing cells for 12 hours. At later times, lysosomes that contain the secretory granule inner cores are seen. Therefore, the cells can remove excess granules by digesting them. Lysosomes containing granule contents are seen less frequently in cells from normal glands.

Degradation of prolactin can be measured biochemically in two ways. One method is to follow the incorporation of amino acids with time; if the rate of accumulation of radioactivity in prolactin decreases with time, newly synthesized prolactin may be getting degraded. The second method is to follow the stability of prolactin that has been previously labeled with radioactive amino acids (if precautions are taken to avoid further incorporation of radioactivity into prolactin). Using both methods, we found no evidence for degradation of prolactin under the conditions we normally use, either in GH cells or in normal cells in cultures (Dannies and Tashjian, 1973; Dannies and Rudnick, 1980); however, in other conditions, degradation does occur and is detectable by both methods. Maurer (1980) found that degradation of prolactin occurs in normal cells in culture. Shenai and Wallis (1979) showed degradation of newly synthesized prolactin in isolated pituitary glands. The degradation of prolactin was specific because growth hormone was not degraded in the same experiments. These experiments indicate that studies in the literature that use long labeling periods to measure prolactin synthesis may actually be measuring a combination of synthesis and degradation.

B. Mechanisms That Control Basal Release

Two factors, calcium and cyclic AMP, have been postulated for years to be involved in prolactin release, and over the last decade a number of laboratories have investigated the role of these compounds.

1. *Calcium*

Douglas (1968) proposed a general model for the role of calcium in secretion from neuronal, exocrine, and endocrine cells. According to this model, depolarization of the cell membrane leads to a calcium influx; the increased intracellular concentrations of calcium trigger hormone release. Several types of observations suggest that this model is true for prolactin release. The first is that calcium in the medium stimulates hormone release. This stimulatory effect of calcium, compared to release in medium with low calcium, was demonstrated in anterior pituitary glands in culture (MacLeod and Fontham, 1970; Parsons, 1970; Wakabayashi *et al.*, 1973) and in dispersed cells from normal pituitary glands (Tam and Dannies, 1981b). Basal release from GH cells does not always appear to be calcium sensitive; Ostlund *et al.* (1978) saw little effect of extracellular calcium after a 10-minute incubation period, and Gautvik and Tashjian (1973) saw no effect on basal release for at least 2 hours. However, Moriarty and Leuschen (1981) and Gautvik and co-workers (1980) saw basal release from GH cells that is dependent on extracellular calcium during a 30-minute incubation. Part of the reason for the variation in results may be caused by the variation of trace quantities of calcium present in buffer or medium; Walker and Hopkins (1978) found 0.2 mM calcium ion (by atomic absorption) in "calcium-free" buffer. In general, basal prolactin release is reduced when calcium in the medium is lowered.

The second type of evidence is that depolarization of the cell membrane by high potassium concentrations causes release of prolactin. Milligan and Kraicer (1970) found that pituitary cells are depolarized by high concentrations of potassium. High potassium levels increase the total calcium concentration in pituitary halves and in GH cells (Eto *et al.*, 1974; Moriarty and Leuschen, 1981) and increase $^{45}Ca^{2+}$ uptake by pituitary halves (Eto *et al.*, 1974). High potassium levels release prolactin from GH cells, and this stimulated release requires the presence of calcium in the medium (Tashjian *et al.*, 1978; Ostlund *et al.*, 1978). An increase in potassium levels was originally reported to have little or no effect on prolactin release from pituitary halves (Parsons, 1970; MacLeod and Fontham, 1970), but later experiments showed that high potassium concentrations cause prolactin release from pituitary halves and dispersed cells in culture and that this release is dependent on the presence of calcium (Wakabayashi *et al.*, 1973; Nakano *et al.*, 1976; Tam and Dannies, 1981a).

The third type of evidence is based on the use of divalent cation ionophores, which can carry calcium through membranes. We showed that A23187 (a commonly used divalent cation ionophore) increases the uptake of $^{45}Ca^{2+}$ in cultures of dispersed pituitary glands (Tam and Dannies, 1980). This ionophore stimulates the release of prolactin from monolayer cultures of anterior pituitary glands and from GH cells (Tam and Dannies, 1980; Gautvik et al., 1980). There is no stimulation of release if calcium is not added to the buffer or if calcium is added together with EGTA. Thorner et al. (1980) obtained different results using perfused columns of freshly dispersed cells. They reported that there is no stimulation caused by the two divalent cation ionophores A23187 and X537A in the presence of calcium; they only saw stimulation in medium to which calcium is not added, when basal prolactin release occurs at a lower level. The difference between the two sets of results may be based on the amount of basal release. If the perfused cells are releasing prolactin at a fully stimulated rate and monolayer cultures are not, then increased calcium will only affect the monolayer cultures. The difference in the ability of ionophore to release prolactin in the absence of added calcium may be due to differences in the stores of intracellular calcium. (Ionophore-induced release of intracellular calcium is presumably what causes prolactin release in the absence of external calcium.) In any case, the ability of several laboratories to obtain ionophore-induced prolactin release under some conditions is consistent with a role of calcium in prolactin release.

Another type of evidence for the involvement of calcium in prolactin release comes from electrophysiological studies. Kidokoro (1975) first reported that GH cells have spontaneous action potentials. Since then several other laboratories have seen action potentials in GH cells (Biales et al., 1977; Dufy et al., 1979a; Ozawa and Kimura, 1979; Taraskevich and Douglas, 1980; Chapter 4) and in dispersed cells from pituitary glands (Taraskevich and Douglas, 1977). Some, but not all, reported evidence for sodium involvement in the action potential, although all laboratories found evidence for calcium involvement. This evidence came from the use of several different drugs. Lanthanum and cobalt (calcium antagonists) block action potentials in GH cells (Kidokoro, 1975; Ozawa and Kimura, 1979) and in normal cells (Taraskevich and Douglas, 1977). Methoxyverapamil (D600), which inhibits voltage-dependent calcium channels, blocks the frequency of the action potentials immediately after its addition in GH cells (Dufy et al., 1979a; Taraskevich and Douglas, 1980) and in normal cells (Taraskevich and Douglas, 1977). Therefore, calcium can enter the cell through action potentials; and it was proposed that such entry triggered prolactin release.

If the entry of calcium through the voltage-dependent calcium channel is the cause of basal release, then calcium channel blockers should blcok basal prolactin release. Several laboratories have tested this hypothesis using the calcium antagonists cobalt, verapamil and methoxyverapamil. These three substances can block the voltage-dependent calcium channel. Tashjian *et al.* (1978) found that 2 mM cobalt reduces basal release to 50–65% of control values in GH cells, but Tan and Tashjian (1981) found that 4 mM cobalt does not reduce basal release, and Ozawa and Kimura found that 2 mM cobalt causes less than a 10% reduction in basal release from GH cells. Thorner and co-workers (1980) have shown that methoxyverapamil causes inhibition of prolactin release from perfused cells; release is reduced to about 65% of control values after 15 minutes. Methoxyverapamil may also block sodium channels, but they saw no effect with tetrodotoxin, which blocks some sodium channels, and therefore they concluded that the sodium channel is not involved. We have found similar results. Verapamil has no significant effect after 10 minutes of incubation, but does produce a 45% decrease in basal prolactin release from cultures of normal cells after 1 hour of incubation (S. W. Tam and P. S. Dannies, unpublished results). Stachura (1982b) found that several doses of verapamil gradually inhibit basal prolactin release from perfused pituitary glands. In contrast to these results, Moriarty and Leuschen (1981) saw no significant inhibition of basal release in one experiment using GH cells and a 30-minute incubation period with methoxyverapamil. More extensive experiments may reveal the causes for the discrepancies. Some questions need to be answered: (1) Do calcium antagonists block prolactin release at concentrations and times consistent with the electrophysiological block of channels? (2) Does the inhibition occur as the result of blocking channels, or through some other toxic side effect? (3) Under what conditions is release independent of the calcium channels?

In summary, several types of evidence indicate a role for calcium in basal release, and calcium can enter the cells through action potentials. It is not yet clear whether calcium entry by this means is always involved in basal prolactin release.

Many effects of calcium have been shown to be mediated through calmodulin; some of these effects are discussed in Chapters 13 and 14 of this book. If calmodulin is involved in prolactin release, inhibitors of the calcium activation of calmodulin should inhibit prolactin release. Some antipsychotic drugs are effective inhibitors of calmodulin activation (Levin and Weiss, 1978). We found that antipsychotic drugs such as butaclamol, haloperidol, and pimozide inhibited prolactin release by a mechanism that does not involve the dopamine receptor (West and Dannies, 1979). These compounds also inhibit calmodulin activation (Levin and Weiss, 1978; Norman and Drummond, 1979). Stereospecificity with the isomers of butaclamol does not exist for either inhibition of prolactin release or inhibition of calmodulin activation (West and Dannies, 1979; Norman and Drummond, 1979). Therefore, a possible mechanism for the inhibition of prolactin release may be the inhibition of calmodulin activation, but there are other possibilities. Fleckman and co-workers (1981) showed that trifluorperazine (a calmodulin inhibitor) inhibits calcium uptake by pituitary glands. This effect might prevent release. If the concentrations of a series of drugs required to inhibit prolactin release correspond to the concentrations of the drugs that inactivate calmodulin, then this correlation would provide support for the role of calmodulin in prolactin release. A study using five drugs has been done by Conn et al. (1981), who showed a reasonable correlation of inhibition of LH release with calmodulin binding properties.

The effect of extracellular calcium on prolactin release from normal perfused cells is biphasic. Thorner and his colleagues (1980) found that prolactin release is inhibited by 10 mM calcium even though lower concentrations stimulate release. Stachura (1982b) found that 5.4 mM calcium inhibits basal prolactin release. It is not known whether this inhibitory effect occurs in GH cells. This information would be of interest because several of the electrophysiological studies with GH cells used 10 mM calcium in the recording solution (Kidokoro, 1975; Taraskevich and Douglas, 1980; Dufy et al., 1980). At present nothing is known about the mechanism of the inhibitory effect.

2. Cyclic AMP

There is less agreement about the role of cAMP in basal prolactin release than there is about the role of calcium. The role of cAMP has been tested by adding agents that increase cAMP or that are cAMP analogs. There are several categories of such agents.

1. Compounds that inhibit phosphodiesterases (the enzymes that degrade cAMP) cause intracellular cAMP levels to rise. Theophylline and isobutylmethylxanthine are two such compounds commonly used, and these compounds have been found to increase prolactin release from GH cells (Dannies et al., 1976), from dispersed cells in culture (Naor et al., 1980; Tam and Dannies, 1981b), and from pituitary halves in culture (Wakabayashi et al., 1973). On the other hand, Thorner and co-workers (1980) saw no stimulation by theophylline in perfused cells, and several laboratories failed to see reproducible increases using

pituitary halves (Bowers, 1971; Cehovic *et al.*, 1972). Ray and Wallis (1981) saw a slight effect with theophylline but no effect with iso-butylmethylxanthine, even though the latter compound causes a greater increase in cAMP levels. One reservation about studies done with phosphodiesterase inhibitors is that they are known to have a wide variety of effects on cells, some of which are apparently unrelated to the inhibition of phosphodiesterase (Appleman *et al.*, 1973). A stimulatory effect of theophylline on $^{45}Ca^{2+}$ efflux from pancreatic islets has been reported (Brisson and Malaisse, 1973).

2. The second class of compounds comprises analogs of cAMP that can penetrate the cell membrane. Dibutyryl cAMP has been shown to increase prolactin release from GH cells (Dannies *et al.*, 1976; Gautvik *et al.*, 1977), from normal cells that are perfused (Thorner *et al.*, 1980; Stern and Conn, 1981) or in monolayer cultures (Naor *et al.*, 1980), and from pituitary halves (Wakabayashi *et al.*, 1973; Hill *et al.*, 1976). The N^6-monobutyryl derivative of cAMP also stimulated release of prolactin from pituitary halves (Pelletier *et al.*, 1972; Labrie and Lemay, 1972). Several laboratories, however, have not seen reproducible stimulation by dibutyryl cAMP in pituitary halves (Bowers, 1971; Cehovic *et al.*, 1972; Ray and Wallis, 1981). We also looked at another analog, 8-Br-cAMP, and found no effect in GH cells but found stimulation in normal cells in culture (Dannies *et al.*, 1976; Tam and Dannies, 1981b). Ray and Wallis (1981) found that this analog stimulates release from pituitary halves. A reasonable interpretation for the difference in stimulation by these compounds, already suggested by Hill *et al.* (1976), is that the glands may sometimes be maximally stimulated with regard to cAMP-induced secretion, so that further increases of cAMP have no effect, but the interpretation of these studies is confused by two other complications. In one study, butyric acid increased prolactin release from GH cells as effectively as dibutyryl cAMP (Dannies *et al.*, 1976). Other studies showed that sodium butyrate can have many dramatic effects on cells in culture (Prasad and Sinha, 1976). Butyric acid is not always a problem. Naor *et al.* (1980) found a smaller stimulation of prolactin release with butyric acid than with dibutyryl cAMP, and later studies with GH cells showed no effect on prolactin release (Yen and Tashjian, 1981). However, most studies using buty-rated analogs have not included butyric acid controls. A second disturbing factor is that Hill *et al.* (1976) found that adenosine and guanosine stimulates release from pituitary halves. Because of these complications, stimulation by cAMP analogs is not sufficient evidence to prove a role for cAMP.

3. The third way of increasing cAMP concentrations in the cell is to

use cholera toxin. The toxin molecule binds to the cell membrane, and part of the molecule enters the cell, where it activates adenylate cyclase by causing ADP ribosylation and inhibition of a GTPase associated with the cyclase (Moss and Vaughn, 1977; Cassel and Selinger, 1977; Gill and Meren, 1978). This method of increasing cAMP levels may be the most specific; however, the results from various laboratories are still not consistent. We saw stimulation both in GH cells and in normal cells in culture using cholera toxin (Tam and Dannies, 1981b; Dannies and Tashjian, 1980), and we showed that cholera toxin increased cAMP levels in GH cells. Rappaport and Grant (1974) found that prolactin release from normal cells in culture is stimulated by cholera toxin in some, but not all, experiments. Growth hormone-producing cells are much more sensitive to cholera toxin. Thorner *et al.* (1980) found that cholera toxin does not stimulate prolactin release from perfused dispersed cells, and Ray and Wallis (1981) found no stimulation using pituitary halves. Botb of these laboratories showed that cAMP levels increased; however, because growth hormone cells are more sensitive, most of the increase may have been in these cells.

In summary, all of the agents that mimic the action of cAMP can stimulate prolactin release some of the time. It is possible to imagine models involving cAMP that can explain the variation in results. For example, cAMP levels may regulate the amount of release that is triggered by another agent (such as calcium); in such a case, cAMP is necessary for prolactin release but is not the sole factor involved.

3. *Interrelations between Calcium and Cyclic AMP*

The interactions between calcium and cAMP can be varied and complex; Rasmussen and Goodman (1977) discussed examples of the different possibilities. The stimulation of prolactin release by cAMP depends on the presence of calcium. Lemay and Labrie (1972) showed that N^6-monobutyryl cAMP does not stimulate prolactin release from pituitary halves if magnesium ions are substituted for calcium ions. Wakabayashi *et al.* (1973) showed that low calcium levels reduce the stimulatory effect of theophylline on prolactin release from pituitary halves, and we showed that the stimulatory effect of 8-Br-cAMP is greater with 1 mM calcium present than in low-calcium medium (Tam and Dannies, 1981b). Kraicer and co-workers have done a series of experiments on growth hormone release using purified somatotrophs to investigate the relationships between calcium and cAMP. They showed that prostaglandin E_2 and isobutylmethylxanthine both increase intracellular cAMP levels; prostaglandin E_2 stimulates adenylate cyclase activity and isobutylmethylxanthine inhibits phosphodiesterase activity (Sheppard *et al.*, 1979). Both agents cause growth hormone release in the presence of calcium, but in the absence of calcium they do not, although cAMP still accumulates in the cells (Spence *et al.*, 1980). The presence of calcium is not necessary for the increase in cAMP, but it is necessary for the stimulation of release; therefore, calcium is necessary at a step other than the increase in cAMP. Gautvik *et al.* (1980) showed that the increase in cAMP seen in GH cells after TRH is added still occurs in the absence of calcium, but prolactin release does not, indicating that mammotrophs may be similar.

Stachura investigated the interactions of cAMP and calcium in another way—by measuring changes in rate of release of prelabeled growth hormone using perfused glands. He found that high potassium levels trigger a rapid release of growth hormone from perfused pituitary glands (presumably by causing calcium entry); the rate of release returns to basal levels quickly with high potassium. Dibutyryl cAMP also triggers a rapid release and, in addition, causes a longer sustained release (Stachura, 1977). When release is blocked by somatostatin, dibutyryl cAMP causes an increase in the rapidly releasable pool, but high potassium levels do not (Stachura, 1977, 1981). He suggested that cAMP can transfer stores of growth hormone to a rapidly releasable pool, which will accumulate if release is prevented or result in sustained release if release occurs. He found similar effects of dibutyryl cAMP on prolactin release in pituitary glands from female rats (M. E. Stachura, unpublished results). The locations in the cell of the rapidly releasable pool and of the pool that causes sustained release have not been determined.

The events that occur after the increase in calcium or cAMP and that lead to the release of prolactin are not known. The microtubules and contractile proteins may play a part in many secretory systems (Butcher, 1978; and Chapters 6 and 7 in this volume). The evidence that microtubules are involved in secretion is that colchicine (a drug that binds to microtubules) inhibits prolactin release and causes accumulation of intracellular prolactin in GH cells, in normal cultures of pituitary cells, and in pituitary glands (Gautvik and Tashjian, 1973; Labrie *et al.*, 1973; Antakly *et al.*, 1979). If colchicine does not inhibit release through side effects, then microtubules are involved. Use of the electron microscope has not provided any clue as to how microtubules are involved or given strong support to their role (Farquhar, 1977). Therefore, at present, steps that occur after elevation of calcium or cAMP are mainly speculative, using analogies with other systems.

II. COMPOUNDS THAT AFFECT PROLACTIN RELEASE

A. Thyrotropin-Releasing Hormone

Thyrotropin-releasing hormone, or TRH, is a tripeptide that was originally isolated by the laboratories of Guillemin (Burges *et al.*, 1969) and Schally (Bøler *et al.*, 1969). The peptide was isolated on the basis of its ability to stimulate the release of thyrotropin. However, when pure TRH became available, it also was found to stimulate prolactin production from GH cells (Tashjian *et al.*, 1971) and later from normal pituitary cells in culture (Vale *et al.*, 1973).

As discussed in the previous section, some prolactin is stored after synthesis and some is released. It is not surprising that TRH releases the stored prolactin from normal cells in culture, because these cells obviously have large stores of prolactin in the secretory granules. Walker and Farquhar (1980) showed that TRH causes preferential release of stored prolactin but does not affect release of prolactin synthesized within the preceding 2 hours. It is perhaps surprising that TRH also causes release of stored prolactin from GH cells because these cells have few secretory granules, and the ones that they do have are small. We showed that TRH stimulates prolactin release within 10 minutes of its addition to GH cells, but that it does not cause detectable increases in prolactin synthesis for 3 to 4 hours (Dannies and Tashjian, 1974; Dannies *et al.*, 1976). Hoyt and Tashjian (1980) did immunocytochemical studies with GH cells; they showed that the amount of intracellular prolactin in GH cells decreases 0.5 hour after the addition of TRH and does not increase until 3–4 hours later. TRH treatment does not change the time (45 minutes) needed for newly synthesized prolactin to be secreted from GH cells (Dannies *et al.*, 1976); therefore the rapid stimulation of release is not caused by increasing the intracellular transit time of the prolactin that is released and not stored. Stachura (1982a) showed that stimulators of secretion release a stored pool of prolactin in perfused GH cells. The few secretory granules that the GH cells have may account for the TRH-induced release.

The mechanism by which TRH stimulates prolactin release has been investigated by many laboratories. The first step in TRH action is the binding of TRH to the cell (TRH binding studies have been reviewed by Martin and Tashjian, 1977). Investigation of subsequent steps has centered around the two components that may have a role in basal prolactin release—calcium and cAMP.

The role of calcium in TRH-induced release is based on several types of evidence. The first type of evidence comprises the electrophysiological findings. When Kidokoro (1975) found calcium action potentials in GH cells, he also found that TRH increases the spike frequency; an analog of TRH that does not release prolactin does not increase the frequency of the spikes. Similar findings were later reported by others. Taraskevich and Douglas (1980) showed that 10 nM TRH increases the frequency of the action potentials within seconds in GH cells, and 50 nM TRH causes induction of action potentials in normal cells within seconds (Taraskevich and Douglas, 1977). Ozawa and Kimura (1979) and Gautvik et al. (1980) also saw an increase in action potentials within seconds. Dufy et al. (1979a) found that 10 μM TRH increases the firing rate, but only after a lag of several minutes. This lag is apparently not related to the time required for TRH to diffuse to the cells (Dufy et al., 1980), so the reason for the lag in this study is not clear. However, TRH increased the frequency of the action potentials in both studies and therefore presumably increased cytosolic calcium. In addition, Maruyama et al. (1981), working with 2B8 cells, which do not show action potentials, found that TRH causes changes in the electrical properties of the cells that can be suppressed by the calcium channel blocker methoxyverapamil and by lanthanum, but not by the sodium channel blocker tetrodotoxin. Therefore, these changes also appear to be caused by the activation of the calcium channel.

The second type of evidence involves direct measurements of calcium or calcium movement. This has been done in several ways. A common technique is to preload the cells with $^{45}Ca^{2+}$ and measure calcium efflux. TRH stimulates $^{45}Ca^{2+}$ efflux from cells and pituitary glands (Williams, 1976; Vale et al, 1976; Schrey et al., 1978; Gershengorn et al., 1981; Tan and Tashjian, 1981). High concentrations of potassium, which depolarize the cell, also cause $^{45}Ca^{2+}$ efflux (Gershengorn et al., 1981). Some laboratories have assumed that calcium efflux represents an increase in cytosolic calcium. The finding that somatostatin (an inhibitory factor) also stimulates calcium efflux from pituitary cells (Bicknell and Schofield, 1981) is difficult to explain based on this simple interpretation. However, Tan and Tashjian (1981) showed that some of the $^{45}Ca^{2+}$ is not intracellular, but is bound to an extracellular site that can be removed by enzymatic digestion. TRH can stimulate release of calcium from this site.

Uptake of calcium by the cells has also been measured. Moriarty and Leuschen (1981) measured calcium uptake by two methods: the determination of intracellular calcium by atomic absorption spectrophotometry and measurements of the disappearance of calcium from the medium using a calcium electrode. They found no detectable uptake of calcium when TRH is added to GH cells, although calcium uptake does increase with high potassium levels. It is clear from these experiments that TRH does not cause an increase of the same magnitude as that caused by high potassium. Moriarty and Leuschen concluded that TRH does not cause calcium uptake, but Tan and Tashjian (1981) measured an increase in intracellular $^{45}Ca^{2+}$ caused by TRH, in addition to the release of $^{45}Ca^{2+}$ from the membrane-bound sites. Tan and Tashjian (1981) showed that the increase can be blocked by cobalt. This intracellular increase must not be large enough to be measured by the techniques of Moriarty and Leuschen.

The third type of evidence for the role of calcium in TRH-induced release is that stimulation by TRH requires the presence of calcium in the medium (Tashjian *et al.*, 1978; Ostlund *et al.*, 1978). Gershengorn *et al.* (1981) showed that the TRH-stimulated release of prolactin is less dependent on extracellular calcium than is release induced by high potassium. When extracellular calcium is reduced to 0.02 μM, TRH-induced release is 35% of that in 1.5 mM calcium, and potassium-induced release is abolished. The authors concluded that only the potassium-induced release is dependent on extracellular calcium; they said that the reduction in TRH-induced release must be caused by calcium leakage from the cell in low-calcium medium. An alternative explanation is suggested by the work of Tan and Tashjian (1981). If high potassium levels do not release the bound extracellular calcium as TRH does, then potassium-induced release would be expected to be more sensitive to calcium in the medium.

If calcium entry through the voltage-dependent calcium channel releases prolactin, agents known to block calcium entry should block TRH-stimulated release. These experiments have been done with conflicting results. Maruyama *et al.* (1981) showed that 1 μM methoxyverapamil inhibits TRH-induced prolactin release from the 2B8 pituitary cell line and that cobalt inhibits TRH-stimulated release from GH cells (Tashjian *et al.* 1978; Ozawa and Kimura 1979; Tan and Tashjian, 1981). However, Moriarty and Leuschen (1981) found that 50 μM methoxyverapamil blocks TRH-stimulated release from GH cells only 23%, which was not significant in this experiment. Potassium-stimulated release is blocked by 50%. Discrepancies also occurred when the stimulation of thyrotropin release by TRH was investigated. Eto *et al.* (1974) found that thyrotropin release is not blocked by verapamil, whereas Schrey *et al.* (1978) and Fleckman *et al.* (1981) found that TRH-induced thyrotropin release is blocked by methoxyverapamil. At present the reason for these differences is not known; possibly TRH-induced release requires voltage-dependent calcium channels in some circumstances and not in others. More extensive studies correlating electrophysiological results with effects on hormone release are needed.

In summary, all evidence supports a role of calcium in TRH-induced release. The electrophysiological findings and the pharmacological studies in some laboratories indicate that TRH causes release by causing entry of extracellular calcium. The strongest evidence that TRH stimulates release by means other than causing entry of calcium is the ability to see stimulated release in the presence of calcium channel blockers. At present, the mechanism by which TRH stimulates release when calcium channels are blocked is not known.

There is agreement about the role of calcium in TRH-induced prolactin release even if there is not agreement about the source of the calcium. There is less agreement about the role of cAMP in TRH-induced release. Textbooks and papers have assumed that TRH requires cAMP as a second messenger (Hardman, 1974; Labrie et al., 1978; Murad and Haynes, 1980). The main evidence for this assumption is that basal release can be stimulated by agents that mimic cAMP, as previously discussed. A second type of evidence is that TRH can increase intracellular cAMP levels. TRH causes increased cAMP levels in GH cells, although we found in our experiments that an increase is not always detectable (Dannies et al., 1976). TRH-induced increases in cAMP were seen in dispersed cells in culture (Naor et al., 1980), but as the authors point out, conclusions from this system are complicated by the presence of three cell types that respond to TRH in the rat: growth hormone-, thyrotropin-, and prolactin-producing cells. Barnes et al. (1978) partially purified mammotrophs on a gradient of bovine serum albumin and found that TRH causes an increase in cAMP in both thyrotrophs and mammotrophs. Increases in cAMP could be a direct effect of TRH or they could be secondary effects as a result of calcium entry or release. Evidence that TRH can directly stimulate adenylate cyclase in pituitary or GH cell membranes has not been found, in spite of extensive studies (Hinkle and Tashjian, 1977). Brozmanová et al. (1980) showed that, when pituitary halves were incubated with TRH and then homogenized, there was a small increase in adenylate cyclase activity, but this effect could be indirect, because the incubation was with the intact gland. Therefore, at the present time, there is no good evidence that TRH uses cAMP as a second messenger, although the presence of cAMP may be necessary to see TRH-induced release.

TRH has many effects on GH cells in addition to the stimulation of prolactin release; these effects include changes in morphology, in membrane properties of the cells, in uridine uptake (Martin and Tashjian, 1978), and in prolactin and growth hormone synthesis. (For reviews, see Martin and Tashjian, 1977; Gourdji, 1980.) More than one mechanism seems to be involved in these changes. We have shown that the structural requirements for increasing prolactin release were different from those for increasing prolactin synthesis in GH cells or for increasing thyrotropin release from normal cells (Dannies and Tashjian, 1976b; Dannies and Markell, 1980). Therefore, the hormone receptor interactions that mediate these processes cannot be identical. We concluded that TRH independently regulates release and synthesis. When the primary actions of TRH on the cell are known, the sensitivity of the actions to various structural analogs will be useful in distinguishing which action is associated with a given effect.

There has been so much argument about the source of calcium and the role of cAMP because the experiments are all indirect. The ability to do direct experiments depends on knowledge of what the primary actions of TRH are, by isolating and characterizing the components involved. A start in this direction has been made by Martin and coworkers. Rapid changes in phosphate incorporation into phospholipids are induced by TRH (Sutton and Martin, 1982). Martin et al. (1981) also demonstrated phosphorylation of specific proteins in GH cells in response to TRH; phosphorylation of one of these proteins is changed by TRH but not by high potassium levels or dibutyryl cAMP. Future studies characterizing how these changes occur should give useful information about the mechanisms of TRH action.

B.   Dopamine

Secretion of prolactin from the rat anterior pituitary gland is primarily under negative control (Meites and Clemens, 1972). Dopamine appears to be a major factor in the inhibition of prolactin release. Dopamine and dopaminergic agonists can inhibit prolactin release directly in isolated rat pituitary glands (MacLeod et al., 1970; Birge et al., 1970), as well as in intact animals (Takahara et al., 1974; Ojeda et al., 1974). Dopamine is present in the hypophyseal portal blood (Ben-Jonathan et al., 1977; Gibbs and Neill, 1978) and in the pituitary gland (Saavedra et al., 1975). It has been reported that dopamine may be associated with prolactin secretory granules on the basis of similar sedimentation properties (Nansel et al., 1979). It will be important to follow this work up by characterizing the fraction containing prolactin and dopamine with electron microscopy and with biochemical markers for cellular organelles to determine the exact location of the intracellular dopamine.

Dopamine-binding sites were detected in pituitary gland membranes and the binding of various dopaminergic analogs were shown to correlate with the ability to inhibit prolactin release (Caron *et al.*, 1978; Cronin *et al.*, 1978). The first step in dopamine action is presumably binding to the membrane receptor. A small amount of soluble receptor with similar characteristics has also been shown to be present; its role is not known (Kerdelhue *et al.*, 1981).

Dopamine causes a detectable inhibition of basal release from perfused cells within 3 minutes and a maximal inhibition by 11 minutes (Thorner *et al.*, 1980). We have also seen a rapid inhibition of basal release from monolayer cells in culture using the dopaminergic agonist bromocriptine. We found that bromocriptine inhibits prolactin release and that the prolactin that is not released accumulates in the cells for at least 8 hours, so that the total amount of prolactin in the cultures is the same in control and treated plates (Dannies and Rudnick, 1980). Antakly *et al.* (1980) showed that prolactin concentrations increase in the cell for up to 16 hours and that during this time secretory granules accumulate in the cell. Initially, bromocriptine inhibits prolactin release without affecting synthesis and stability; therefore, prolactin accumulates in the cell. After longer periods of time, other processes are affected. Control cultures accumulate prolactin for 4 days, but bromocriptine largely inhibits secretion when present during this time period (Dannies and Rudnick, 1980). During this longer time of treatment, the prolactin that is not released does not accumulate in the cells; therefore, the total amount in the bromocriptine cultures is much less. We found that the rate of accumulation of prolactin in the treated cultures varies from 6-fold less than controls to no accumulation at all. Evidence from two laboratories using pulse–chase and continuous labeling techniques indicates that at least part of the lack of accumulation is caused by degradation of prolactin (Dannies and Rudnick, 1980; Maurer, 1980). When cells are continuously labeled, incorporation of radioactive amino acids into protein will first reflect synthesis, but after longer intervals, labeling may represent a combination of synthesis and degradation. The rate of accumulation of [^{3}H]prolactin decreases with time in bromocriptine-treated cells but not in controls, indicating that radioactive prolactin is being degraded in the treated cultures. The increased degradation by bromocriptine-treated cells was confirmed in pulse–chase experiments, in which the stability of labeled prolactin was followed, using excess nonradioactive amino acids, cycloheximide, or both, to prevent further incorporation of radioactive amino acids into prolactin. Both laboratories found degradation of prolactin caused by bromocriptine with this technique. In addition,

Maurer (1980) demonstrated that cycloheximide prevents the degradation of prolactin if it is added with bromocriptine, but not if the cells are pretreated with bromocriptine, suggesting that protein synthesis may be necessary for the induction of prolactin degradation. The basic findings of the two laboratories are similar; bromocriptine can cause cells to degrade prolactin.

Although the basic findings were the same, there are several differences between Maurer's results and our results. The first is the stability of prolactin in the control cells; as mentioned earlier, Shenai and Wallis (1979) and Maurer (1980) did see degradation in control cultures and we did not. Either prolactin was stable in the cells under our culture conditions, or cells were still able to incorporate radioactive leucine into prolactin in spite of the excess unlabeled leucine and cycloheximide. Maurer's conditions appear better for pulse–chase experiments because he did not have to use cycloheximide and we did. The other differences must also be a result of culture conditions. One difference is the rapidity of the effect; we saw no effect on prolactin accumulation at 8 hours, but at this time Maurer saw effects on degradation and synthesis. Another difference is the effect on prolactin synthesis measured by amino acid incorporation; we saw smaller effects than Maurer. The most obvious differences between the two sets of experimental conditions are that Maurer used pituitary glands from retired breeders and did the experiments in serum-free medium; we used male rats and used serum in the medium. We do not yet know which factors are responsible for the variation, but it is clear that the time course and magnitude of the effects can be varied.

It is not yet known at what stage in the processing prolactin is degraded; it may occur before or after prolactin is packaged into granules. Excess granules can be degraded by lysosomes (Smith and Farquhar, 1966); these experiments were described in the first section. It has not yet been determined whether this process, which was seen after heavily secreting cells were turned off, applies to chronic treatment with dopaminergic agents. In our experiments, the amount of intracellular prolactin is about the same in treated and control cells after 3 or 4 days of treatment. If degradation occurs after the prolactin is packaged, the cells must have some way of regulating the number of granules. On the other hand, degradation may occur before the hormone is packaged into granules. The formation of new granules may become rate-limiting if old granule components are not recycled when release is prevented; the extra hormone may then be degraded because it is not protected. Other models are also possible; for example, bromocriptine could induce synthesis of a protease. Experiments following the course of incorporated leucine through the cell, such as those by Farquhar and co-workers described earlier, will distinguish at what stage the degradation occurs in the processing of prolactin.

The mechanisms by which dopamine inhibits prolactin release have been studied by examining the role of calcium and cAMP. Taraskevich and Douglas (1978) showed that dopamine inhibited the generation of spontaneous action potentials within seconds in the prolactin-secreting cells of the fish pituitary. These action potentials, like those in the rat pituitary cells, contain a calcium component. Dufy *et al.* (1979b) found that dopamine inhibits the generation of action potentials in a clone of GH cells. This effect is somewhat surprising because GH cells have been shown not to have detectable dopamine receptors nor to respond to dopamine (Cronin *et al.*, 1980a). The clone used by Dufy and co-workers must have unusual properties.

The inhibition of action potentials, which would prevent the entry of calcium into the cell through voltage-dependent channels, may be a mechanism of preventing prolactin release. If it were the only mechanism for inhibiting release, then causing calcium to enter the cytoplasm by a means other than the calcium channel should cause release in the presence of dopamine. We used the divalent cation ionophore A23187 to bypass the voltage-dependent calcium channels in monolayer pituitary cultures and found that bromocriptine is still able to block the ionophore-induced release of prolactin at doses that correspond to the inhibition of basal prolactin release (Tam and Dannies, 1980). Bromocriptine does not interfere with ionophore-induced uptake of $^{45}Ca^{2+}$. The inhibition of ionophore-induced release appears to be mediated through the dopamine receptor for the following reasons: (1) Dopamine and another dopaminergic agonist (dihydroergocryptine) also block this stimulated release. (2) The dopaminergic antagonists (+)-butaclamol and *cis*-flupenthixol block the inhibition by bromocriptine. (3) A23187-induced release of prolactin in GH cells is not blocked by bromocriptine. GH cells in our hands also do not bind dopamine, as Cronin *et al.* (1980a). We, therefore, concluded that dopamine can block prolactin release at a step after the increase in intracellular calcium.

Thorner *et al.* (1980) did the same experiment in perfused cells and obtained different results; they found that ionophore A23187 reverses the inhibiton by dopamine. Two possible explanations for the difference in results are that (1) dopamine can block prolactin release both before and after calcium entry; however, in the perfused cells, only the block before calcium entry is operating; (2) the reversal is a toxic effect; A23187 is a toxic compound that is an uncoupler of oxidative phosphorylation in the mitochondria and has other side effects. We therefore looked at short time periods in our experiments (usually 10 minutes) and found no evidence of cell lysis. Thorner and co-workers found a reversal of dopamine inhibition after exposure of the cells to low concentrations of ionophore, which they gradually increased for over 1 hour. Low concentrations of ionophore preferentially localize in mitochondrial membranes (Babcock *et al.*, 1976) and so the reversal of dopamine inhibition after that length of time might be a toxic effect.

Dopamine has effects on cAMP accumulation. Barnes *et al.* (1978) showed that dopamine decreases the rise in cAMP levels induced by TRH in partially purified mammotrophs, and DeCamilli *et al.* (1979) showed that dopamine can inhibit adenylate cyclase activity in human tumor cell membranes. A possible site for the block after the entry of calcium is the inhibition of adenylate cyclase. Isobutylmethylxanthine and 8-Br-cAMP increase cAMP by means other than activation of adenylate cyclase. If the only block is at the activation of cyclase, then dopaminergic agonists should not block release induced by these agents. We have shown that this suggestion is not true; the increase in prolactin release caused by 8-Br-cAMP and isobutylmethylxanthine is blocked by bromocriptine (Tam and Dannies, 1981b). We found that release induced by cholera toxin is also blocked. Other laboratories have found similar results. Stern and Conn (1981) showed that dibutyryl cAMP-induced release was blocked by dopamine. Ray and Wallis (1981) found that isobutylmethylxanthine, theophylline, and cholera toxin increase cAMP levels in the pituitary gland but do not affect the dopamine inhibition of prolactin release.

Another possible model is that certain levels of both calcium and cAMP are needed in the cytoplasm in order to cause prolactin release. If dopamine blocks both calcium entry and adenylate cyclase, replacing either calcium or cAMP would not be sufficient. To test this model, we added both ionophore A23187 and 8-Br-cAMP to cultures of cells. Release in the presence of the two compounds together is greater than either alone, but this stimulated release of prolactin is still blocked by the same concentrations of bromocriptine that blocks basal release (S. W. Tam and P. S. Dannies, unpublished results). This experiment suggests that dopamine may also block release at a step or steps other than calcium entry or adenylate cyclase activation, but like all the drug experiments cited in this chapter, this conclusion is subject to the reservation that there may be unknown side effects.

Estrogen treatment makes cells much less sensitive to the dopaminergic inhibition of prolactin release (Raymond *et al.*, 1978; West and Dannies, 1980). The effect of estradiol does not appear to be caused by decreasing the number of dopamine receptors (DiPaolo *et al.*, 1979; Cronin *et al.*, 1980b). We have shown that the effect is not caused by increased metabolism of dopaminergic agonists in the presence of estrogen (West and Dannies, unpublished results). The antidopaminergic effect of estrogen therefore occurs after the binding of dopamine to the cell. The effects of long-term estradiol treatment on the dopaminergic inhibition of action potentials and of adenylate cyclase should be investigated to see if estradiol acts at these levels.

Dopamine affects more than just prolactin production in the pituitary gland. Porter and colleagues have done a series of experiments looking at β-glucuronidase activity. Dopamine added to pieces of pituitary tissue causes a 75% increase in β-glucuronidase activity, which reaches an apparent maximum 30 minutes after dopamine addition. L-Dopa (a dopamine precursor) given to intact rats causes a rise in the activity of the enzyme, which continues for at least 8 hours (Nansel *et al.*, 1981). They presented two kinds of evidence that this activation occurs through the dopamine receptor that inhibits prolactin release: (1) The dose response curve for the inhibition of release and activation of β-glucuronidase are not distinguishable, and (2) 10 nM *cis*-flupenthixol (a dopamine antagonist) blocks both effects.

The activation of β-glucuronidase raises several questions. First, is the increase in β-glucuronidase activity occurring in the lysosomes or elsewhere in the cell? β-Glucuronidase occurs not only in the lysosomes but also in the microsomes, and the properties of the two enzymes are very similar (Holtzman, 1976). Nansel *et al.* (1981) suggest that the activity is in the lysosomes for two reasons: (1) The enzyme is in the particles that have a density similar to lysosomes in other tissues. They show one peak of activity and have not shown that the microsomes and lysosomes have been separated. (2) They found that acid phosphatase (another lysosomal enzyme) is also in that peak, and the activity is increased by treating rats with L-dopa. Acid phosphatase is also in other locations in the cells, including the microsomes and the secretory granules (Smith and Farquhar, 1966). Therefore, biochemical and morphological characterization of the purity of the lysosomal fraction is important. A second question raised by the work concerns which cells are involved. Is the activated enzyme in the mammotrophs of the pituitary gland or elsewhere? The question is important because others have shown increases in acid phosphatase that correspond to increases in rates of pituitary secretion rather than to decreases in secretion (see Smith and Farquhar, 1966, for a review of this work). In addition, L-dopa stimulates lysosomal activity of all pituitary cell types in the quail (Harrison, 1979). A third question is what does activation represent? The stimulation could reflect increased synthesis, removal of an inhibitor of activity, stabilization of the enzyme, or activation of a less active form. Finally, is the activation of β-glucuronidase an event that occurs in parallel with prolactin release, or are the two events related? Nansel and co-workers (1981) showed that when the lysosomal inhibitory agents chloroquin and ammonium chloride are incubated with pituitary pieces, the inhibition of prolactin release by dopamine is prevented. When enzyme activity is measured in the pituitary homogenate, activity of the enzyme is not increased either. This result is somewhat surprising because chloroquin and ammonium chloride are thought to inhibit lysosomal enzymes by changing the pH of the interior of the lysosomes. Such an effect should not be seen in a homogenate. Therefore, the activation of β-glucuronidase and the inhibition of prolactin release must both require functional lysosomes, or else the inhibitors are exerting their effects through a separate mechanism. This experiment does not give information as to whether the events are related causally or in parallel; it says both processes are prevented by the two bases.

Nansel et al. (1981) suggest that lysosomes may sequester the granules, preventing their release. If this mechanism of inhibiting prolactin release operates in some circumstances, it clearly is not the only mechanism that inhibits release. Smith and Farquhar (1966) reported that granules accumulate in the pituitary cell for 12 hours after prolactin release is inhibited in intact animals and that there is little increase in lysosomes in the cell 12 to 14 hours after secretion is suppressed. Antakly et al. (1980) also reported that granules accumulate in the cell after incubation with bromocriptine; they found that the intracellular prolactin increases, as we found (Dannies and Rudnick, 1980). Because granules accumulate without being sequestered in lysosomes, release of these granules must be inhibited by some other mechanism.

One other effect of dopamine on pituitary glands has been reported; this is a stimulation of prolactin release at concentrations of dopamine lower than those that inhibit prolactin release. Denef et al. (1980) found that 10^{-10} M dopamine stimulates prolactin release 50% and that bromocriptine also stimulates release when it is added with dopamine antagonists. In these studies, bromocriptine alone inhibits prolactin release at 10^{-18} M. An effect at this concentration is much lower than anyone else has found, and it is surprising, because in his experiment at this concentration there is less than one molecule for every hundred cells. Other laboratories have not reported the effects he described (for example, Caron et al., 1978; West and Dannies, 1979) but most laboratories have not used such low doses.

C. Other Inhibitory Factors

There are several other compounds that have been shown to affect prolactin release directly in either normal cells or GH cells or both. Although some of these effects may have no physiological relevance, they may prove to be useful tools for elucidating the mechanisms by which prolactin release can be controlled.

1. γ-*Aminobutyric Acid*

γ-Aminobutyric acid (GABA), which is an inhibitory neurotransmitter in the brain, also inhibits prolactin release by a direct action on the pituitary gland that is separate from the dopaminergic inhibition (Grandison and Guidotti, 1979; Enjalbert *et al.,* 1979a; Racagni *et al.,* 1979). The effect is blocked by picrotoxin, a GABA antagonist, and mimicked by muscimol, a GABA agonist. GABA-binding sites similar to those in the brain have been measured in the pituitary gland (Grandison and Guidotti, 1979).

As a neurotransmitter in the brain, GABA causes an increase in chloride conductance that sometimes leads to hyperpolarization. It is easy to imagine how such a mechanism could be incorporated into a model in which action potentials are responsible for prolactin release, but whether GABA has the same action in the pituitary gland as it does in the brain must be shown.

2. *Acetylcholine*

Acetylcholine inhibits prolactin release from normal pituitary cells and from GH cells (Vale *et al.,* 1976; Rudnick and Dannies, 1981); the inhibition has the characteristics of a muscarinic receptor. Muscarinic binding sites have been detected in the anterior pituitary gland (Mukhejee *et al.,* 1980). The mechanism of inhibition of prolactin secretion is not known; activation of muscarinic receptors can inhibit adenylate cyclase in tissues such as heart (Rodbell, 1980) and this inhibition may also occur in prolactin-producing cells. Acetylcholine does not affect cAMP levels in the pituitary gland (Young *et al.,* 1979), but the lack of detectable effect may be caused by heterogeneity of cell types in the gland.

3. *Somatostatin*

Somatostatin inhibits prolactin and growth hormone release from GH cells and from cultures of normal pituitary cells (Vale *et al.,* 1974; Grant *et al.,* 1974; Drouin *et al.,* 1976; Schonbrunn and Tashjian, 1978). The mechanisms for inhibiting growth hormone release have been investigated by several laboratories and the results are quite similar to those found for dopamine inhibition of prolactin release. Somatostatin inhibits secretion stimulated by high potassium concentrations (Stachura, 1977; Schofield and Bicknell, 1978) as well as release induced by the ionophore A23187 (Bicknell and Schofield, 1976). Somatostatin decreases cAMP levels in pituitary glands (Kaneko *et al.*, 1973; Borgeat *et al.*, 1974). Using purified somatotrophs, Sheppard *et al.* (1979) found no effect on basal cAMP levels, but they did see some inhibition of the increases in cAMP induced by prostaglandin E_2 or isobutylmethylxanthine. The rise in cAMP is not completely prevented but the increase in growth hormone release is. In addition, somatostatin blocks release induced by dibutyryl cAMP. It seems likely that the mechanisms by which somatostatin inhibits prolactin release will be similar to the effects on growth hormone release.

4. Histidyl-Proline-Diketopiperazine

Histidyl-proline-diketopiperazine [cyclo (His-Pro)] is a product of the metabolism of TRH (Prasad and Peterkofsky, 1976). Bauer *et al.* (1978) showed that this compound inhibits prolactin release from GH cells and proestrous rats, and Enjalbert *et al.* (1979b) and Prasad *et al.* (1980) showed inhibition from pituitary halves. The work that has been done with this compound is discussed in a review by Peterkofsky *et al.* (1981). Not all laboratories found inhibition using cyclo(His-Pro). The mechanisms by which cyclo(His-Pro) inhibits prolactin release, when it does, are not known.

D. Other Stimulatory Factors

1. Vasoactive Intestinal Peptide

Vasoactive intestinal peptide (VIP) stimulates prolactin release directly from pituitary glands, pituitary cells in culture, and GH cells (Ruberg *et al.*, 1978; Kato *et al.*, 1978; Gourdji *et al.*, 1979; Shaar *et al.*, 1979; Enjalbert *et al.*, 1980). Release occurs with nanomolar concentrations of VIP; secretin, a structurally similar peptide, was active at higher concentrations. VIP stimulates adenylate cyclase in systems other than the pituitary gland. The pituitary gland appears similar, because a direct effect of VIP on cyclase activity was shown in membranes from a human prolactin-secreting pituitary tumor (Bataille *et al.*, 1979). In addition Gourdji *et al.* (1979) demonstrated VIP-stimulated cAMP levels in intact GH cells. The first step in the mechanism of VIP-induced prolactin release therefore appears relatively straightforward—VIP stimulates adenylate cyclase activity.

2. Epidermal Growth Factor

EGF causes an increase in prolactin release in GH cells in addition to an increase in prolactin synthesis (Schonbrunn *et al.*, 1980). The effects on prolactin release are small, but the EGF effects are interesting because EGF is the only factor other than TRH to increase prolactin synthesis and decrease growth hormone synthesis in GH cells. EGF stimulates phosphorylation of membrane proteins in membranes isolated from A-431 human epidermal carcinoma cells, and the phosphorylation is on tyrosine residues (Carpenter *et al.*, 1979; Ushiro and Cohen, 1980). It is not known whether similar stimulations of phosphorylations are induced by EGF in GH cell membranes.

3. Endorphins

Lien *et al.* (1976) found that Met-enkephalin has a stimulatory effect on prolactin release in cultures of rat pituitary cells, but other laboratories have found no direct effects of opiate-like peptides on prolactin release (Shaar *et al.*, 1977; Rivier *et al.*, 1977). However, Enjalbert *et al.* (1979c) found that enkephalin and opiates can block the dopamine-induced inhibition of prolactin release from pituitary halves, indicating that a stimulatory effect of opiate-like peptides can be seen under some circumstances. The exact conditions are not clear; Wardlaw *et al.* (1980) and Grandison *et al.* (1980) could not show a reversal of dopaminergic inhibition. The mechanisms by which opiates reverse the inhibition of dopamine and stimulate prolactin secretion are not known.

4. Bombesin

Bombesin was originally isolated from amphibians, and later similar peptides were found in mammalian brains. Bombesin stimulates prolactin secretion in intact rats (Rivier *et al.*, 1978). The peptide causes prolactin release from GH cells in culture (Westendorf and Schonbrunn, 1982); no studies have been done yet on the mechanisms involved.

III. RELEASE IN INTACT ANIMALS

Prolactin release in the intact animal appears to go through two stages. The first is called "depletion" or transformation and occurs in the pituitary gland. The second step is release from the gland. This process has been investigated by Grosvenor and colleagues in a series of experiments. There are two kinds of evidence that the first step exists. The first is that the amount of prolactin in the pituitary gland decreases within minutes after rats begin to suckle, and the amount of prolactin that appears in the serum within that time does not reflect the apparent decrease in the gland (Nicoll, 1972; Grosvenor *et al.,* 1979). Observation of this effect is probably dependent on the way in which the glands are prepared for prolactin assay; when the effect was seen, the glands were homogenized at neutral pH. As Giannattasio *et al.* (1975) showed, this procedure may not give complete solubilization of prolactin. The apparent "depletion" may be a change in the recovery of prolactin from the cell. This interpretation is supported by the results of Nicoll *et al.* (1976), who did not see reproducible depletion when glands were homogenized at high pH. Therefore, the term transformation, which has been used by Grosvenor and co-workers to describe this effect, seems more appropriate than depletion.

The second kind of evidence for a process besides release is based on the change in the response of the pituitary gland before and after a brief period of suckling. The system Grosvenor and co-workers used was suckling rats that had been deprived of their young for hours and therefore had built up large stores of untransformed prolactin. Compounds were tested when rats were in this state or after the rats had been allowed to suckle their young for 10 minutes. Prolactin release rises during suckling but drops to basal levels when suckling is discontinued. Grosvenor and Mena (1980) found that TRH stimulates prolactin release only slightly in rats that have not suckled. However, there is a larger elevation in release from rats that have first suckled for 10 minutes and then received TRH. They also found that TRH does not cause the apparent depletion from the pituitary gland. They suggest that TRH can only release prolactin after the prolactin stores are transformed by suckling. Dopamine and bromocriptine inhibit the suckling-induced rise if given to rats before suckling, but bromocriptine does not inhibit release induced by further suckling when it is given after a brief suckling period (Grosvenor *et al.,* 1980). Therefore, they suggest that dopamine can inhibit the transformation step but not the subsequent stimulation of release. This series of experiments raises several questions:

1. What is the factor that causes transformation? Suckling, mammary nerve stimulation, or exposure to the pups without suckling can cause transformation (Mena *et al.,* 1980; Grosvenor *et al.,* 1981), but the factor or factors that mediate this response are not known. TRH does not cause transformation, and they did not find any such activity in extracts of stalk median eminence, although these extracts can stimulate release after transformation as TRH does (Grosvenor and

Mena, 1980). The factors and the pathways involved are unknown at this time.

2. Several related questions can be raised about the transformation step itself. What physical change occurs when pituitary prolactin is apparently depleted? Is it a change in recovery, and if so, what is causing the change? Does calcium or cAMP induce the change? Does the change occur only to prolactin in secretory granules; if so, are all types of granules, mature and immature, involved?

3. How do these experiments relate to those performed in cultures of cells? Cells in culture in our hands do not release a large portion of their intracellular prolactin no matter what stimulus is used—is this because transformation is necessary?

It is tempting to relate Stachura's results (mentioned previously) with these results and to suggest that the ability of cAMP to stimulate accumulation of prolactin in a readily releasable pool is transformation. However, somatostatin does not inhibit transfer of growth hormone into a releasable pool but only inhibits release (Stachura, 1981); and dopamine does inhibit transformation of prolactin and not subsequent release (Grosvenor *et al.*, 1980). If somatostatin and dopamine have the same mechanism, then the releasable pool is not transformed prolactin. More experiments will have to be done to determine the relation of the rapidly releasable pool *in vitro* to the transformed pool *in vivo*.

IV. CONCLUDING REMARKS

Investigations of the mechanisms of regulation of prolactin release have used many different approaches, and it is still not clear how some of the findings using different approaches are related to each other. The regulation of release is obviously complex, and the two factors studied in the most detail, dopamine and TRH, appear to have more than one mechanism of action. Many of the models tested in the past may have been too simple to fully explain the processes involved. The amount of interest in prolactin release and the number of laboratories working in the field should mean that experiments that expand and relate the various approaches discussed here will be appearing soon.

ACKNOWLEDGMENTS

We thank Drs. Agnes Schonbrunn and Max Stachura for allowing us to see unpublished data, and Dr. Jonathan Scammell, Diane Kiino, and Jane Amara for useful discussions. This work was supported by NIH grant HD11487 and Research Career Development Award HD00272.

REFERENCES

Antakly, T., Pelletier, G., Zeytinoglu, F., and Labrie, F. (1979). Effects of colchicine on the morphology and prolactin secretion of rat anterior pituitary cells in monolayer culture. *Am. J. Anat.* **156,** 353–372.

Antakly, T., Pelletier, G., Zeytinoglu, F., and Labrie, F. (1980). Changes of cell morphology and prolactin secretion induced by 2-Br-α-ergocryptine, estradiol, and thyrotropin-releasing hormone in rat anterior pituitary cells in culture. *J. Cell Biol.* **86,** 377–387.

Appleman, M. M., Thompson, W. J., and Russell, T. R. (1973). Cyclic nucleotide phosphodiesterases. *Adv. Cyclic Nucleotide Res.* **3,** 65–98.

Babcock, D. F., First, N. L., and Lardy, H. A. (1976). Action of ionophore A23187 at the cellular level; separation of effects at the plasma and mitochondrial membranes. *J. Biol. Chem.* **251,** 3881–3886.

Baker, B. L. (1970). Studies on hormone localization with emphasis on the hypophysis. *J. Histochem. Cytochem.* **18,** 1–8.

Barnes, G. D., Brown, B. L., Gard, T. G., Atkinson, D., and Ekins, R. P. (1978). Effect of TRH and dopamine on cyclic AMP levels in enriched mammotrophs and thyrotroph cells. *Mol. Cell. Endocrinol.* **12,** 273–284.

Bataille, D., Peillon, F., Besson, J., and Rosselin, G. (1979). Vasoactive intestinal peptide (VIP) récepteurs spécifiques et activation de l'adénylate cyclase dans une tumeur hypophysaire humaine à prolactine. *C.R. Acad. Sci., Ser. D* **288,** 1315–1317.

Bauer, K., Gräf, K. J., Faivre-Bauman, A., Beier, S., Tixier-Vidal, A., and Kleinkauf, H. (1978). Inhibition of prolactin secretion by histidyl-proline-diketopiperazine. *Nature (London)* **274,** 174–175.

Ben-Jonathan, N., Oliver, C., Wiener, H. J., Mical, R. S., and Porter, J. C. (1977). Dopamine in hypophysial portal plasma of the rat during the estrous cycle and throughout pregnancy. *Endocrinology (Baltimore)* **100,** 452–458.

Biales, B., Dichter, M. A., and Tischler, A. (1977). Sodium and calcium action potential in pituitary cells. *Nature (London)* **267,** 172–173.

Bicknell, R. J., and Schofield, J. G. (1976). Mechanism of action of somatostain: Inhibition of ionophore A23187-induced release of growth hormone from dispersed bovine pituitary cells. *FEBS Lett.* **68,** 23–26.

Bicknell, R. J., and Schofield, J. G. (1981). Inhibition by somatostatin of bovine growth hormone secretion following sodium channel activation. *J. Physiol. (London)* **316,** 85–96.

Birge, C. A., Jacobs, L. S., Hammer, C. T., and Daughaday, W. H. (1970). Catecholamine inhibition of prolactin secretion by isolated rat adenohypophyses. *Endocrinology (Baltimore)* **86,** 120–130.

Biswas, D. K., and Tashjian, A. H., Jr. (1974). Intracellular site of prolactin synthesis in rat pituitary cells in culture. *Biochem. Biophys. Res. Commun.* **60,** 241–248.

Bøler, J., Enzmann, F., Folkers, K., Bowers, C. Y., and Schally, A. V. (1969). The identity of chemical and hormonal properties of the thyrotropin releasing hormone and pyroglutamyl-histidyl-proline amide. *Biochem. Biophys. Res. Commun.* **37,** 705–710.

Borgeat, P., Labrie, F., Drouin, J., Bélanger, A., Immer, H., Sestanj, K., Nelson, V., Gotz,

M., Schally, A. V., Coy, D. H., and Coy, E. J. (1974). Inhibition of adenosine
3',5'-monophosphate accumulation in anterior pituitary gland *in vitro* by growth
hormone-release inhibiting hormone. *Biochem. Biophys. Res. Commun.* **56,**
1052–1059.

Bowers, C. Y. (1971). Studies on the role of cyclic AMP in the release of anterior pituitary hormones. *Ann. N. Y. Acad. Sci.* **185,** 263–290.

Brisson, G. R., and Malaisse, W. J. (1973). The stimulus-secretion coupling of glucose-
induced insulin release. XI. Effects of theophylline and epinephrine on ^{45}Ca efflux
from perifused islets. *Metab. Clin. Exp.* **22,** 455–465.

Brozmanová, H., Langer, P., Földes, O., Kolena, J., and Knopp, J. (1980). *In vitro* effect of
TRH on adenylate cyclase and cAMP in rat anterior pituitary and on TSH and PRL
release into incubation medium. *Endocrinol. Exp.* **14,** 291–296.

Burgus, R., Dunn, T. F., Desiderio, D., and Guillemin, R. (1969). Structure moléculaire
du facteur hypothalamique hypophysiotrope TRH d'origine ovine; mise én évidence
par spectrométrie de masse de la séquence PCA-His-Pro-NH_2. *C. R. Acad. Sci. Ser.*
D **269,** 1870–1873.

Butcher, F. R. (1978). Regulation of exocytosis. *In* "Biochemical Actions of Hormones"
(G. Litwack, ed.), Vol. V, pp. 54–99. Academic Press, New York.

Caron, M. G., Beaulieu, M., Raymond, V., Gagné, B., Drouin, J., Lefkowitz, R. J., and
Labrie, F. (1978). Dopaminergic receptors in the anterior pituitary gland: Correlation of [^{3}H]dihydroergocryptine binding with the dopaminergic control of prolactin
relase. *J. Biol. Chem.* **253,** 2244–2253.

Carpenter, G., King, L., Jr., and Cohen, S. (1979). Rapid enhancement of protein phosphorylation in A-431 cell membrane preparations by epidermal growth factor. *J.*
Biol. Chem. **254,** 4884–4891.

Cassel, D., and Selinger, Z. (1977). Mechanism of adenylate cyclase activation by cholera
toxin: Inhibition of GTP hydrolysis at the regulatory site. *Proc. Natl. Acad. Sci.*
U.S.A. **74,** 3307–3311.

Cehovic, G., Posternak, T., and Charollais, E. (1972). A study of the biological activity
and resistance to phosphodiesterase of some derivatives and analogues of cAMP.
Adv. Cyclic Nucleotide Res. **1,** 521–540.

Conn, P. M., Rogers, D. C., and Sheffield, T. (1981). Inhibition of gonadotropin-releasing
hormone-stimulated luteinizing hormone release by pimozide: Evidence for a site
of action after calcium mobilization. *Endocrinology (Baltimore)* **109** 1122–1126.

Cronin, M. J., Roberts, J. M., and Weiner, R. I. (1978). Dopamine and dihydroergocryptine binding to the anterior pituitary and other brain areas of the rat and sheep.
Endocrinology (Baltimore) **103,** 302–309.

Cronin, M. J., Faure, N., Martial, J. A., and Weiner, R. I. (1980a). Absence of high
affinity dopamine receptors in GH_3 cells: A prolactin-secreting clone resistant to
the inhibitory action of dopamine. *Endocrinology (Baltimore)* **106,** 718–723.

Cronin, M. J., Cheung, C. Y., and Weiner, R. I. (1980b). Dopamine receptor in the
pituitary of medial basal hypothalamic lesioned rats. *Int. Cong. Endocrinol. 6th,* p.
645. (Abstr. 871.)

Dannies, P. S., and Markell, M. S. (1980). Differential ability of thyrotropin-releasing
hormone and N^{3im}-methyl-thyrotropin-releasing hormone to affect prolactin and
thyrotropin production in primary rat pituitary cell cultures. *Endocrinology (Baltimore)* **106,** 107–112.

Dannies, P. S., and Rudnick, M. S. (1980). 2-Bromo-α-ergocryptine causes degradation of
prolactin in primary cultures of rat pituitary cells after chronic treatment. *J. Biol.*
Chem. **255,** 2776–2781.

Dannies, P. S., and Tashjian, A. H., Jr. (1973). Effects of thyrotropin-releasing hormone and hydrocortisone on synthesis and degradation of prolactin in a rat pituitary cell strain. *J. Biol. Chem.* **248**, 6174–6179.

Dannies, P. S., and Tashjian, A. H., Jr. (1974). Pyroglutamyl-histidyl-prolineamide (TRH): A neurohormone which affects the release and synthesis of prolactin and thyrotropin. *Isr. J. Med. Sci.* **10**, 1294–1304.

Dannies, P. S., and Tashjian, A. H., Jr. (1976a). Thyrotropin-releasing hormone increases prolactin mRNA activity in the cytoplasm of GH-cells as measured by translation in a wheat germ cell-free system. *Biochem. Biophys. Res. Commun.* **70**, 1180–1189.

Dannies, P. S., and Tashjian, A. H., Jr. (1976b). Release and synthesis of prolactin by rat pituitary cell strains are regulated independently by thyrotropin-releasing hormone. *Nature (London)* **261**, 707–710.

Dannies, P. S., and Tashjian, A. H., Jr. (1980). Action of cholera toxin on hormone synthesis and release in GH cells: Evidence that adenosine 3′,5′-monophosphate does not mediate the decrease in growth hormone synthesis caused by thyrotropin-releasing hormone. *Endocrinology (Baltimore)* **106**, 1532–1536.

Dannies, P. S., Gautvik, K. M., and Tashjian, A. H., Jr. (1976). A possible role for cyclic AMP in mediating the effects of thyrotropin-releasing hormone on prolactin release and on prolactin and growth hormone synthesis in pituitary cells in culture. *Endocrinology (Baltimore)* **98**, 1147–1159.

DeCamilli, P., Macconi, D., and Spada, A. (1979). Dopamine inhibits adenylate cyclase in human prolactin-secreting pituitary adenomas. *Nature (London)* **278**, 252–254.

Denef, C. (1980). Functional heterogeneity of separated dispersed gonadotrophic cells. *In* "Synthesis and Release of Adenohypophyseal Hormones" (M. Jutisz and K. W. McKerns, eds.), pp. 659–676. Plenum, New York.

Denef, C., Manet, D., and Dewals, R. (1980). Dopaminergic stimulation of prolactin release. *Nature (London)* **285**, 243–246.

DiPaolo, T., Carmichael, R., Labrie, F., and Raynaud, J. P. (1979). Effects of estrogens on the characteristics of [3H]-spiroperidol and [3H]-RU24213 binding in rat anterior pituitary gland and brain. *Mol. Cell. Endocrinol.* **16**, 99–112.

Douglas, W. W. (1968). Stimulus-secretion coupling: The concept and clues from chromaffin and other cells. *Br. J. Pharmacol.* **34**, 451–474.

Drouin, J., DeLean, A., Rainville, D., Lachance, R., and Labrie, F. (1976). Characteristics of the interaction between thyrotropin-releasing hormone and somatostatin for thyrotropin and prolactin release. *Endocrinology (Baltimore)* **98**, 514–521.

Dufy, B., Vincent, J. D., Fleury, H., Du Pasquier, P. D., Gourdji, D., and Tixier-Vidal, A. (1979a). Membrane effects of thyrotropin-releasing hormone and estrogen shown by intracellular recording from pituitary cells. *Science* **204**, 509–511.

Dufy, B., Vincent, J. D., Fleury, H., Du Pasquier, P. D., Gourdji, D., and Tixier-Vidal, A. (1979b). Dopamine inhibition of action potentials in a prolactin secreting cell line is modulated by oestrogen. *Nature (London)* **282**, 855–857.

Dufy, B., Fleury, H., Gourdji, D., Tixier-Vidal, A., Du Pasquier, P., and Vincent, J. D. (1980). Intracellular recordings from prolactin-secreting pituitary cells in culture: Evidence for a direct action of estrogen on the cell membrane. *In* "Synthesis and Release of Adenohypophyseal Hormones" (J. M. Jutisz and K. W. McKerns, eds.), pp. 765–773. Plenum, New York.

Enjalbert, A., Ruberg, M., Arancibia, S., Fiore, L., Priam, M., and Kordon, C. (1979a). Independent inhibition of prolactin secretion by dopamine and γ-aminobutyric acid *in vitro. Endocrinology (Baltimore)* **105**, 823–826.

Enjalbert, A., Ruberg, M., Arancibia, S., Priam, M., Bauer, K., and Kordon, C. (1979b).

Inhibition of in vitro prolactin secretion by histidyl-proline-diketopiperazine, a degradation product of TRH. Eur. J. Pharmacol. 58, 97–98.

Enjalbert, A., Ruberg, M., Arancibia, S., Priam, M., and Kordon, C. (1979c). Endogenous opiates block dopamine inhibition of prolactin secretion in vitro. Nature (London) 280, 595–596.

Enjalbert, A., Arancibia, S., Ruberg, M., Priam, M., Bluet-Pajot, M. T., Rotsztejn, W. H., and Kordon, C. (1980). Stimulation of in vitro prolactin release by vasoactive intestinal peptide. Neuroendocrinology 31, 200–204.

Eto, S., Wood, J. M., Hutchins, M., and Fleischer, N. (1974). Pituitary $^{45}Ca^{++}$ uptake and release of ACTH, GH and TSH: Effect of verapamil. Am. J. Physiol. 226, 1315–1320.

Evans, G. A., and Rosenfeld, M. G. (1976). Cell-free synthesis of a prolactin precursor directed by mRNA from cultured rat pituitary cells. J. Biol. Chem. 251, 2842–2847.

Farquhar, M. G. (1977). Secretion and Crinophagy in Prolactin Cells. In "Comparative Endocrinology of Prolactin" (H. D. Dellman, J. A. Johnson, and D. M. Klachko, eds.), pp. 37–94. Plenum, New York.

Farquhar, M. G., Reid, J. J., and Daniell, L. W. (1978). Intracellular transport and packaging of prolactin: A quantitative electron microscope autoradiographic study of mammotrophs dissociated from rat pituitaries. Endocrinology (Baltimore) 102, 296–311.

Fleckman, A., Erlichman, J., Schubart, U. K., and Fleischer, N. (1981). Effect of tri-fluoperazine, D600, and phenytoin on depolarization- and thyrotropin-releasing hormone-induced thyrotropin release from rat pituitary tissue. Endocrinology (Baltimore) 108, 2072–2077.

Gautvik, K. M., and Tashjian, A. H. Jr. (1973). Effects of cations and colchicine on the release of prolactin and growth hormone by functional pituitary tumors in culture. Endocrinology (Baltimore) 93, 793–799.

Gautvik, K. M., Walaas, E., and Walaas, O. (1977). Effect of thyroliberin on the concentration of adenosine 3':5'-phosphate and on the activity of adenosine 3':5'-phosphate dependent protein kinase in prolactin-producing cells in culture. Biochem. J. 162, 379–386.

Gautvik, K. M., Iversen, J. G., and Sand, O. (1980). On the role of extracellular Ca^{+2} for prolactin release and adenosine 3':5'-monophosphate formation induced by thyroliberin in cultured rat pituitary cells. Life Sci. 26, 995–1005.

Gershengorn, M. C., Hoffstein, S. T., Rebecchi, M. J., Geras, E., and Rubin, B. G. (1981). Thyrotropin-releasing hormone stimulation of prolactin release from clonal rat pituitary cells. J. Clin. Invest. 67, 1769–1776.

Giannattasio, G., and Zanini, A. (1976). Presence of sulfated proteoglycans in prolactin secretory granules isolated from the rat pituitary gland. Biochim. Biophys. Acta 439, 349–357.

Giannattasio, G., Zanini, A., and Meldolesi, J. (1975). Molecular organization of rat prolactin granules. I. In vitro stability of intact and "membraneless" granules. J. Cell Biol. 64, 246–251.

Gibbs, D. M., and Neill, J. D. (1978). Dopamine levels in hypophysial stalk blood in the rat are sufficient to inhibit prolactin secretion in vivo. Endocrinology (Baltimore) 102, 1895–1900.

Gill, D. M., and Meren, R. (1978). ADP-ribosylation of membrane proteins catalyzed by cholera toxin: Basis of the activation of adenylate cyclase. Proc. Natl. Acad. Sci. U.S.A. 75, 3050–3054.

Gourdji, D. (1980). Characterization of thyroliberin (TRH) binding sites and coupling

with prolactin and growth hormone secretion in rat pituitary cell lines. In "Synthesis and Release of Adenohypophyseal Hormones" (M. Jutisz and K. W. McKerns, eds.), pp. 463–494. Plenum, New York.

Gourdji, D., Bataille, D., Vauclin, N., Grouselle, D., Rosselin, G., and Tixier-Vidal, A. (1979). Vasoactive intestinal peptide (VIP) stimulates prolactin (PRL) release and cAMP production in a rat pituitary cell line (GH3/B6). Additive effects of VIP and TRH on PRL release. FEBS Lett. 104, 165–168.

Grandison, L., and Guidotti, A. (1979). γ-Aminobutyric acid receptor function in rat anterior pituitary: Evidence for control of prolactin release. Endocrinology (Baltimore) 105, 754–759.

Grandison, L., Fratta, W., and Guidotti, A. (1980). Location and characterization of opiate receptors regulating pituitary secretion. Life Sci. 26, 1633–1642.

Grant, N. H., Sarantakis, D., and Yardley, J. P. (1974). Action of growth hormone release inhibitory hormone on prolactin release in rat pituitary cell cultures. J. Endocrinol. 61, 163–164.

Grosvenor, C. E., and Mena, F. (1980). Evidence that thyrotropin-releasing hormone and a hypothalamic prolactin-releasing factor may function in the release of prolactin in the lactating rat. Endocrinology (Baltimore) 107, 863–868.

Grosvenor, C. E., Mena, F., and Whitworth, N. S. (1979). The secretion rate of prolactin in the rat during suckling and its metabolic clearance rate following increasing intervals of non-suckling. Endocrinology (Baltimore) 104, 372–376.

Grosvenor, C. E., Mena, F., and Whitworth, N. S. (1980). Evidence that dopaminergic prolactin-inhibiting factor mechanism regulates only the depletion-transformation phase and not the release phase of prolactin secretion during suckling in the rat. Endocrinology (Baltimore) 106, 481–485.

Grosvenor, C. E., Whitworth, N. S., and Mena, F. (1981). Evidence that the depletion and release phases of prolactin secretion in the lactating rat have different activation thresholds in response to exteroceptive stimulation from rat pups. Endocrinology (Baltimore) 108, 820–824.

Hardman, J. G. (1974). Cyclic nucleotides and hormone action. In "Textbook of Endocrinology" (R. H. Williams, ed.), p. 875. Saunders, Philadelphia, Pennsylvania.

Harrison, F. (1979). The effect of L-DOPA on the ultrastructure of the adenohypophysis of the Chinese quail, Excalfactoria chinensis. Cell Tissue Res. 198, 521–533.

Hill, M. K., MacLeod, R. M., and Orcutt, P. (1976). Dibutyryl cyclic AMP, adenosine and guanosine blockade of the dopamine, ergocryptine and apomorphine inhibition of prolactin release in vitro. Endocrinology (Baltimore) 99, 1612–1617.

Hinkle, P. M., and Tashjian, A. H., Jr. (1977). Adenylyl cyclase and cyclic nucleotide phosphodiesterases in GH-strains of rat pituitary cells. Endocrinology (Baltimore) 100, 934–944.

Holtzman, E. (1976) "Lysosomes: A Survey," p. 62. Springer-Verlag, Berlin and New York.

Hopkins, C. R., and Farquhar, M. G. (1973). Hormone secretion by cells dissociated from rat anterior pituitaries. J. Cell Biol. 59, 276–303.

Hortin, G., and Boime, I. (1980). Pre-prolactin accumulates in rat pituitary cells incubated with a threonine analog. J. Biol. Chem. 255, 7051–7054.

Hoyt, R. F., and Tashjian, A. H., Jr. (1980). Immunocytochemical analysis of prolactin production by monolayer cultures of GH3 rat anterior pituitary tumor cells: II. Variation in prolactin content of individual cell colonies, and dynamics of stimulation with thyrotropin-releasing hormone (TRH). Anat. Rec. 197, 163–181.

Hymer, W. C., Snyder, J., Wilfinger, W., Swanson, N., and Davis, J. A. (1974). Separa-

tion of pituitary mammotrophs from the female rat by velocity sedimentation at unit gravity. *Endocrinology (Baltimore)* **95**, 107–122.

Jackson, R. C., and Blobel, G. (1977). Post-translational cleavage of presecretory proteins with an extract of rough microsomes from dog pancreas containing signal peptidase activity. *Proc. Natl. Acad. Sci. U.S.A.* **74**, 5598–5602.

Kaneko, T., Oka, H., Saito, S., Munemura, M., Musa, K., Oda, T., Yanahara, N., and Yanahara, C. (1973). *In vitro* effects of synthetic somatotropin-release inhibiting factor on cyclic AMP level and GH release in rat anterior pituitary gland. *Endocrinol. Jpn.* **20**, 535–544.

Kato, Y., Iwasaki, Y., Iwasaki, J., Abe, H., Yanaihara, N., and Imura, H. (1978). Prolactin release by vasoactive intestinal polypeptide in rats. *Endocrinology (Baltimore)* **103**, 554–558.

Kerdelhue, B., Weisman, A. S., and Weiner, R. I. (1981). A dopaminergic binding site in the high speed supernatant of steer anterior pituitary homogenates. *Endocrinology (Baltimore)* **109**, 307–309.

Kidokoro, Y. (1975). Spontaneous calcium action potentials in a clonal pituitary cell strain and their relationship to prolactin secretion. *Nature (London)* **258**, 741–742.

Kiino, D. R., and Dannies, P. S. (1981). Insulin and 17 β-estradiol increase prolactin content of GH cells. *Endocrinology (Baltimore)* **109**, 1264–1269.

Labrie, F., Gauthier, M., Pelletier, G., Borgeat, P., Lemay, A., and Gouge, J. J. (1973). Role of microtubules in basal and stimulated release of growth hormone and prolactin in rat adenohypophysis *in vitro*. *Endocrinology (Baltimore)* **93**, 903–914.

Labrie, F., Drouin, J., Ferland, L., Lagacé, L., Beaulieu, M., DeLean, A., Kelly, P. A., Caron, M. G., and Raymond, V. (1978). Mechanism of action of hypothalamic hormones in the anterior pituitary gland and specific modulation of their activity by sex steroids and thyroid hormones. *Recent Prog. Horm. Res.* **34**, 25–93.

Lemay, A., and Labrie, F. (1972). Calcium-dependent stimulation of prolactin release in rat anterior pituitary *in vitro* by N6-monobutyryl adenosine 3',5'-monophosphate. *FEBS Lett.* **20**, 7–10.

Levin, R. M., and Weiss, B. (1978). Selective binding of antipsychotics and other psychoactive agents to the calcium-dependent activator of cyclic nucleotide phosphodiesterase. *J. Pharmacol. Exp. Ther.* **208**, 454–459.

Lien, E. L., Fenichel, R. L., Garsky, V., Sarantakis, D., and Grant, N. H. (1976). Enkephalin-stimulated prolactin release. *Life Sci.* **19**, 837–840.

Lingappa, V. R., Devillers-Thiery, A., and Blobel, G. (1977). Nascent prehormones are intermediates in the biosynthesis of authentic bovine pituitary growth hormone and prolactin. *Proc. Natl. Acad. Sci. U.S.A.* **74**, 2432–2436.

MacLeod, R. M., and Fontham, E. H. (1970). Influence of ionic environment on the *in vitro* synthesis and release of pituitary hormones. *Endocrinology (Baltimore)* **86**, 863–869.

MacLeod, R. M., Fontham, E. H., and Lehmeyer, J. E. (1970). Prolactin and growth hormone production as influenced by catecholamines and agents that affect brain catecholamines. *Neuroendocrinology* **6**, 283–294.

Martin, T. F. J., and Tashjian, A. H., Jr. (1977). Cell culture studies of thyrotropin-releasing hormone action. *In* "Biochemical Actions of Hormones" (G. Litwack, ed.), Vol. IV, pp. 270–312. Academic Press, New York.

Martin, T. F. J., and Tashjian, A. H., Jr. (1978). Thyrotropin-releasing hormone modulation of uridine uptake in rat pituitary cells. *J. Biol. Chem.* **253**, 106–115.

Martin, T. F. J., Sutton, C. A., and Drust, D. S. (1981). Thyrotropin-releasing hormone (TRH), vasoactive intestinal peptide (VIP) and 50 mM K⁺ activate distinctive

pathways of protein phosphorylation in GH pituitary cell cultures: Evidence for cAMP-independent action of TRH. Annu. Meet. Endocr. Soc., 63rd, June 17-19, Cincinnati, Ohio (Abstr. 951), p. 320.

Maruyama, T., Shiino, M., and Rennels, E. G. (1981). Calcium-dependent changes in electrical properties of prolactin-secreting anterior pituitary (2B8) clonal cells. Neuroendocrinology 32, 28-32.

Maurer, R. A. (1980). Bromocryptine-induced prolactin degradation in cultured pituitary cells. Biochemistry 19, 3573-3579.

Maurer, R. A., and McKean, D. J. (1978). Synthesis of preprolactin and conversion to prolactin in intact cells and a cell-free system. J. Biol. Chem. 253, 6315-6319.

Maurer, R. A., Stone, R., and Gorski, J. (1976). Cell-free synthesis of a large translation product of prolactin messenger RNA. J. Biol. Chem. 251, 2801-2807.

Meites, J., and Clemens, J. A. (1972). Hypothalamic control of prolactin secretion. Recent Prog. Horm. Res. 28, 165-221.

Mena, F., Pacheco, P., and Grosvenor, C. E. (1980). Effect of electrical stimulation of mammary nerve upon pituitary and plasma production concentrations in anesthetized lactating rats. Endocrinology (Baltimore) 106, 458-462.

Milligan, J. V., and Kraicer, J. (1970). Adenohypophyseal transmembrane potentials: Polarity reversal by elevated potassium ion concentration. Science 167, 182-184.

Moriarty, C. M., and Leuschen, M. P. (1981). Role of calcium in acute stimulated release of prolactin from neoplastic GH_3 cells. Am. J. Physiol. 240, E705-E711.

Moss, J., and Vaughn, M. (1977). Mechanism of action of choleragen: Evidence for ADP-ribosyltransferase activity with arginine as an acceptor. J. Biol. Chem. 252, 2455-2457.

Mukherjee, A., Snyder, G., and McCann, S. M. (1980). Characterization of muscarinic cholinergic receptors on intact rat anterior pituitary cells. Life Sci. 27, 475-482.

Murad, F., and Haynes, R. C., Jr. (1980). Adenohypophyseal hormones and related substances. In "The Pharmacological Basis of Therapeutics" (A. G. Gilman, L. S. Goodman, and A. Gilman, eds.), p. 1390. MacMillan, New York.

Nakano, H., Fawcett, C. P., and McCann, S. M. (1976). Enzymatic dissociation and short-term culture of isolated anterior pituitary cells for studies on the control of hormone secretion. Endocrinology (Baltimore) 98, 278-288.

Nansel, D. D., Gudelsky, G. A., and Porter, J. C. (1979). Subcellular localization of dopamine in the anterior pituitary gland of the rat: apparent association of dopamine with prolactin secretory granules. Endocrinology (Baltimore) 105, 1073-1077.

Nansel, D. D., Gudelsky, G. A., Reymond, M. J., Neaves, W. B., and Porter, J. C. (1981). A possible role for lysosomes in the inhibitory action of dopamine on prolactin release. Endocrinology (Baltimore) 108, 896-902.

Naor, Z., Snyder, G., Fawcett, C. P., and McCann, S. M. (1980). Pituitary cyclic nucleotides and thyrotropin-releasing harmone action: The relationship of adenosine 3',5'-monophosphate and guanosine 3',5'-monophosphate to the release of thyrotropin and prolactin. Endocrinology (Baltimore) 106, 1304-1310.

Nicoll, C. S. (1972). Some observations and speculation on the mechanism of "depletion", "repletion" and release of adenohypophyseal hormones. Gen. Comp. Endocrinol. Suppl. No. 3, pp. 86-96.

Nicoll, C. S., Mena, F., Nichols, C. W., Jr., Green, S. H., Tai, M., and Russell, S. M. (1976). Analysis of suckling-induced changes in adenohypophyseal prolactin concentration in the lactating rat by three assay methods. Acta Endocrinol. (Copenhagen) 83, 512-521.

Norman, J. A., and Drummond, A. H. (1979). Inhibition of calcium-dependent regulator-stimulated phosphodiesterase activity by neuroleptic drugs is unrelated to their clinical efficacy. *Mol. Pharmacol.* **16,** 1089–1094.

Ojeda, S. R., Harms, P. G., and McCann, S. M. (1974). Effect of blockade of dopaminergic receptors on prolactin and LH release: median eminence and pituitary sites of action. *Endocrinology (Baltimore)* **94,** 1650–1657.

Ostlund, R. E., Jr., Leung, J. T., Hajek, S. V., Winokur, T., and Melman, M. (1978). Acute stimulated hormone release from cultured GH₃ pituitary cells. *Endocrinology (Baltimore)* **103,** 1245–1252.

Ozawa, S., and Kimura, N. (1979). Membrane potential changes caused by thyrotropin-releasing hormone in the clonal GH₃ cell and their relationship to secretion of pituitary hormone. *Proc. Natl. Acad. Sci. U.S.A.* **76,** 6017–6020.

Parsons, J. A. (1970). Effects of cations on prolactin and growth hormone secretion by rat adenohypophyses *in vitro*. *J. Physiol. (London)* **210,** 973–987.

Pelletier, G., Lemay, A., Béraud, G., and Labrie, F. (1972). Ultrastructural changes accompanying the stimulatory effect of N^6-monobutyryl adenosine 3′,5′ monophosphate on the release of prolactin, growth hormone and adrenocorticotropic hormone in rat anterior pituitary gland *in vitro*. *Endocrinology (Baltimore)* **91,** 1355–1371.

Peterkofsky, A., Battaini, F., Koch, Y., Takahara, Y., and Dannies, P. (1981). Histidyl-proline-diketopiperazine: Its biological role as a regulatory peptide. *Mol. Cell. Biochem.,* **42,** 45–63.

Prasad, C., and Peterkofsky, A. (1976). Demonstration of pyroglutamylpeptidase and amidase activities toward thyrotropin-releasing hormone in hamster hypothalamic extracts. *J. Biol. Chem.* **251,** 3229–3234.

Prasad, K. N., and Sinha, P. K. (1976). Effect of sodium butyrate on mammalian cells in culture: A review. *In Vitro* **12,** 125–132.

Prasad, C., Wilber, J. F., Akerstrom, V., and Banerji, A. (1980). Cyclo (his-pro): A selective inhibitor of rat prolactin secretion *in vitro*. *Life Sci.* **27,** 1979–1983.

Racagni, C., Apud, J. A., Locatelli, V., Cocchi, D., Nistico', G., di Giorgio, R. M., and Müller, E. E. (1979). GABA of CNS origin in the rat anterior pituitary inhibits prolactin secretion. *Nature (London)* **281,** 575–578.

Rappaport, R. S., and Grant, N. H. (1974). Growth hormone releasing factor of microbial origin. *Nature (London)* **248,** 73–74.

Rasmussen, H., and Goodman, D. B. P. (1977). Relationships between calcium and cyclic nucleotides in cell activation. *Physiol. Rev.* **57,** 421–509.

Ray, K. P., and Wallis, M. (1981). Effects of dopamine on prolactin secretion and cyclic AMP accumulation in the rat anterior pituitary gland. *Biochem. J.* **194,** 119–128.

Raymond, V., Beaulieu, M., Labrie, F., and Boissier, J. (1978). Potent antidopaminergic activity of estradiol at the pituitary level on prolactin release. *Science* **200,** 1173–1175.

Rivier, C., Vale, W., Ling, N., Brown, M., and Guillemin, R. (1977). Stimulation *in vivo* of the secretion of prolactin and growth hormone by β-endorphin. *Endocrinology (Baltimore)* **100,** 238–241.

Rivier, C., Rivier, J., and Vale, W. (1978). The effect of bombesin and related peptides on prolactin and growth hormone secretion in the rat. *Endocrinology (Baltimore)* **102,** 519–522.

Rodbell, M. (1980). The role of hormone receptors and GTP-regulatory proteins in membrane transduction. *Nature (London)* **284,** 17–22.

Ruberg, M., Rotsztejn, W. H., Arancibia, S., Besson, J., and Enjalbert, A. (1978). Stimulation of prolactin release by vasoactive intestinal peptide (VIP). *Eur. J. Pharmacol.* **51**, 319–320.

Rudnick, M. S., and Dannies, P. S. (1981). Muscarinic inhibition of prolactin production in cultures of rat pituitary cells. *Biochem. Biophys. Res. Commun.* **101**, 689–696.

Saavedra, J. M., Palkovits, M., Kizer, J. S., Brownstein, M., and Zivin, J. A. (1975). Distribution of biogenic amines and related enzymes in the rat pituitary gland. *J. Neurochem.* **25**, 257–260.

Schofield, J. G., and Bicknell, R. J. (1978). Effects of somatostatin and verapamil on growth hormone release and ^{45}Ca fluxes. *Mol. Cell. Endocrinol.* **9**, 255–268.

Schonbrunn, A., and Tashjian, A. H., Jr. (1978). Characterization of functional receptors for somatostatin in rat pituitary cells in culture. *J. Biol. Chem.* **253**, 6473–6483.

Schonbrunn, A., Krasnoff, M., Westendorf, J. M., and Tashjian, A. H., Jr. (1980). Epidermal growth factor and thyrotropin-releasing hormone act similarly on a clonal pituitary cell strain. *J. Cell Biol.* **85**, 786–797.

Schrey, M. P., Brown, B. L., and Ekins, R. P. (1978). Studies on the role of calcium and cyclic nucleotides in the control of TSH secretion. *Mol. Cell. Endocrinol.* **11**, 249–264.

Shaar, C. J., Frederickson, R. C., Dininger, N. B. and Jackson, L. (1977). Enkephalin analogues and naloxone modulate the release of growth hormone and prolactin-evidence for regulation by an endognous opioid peptide in brain. *Life Sci.* **21**, 853–860.

Shaar, C. J., Clemens, J. A., and Dininger, N. B. (1979). Effect of vasoactive intestinal polypeptide on prolactin release *in vitro. Life Sci.* **25**, 2071–2074.

Shenai, R., and Wallis, M. (1979). Biosynthesis and degradation of prolactin in the rat anterior pituitary gland: Time course of incorporation of label *in vitro* and evidence for rapid degradation. *Biochem. J.* **182**, 735–743.

Sheppard, M. S., Spence, J. W., and Kraicer, J. (1979). Release of growth hormone from purified somatotrophs: Role of adenosine 3′,5′-monophosphate and guanosine 3′,5′-monophosphate. *Endocrinology (Baltimore)* **105**, 261–268.

Shiino, M., Williams, G., and Rennels, E. G. (1972). Ultrastructural observation of pituitary release of prolactin in the rat by suckling stimulus. *Endocrinology (Baltimore)* **90**, 176–187.

Slaby, F., and Farquhar, M. G. (1980). Characterization of rat somatotroph and mammotroph secretory granules: presence of sulfated molecules. *Mol. Cell. Endocrinol.* **18**, 33–48.

Smith, R. E., and Farquhar, M. G. (1966). Lysosome function in the regulation of the secretory process in cells of the anterior pituitary gland. *J. Cell Biol.* **31**, 319–347.

Snyder, J., Wilfinger, W., and Hymer, W. C. (1976). Maintenance of separated rat pituitary mammotrophs in cell culture. *Endocrinology (Baltimore)* **98**, 25–32.

Spence, J. W., Sheppard, M. S., and Kraicer, J. (1980). Release of growth hormone from purified somatotrophs: Interrelation between Ca^{++} and adenosine 3′,5′-monophosphate. *Endocrinology (Baltimore)* **106**, 764–769.

Stachura, M. E. (1977). Interaction of somatostatin inhibition and dibutylryl cyclic AMP or K^+ stimulation of growth hormone release from perfused rat pituitaries. *Endocrinology (Baltimore)* **101**, 1044–1053.

Stachura, M. E. (1982a). Sequestration of an early releasable pool of GH and PRL in GH_3 rat pituitary tumor cells. In press.

Stachura, M. E. (1982b). Verapamil: Influence upon basal and stimulated rat growth hormone and prolactin release *in vitro*. In press.

Stachura, M. E. (1981). Potassium modification of the somatostatin effect on stimulated rat growth hormone release. *Endocrinology (Baltimore)* **108**, 1027–1034.

Stern, J. E., and Conn, P. M. (1981). Perfusion of rat hemipituitaries: Requirements for optimal GnRH-stimulated LH release *Am. J. Physiol.* **240**, E204–E509.

Sutton, C. A., and Martin, T. F. J. (1982). Thyrotropin-releasing hormone (TRH) selectively and rapidly stimulates phosphatidylinositol turnover in GH pituitary cells: a possible second step of TRH action. *Endocrinology* **110**, 1273–1280.

Swearingen, K. C. (1971). Heterogeneous turnover of adenohypophysial prolactin. *Endocrinology (Baltimore)* **89**, 1380–1388.

Takahara, J., Arimura, A., and Schally, A. V. (1974). Suppression of prolactin release by a purified porcine PIF preparation and catecholamines infused into a rat hypophysial portal vessel. *Endocrinology (Baltimore)* **95**, 462–465.

Tam, S. W., and Dannies, P. S. (1980). Dopaminergic inhibition of ionophore A23187-stimulated release of prolactin from rat anterior pituitary cells. *J. Biol. Chem.* **255**, 6595–6599.

Tam, S. W., and Dannies, P. S. (1981a). Dopamine inhibition of calcium- and cAMP-stimulated release of prolactin in anterior pituitary cell cultures. *Annu. Meet. Endocr. Soc., 63rd, June 17–19, Cincinnati, Ohio.* (Abstr. 545), p. 219.

Tam, S. W., and Dannies, P. S. (1981a). Dopamine inhibition of calcium- and cAMP-stimulated release of prolactin in anterior pituitary cell cultures. *Annu. Meet. Endocr. Soc., 63rd, June 17–19, Cincinnati, Ohio.* (Abstr. 545), p. 219.

Tan, K. N., and Tashjian, A. H., Jr. (1981). Receptor-mediated release of plasma membrane-associated calcium and stimulation of calcium uptake by thyrotropin-releasing hormone in pituitary cells in culture. *J. Biol. Chem.* **256**, 8994–9002.

Taraskevich, P. S., and Douglas, W. W. (1977). Action potentials occur in cells of the normal anterior pituitary gland and are stimulated by the hypophysiotropic peptide thyrotropin-releasing hormone. *Proc. Natl. Acad. Sci. U.S.A.* **74**, 4064–4067.

Taraskevich, P. S., and Douglas, W. W. (1978). Catecholamines of supposed inhibitory hypophysiotrophic function suppress action potentials in prolactin cells. *Nature (London)* **276**, 832–834.

Taraskevich, P. S., and Douglas, W. W. (1980). Electrical behaviour in a line of anterior pituitary cells (GH cells) and the influence of the hypothalamic peptide, thyrotropin releasing factor. *Neuroscience* **5**, 421–431.

Tashjian, A. H., Jr., Bancroft, F. C., and Levine, L. (1970). Production of both prolactin and growth hormone by clonal strains of rat pituitary tumor cells: Differential effects of hydrocortisone and tissue extracts. *J. Cell Biol.* **47**, 61–70.

Tashjian, A. H., Jr., Barowsky, N. J., and Jensen, D. K. (1971). Thyrotropin releasing hormone: Direct evidence for stimulation of prolactin production by pituitary cells in culture. *Biochem. Biophys. Res. Commun.* **43**, 516–523.

Tashjian, A. H., Jr., Lomedico, M. E., and Mains, D. (1978). Role of calcium in the thyrotropin-releasing hormone-stimulated release of prolactin from pituitary cells in culture. *Biochem. Biophys. Res. Commun.* **81**, 798–806.

Thorner, M. O., Hackett, J. T., Murad, F., and MacLeod, R. M. (1980). Calcium rather than cyclic AMP as the physiological intracellular regulator of prolactin release. *Neuroendocrinology* **31**, 390–402.

Tixier-Vidal, A. (1975). Ultrastructure of anterior pituitary cells in culture. *In* "The Anterior Pituitary Gland" (A. Tixier-Vidal and M. G. Farquhar, eds.), p. 181. Academic Press, New York.

Tougard, C., Picart, R., and Tixier-Vidal, A. (1980). Electronmicroscopic cytochemical studies on the secretory process in rat prolactin cells in primary culture. *Am. J. Anat.* **158**, 471–490.

Ushiro, H., and Cohen, S. (1980). Identification of phosphotyrosine as a product of epidermal growth factor-activated protein kinase in A-431 cell membranes. *J. Biol. Chem.* **255**, 8363–8365.

Vale, W., Blackwell, R., Grant, G., and Guillemin, R. (1973). TRF and thyroid hormones on prolactin secretion by rat anterior pituitary cells *in vitro*. *Endocrinology (Baltimore)* **93**, 26–33.

Vale, W., Rivier, C., Brazeau, P., and Guillemin, R. (1974). Effects of somatostatin on the secretion of thyrotropin and prolactin. *Endocrinology (Baltimore)* **95**, 968–977.

Vale, W., Rivier, C., Brown, M., Chan, L., Ling, N., and Rivier, J. (1976). Applications of adenohypophyseal cell cultures to neuroendocrine studies. *In* "Hypothalamus and Endocrine Functions" (F. Labrie, J. Meites, and G. Pelletier, eds.), pp. 397–432. Plenum, New York.

Wakabayashi, K., Date, Y., and Tamaoki, B. I. (1973). On the mechanism of action of luteinizing hormone-releasing factor and prolactin release inhibiting factor. *Endocrinology (Baltimore)* **92**, 698–704.

Walker, A. M., and Farquhar, M. G. (1980). Preferential release of newly synthesized prolactin granules is the result of functional heterogeneity among mammotrophs. *Endocrinology (Baltimore)* **107**, 1095–1104.

Walker, A. M., and Hopkins, C. R. (1978). Calcium as a second messenger in the stimulation of luteinizing hormone secretion. *Mol. Cell. Endocrinol.* **12**, 189–208.

Walter, P., and Blobel, G. (1980). Purification of a membrane-associated protein complex required for protein translocation across the endoplasmic reticulum. *Proc. Natl. Acad. Sci. U.S.A.* **77**, 7112–7116.

Wardlaw, S. L., Wehrenberg, W. B., Ferin, M., and Frantz, A. G. (1980). Failure of a β-endorphin to stimulate prolactin release in the pituitary stalk-sectioned monkey. *Endocrinology (Baltimore)* **107**, 1663–1666.

West, B., and Dannies, P. S. (1979). Antipsychotic drugs inhibit prolactin release from anterior pituitary cells in culture by a mechanism not involving the dopamine receptor. *Endocrinology (Baltimore)* **104**, 877–880.

West, B., and Dannies, P. S. (1980). Effects of estradiol on prolactin production and dihydroergocryptine-induced inhibition of prolactin production in primary cultures of rat pituitary cells. *Endocrinology (Baltimore)* **106**, 1108–1113.

Westendorf, J. M., and Schonbrunn, A. (1982). Bombesin stimulates prolactin and growth hormone release by pituitary cells in culture. *Endocrinology (Baltimore)* **110**, 352–358.

Williams, J. A. (1976). Stimulation of $^{45}Ca^{2+}$ efflux from rat pituitary by luteinizing hormone-releasing hormone and other pituitary stimulants. *J. Physiol. (London)* **260**, 105–115.

Yen, P. M., and Tashjian, A. H., Jr. (1981). Short chain fatty acids increase prolactin and growth hormone production and alter cell morphology in the GH_3 strain of rat pituitary cells. *Endocrinology (Baltimore)* **109**, 17–22.

Young, P. W., Bicknell, R. J., and Schofield, J. G. (1979). Acetylcholine stimulates growth hormone secretion, phosphatidyl inositol labelling, $^{45}Ca^{+2}$ efflux and cGMP accumulation in bovine anterior pituitary glands. *J. Endocrinol.* **80**, 203–213.

Index

L

Lactation
  in cystic fibrosis, 339
  prolactin secretion during, 532, 533, 534
Lactotrope, 475
Leader peptide
  amino acid composition, 303, 314, 315
  β-turn, 303, 306, 307
  helix formation, 302–307, 309–310, 315–316
  hydrophobicity, 302–303, 307, 310
  membrane interaction, 307–308
  model systems, 308–310
  in prolactin secretion, 530
  in protein transmembrane translocation, 302, 303
  structural features, 302–307
Leukocyte
  chemotaxis, 183
  protein-carboxyl methylase in, 161
Leukotriene, 82, 83, 84, 89
Leydig cell
  I, 361, 362–367, 368–371, 373, 383–384, 385–386, 398
  II, 361, 362–367, 368–371, 373, 383–384, 385–386, 398
  aromatization, 384–386
  cholesterol in, 372–373
  gonadotropin
    binding, 359, 360, 361, 362, 363, 364, 373, 376, 386–389, 396–397
    stimulation, 390, 393–393
  luteinizing hormone receptors, 356, 357, 367–373, 389–390
  pituitary hormone regulation, 356–357
  purification, 357–362
  during sexual maturation, 386–397
    hormonal regulation, 393–397
    numbers, 386–389, 393
  steroid hormone secretion, 208, 355–408
  testerone secretion
    gonadotropin stimulation, 367–372, 374–375, 385, 386
    luteinizing hormone stimulation, 362–372
    steroidogenic enzyme stimulation, 373–386

tumor
  deoxyribonucleic acid synthesis in, 431–432
  gonadotropin binding, 422–423
  steroid hormone secretion, 412–414, 417–419, 427–428
Lipid, fusogenic, 56–57
Lipolysis, 24
Lipophilic hormone, 116
Lipoprotein
  high-density, 373, 426
  low-density, 15, 373, 426–427
  receptor, 426
Lipoxygenase, 57, 69, 79, 80, 82, 83, 86, 87, 89
Liver
  calcium mobilization in, 68–69
  in cystic fibrosis, 330–331
Luminal membrane, 209
Luteinizing hormone
  in cholesterol transport, 430
  pituitary, 7–8
  receptor
    follicle-stimulating hormone interaction, 357, 394–395, 397, 398
  receptor
    gonadotropin interaction, 367–373, 395–397
    in Leydig cell, 356–357, 363–373, 375, 389–390, 394, 395–397
    prolactin interaction, 356–357
  secretion regulation
    of androgen, 410
    by calcium, 470–471, 472–474, 479–480
    by calmodulin, 448
    by Clomid, 507–510, 513–514
    by estrogen, 500–504
    of estrogen, 410
    by gonadotropin-releasing hormone, 7–8, 448, 463, 467–469, 479–480, 486, 495, 497–504, 519–522
    by progesterone, 504–507
    of progestin, 410
    of steroid hormones, 206, 208, 356, 367–372, 390–393, 420–421
Lyase, C_{17}-C_{20}, 374, 376, 377, 378–379, 380–381, 391
Lysophophatide, 54

CELL BIOLOGY: A Series of Monographs

EDITORS

D. E. BUETOW

*Department of Physiology
and Biophysics
University of Illinois
Urbana, Illinois*

I. L. CAMERON

*Department of Anatomy
University of Texas
Health Science Center at San Antonio
San Antonio, Texas*

G. M. PADILLA

*Department of Physiology
Duke University Medical Center
Durham, North Carolina*

A. M. ZIMMERMAN

*Department of Zoology
University of Toronto
Toronto, Ontario, Canada*

Stuart Coward (editor). DEVELOPMENTAL REGULATION: Aspects of Cell Differentiation, 1973

I. L. Cameron and J. R. Jeter, Jr. (editors). ACIDIC PROTEINS OF THE NUCLEUS, 1974

Govindjee (editor). BIOENERGETICS OF PHOTOSYNTHESIS, 1975

James R. Jeter, Jr., Ivan L. Cameron, George M. Padilla, and Arthur M. Zimmerman (editors). CELL CYCLE REGULATION, 1978

Gary L. Whitson (editor). NUCLEAR–CYTOPLASMIC INTERACTIONS IN THE CELL CYCLE, 1980

Danton H. O'Day and Paul A. Horgen (editors). SEXUAL INTERACTIONS IN EUKARYOTIC MICROBES, 1981

Ivan L. Cameron and Thomas B. Pool (editors). THE TRANSFORMED CELL, 1981

Arthur M. Zimmerman and Arthur Forer (editors). MITOSIS/CYTOKINESIS, 1981

Ian R. Brown (editor). MOLECULAR APPROACHES TO NEUROBIOLOGY, 1982

Henry C. Aldrich and John W. Daniel (editors). CELL BIOLOGY OF *PHYSARUM* AND *DIDYMIUM*, Volume I: Organisms, Nucleus, and Cell Cycle, 1982; Volume II: Differentiation, Metabolism, and Methodology, 1982

John A. Heddle (editor). MUTAGENICITY: New Horizons in Genetic Toxicology, 1982

Potu N. Rao, Robert T. Johnson, and Karl Sperling (editors). PREMATURE CHROMOSOME CONDENSATION: Application in Basic, Clinical, and Mutation Research, 1982

George M. Padilla and Kenneth S. McCarty, Sr. (editors). GENETIC EXPRESSION IN THE CELL CYCLE, 1982

David S. McDevitt (editor). CELL BIOLOGY OF THE EYE, 1982

P. Michael Conn (editor). CELLULAR REGULATION OF SECRETION AND RELEASE, 1982

In preparation

Govindjee (editor). PHOTOSYNTHESIS, Volume I: Energy Conversion by Plants and Bacteria, 1982; Volume II: Development, Carbon Metabolism, and Plant Productivity, 1982

John Morrow. EUKARYOTIC CELL GENETICS, 1983

John F. Hartmann (editor). MECHANISM AND CONTROL OF ANIMAL FERTILIZATION, 1983